Bioactive Compounds and Functional Foods in Human Health

Bioactive Compounds and Functional Foods in Human Health

Guest Editors

Vassilis Athanasiadis
Stavros I. Lalas
Theodoros G. Chatzimitakos

MDPI

Basel • Beijing • Wuhan • Barcelona • Belgrade • Novi Sad • Cluj • Manchester

Guest Editors
Vassilis Athanasiadis
Department of Food Science and Nutrition
University of Thessaly
Karditsa
Greece

Stavros I. Lalas
Department of Food Science and Nutrition
University of Thessaly
Karditsa
Greece

Theodoros G. Chatzimitakos
Department of Food Science and Nutrition
University of Thessaly
Karditsa
Greece

Editorial Office
MDPI AG
Grosspeteranlage 5
4052 Basel, Switzerland

This is a reprint of the Special Issue, published open access by the journal *Nutrients* (ISSN 2072-6643), freely accessible at: https://www.mdpi.com/journal/nutrients/special_issues/9B524TEG6P.

For citation purposes, cite each article independently as indicated on the article page online and as indicated below:

Lastname, A.A.; Lastname, B.B. Article Title. *Journal Name* **Year**, *Volume Number*, Page Range.

ISBN 978-3-7258-6406-5 (Hbk)
ISBN 978-3-7258-6407-2 (PDF)
https://doi.org/10.3390/books978-3-7258-6407-2

Contents

About the Editors

Vassilis Athanasiadis

Vassilis Athanasiadis is a Postdoctoral Researcher at the Department of Food Science and Nutrition, University of Thessaly, Greece. His work focuses on functional foods, polyphenols, antioxidants, and nutritional evaluation of natural product extracts. He has contributed extensively to the study of bioactive compounds and their role in public health, while also serving as Guest Editor and reviewer for international journals. His academic interests include experimental design, statistical modeling, and mentoring students in scientific writing and laboratory practice.

Stavros I. Lalas

Stavros I. Lalas is a Professor at the Department of Food Science and Nutrition, University of Thessaly, Greece. His research spans food analysis, food antioxidants, pulsed electric field applications, and extraction techniques. He has published widely on the chemistry and functionality of bioactive compounds and has coordinated numerous projects in food science and technology. As Guest Editor, he promotes interdisciplinary collaboration and advances in functional food research.

Theodoros G. Chatzimitakos

Theodoros G. Chatzimitakos is a Researcher at the Department of Food Science and Nutrition, University of Thessaly, Greece. His scientific work focuses on analytical chemistry, bioactive compounds, and the development of innovative methodologies for food analysis and natural product characterization. He has contributed to several research projects and publications in the fields of food chemistry and functional ingredients. His interests include method development, chromatographic techniques, and the study of bioactive molecules in relation to human health.

Preface

The Reprint "Bioactive Compounds and Functional Foods in Human Health" aims to provide a consolidated reference for scientists, nutritionists, and students interested in the intersection of food science and public health. Our motivation was to highlight the growing importance of bioactive compounds and functional foods in addressing modern health challenges. This Reprint is addressed to researchers and practitioners who seek to understand both mechanistic insights and practical applications of these compounds. We hope it will serve as a valuable resource for advancing knowledge, fostering innovation, and supporting the development of functional foods that contribute to healthier societies.

Vassilis Athanasiadis, Stavros I. Lalas, and Theodoros G. Chatzimitakos
Guest Editors

nutrients

MDPI

Editorial

Bioactive Compounds and Functional Foods in Human Health—Bridging Mechanisms and Applications for Future Nutrition

Vassilis Athanasiadis * and Stavros I. Lalas

Department of Food Science and Nutrition, University of Thessaly, Terma N. Temponera Street, 43100 Karditsa, Greece; slalas@uth.gr
* Correspondence: vaathanasiadis@uth.gr

The role of bioactive compounds in the diet has moved from the periphery to the center of scientific and societal debate in both research and public health. Over the past decade, evidence has accumulated showing that polyphenols, carotenoids, and other bioactive molecules can influence inflammation, oxidative stress, and metabolic regulation. These findings are particularly important for chronic diseases such as cardiovascular disease and type 2 diabetes, where proper nutrition continues to act as an adjunct to medical therapy [1,2]. However, the benefits of these compounds are not guaranteed. Their efficacy depends on bioavailability, which is shaped by food structure and, increasingly, by interactions with the gut microbiota [1–3].

Despite this progress, many questions remain unanswered. We still lack a clear picture of how phytochemicals are absorbed and metabolized in real-world dietary contexts. Food matrices, preparation methods, and microbial interactions can alter outcomes in ways that are difficult to predict [2]. These uncertainties explain why clinical outcomes are sometimes inconsistent and highlight the need for more integrated approaches. Exploring these mechanisms is not only scientifically demanding, but also provides a foundation for translating laboratory data into realistic dietary practices [2,4].

The contributions to this Special Issue make important steps toward filling these gaps. Several publications examine how bioactive compounds interact with the microbiome [5], mitochondrial function [6], and lipid metabolism [7]. Together, they demonstrate a shift in the field—from isolated biochemical observations to a system-level understanding of nutrition. This approach is a necessary condition for the practical application of functional foods. A clear understanding of the mechanisms, especially biomolecular interactions, is essential for the reproducibility and clinical validity of the results [1,8].

Personalized nutrition is expected to be a central focus of future research and clinical activity. Genetic diversity, microbiome composition, and lifestyle factors all shape individual responses to nutrition. Although personalized nutrition is of particular interest, its implementation must be based on documented scientific and functional data [5,9]. Without a scientific basis, personalized nutrition may become a marketing fad rather than a meaningful therapeutic approach. Current research on nutrient–genotype interactions and microbiome-based nutritional strategies suggests that personalized recommendations could ultimately improve therapeutic outcomes [4,9,10].

The need for sustainable solutions makes it imperative to exploit alternative sources of bioactive compounds, such as neglected crops and agro-industrial by-products, placing nutritional research in the broader context of ecological responsibility. For example, olive leaves and citrus peels—by-products of the olive oil and juice industries, respectively—have emerged as promising sources of polyphenols with antioxidant and anti-inflammatory properties [11,12]. Similarly, underutilized crops such as amaranth and *Moringa oleifera* offer bioactive profiles that support both nutritional and ecological goals [13]. Advances in extraction and processing will be crucial to ensure that functional foods contribute not only to human health but also to ecological resilience [14]. In parallel, regulatory frameworks need to evolve, aiming to establish internationally harmonized standards, so that functional foods can gain consumer trust and be widely integrated into the market [9]. Looking ahead, several challenges remain in translating mechanistic insights into actionable dietary recommendations. Key questions include how to account for individual variability in microbiome composition, how to ensure reproducibility across diverse populations, and how to integrate emerging molecular data into practical guidelines. Addressing these issues will require coordinated efforts across nutrition science, clinical research, and regulatory policy [15,16].

In conclusion, bioactive compounds and functional foods have significant potential, the exploitation of which requires, beyond laboratory documentation, interdisciplinary collaboration and applied research. The transition from theory to practice requires interdisciplinary synergy and institutional alignment, with particular attention to environmental and regulatory parameters. If these elements are aligned, functional nutrition could become one of the defining public health strategies of the coming decades.

Conflicts of Interest: The authors declare no conflicts of interest.

References

1. Aydın, E. The Impact of Raisin Consumption on Quercetin Bioavailability: An In Vivo Approach In Vivo. *Gida J. Food* **2024**, *49*, 741–750. [CrossRef]
2. Bohn, T.; McDougall, G.J.; Alegría, A.; Alminger, M.; Arrigoni, E.; Aura, A.; Brito, C.; Cilla, A.; El, S.N.; Karakaya, S.; et al. Mind the Gap—Deficits in Our Knowledge of Aspects Impacting the Bioavailability of Phytochemicals and Their Metabolites—A Position Paper Focusing on Carotenoids and Polyphenols. *Mol. Nutr. Food Res.* **2015**, *59*, 1307–1323. [CrossRef] [PubMed]
3. Danesi, F.; Calani, L.; Valli, V.; Bresciani, L.; Rio, D.D.; Bordoni, A. (Poly)phenolic Content and Profile and Antioxidant Capacity of Whole-Grain Cookies Are Better Estimated by Simulated Digestion Than Chemical Extraction. *Molecules* **2020**, *25*, 2792. [CrossRef] [PubMed]
4. Goñi, L.; Cuervo, M.; Milagro, F.I.; Martínéz, J.A. Future Perspectives of Personalized Weight Loss Interventions Based on Nutrigenetic, Epigenetic, and Metagenomic Data. *J. Nutr.* **2016**, *146*, 905S–912S. [CrossRef] [PubMed]
5. Zancarini, A.; Signor, C.L.; Terrat, S.; Aubert, J.; Salon, C.; Munier-Jolain, N.; Mougel, C. Medicago Truncatula Genotype Drives the Plant Nutritional Strategy and Its Associated Rhizosphere Bacterial Communities. *New Phytol.* **2024**, *245*, 767–784. [CrossRef] [PubMed]
6. Zancarini, A.; Mougel, C.; Voisin, A.-S.; Prudent, M.; Salon, C.; Munier-Jolain, N. Soil Nitrogen Availability and Plant Genotype Modify the Nutrition Strategies of M. Truncatula and the Associated Rhizosphere Microbial Communities. *PLoS ONE* **2012**, *7*, e47096. [CrossRef] [PubMed]
7. O'Brien, A.; Laurich, J.R.; Frederickson, M.E. Having the 'Right' Microbiome Matters for Host Trait Expression and the Strength of Mutualism Between Duckweeds and Microbes. *bioRxiv* **2022**. [CrossRef]
8. Hamonts, K.; Trivedi, P.; Garg, A.; Janitz, C.; Grinyer, J.; Holford, P.; Botha, F.C.; Anderson, I.C.; Singh, B.K. Field Study Reveals Core Plant Microbiota and Relative Importance of Their Drivers. *Environ. Microbiol.* **2018**, *20*, 124–140. [CrossRef] [PubMed]
9. Celis-Morales, C.; Livingstone, K.M.; Marsaux, C.F.M.; Macready, A.L.; Fallaize, R.; O'Donovan, C.B.; Woolhead, C.; Forster, H.; Walsh, M.C.; Navas-Carretero, S.; et al. Effect of Personalized Nutrition on Health-Related Behaviour Change: Evidence from the Food4me European Randomized Controlled Trial. *Int. J. Epidemiol.* **2017**, *46*, 578–588. [CrossRef] [PubMed]
10. Song, E.; Shin, J. Personalized Diets Based on the Gut Microbiome as a Target for Health Maintenance: From Current Evidence to Future Possibilities. *J. Microbiol. Biotechnol.* **2022**, *32*, 1497–1505. [CrossRef] [PubMed]
11. Athanasiadis, V.; Grigorakis, S.; Lalas, S.; Makris, D.P. Highly Efficient Extraction of Antioxidant Polyphenols from *Olea europaea* Leaves Using an Eco-friendly Glycerol/Glycine Deep Eutectic Solvent. *Waste Biomass Valor.* **2018**, *9*, 1985–1992. [CrossRef]

12. Athanasiadis, V.; Chatzimitakos, T.; Mantiniotou, M.; Bozinou, E.; Lalas, S.I. Exploring the Antioxidant Properties of *Citrus limon* (Lemon) Peel Ultrasound Extract after the Cloud Point Extraction Method. *Biomass* **2024**, *4*, 202–216. [CrossRef]
13. Wani, S.A. Utilization of Underutilized Vegetables. In *Sustainable Plant Foods*; Academic Press: Cambridge, MA, USA, 2025; pp. 97–110, ISBN 978-0-443-31652-4.
14. Lailheugue, V.; Darriaut, R.; Tran, J.; Morel, M.; Marguerit, E.; Lauvergeat, V. Both the Scion and Rootstock of Grafted Grapevines Influence the Rhizosphere and Root Endophyte Microbiomes, but Rootstocks Have a Greater Impact. *Environ. Microbiome* **2024**, *19*, 24. [CrossRef] [PubMed]
15. Rashidinejad, A. The road ahead for functional foods: Promising opportunities amidst industry challenges. *Future Postharvest Food* **2024**, *1*, 266–273. [CrossRef]
16. Phung, N.T.K.; Anh, N.C.H.; Thy, N.Q.; Anh, T.P.P.; Vinh, V.M.; Nhu, L.N.H. Economic Implications of Biotech-Driven Functional Foods: The Role of Consumer Trust and Scientific Validation, Moderated by Health Awareness. *J. Econ. Financ. Manag. Stud.* **2025**, *08*, 6360–6373. [CrossRef]

nutrients

MDPI

Article

Biological Effect of Mycosporine-Gly-Ser (Shinorine) Against Bis-Retinoid *N*-Retinyl-*N*-Retinylidene Ethanolamine- and Blue-Light-Induced Retinal Pigment Epithelium Cell Damage

Seung-Yub Song [1,2,†], Jeong-Yong Cho [3,†], Dae-Hun Park [4,†], Si-Hun Song [3], Sung-Ho Lee [1,2], Jin-Woo Park [1,2], Han-Kyu Lim [2,5] and Seung-Sik Cho [1,2,*]

1 Department of Pharmacy, College of Pharmacy, Mokpo National University, Muan 58554, Jeonnam, Republic of Korea
2 Biomedicine, Health & Life Convergence Sciences, BK21 Four, College of Pharmacy, Mokpo National University, Muan-gun 58554, Jeonnam, Republic of Korea
3 Department of Integrative Food, Bioscience and Biotechnology, Chonnam National University, Gwangju 61186, Jeollanam-do, Republic of Korea
4 College of Oriental Medicine, Dongshin University, Naju-si 58245, Jeonnam, Republic of Korea; dhj1221@hanmail.net
5 Department of Marine and Fisheries Resources, Mokpo National University, Muan 58554, Jeonnam, Republic of Korea
* Correspondence: sjason1@naver.com; Tel.: +82-10-3606-5801
† These authors contributed equally to this work.

Abstract: Shinorine is a mycosporine-like amino acid isolated from laver (*Porphyra dentata*), and interest in its functionality has increased recently due to increased production using yeast. There have been few reports on the pharmacological activity of shinorine, and we sought to find the pharmacological significance of shinorine. In the present study, we investigated the pharmacological effects of shinorine purified from *Porphyra dentata* on ARPE-19 cells. First, when ARPE-19 cells were treated with bis-retinoid *N*-retinyl-*N*-retinylidene ethanolamine (A2E) and blue light (BL), cytotoxicity increased, and apoptosis was observed. We investigated the effects of shinorine on A2E- and BL-induced cytotoxicity and changes in apoptotic factors, inflammation, and carbonyl stress. A2E and BL exposure increased ARPE-19 cell apoptosis, but this increase was attenuated by shinorine in a concentration-dependent manner. Treatment with A2E and BL induced ARPE-19 cell apoptosis, but treatment with shinorine decreased the apoptotic factors, such as MAPKs. Shinorine reduced *p*-JNK and *p*-P38, which were increased by A2E and BL. In addition, shinorine was found to regulate inflammatory proteins and proteins associated with carbonyl stress. In conclusion, shinorine may suppress cell damage caused by A2E treatment and BL exposure at the cellular level by regulating various cell death and inflammatory response pathways.

Keywords: mycosporine-like amino acid; black paper; *Porphyra dentata*; eye health; ARPE-19

1. Introduction

Mycosporine-like amino acids (MAAs) are metabolites derived by various marine organisms. In particular, MAAs are secondary metabolites to protect against light, such as ultraviolet (UV) light [1]. Microorganisms, such as cyanobacteria and *Microcystis aeruginosa*, produce MAAs, such as asterina-330 and shinorine, for photoprotection [2,3].

MAAs typically contain cyclohexenone or cyclohexenimine bonded to one or two amino acids or alcohols at the C1 and C3 positions [4]. To date, approximately 35 MAAs have been identified. One biological effect of MAA is its UV-blocking capability [5].

Recently, MAAs were reported to exert various biological effects. Shinorine is an MAA that is used for its varying biological effects. According to Fernandes et al., shinorine, porphyra-334, and mycosporine-glycine exhibit low toxicity in mouse fibroblasts [6]. Porphyra-334 and shinorine have also been reported to alleviate oxidative stress caused by ultraviolet rays by regulating the Nrf2 pathway [7]. Becker et al. revealed that shinorine and porphyra-334 affect the NF-κB pathway in vitro [8]. Shinorine and porphyra-334 regulate genes involved in inflammation, oxidative stress, and skin aging [9]. Recently, some MAAs have been reported to exhibit anticancer and wound-healing effects. Therefore, besides alleviating UV-induced damage, MAAs may be used in different pharmaceutical applications [10,11].

Shinorine is found in *Chordata, Cyanobacteria, Dinofluagellata, Lichen, Miozoa, Mollusca, Ochrophyta, Phaeophyta, Porifera*, and *Rhodophyta* [12,13]. Recently, 68 mg/L of shinorine were produced by manipulating a *Saccharomyces cerevisiae* strain. Therefore, further studies must be conducted to confirm the various functions and commercial applications of shinorine [14].

We found no studies on the effects of shinorine on eye health. The importance of eye protection due to consistent use of electronic devices is increasing. Excessive use of video equipment was found to increase the risk of macular degeneration and dry eye syndrome [15]. Long-term exposure to electronic devices has been linked to age-related macular degeneration (AMD) [16]. The BL from cellular phones comprises visible light ranging from 380 to 500 nm. Upon energy accumulation, substantial damage to retinal cells is induced [17]. Short wavelengths can increase intracellular free radical levels and induce cell damage. Exposure to short wavelengths is a known risk factor for uveal melanoma.

In our experiment, we aimed to investigate the preventive effect of shinorine against eye diseases and its effect on ocular cell damage induced by blue light (BL) and ultraviolet rays.

In a previous report, BL caused oxidative stress in dry AMD. BL has been reported to cause mitochondrial damage, such as weakening of the retinal layer and retinal cell death. In particular, mitochondrial functions were reported to deteriorate [18].

In the present study, shinorine at micromolar levels was found to efficiently reduce retinal pigment epithelial (RPE) cell damage caused by BL and reactive oxidants. In addition, the mechanism of action of shinorine was confirmed at the cellular level. Collectively, the results provide evidence supporting the development of shinorine as an effective functional material for the curation/prevention of macular disease.

2. Materials and Methods

2.1. Cytotoxocity

ARPE-19 cells (retinal pigment epithelium cells, from human) were used in vitro (ATCC, Manassas, VA, USA). The cells were maintained with Dulbecco's Modified Eagle's Medium containing 10% fetal bovine serum. The cells were cultured at 37 °C with 5% CO_2.

Shinorine was isolated according to a previously reported method. Shinorine was purified from laver by organic solvent extraction, RP-18 silica gel column, and Prep-LC, and the purity was 100%. The molecular structure was determined by NMR [19]. The ARPE-19 cells were treated with lutein and shinorine. Cell damage was induced using A2E (10 μM) and BL (20 mW/cm^2, 15 min). The ARPE-19 cells were seeded in a 96-well plate (5×10^3 cells/well). Then, the cells were continuously treated with lutein (10 μM) and shinorine (1.25–5 μM) for 24 h, and an MTT assay was performed according to previous reference [20]. When evaluating cytotoxicity, the lutein showed no toxicity below 10 μM, and the shinorine also showed no toxicity below 5 μM. Therefore, the maximum treatment concentration of the test substance was set at 10.5 μM.

2.2. Fluorescence-Activated Cell-Sorting (FACS) Assay

We aimed to determine the ratio of live cells and apoptotic cells after treatment with A2E and BL and the cellular patterns that changed after treatment with lutein and shinorine.

The ARPE-19 cells were seeded in a 6-well plate (2×10^5 cells/well) for 24 h. The treatment substances were shinorine and lutein, and shinorine was treated in the range of 1.25–5 μM and lutein at 10 μM. The cells were treated with A2E (10 μM) and then exposed to BL (20 mW/cm^2) for 15 min. After 24 h, the cells were washed with PBS, harvested using trypsin, and centrifuged. The cells were suspended with binding buffer and were treated with Alexa Fluor 488 annexin V (5 μL) and PI (1 mg/mL, 1 μL). A Guava easyCyte instrument (Millipore, Burlington, MA, USA) was used for cell sorting.

2.3. TUNEL Assay

The ARPE-19 cells were seeded at a density of 1×10^4 cells/well in a 4-chamber apparatus. After 24 h, the medium was removed, and the cells were treated with shinorine (1.25–5 μM) and lutein (10 μM). Then, the cells were co-treated with A2E and BL. Following medium removal, the cells were fixed with 4% formaldehyde and incubated with 0.25% Triton X-100. The cells were treated with TdT for one hour at 37 °C. Following nuclear staining with DAPI, a confocal microscope was used for imaging.

2.4. Western Blot

The ARPE-19 cells were co-treated with A2E and BL exposure. The cells were harvested using protease inhibitors and an RIPA buffer, and then, they were centrifuged for 20 min. The proteins were transferred to PVDF membranes and incubated with 5% skim milk for
2 h at 4 °C and then incubated with primary antibodies (1/100–1/500 dilution) overnight at 4 °C. Bcl-xL, Bcl-2, and GADPH were purchased from Invitrogen, and Bax and Bim were purchased from Santa Cruz Biotechnology. *p*-JNK, JNK, and *p*-P38 were purchased from Cell Signaling Technology. *p*-NF-κB, NF-κB, *p*-IκBα, and IκBα were purchased from Thermo Fisher Scientific Inc. (Waltham, MA, USA). PGE_2, COX-2, 4-HNE, and malondialdehyde were purchased from Abcam. The membrane was incubated with secondary antibodies (~1/200 dilution).

2.5. ELISA Analysis

Human ELISA kits for interleukin tumor necrosis factor alpha (TNF-α) and interleukin-6 (IL-6) and 1-beta (IL-1β) were purchased from the Thermo Fisher Scientific corporation. The samples were incubated with capture antibodies overnight at 4 °C. Following three washes with 0.05% Tween-20, the standards and samples were incubated for 2 h at 4 °C, followed by 1 h at room temperature. Following the addition of a stop solution, the sample was measured at 450 nm.

2.6. Immunofluorescence (IF) Analysis

The levels of *p*-NF-κB and COX-2 were determined via immunofluorescence analysis. The ARPE-19 cells were seeded at 1×10^4 cells/well in a 4-chamber apparatus. After 24 h, the medium was removed, and the cells were treated with shinorine (1.25–5 μM) and lutein (10 μM). The cells were treated with A2E (10 μM) after 24 h and exposed to BL (20 mW/cm^2) for 15 min. The cells were washed with PBS, fixed with 4% formaldehyde, and incubated with Triton X-100 (Thermo Fisher Scientific Inc.). The cells were blocked using 1% bovine serum albumin (BSA), incubated with primary antibodies overnight at 4 °C, washed thrice with PBS, and incubated with secondary antibodies. Following nuclear staining with DAPI, *p*-NF-Kb, COX-2, Alexa Fluor 488-conjugated anti-rabbit IgG, or Alexa Fluor 555-conjugated anti-goat IgG was employed.

2.7. Statistical Analysis

The experimental results are expressed as the mean ± standard deviation (SD). Statistical significance was determined using one-way analysis of variance (ANOVA) and Dunnett's multiple comparison test. Excel software was used. The p value was set at $p < 0.05$. All the tests were repeated three times.

3. Results and Discussion

3.1. Cytotoxicity

As presented in Figure 1A, lutein and shinorine are considered safe when used at concentrations of up to 5 μM. Thus, subsequent experiments were performed with up to 5 μM of these compounds. Cytotoxicity was found to be reduced due to the A2E and BL doses dependently. The cell survival rate was approximately 76% following treatment with A2E and BL. Treatment with 10 μM of lutein resulted in a cell survival rate of 89%, while treatment with 5 μM of shinorine resulted in a survival rate of 92% (Figure 1B).

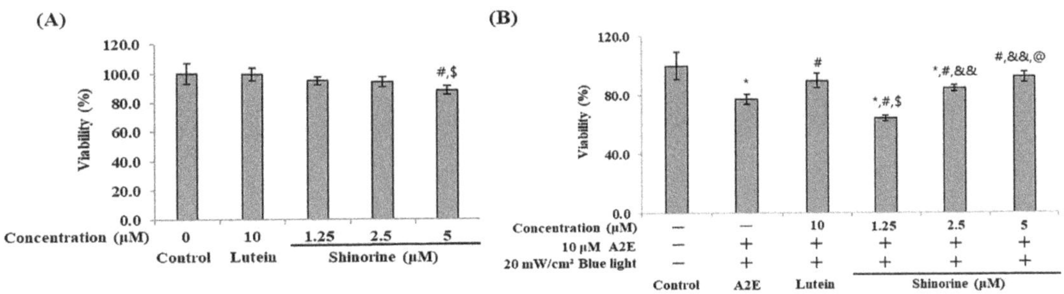

Figure 1. Cytotoxicity of shinorine on ARPE-19. (**A**) ARPE-19 cells treated with lutein (10 μM) and shinorine (1.25–5 μM); (**B**) shinorin attenuated A2E- and BL-induced cytotoxicity. Mean ± S.D. ($n = 3$) triplicate. * $p < 0.05$ vs. CON; # $p < 0.05$ vs. A2E; $ $p < 0.05$ vs. Lutein; && $p < 0.001$ vs. 1.25 μM; @ $p < 0.05$ vs. 2.5 μM.

3.2. Shinorine Regulated the Apoptotic Factors in ARPE-19

When A2E and BL were simultaneously administered, the number of apoptotic cells increased in the order of 10% (Figure 2). In the lutein treatment group, the apoptotic cells decreased to approximately 6.7%. Shinorine reduced the number of apoptotic cells in a concentration-dependent manner (Figure 2A). In fact, 5 μM of shinorine decreased the number of apoptotic cells to approximately 5.8%, which aligns with the percentage of apoptotic cells found in the untreated group. As shown in Figure 2B, in particular, shinorine also reduced A2E- and BL-induced cell death in a concentration-dependent manner.

Figure 3 shows the expression patterns of apoptosis. When A2E and BL were co-treated, the expression of Bcl-2 decreased. However, in the groups treated with 10 μM lutein and 5 μM shinorine, the Bcl-2 expression was almost restored to the control level. The Bcl-xL expression did not reveal significant changes following treatment with A2E and BL; however, treatment with lutein and shinorine increased the expression of Bcl-xL. In terms of Bax and Bim, lutein (10 μM) could not reduce the expression induced by A2E and BL; however, shinorine reduced the expression of Bax, Bad, and Bim.

(A)

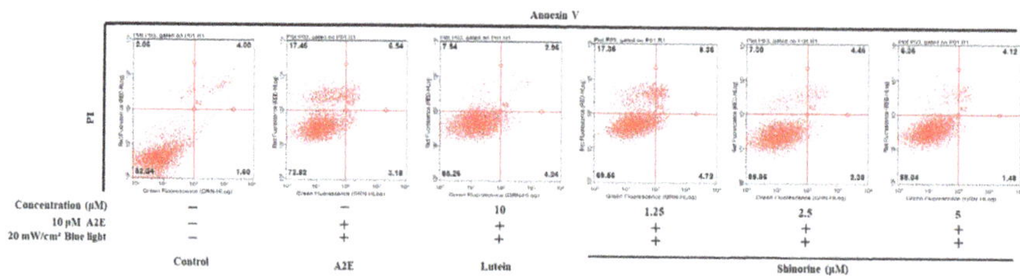

(B)

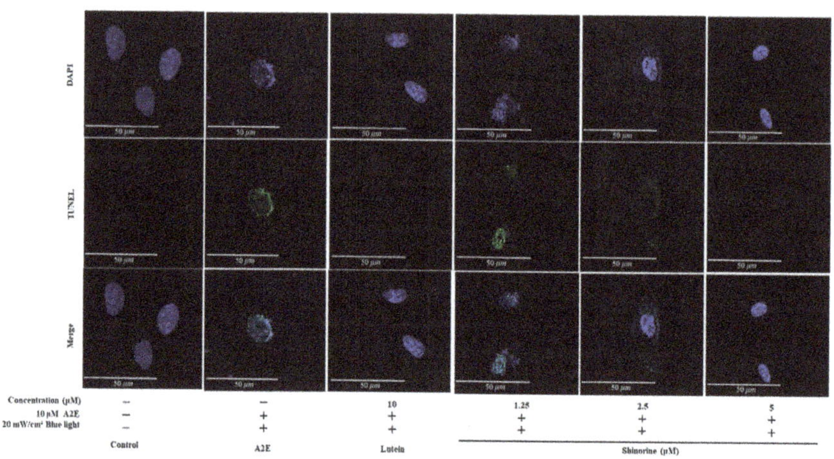

Figure 2. Shinorine reduces apoptosis induced by A2E and BL. (**A**) Annexin V/PI staining and flow cytometry. Q1: Necroptotic cells; Q2: Late apoptotic cells; Q3: Early apoptosis; Q4: Live cells. (**B**) TUNEL results indicating a decrease in apoptosis with an increase in shinorine concentration. α-tubulin (green) and DAPI (blue) were visualized using a confocal microscope. Magnification 10×; Scale bar, 50 μm.

3.3. *Shinorine Regulated the p38 and JNK in ARPE-19*

As shown in Figure 4, by determining the expression of MAPKs related to apoptosis, the phosphorylation levels of JNK and p38 were found to increase following the simultaneous administration of A2E and BL (Figure 4A). Notably, shinorine reduced the expression of *p*-JNK and weakly inhibited that of *p*-p38 in a dose-dependent manner. Compared to lutein (10 μM), shinorine (5 μM) exhibited a marked inhibition of *p*-JNK expression. Treatment with lutein markedly inhibited the expression of *p*-p38 (Figure 4B).

3.4. *Shinorine Regulated the Inflammatory Response in ARPE-19 Cells*

Shinorine was effective in regulating the inflammatory proteins that were increased by the A2E and BL treatments. As shown in Figure 5A–C, Shinorine reduced the expression levels of *p*-NF-kB, COX-2, and PGE2 that were increased by A2E and BL. In addition, shinorine regulated the production of pro-inflammatory cytokines (Figure 5D).

3.5. Shinorine Regulated the Carbonyl Stress Induced by A2E and BL

We investigated whether A2E- and BL-induced apoptosis and inflammation were associated with carbonyl stress. Shinorine decreased the expression levels of 4-HNE and MDA, which were induced by A2E and BL (Figure 6A,B).

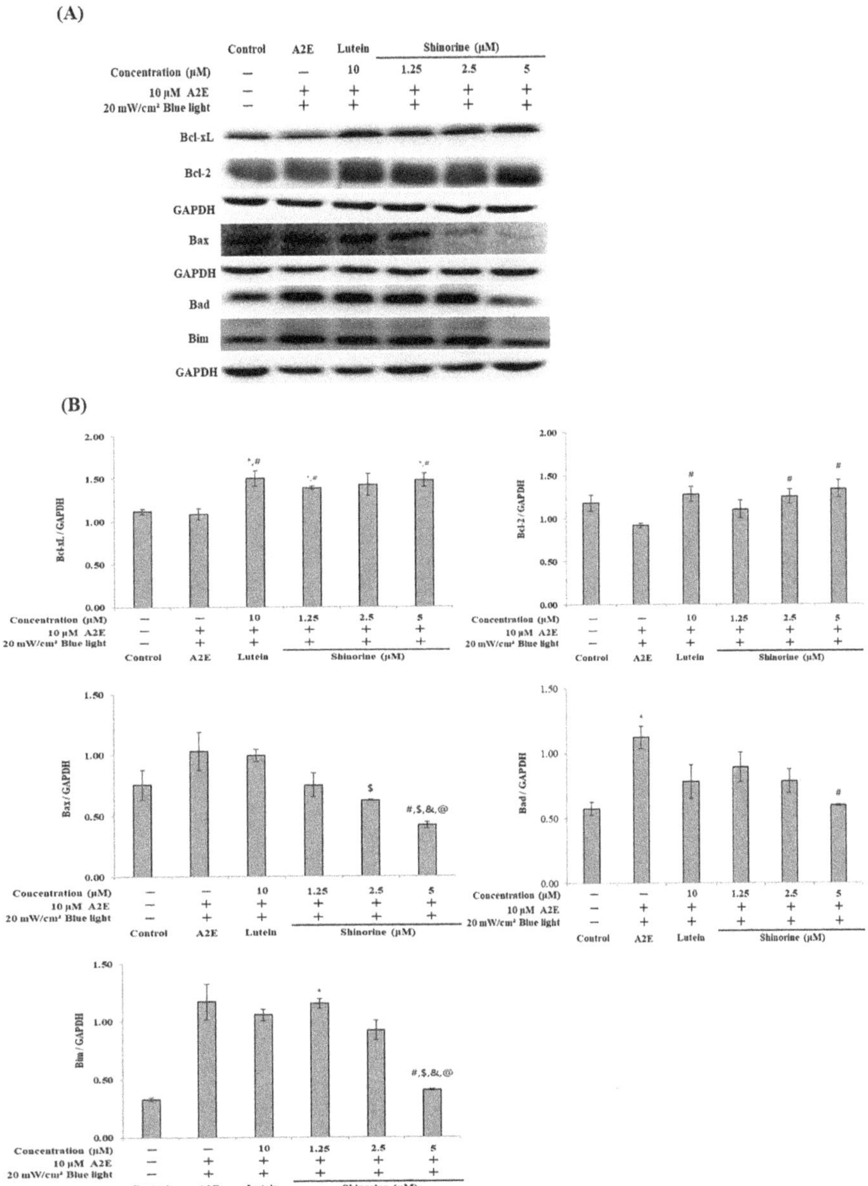

Figure 3. Expression of Bcl family induced by A2E plus BL. (**A**) Western blot of Bcl proteins. (**B**) Densitometry (Image J 1.54 software) of expressed Bcl proteins. Mean ± S.D. (n = 3), triplicate. * $p < 0.05$ vs. CON; # $p < 0.05$ vs. A2E; $ $p < 0.05$ vs. Lutein; & $p < 0.05$ vs. 1.25 μM; @ $p < 0.05$ vs. 2.5 μM.

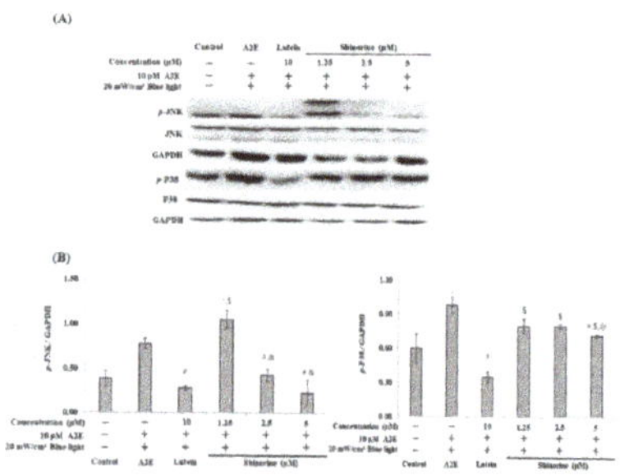

Figure 4. Expression of of MAPKs induced by A2E plus BL. (**A**) Western blots of *p*-JNK, JNK, *p*-P38, P38, and GAPDH. (**B**) Densitometry (Image J software) of expressed MAPKs. Mean ± S.D (n = 3). Triplicate, * $p < 0.05$ vs. CON; # $p < 0.05$ vs. A2E; $ $p < 0.05$ vs. Lutein; & $p < 0.05$ vs. 1.25 μm; @ $p < 0.05$ vs. 2.5 μM.

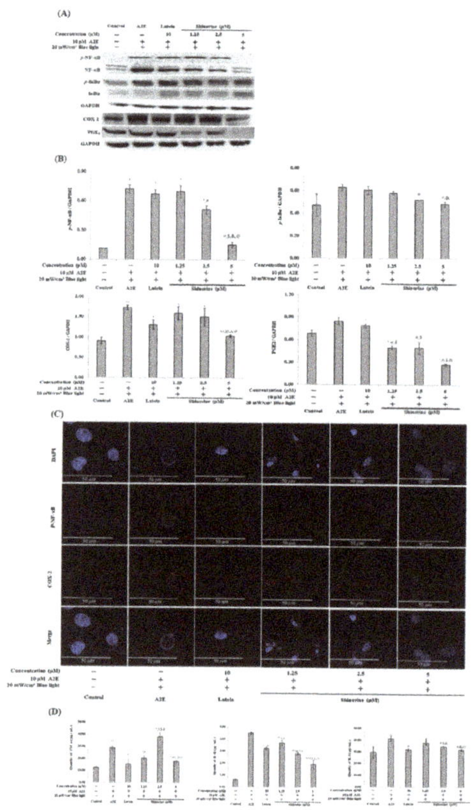

Figure 5. Shinorine has anti-inflammatory effect in ARPE-19. (**A**) Expression of inflammatory biomarkers; (**B**) densitometry (Image J software) of expressed inflammatory biomarkers; (**C**) immunofluorescence images of *p*-NF-κB and COX-2. DAPI (blue) was visualized using a confocal microscope. Magnification 10×; Scale bar, 50 μm; (**D**) ELISA assay of pro-inflammatory cytokines. Mean ± S.D. (n = 3). * $p < 0.05$ vs. CON; ** $p < 0.001$ vs. CON; # $p < 0.05$ vs. A2E; ## $p < 0.001$ vs. A2E; $ $p < 0.05$ vs. Lutein; $$ $p < 0.001$ vs. Lutein; & $p < 0.05$ vs. 1.25 μM; @ $p < 0.05$ vs. 2.5 μM; @@ $p < 0.001$ vs. 2.5 μM.

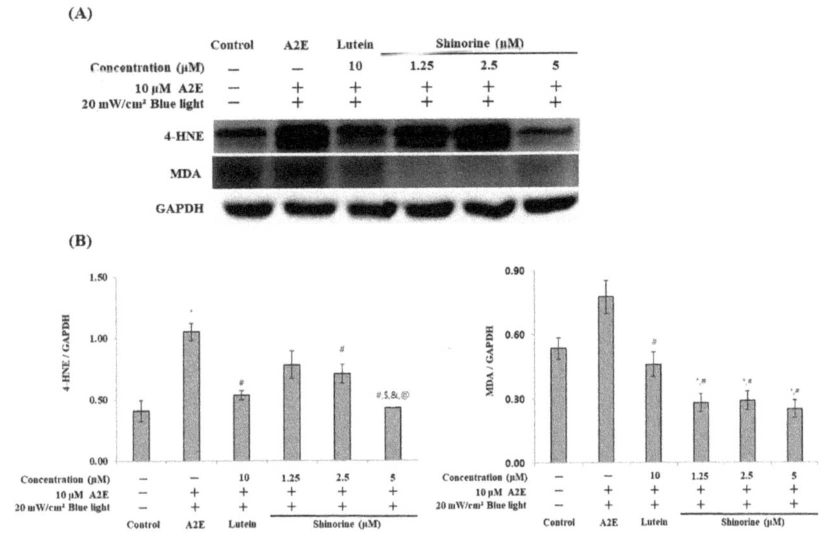

Figure 6. Shinorine decreases carbonyl stress induced by BL plus A2E. (**A**) Expression of 4-HNE, MDA, and GAPDH; (**B**) densitometry (Image J software) of 4-HNE, MDA. Mean ± S.D. ($n = 3$). * $p < 0.05$ vs. CON; # $p < 0.05$ vs. A2E; $ $p < 0.05$ vs. Lutein; & $p < 0.05$ vs. 1.25 μM; @ $p < 0.05$ vs. 2.5 μM.

4. Discussion

In the present study, treatment with A2E and BL was found to induce cytotoxicity in RPE cells. Lutein and shinorine regulated increased inflammatory and apoptotic biomarkers induced by A2E and BL.

BL has been reported to cause damage to eye cells and is linked to diseases such as macular degeneration [21]. In a previous report, cell damage was induced by treatment with A2E and BL. BL causes extreme oxidative stress in dry AMD. In vivo, BL was found to induce apoptosis in the retinal layer and reduce mitochondrial function. In particular, mitochondrial function was found to be clearly weakened by long-term BL exposure [21].

As MAAs, such as shinorine, protect against UV-induced damage [14], we decided to determine whether MAAs can inhibit UV and other types of light-induced damage. We confirmed that 5 μM of shinorine could regulate A2E-induced and BL-induced apoptosis and inflammation in RPE cells. Lutein is a representative eye drug that is broadly used as an ingredient in functional foods and is broadly used worldwide to prevent retinal degeneration [22]. The protective effects of lutein have been demonstrated using RPE cells and mouse models [23]. Therefore, lutein was employed as a control. In this study, 10 μM of lutein were found to alleviate RPE cell damage.

Studies have revealed the UV-protective and wound-healing effect of shinorine [11,14]. To our knowledge, we are the first to report the protective effect of MMA(shinorine) relative to the eye. According to previous studies, MAA is involved in DNA damage, the inhibition of reactive oxygen species (ROS) production, and thymine dimer formation [24]. The activity of MAAs may be based on their respective residue. By comparing shinorine and porphyra-334 residues, shinorine was found to contain serine residue, whereas porphyra-334 exhibited threonine residue. In our preliminary study, when the same concentrations of shinorine and porphyra-334 were administered to cells that were subsequently exposed to A2E and BL, we confirmed that shinorine further reduced the number of apoptotic cells. Therefore, we speculate that serine residue is responsible for the biological difference between shinorine and porphyra-334.

In a previous paper, BL was reported to increase the production of oxi-A2E in RPE cells treated with A2E and induce apoptosis and inflammation. As a result, photoreceptor cells are damaged by lipofuscin and die [25]. Therefore, we sought to elucidate how MAAs such as shinorine protect against inflammation and/or apoptosis of RPE cells induced by A2E and BL. As shown in Figure 1, lutein (10 μM) and shinorine (5 μM) attenuated A2E- and BL-induced cytotoxicity. Therefore, subsequent experiments were performed using concentrations less than 10 μM and 5 μM, respectively (Figure 1).

MAPKs are widely studied and are associated with various processes and diseases, such as inflammation and cancer [26]. MAPKs are closely related to RPE cell differentiation, and they seem to be particularly associated with p38 and JNK [27].

We found that A2E and BL induced the phosphorylation of p38 and JNK in RPE cells, suggesting that apoptosis and inflammatory responses may be induced. UV has an effect on ocular cells, and our results are similar to studies that report that UV increases the expression of ERK1/2, p38, and JNK in RPE cells [28]. Therefore, it can be observed that MAAs such as shinorine regulate ARPE-19 cell damage induced by A2E and BL by regulating the MAPK pathway.

Tsao et al. revealed that the death of RPE cells treated with H_2O_2 does not involve ERK1/2 but is affected by JNK and p38 activation [29]. According to Sawyer et al., the activation of ERK1/2 induces apoptosis [30]. In our results, A2E and BL induced p38 and JNK expression, aligning with the results of Tsao et al. Shinorine downregulated A2E-induced and BL-induced JNK activation but only weakly regulated p38 (Figure 4).

Bcl-xL and BCL-2 are apoptotic factors, and cytochrome C is closely related to the BCL family [31]. Treatment with 5 μM of shinorine induced an increase in Bcl-xL and Bcl-2 expression, similarly to that obtained following treatment with 10 μM of lutein. In addition, the expression levels of Bax, Bad, and Bim, which are pro-apoptotic protein-induced by A2E and BL, were suppressed by lutein and shinorine. Such findings align with that of a previous study, in which factors, such as Bad, were found to form dimers with Bcl-xL. Taken together, shinorine inhibits RPE cell death by controlling the apoptotic pathway (Figure 3).

BL has been reported to induce oxidized A2E and ROS production [32]. ROS are known to induce cell death by causing oxidative stress. [33]. Wang et al. described that oxidative stress-induced inflammation is also closely associated with apoptosis of RPE cells [34].

Continuously exposing RPE cells to oxidative stress can damage the mitochondria [35], which eventually worsens macular degeneration. Thus, RPE damage induced by oxidative stress is considered one of the main factors of eye diseases. Fiorani et al. revealed that light exposure activates microglia and induces an inflammatory response. In a similar study, Guillonneau reported that if microglia activate and accumulate in the subretinal space, activated cells release inflammatory cytokines [36]. Therefore, the simultaneous treatment of RPE cells with A2E and BL may be an important factor in inducing ocular diseases through apoptosis and inflammatory responses.

Few reports have been described regarding the mechanisms of action between inflammation and carbonyl/oxidative stress in RPE cells. Yang et al. reported that 4-HNE induces the production of inflammatory cytokines and modified the HSP70 in RPE cells [37].

In the present study, A2E and BL treatments resulted in the increased expression of 4-HNE and MDA; however, treatment with shinorine regulated this effect (Figure 6). This result is associated with the data presented in Figure 5, in which the levels of pro-inflammatory cytokines that were increased following treatments with A2E and BL were downregulated by treatments with shinorine. Thus, it was found that shinorine effectively attenuates the apoptosis and inflammatory response of ARPE-19 cells induced by A2E and BL and is considered an appropriate functional material for the treatment of AMD.

5. Conclusions

In the present study, we obtained shinorine from the main component of *Porphyra dentata* in order to verify its pharmacological effect in RPE cells. It was confirmed that apoptosis and inflammatory responses induced by A2E and BL are regulated by shinorine. In addition, apoptosis and inflammatory reactions were found to be associated with carbonyl stress. The results of our study suggest that *Porphyra dentata* and its major constituent, shinorine, have a curative effect on eye health and/or disease, and it is thought that future studies on the safety of shinorine should be combined with in vivo studies.

Author Contributions: Conceptualization and methodology, S.-Y.S., J.-Y.C. and S.-H.S.; investigation and data curation, S.-H.L., J.-Y.C., S.-H.S., H.-K.L., J.-W.P. and D.-H.P.; writing—original draft preparation, S.-S.C. All authors have read and agreed to the published version of the manuscript.

Funding: This work was supported by the National Research Foundation of Korea (NRF) grant, funded by the Korea government (MSIT) (RS-2022-NR070862) and was supported by the Korea Institute of Marine Science & Technology Promotion (KIMST), funded by the Ministry of Oceans and Fisheries (RS-2022-KS221671).

Institutional Review Board Statement: Not applicable.

Informed Consent Statement: Not applicable.

Data Availability Statement: Should any raw data files be needed, they are available from the corresponding author upon reasonable request.

Conflicts of Interest: The authors declare no conflicts of interest.

References

1. Peng, J.; Guo, F.; Liu, S.; Fang, H.; Xu, Z.; Wang, T. Recent Advances and Future Prospects of Mycosporine-like Amino Acids. *Molecules* **2023**, *28*, 5588. [CrossRef] [PubMed]
2. Ficek, D.; Dera, J.; Woźniak, B. UV absorption reveals mycosporine-like amino acids (MAAs) in Tatra mountain lake phytoplankton. *Oceanologia* **2013**, *55*, 599–609. [CrossRef]
3. Babele, P.K.; Singh, G.; Singh, A.; Kumar, A.; Tyagi, M.B.; Sinha, R.P. UV-B radiation and temperature stress-induced alterations in metabolic events and defense mechanisms in a bloom-forming cyanobacterium Microcystis aeruginosa. *Acta Physiol. Plant.* **2017**, *39*, 248. [CrossRef]
4. Carreto, J.I.; Carignan, M.O. Mycosporine-like amino acids: Relevant secondary metabolites. Chemical and ecological aspects. *Mar. Drugs* **2011**, *9*, 387–446. [CrossRef]
5. Hartmann, A.; Gostner, J.; Fuchs, J.E.; Chaita, E.; Aligiannis, N.; Skaltsounis, L.; Ganzera, M. Inhibition of Collagenase by Mycosporine-like Amino Acids from Marine Sources. *Planta Medica* **2015**, *81*, 813–820. [CrossRef]
6. Fernandes, S.C.; Alonso-Varona, A.; Palomares, T.; Zubillaga, V.; Labidi, J.; Bulone, V. Exploiting Mycosporines as Natural Molecular Sunscreens for the Fabrication of UV-Absorbing Green Materials. *ACS Appl. Mater. Interfaces* **2015**, *7*, 16558–16564. [CrossRef]
7. Gacesa, R.; Lawrence, K.P.; Georgakopoulos, N.D.; Yabe, K.; Dunlap, W.C.; Barlow, D.J.; Wells, G.; Young, A.R.; Long, P.F. The mycosporine-like amino acids porphyra-334 and shinorine are antioxidants and direct antagonists of Keap1-Nrf2 binding. *Biochimie* **2018**, *154*, 35–44. [CrossRef]
8. Becker, K.; Hartmann, A.; Ganzera, M.; Fuchs, D.; Gostner, J.M. Immunomodulatory Effects of the Mycosporine-Like Amino Acids Shinorine and Porphyra-334. *Mar. Drugs* **2016**, *14*, 119. [CrossRef]
9. Suh, S.S.; Hwang, J.; Park, M.; Seo, H.H.; Kim, H.S.; Lee, J.H.; Moh, S.H.; Lee, T.K. Anti-inflammation activities of mycosporine-like amino acids (MAAs) in response to UV radiation suggest potential anti-skin aging activity. *Mar. Drugs* **2014**, *12*, 5174–5187. [CrossRef]

10. Yuan, Y.V.; Westcott, N.D.; Hu, C.; Kitts, D.D. Mycosporine-like amino acid composition of the edible red alga, Palmaria palmata (dulse) harvested from the west and east coasts of Grand Manan Island, New Brunswick. *Food Chem.* **2009**, *112*, 321–328. [CrossRef]
11. Choi, Y.H.; Yang, D.J.; Kulkarni, A.; Moh, S.H.; Kim, K.W. Mycosporine-Like Amino Acids Promote Wound Healing through Focal Adhesion Kinase (FAK) and Mitogen-Activated Protein Kinases (MAP Kinases) Signaling Pathway in Keratinocytes. *Mar. Drugs* **2015**, *13*, 7055–7066. [CrossRef] [PubMed]
12. Carignan, M.O.; Cardozo, K.H.; Oliveira-Silva, D.; Colepicolo, P.; Carreto, J.I. Palythine-threonine, a major novel mycosporine-like amino acid (MAA) isolated from the hermatypic coral Pocillopora capitata. *J. Photochem. Photobiol. B Biol.* **2009**, *94*, 191–200. [CrossRef] [PubMed]
13. Rastogi, R.P.; Sinha, R.P. Biotechnological and industrial significance of cyanobacterial secondary metabolites. *Biotechnol. Adv.* **2009**, *27*, 521–539. [CrossRef] [PubMed]
14. Jin, C.; Kim, S.; Moon, S.; Jin, H.; Hahn, J.S. Efficient production of shinorine, a natural sunscreen material, from glucose and xylose by deleting HXK2 encoding hexokinase in Saccharomyces cerevisiae. *FEMS Yeast Res.* **2021**, *21*, foab053. [CrossRef]
15. Chidi-Egboka, N.C.; Jalbert, I.; Golebiowski, B. Smartphone gaming induces dry eye symptoms and reduces blinking in school-aged children. *Eye* **2023**, *37*, 1342–1349. [CrossRef]
16. Zhao, Z.C.; Zhou, Y.; Tan, G.; Li, J. Research progress about the effect and prevention of blue light on eyes. *Int. J. Ophthalmol.* **2018**, *11*, 1999–2003. [CrossRef]
17. Theruveethi, N.; Bui, B.V.; Joshi, M.B.; Valiathan, M.; Ganeshrao, S.B.; Gopalakrishnan, S.; Kabekkodu, S.P.; Bhat, S.S.; Surendran, S. Blue Light-Induced Retinal Neuronal Injury and Amelioration by Commercially Available Blue Light-Blocking Lenses. *Life* **2022**, *12*, 243. [CrossRef]
18. Wang, L.; Yu, X.; Zhang, D.; Wen, Y.; Zhang, L.; Xia, Y.; Chen, J.; Xie, C.; Zhu, H.; Tong, J.; et al. Long-term blue light exposure impairs mitochondrial dynamics in the retina in light-induced retinal degeneration in vivo and in vitro. *J. Photochem. Photobiol. B Biol.* **2023**, *240*, 112654. [CrossRef]
19. Choi, S.Y.; Lee, S.Y.; Kim, H.G.; Jeong, J.C.; Batara, D.C.; Kim, S.H.; Cho, J.Y. Shinorine and porphyra-334 isolated from laver (Porphyra dentata) inhibit adipogenesis in 3T3-L1 cells. *Food Sci. Biotechnol.* **2022**, *31*, 617–625. [CrossRef]
20. Song, S.Y.; Park, D.H.; Lee, S.H.; Lim, H.K.; Park, J.W.; Seo, J.W.; Cho, S.S. Protective Effects of 7S,15R-Dihydroxy-16S,17S-Epoxy-Docosapentaenoic Acid (diHEP-DPA) against Blue Light-Induced Retinal Damages in A2E-Laden ARPE-19 Cells. *Antioxidants* **2024**, *13*, 982. [CrossRef]
21. Wu, J.; Seregard, S.; Algvere, P.V. Photochemical damage of the retina. *Surv. Ophthalmol.* **2006**, *51*, 461–481. [CrossRef] [PubMed]
22. Agrón, E.; Mares, J.; Clemons, T.E.; Swaroop, A.; Chew, E.Y.; Keenan, T.D.L. Dietary Nutrient Intake and Progression to Late Age-Related Macular Degeneration in the Age-Related Eye Disease Studies 1 and 2. *Ophthalmology* **2021**, *128*, 425–442. [CrossRef] [PubMed]
23. Jo, Y.-D.; Kim, J.; Choung, S.-Y. Protective effects of quercetin-3-O-α-l-arabinopyranoside against UVA induced apoptosis via regulating inflammatory pathways in ARPE-19 cells and Balb/c mice. *J. Funct. Foods* **2019**, *62*, 103541. [CrossRef]
24. Kasanah, N.; Ulfah, M.; Imania, O.; Hanifah, A.N.; Marjan, M.I.D. Rhodophyta as Potential Sources of Photoprotectants, Antiphotoaging Compounds, and Hydrogels for Cosmeceutical Application. *Molecules* **2022**, *27*, 7788. [CrossRef]
25. Marie, M.; Gondouin, P.; Pagan, D.; Barrau, C.; Villette, T.; Sahel, J.; Picaud, S. Blue-violet light decreases VEGFa production in an in vitro model of AMD. *PLoS ONE* **2019**, *14*, e0223839. [CrossRef]
26. Kyosseva, S.V. Targeting MAPK Signaling in Age-Related Macular Degeneration. *Ophthalmol. Eye Dis.* **2016**, *8*, 23–30. [CrossRef]
27. Zhang, W.; Liu, H.T. MAPK signal pathways in the regulation of cell proliferation in mammalian cells. *Cell Res.* **2002**, *12*, 9–18. [CrossRef]
28. Roduit, R.; Schorderet, D.F. MAP kinase pathways in UV-induced apoptosis of retinal pigment epithelium ARPE19 cells. *Apoptosis* **2008**, *13*, 343–353. [CrossRef]
29. Tsao, Y.P.; Ho, T.C.; Chen, S.L.; Cheng, H.C. Pigment epithelium-derived factor inhibits oxidative stress-induced cell death by activation of extracellular signal-regulated kinases in cultured retinal pigment epithelial cells. *Life Sci.* **2006**, *79*, 545–550. [CrossRef]
30. Sawyer, R.T. Thrombolytics and Anticoagulants from Leeches. *Bio/Technology* **1991**, *9*, 513–518. [CrossRef]
31. Jürgensmeier, J.M.; Xie, Z.; Deveraux, Q.; Ellerby, L.; Bredesen, D.; Reed, J.C. Bax directly induces release of cytochrome c from isolated mitochondria. *Proc. Natl. Acad. Sci. USA* **1998**, *95*, 4997–5002. [CrossRef] [PubMed]
32. Sparrow, J.R.; Zhou, J.; Ben-Shabat, S.; Vollmer, H.; Itagaki, Y.; Nakanishi, K. Involvement of oxidative mechanisms in blue-light-induced damage to A2E-laden RPE. *Investig. Ophthalmol. Vis. Sci.* **2002**, *43*, 1222–1227.
33. Fang, Y.; Su, T.; Qiu, X.; Mao, P.; Xu, Y.; Hu, Z.; Zhang, Y.; Zheng, X.; Xie, P.; Liu, Q. Protective effect of alpha-mangostin against oxidative stress induced-retinal cell death. *Sci. Rep.* **2016**, *6*, 21018. [CrossRef] [PubMed]

34. Wang, Y.; Shen, D.; Wang, V.M.; Yu, C.R.; Wang, R.X.; Tuo, J.; Chan, C.C. Enhanced apoptosis in retinal pigment epithelium under inflammatory stimuli and oxidative stress. *Apoptosis* **2012**, *17*, 1144–1155. [CrossRef]
35. Kaarniranta, K.; Uusitalo, H.; Blasiak, J.; Felszeghy, S.; Kannan, R.; Kauppinen, A.; Salminen, A.; Sinha, D.; Ferrington, D. Mechanisms of mitochondrial dysfunction and their impact on age-related macular degeneration. *Prog. Retin. Eye Res.* **2020**, *79*, 100858. [CrossRef]
36. Guillonneau, X.; Eandi, C.M.; Paques, M.; Sahel, J.A.; Sapieha, P.; Sennlaub, F. On phagocytes and macular degeneration. *Prog. Retin. Eye Res.* **2017**, *61*, 98–128. [CrossRef]
37. Yang, H.J.; Hu, R.; Sun, H.; Bo, C.; Li, X.; Chen, J.B. 4-HNE induces proinflammatory cytokines of human retinal pigment epithelial cells by promoting extracellular efflux of HSP70. *Exp. Eye Res.* **2019**, *188*, 107792. [CrossRef]

nutrients

Article

Evaluation of Metabolic Dysfunction-Associated Fatty Liver Disease-Related Pathogenic Mechanisms in Human Steatotic Liver Cell-Based Model: Beneficial Effects of *Prunus domestica* L. subsp. *syriaca* Extract

Laura Comi [1,†], Claudia Giglione [1,†], Fationa Tolaj Klinaku [1], Lorenzo Da Dalt [1], Hammad Ullah [2], Maria Daglia [3,4] and Paolo Magni [1,5,*]

1 Department of Pharmacological and Biomolecular Sciences, Università degli Studi di Milano, 20133 Milan, Italy; laura.comi1@unimi.it (L.C.); claudia.giglione@unimi.it (C.G.); fationa.tolaj@unimi.it (F.T.K.); lorenzo.dadalt@unimi.it (L.D.D.)
2 School of Pharmacy, University of Management and Technology, Lahore 54000, Pakistan; hammadrph@gmail.com
3 Department of Pharmacy, University of Naples Federico II, 80168 Naples, Italy; maria.daglia@unina.it
4 International Research Center for Food Nutrition and Safety, Jiangsu University, Zhenjiang 212013, China
5 IRCCS MultiMedica, 20099 Sesto San Giovanni, Milan, Italy
* Correspondence: paolo.magni@unimi.it; Tel.: +39-0250318229
† These authors equally contributed as first author.

Abstract: Background/Objectives: Disrupted glucose uptake, oxidative stress, and increased de novo lipogenesis are some of the key features of metabolic dysfunction-associated fatty liver disease (MASLD). The modulation of these pathogenic mechanisms using extracts from natural and sustainable sources is a promising strategy to mitigate disease progression. This study aimed to evaluate the effects of *Prunus domestica* L. subsp. syriaca extract on these processes, taking advantage of a cell-based model of steatotic hepatocytes (HepG2-OA) that recapitulates some key pathophysiological features of MASLD. **Methods**: The HepG2-OA cell model was generated by treating cells for 7 days with 100 μM oleic acid (OA). The effect of different concentrations (0.01, 0.1, 0.5, and 1 mg/mL) of *P. domestica* extract was assessed through MTT assay (cell viability), flow cytometry (glucose uptake and reactive oxygen species, ROS, production), spectrophotometry (lipid accumulation), and qRT-PCR (expression of selected genes). **Results**: *P. domestica* extract exhibited no cytotoxicity at any tested concentration after 24 and 48 h in the HepG2-OA cells. The extract increased glucose uptake in a dose-dependent fashion after both 6 and 24 h. Additionally, the extract reduced lipid accumulation and downregulated the expression of key lipogenic genes (DGAT1 and FASN). Furthermore, in the HepG2-OA cells, *P. domestica* extract reduced ROS production and downregulated the expression of oxidative stress-related genes (SOD and CAT). **Conclusions**: *P. domestica* extract positively modulated some key molecular mechanisms associated with glucose metabolism, lipogenesis, and oxidative stress, supporting its potential as a nutraceutical candidate for MASLD management.

Keywords: metabolic dysfunction-associated fatty liver disease (MASLD); HepG2 hepatocytes; oleic acid; glucose uptake; oxidative stress; lipid accumulation; *Prunus domestica* L. subsp. *syriaca*; natural extract; agro-food waste

1. Introduction

Metabolic dysfunction-associated fatty liver disease (MASLD) has emerged as the most prevalent chronic liver condition worldwide [1], affecting approximately one in four individuals [2]. Closely linked to obesity and type 2 diabetes mellitus (T2DM), MASLD represents a critical component of metabolic syndrome and is projected to rise in prevalence alongside these conditions [3]. While often asymptomatic in its early stages, MASLD can progress to metabolic dysfunction-associated steatohepatitis (MASH), a more severe form characterized by inflammation, hepatocellular damage, and fibrosis, increasing the risk of cirrhosis and hepatocellular carcinoma (HCC) [4].

In this context, cell-based in vitro models are crucial for evaluating the effect of potential treatments for MASLD on specific pathogenetic mechanisms. Interestingly, when exposed to the fatty acid oleic acid (OA), human HepG2 cells, a widely used cell model able to mimic some hepatocyte features [5], develop intracellular lipid accumulation and cytotoxic responses, closely recapitulating some key features of MASLD [6]. Specifically, this cell-based model, defined here as HepG2-OA, recapitulates the relevant disease's molecular hallmarks, including fat accumulation [7], driven by de novo lipogenesis, insulin resistance, oxidative stress, and inflammation [8].

Current MASLD management relies on lifestyle modifications, particularly the adoption of a Mediterranean diet [9] and regular physical activity, which improve insulin sensitivity and reduce liver fat [10]. Given the absence of approved pharmacological treatments [11], nutraceuticals, derived from food sources, are being explored for their potential hepatoprotective effects [12]. Polyphenols [13], omega-3 fatty acids, probiotics, prebiotics [14], and silymarin [15] have demonstrated antioxidant and anti-inflammatory properties on HepG2 steatotic cells, proving effective for MASLD management [16].

Prunus domestica L. subsp. *syriaca* (*P. domestica*; Mirabelle plum) extract is a promising nutraceutical candidate in this field due to its rich composition of hydroxycinnamic acids, flavanols, and glycoside flavonols, which contribute to its antioxidant and anti-inflammatory activities [17]. Various *Prunus* species have been shown to positively regulate body weight, glucose and lipid homeostasis, insulin resistance, prothrombin state, and chronic inflammation, as well as improve hypertension-related signaling pathways [18]. Furthermore, since the plum production chain features a relevant amount of agro-food waste, utilizing *Prunus* extracts aligns with sustainable agro-food waste valorization, adding economic and environmental benefits [19].

This study aimed to test the effect of *P. domestica* extract on the modulation of lipid accumulation, the reduction in glucose uptake, and the increase in oxidative stress, taking advantage of the HepG2-OA cell model.

2. Materials and Methods

2.1. Chemicals

Dulbecco's Phosphate-Buffered Saline (DPBS), Fetal Bovine Serum (FBS), L-Glutamine, non-essential amino acids, dimethyl sulfoxide (DMSO), and isopropanol (99.5%) were obtained from Gibco ThermoFisher (Waltham, MA, USA). Oleic Acid-Water Soluble, hydrogen peroxide (H_2O_2), 6-Hydroxy-2,5,7,8-tetramethylchroman-2-carboxylic acid (Trolox), Lipid (Oil Red O) Staining kit, and dextran-coated charcoal (DCC) were obtained from Sigma-Aldrich (Milan, Italy). A total of 100 mM sodium pyruvate, 1X Trypsin–EDTA in PBS, Eagle's Minimum Essential Medium (MEM), 100X penicillin–streptomycin solution, and Moon kit's Universal One-Step RT-qPCR Kit (E3005) were obtained from EuroClone (Milan, Italy). 3-(4,5-dimethylthiazol-2-yl)–2,5-diphenyl tetrazolium bromide (MTT), CellROX^{TM} Green Reagent for oxidative stress detection (C10444), and 6-(*N*-(7-Nitrobenz-2-oxa-1,3-

diazol-4-yl)amino)-6-Deoxyglucose (6-NBDG) were obtained from Invitrogen (Waltham, MA, USA). Direct-zol RNA Miniprep Kit and TRI Reagent® were obtained from Zymo Research (Irvine, CA, USA).

2.2. Cell Cultures and Differentiation

The human HepG2 hepatocellular carcinoma cell line (ATCC® HTB-92™) was obtained from the American Type Culture Collection (ATCC®, Manassas, VA, USA) and cultured according to the recommended protocols. The cells were grown and maintained in MEM supplemented with 2.0 mM L-Glutamine, 0.1 mM non-essential amino acids, 1.0 mM sodium pyruvate, 10,000 U/mL penicillin, 10 mg/mL streptomycin, and 10% FBS.

To obtain a steatotic in vitro model mimicking some MASLD features, HepG2 cells were treated with 100 μM OA for 7 days, following the guidelines in the literature [20]. Specifically, OA was added 24 h after cell seeding in multiwell plates and was replenished with every medium change (occurring every 2 or 3 days). After 7 days of OA treatment, the cells (designated as HepG2-OA) were considered fully differentiated into the steatotic phenotype, making them suitable for subsequent experiments. During the experimental exposure to *P. domestica* extract, H_2O_2, or Trolox, OA was not added, as the cells had already undergone full steatotic differentiation. The cells were cultured in 100 mm Petri dishes or in 96-, 24-, or 6-multiwell plates at 37 °C in a humidified atmosphere with 5% CO_2.

2.3. Preparation of Prunus domestica L. subsp. syriaca Extract

The *P. domestica* extract was prepared following the method described by Ullah et al. [17]. Briefly, fruit samples were sourced from a local farm in the Campania Region, Italy. The fruits were thoroughly washed with water to remove any dirt or residues. The skins were peeled off, and the pulp was cut into small pieces with a ceramic knife. To prevent oxidation during preparation, the samples were cut in an ice bath. The prepared pulp was freeze-dried and ground into a fine powder using a mortar and pestle. Aliquots of 2 g of the powdered pulp were added to 40 mL of 50% hydroethanolic solution acidified with a 0.1% HCl solution (adjusted to pH 2.0). The mixture was subjected to magnetic stirring for 3 h at room temperature, followed by centrifugation at 6000 rpm for 10 min. The precipitate was separated from the supernatant, and the extraction process was repeated three times. The collected supernatants were filtered through Whatman cellulose filter paper. The filtrate was then concentrated using a rotary evaporator and was subsequently freeze-dried. Given the high glucose and sucrose content identified via nuclear magnetic resonance (NMR) spectroscopy [17], the dry extract underwent a chemical precipitation of its sugars. This was achieved by a treatment with absolute ethanol, followed by ultra-freezing temperatures. The organic solvent was then removed under reduced pressure using a rotary evaporator. The resulting sugar-free dry extract of the *P. domestica* fruit pulp was stored at −20 °C for subsequent biological assays.

For the cell treatment experiments, the *P. domestica* extract was reconstituted in DMSO to a stock concentration of 200 mg/mL. Serial dilutions were prepared to achieve concentrations of 100, 20, and 2 mg/mL in DMSO. These diluted solutions were then added to a DCC-treated culture medium, resulting in final working concentrations of 1, 0.5, 0.1, and 0.01 mg/mL, which were used across all experiments.

2.4. 3-(4,5-Dimethylthiazol-2-yl)-2,5-diphenyltetrazolium Bromide MTT Cell Vitality Assay

Cell viability was assessed using the MTT proliferation assay, following a previously established protocol [21]. This colorimetric assay relies on the reduction of yellow tetrazolium salt (MTT) to insoluble purple formazan via metabolically active cells. HepG2-OA cells were treated with *P. domestica* at specified concentrations. After 24 and 48 h, MTT was added directly to each well. The resulting formazan crystals were then dissolved by adding DMSO. Absorbance was measured at 570 nm using an EnSpire Multimode Plate Reader spectrophotometer (PerkinElmer Italia, Milano, Italy) with a dynamic range from 0.000 to 0.200 O.D. Cell viability was calculated using the following formula:

$$\text{Cell Viability \%} = \frac{(\text{Average ABS Samples} - \text{Average ABS Blank})}{(\text{Average ABS Controls} - \text{Average ABS Blank})} \times 100$$

2.5. Lipid (Oil Red O) Quantification

The assay was performed using Oil Red O staining, a dye that selectively binds to neutral lipids, allowing for their visualization and quantification. Oil Red O staining was used for the morphological staining of the control HepG2-OA cells and cells treated with *P. domestica* at the concentration of 1 mg/mL (grown on cover glass and stained as described below), as well as for lipid quantification in the HepG2-OA cells. To this aim, the cells were seeded in a 12-well plate for morphological staining and in a 96-well plate for lipid quantification and treated with *P. domestica* extract at the specified concentrations. After 24 h, the cells were fixed with 10% formalin, followed by staining with an Oil Red O working solution. The excess stain was removed with 60% isopropanol, and hematoxylin was used for counterstaining. The images were obtained using a phase contrast optical microscope at 40× magnification. Absorbance was measured at 492 nm using an EnSpire PerkinElmer Multimode Plate Reader spectrophotometer, with a dynamic range from 0.000 to 0.200 O.D.

2.6. Glucose Uptake NovoCyte3000 Flow Cytometer Analysis

Glucose uptake in the HepG2-OA cells was assessed using 6-NBDG, a fluorescent glucose analog that allows for the quantification of cellular glucose uptake via flow cytometry. A total of 72 and 96 h after seeding, the cells were treated with *P. domestica* extract at the various concentrations. Following 6 or 24 h of treatment, the cells were incubated with 20 μM 6-NBDG for 30 min. After incubation, the cells were collected and analyzed using a NovoCyte 3000 flow cytometer (Agilent Technologies Italia, Milano, Italy) [22].

2.7. Reactive Oxygen Species (ROS) NovoCyte3000 Flow Cytometer Analysis

ROS production in the HepG2-OA cells was evaluated using the fluorogenic probe CellROX^{TM} Green Reagent (Thermo Fisher Scientific, Milano, Italy), which detects oxidative stress by binding to DNA in the presence of reactive oxygen species (ROS), resulting in a strong green fluorescence signal. The HepG2-OA cells were treated with *P. domestica* extract at various concentrations, as well as with Trolox (500 μM) as a positive control. After 24 h of treatment, the cells were incubated with 5 μM CellROX^{TM} Green Reagent, followed by 500 μM H_2O_2 for 30 min, to induce oxidative stress. The cells were then collected for analysis using a NovoCyte3000 flow cytometer.

2.8. Reverse Transcription–Quantitative Polymerase Chain Reaction (RT-qPCR)

To evaluate the expression of the genes involved in lipid metabolism (DGAT1, diacylglycerol acyltransferase-1, and FASN, fatty acid synthase) and oxidative stress (SOD, superoxide dismutase, and CAT, catalase), RT-qPCR was performed. HepG2-OA cells were treated with different concentrations of *P. domestica* extract for 6 or 24 h. After treatment, the cells were collected for RNA extraction and purification using a Direct-zol RNA kit (Minipreps; Zymo Research, Irvine, CA, USA). RNA purity and concentration were assessed using a NanoDrop spectrophotometer (Thermo Fisher Scientific, Milano, Italy). The mRNA levels of the target genes listed in Table 1 were measured using a Luna Universal One-Step RT-qPCR kit (E3005; EuroClone, Milano, Italy) according to the provided protocol. ACTB, β-actin, was used as the housekeeping gene for normalization.

Table 1. Forward and reverse sequences of the primers used.

Gene	Forward Sequence (5′→3′)	Reverse Sequence (3′→5′)
ACTB	CACCATTGGCAATGAGCGGTTC	AGGTCTTTGCGGATGTCCACGT
FASN	TATGCTTCTTCGTGCAGCAGTT	GCTGCCACACGCTCCTCTAG
DGAT1	AACTGGTGTGTGGTGATGCT	CCTTCAGGAACAGAGAAACC
SOD	GGTGTGGGGAAGCATTAAAGG	CAAGTCTCCAACATGCCTCTC
CAT	TTTAACGCCATTGCCACAGG	TGAGGCCAAACCTTGGTGA

2.9. Statistical Analysis

The results from three independent experiments carried out in triplicate were expressed as the mean percentage (%) ±SD (standard deviation) compared to a control. The graphs and data were analyzed using GraphPad Prism version 9.0.2. The statistical analysis was conducted with One-Way ANOVA or Two-Way ANOVA multiple comparisons, followed by a Dunnett test, considered statistically significant at $p < 0.05$.

3. Results

3.1. HepG2-OA Cell Viability Was Not Affected by P. domestica Extract Treatment (24 and 48 h)

The MTT cell viability assay was conducted to evaluate the potential cytotoxic effects of different concentrations of *P. domestica* treatments on HepG2-OA cells. The concentrations tested were 0.01, 0.1, 0.5, and 1 mg/mL. The main objective was to determine the appropriate concentrations for further experimental assays while maintaining cell viability. Following previous validation studies [21], concentrations that caused a reduction in cell viability below 80% compared to control cells (CTRs), which were untreated and assumed to have 100% viability, were considered toxic. The MTT assay measures cell metabolic activity as an indicator of viability, where live cells convert the MTT reagent into formazan crystals, resulting in a color change that is spectrophotometrically measurable.

The results showed that none of the *P. domestica* treatments at the tested concentrations caused a significant decrease in cell viability below the 80% threshold, even after 24 and 48 h of exposure in HepG2-OA (Figure 1). Specifically, after 48 h of treatment at the 0.01 mg/mL *P. domestica* concentration, a significant reduction in cell viability was observed ($p < 0.05$), although viability remained above the 80% threshold. In contrast, the 1 mg/mL treatment at the same time point resulted in a significant increase in cell viability ($p < 0.01$), suggesting a positive effect at this concentration. These findings indicate that the tested concentrations of *P. domestica* are non-toxic and suitable for further experiments. This provides a solid foundation for the exploration of the potential therapeutic effects of *P. domestica* in future assays.

3.2. Lipid Content and Expression of Genes Involved in Lipid Metabolism in HepG2-OA Were Reduced by P. domestica Extract

Lipid accumulation, a hallmark of MASLD, was assessed in HepG2-OA cells using Oil Red O staining, comparing control cells with those treated with *P. domestica* extract at a concentration of 1 mg/mL. As shown in Figure 2a, HepG2-OA showed a high basal high intracellular lipid content, as evidenced by the intense red staining of lipid droplets, corresponding to a lipid concentration of 199.1 ng/µL. Figure 2b shows that treatment with

1 mg/mL of *P. domestica* extract significantly reduced lipid droplet accumulation compared to the control.

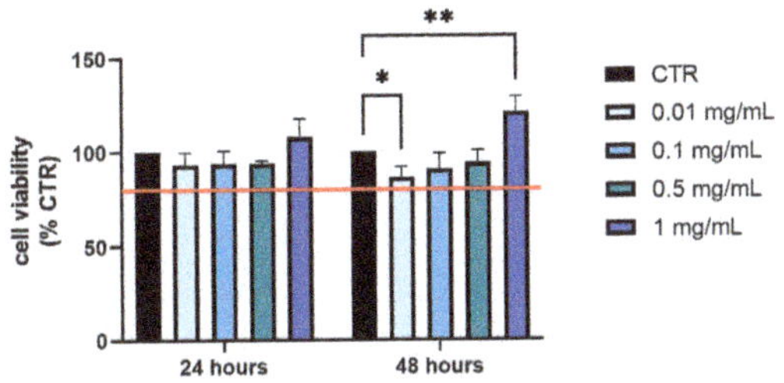

Figure 1. Effect of treatment with *P. domestica* at concentrations of 0.01, 0.1, 0.5, and 1 mg/mL for 24 and 48 h on HepG2-OA cell viability. The red line at 80% indicates the threshold above which cells can be considered viable. The data are expressed as a percentage, representing the mean ± SD (standard deviation), and normalized to the control (CTR = 100%). The graph was obtained from the average of three separate experiments, each performed in quadruplicate. * $p < 0.05$; ** $p < 0.01$ (Two-Way ANOVA multiple comparison, Dunnett test).

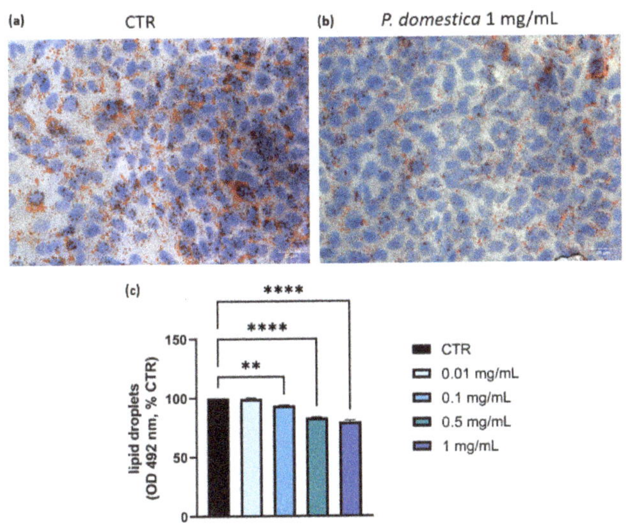

Figure 2. Oil Red O staining in HepG2-OA control cells and in HepG2-OA cells treated with 1 mg/mL of *P. domestica* extract for 24 h, and effect of 24 h treatment with *P. domestica* extract on lipid accumulation in HepG2-OA cells. (**a**) Oil Red O staining of control (CTR) HepG2-OA, showing a marked lipid accumulation after OA treatment (40× magnification). Nuclei were stained in blue with hematoxylin. (**b**) Oil Red O staining of HepG2-OA cells treated with 1 mg/mL of *P. domestica* extract (40× magnification). Nuclei were stained in blue with hematoxylin. (**c**) Effect of treatment with *P. domestica* on lipid accumulation in HepG2-OA cell line. Quantification of lipids was performed using "EnSpire PerkinElmer Multimode Plate Reader" spectrophotometer. Data are presented as mean ± SD (standard deviation) and normalized to control (CTR = 100%, corresponding to 199.1 ng/µL). Graph represents average of three separate experiments, each conducted in triplicate. ** $p < 0.01$; **** $p < 0.0001$ (One-Way ANOVA multiple comparison, Dunnett test).

Following a 24 h treatment with *P. domestica* extract, a dose-dependent reduction in lipid content was observed in the HepG2-OA cells (Figure 2c). Specifically, lipid accumulation decreased by 6.4% at 0.1 mg/mL ($p < 0.01$), reaching a maximum reduction of 20.3% at 1 mg/mL ($p < 0.0001$), indicating a partial recovery from OA-induced steatosis.

These findings suggest that *P. domestica* extract partially counteracts OA-induced lipid accumulation, supporting its potential role in mitigating this process.

The potential modulation of gene expression following exposure to *P. domestica* extract at different concentrations for 6 and 24 h was assessed using RT-qPCR in HepG2-OA cells. The analysis specifically focused on the expression of the DGAT1 gene, a key enzyme involved in triglyceride synthesis, and the FASN gene, which plays a central role in lipogenesis. The gene expression levels were normalized to the housekeeping gene ACTB.

Following treatment with *P. domestica* extract, the DGAT1 expression in HepG2-OA cells decreased in a dose-dependent manner, with a significant reduction observed after both 6 and 24 h (Figure 3a). After 6 h, DGAT1 gene expression was significantly reduced by 12.6% (0.1 mg/mL; $p < 0.01$), reaching a maximum decrease of 23.6% (1 mg/mL; $p < 0.0001$), compared to the control. After 24 h, the reduction ranged from 6.5% (0.01 mg/mL; $p < 0.05$) to 23.7% (1 mg/mL; $p < 0.0001$) compared to the control.

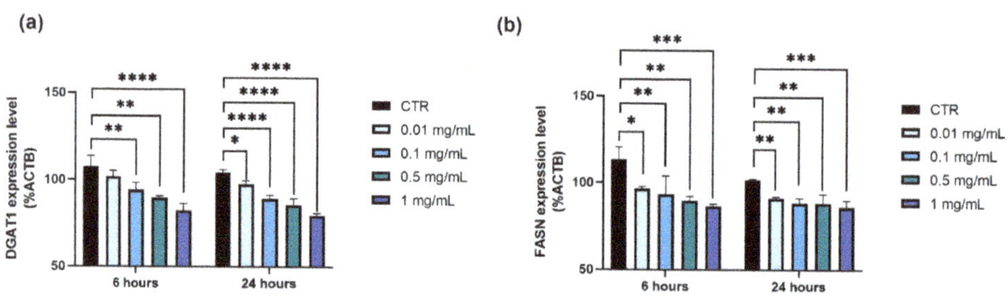

Figure 3. Lipid metabolism-related gene expression in HepG2-OA cells treated for 6 or 24 h with *P. domestica* extract. (**a**) Expression levels of diacylglycerol O-acyltransferase 1 (DGAT1) after 6 and 24 h of treatment with *P. domestica* in HepG2-OA cells. (**b**) Expression levels of fatty acid synthase (FASN) after 6 and 24 h of treatment with *P. domestica* in HepG2-OA cells. Experiments were conducted using RT-qPCR, and results are expressed as percentages, representing mean of three separate experiments, each performed in triplicate. Values are normalized against expression levels of housekeeping gene β-actin (ACTB) (ACTB = 100%). * $p < 0.05$; ** $p < 0.01$; *** $p < 0.001$; **** $p < 0.0001$ (Two-Way ANOVA multiple comparison, Dunnett test).

Similarly, the FASN gene expression in HepG2-OA cells (Figure 3b) was significantly downregulated in a dose-dependent manner at both 6 and 24 h of exposure to *P. domestica* extract. After 6 h, the reduction ranged from 14.9% (0.01 mg/mL; $p < 0.05$) to 23.7% (1 mg/mL; $p < 0.001$), while after 24 h, it varied between 10.4% ($p < 0.01$) and 15.3% ($p < 0.001$) at the same concentrations.

3.3. *HepG2-OA Glucose Uptake Increased in a Dose-Dependent Fashion After 6 and 24 h P. domestica Extract Treatments*

The impact of *P. domestica* treatment on the glucose uptake in HepG2-OA cells was assessed. A quantitative analysis was performed using a flow cytometer, which measures the fluorescent signal emitted by the glucose labeled with the fluorophore 6-NBDG that was absorbed by the cells. The cells were exposed to different concentrations of *P. domestica* extract for 6 and 24 h.

Upon treatment with the *P. domestica* extract, these cells showed a dose-dependent increase in glucose uptake (Figure 4). Compared to the control, glucose uptake increased by 19.7% after 6 h of treatment at the highest concentration tested (1 mg/mL; $p < 0.05$) and by 20.4% ($p < 0.01$) and 39.1% ($p < 0.0001$) at concentrations of 0.5 mg/mL and 1 mg/mL, respectively, after 24 h.

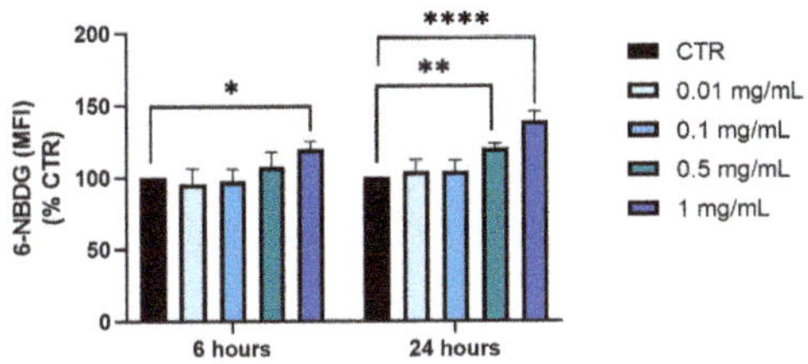

Figure 4. Glucose uptake in HepG2-OA cells following treatment with *P. domestica* extract at concentrations of 0.01, 0.1, 0.5, and 1 mg/mL for 6 and 24 h. The evaluations were conducted using the NovoCyte3000 flow cytometer. The graph represents the mean of three separate experiments, each performed in triplicate. The data are expressed as mean fluorescent intensity (MFI) percentages. Each bar indicates the mean ± SD (standard deviation), with the control set at 100%. * $p < 0.05$, ** $p < 0.01$; **** $p < 0.0001$ (Two-Way ANOVA multiple comparison, Dunnett test).

3.4. Reactive Oxygen Species (ROS) Production and the Expression of Genes Involved in Oxidative Stress Were Reduced by P. domestica Extract in HepG2-OA Cells

This study also explored the potential impact of *P. domestica* extract on ROS production and the expression of genes related to oxidative stress in HepG2-OA cells due to their relevance in MASLD. ROS production was quantitatively measured using flow cytometry after treatment with *P. domestica* extract at the concentrations of 0.01, 0.1, 0.5, and 1 mg/mL.

In the HepG2-OA cells, a 500 µM H_2O_2 treatment was used as a pro-oxidant control, resulting in a 65.2% ($p < 0.0001$) increase in ROS production compared to the control cells. Trolox, a potent antioxidant, was able to only partially restore the control ROS levels upon H_2O_2 challenge (−23.7%, $p < 0.001$). Interestingly, the treatments with *P. domestica* at various concentrations resulted in a significant reduction in ROS production, with a decrease ranging from 16.4% at 0.01 mg/mL ($p < 0.01$) to 22.9% at 1 mg/mL ($p < 0.001$) (Figure 5), suggesting that the extract was unable to fully quench the H_2O_2-induced ROS production in this cell model.

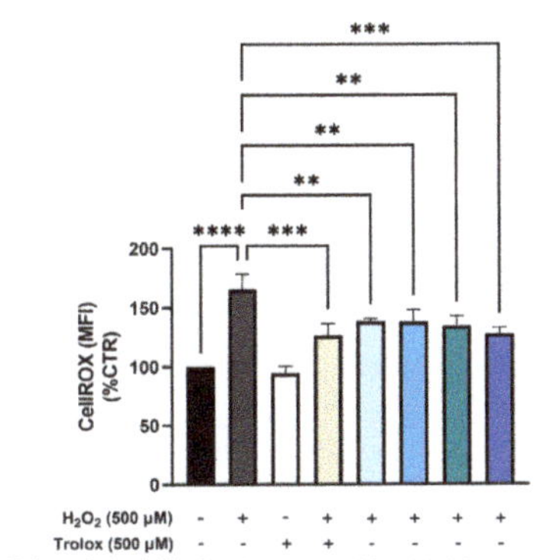

Figure 5. Intracellular formation of reactive oxygen species (ROS) in HepG2-OA cells treated with *P. domestica* extract for 24 h at different concentrations. The quantification of ROS was performed using a NovoCyte3000 flow cytometer. The data are presented as mean fluorescent intensity (MFI) and are normalized to the control (CTR = 100%). This Figure shows the average of three separate experiments, each conducted in triplicate. ** $p < 0.01$; *** $p < 0.001$; **** $p < 0.0001$ (One-Way ANOVA multiple comparison, Dunnett test).

To further investigate the effects of *P. domestica* extract, RT-qPCR was used to assess the expression of genes related to oxidative stress, specifically SOD and CAT, in response to *P. domestica* treatment. The expression levels of these genes were normalized to ACTB as a housekeeping gene.

In the HepG2-OA cells, *P. domestica* treatment resulted in a significant, dose-dependent decrease in SOD gene expression at both 6 and 24 h. After 6 h, reductions ranged from 12.6% at 0.1 mg/mL ($p < 0.05$) to 19.8% at 1 mg/mL ($p < 0.001$), and after 24 h, reductions of 10.2% ($p < 0.05$) and 16.9% ($p < 0.001$) were observed at the same concentrations, respectively (Figure 6a).

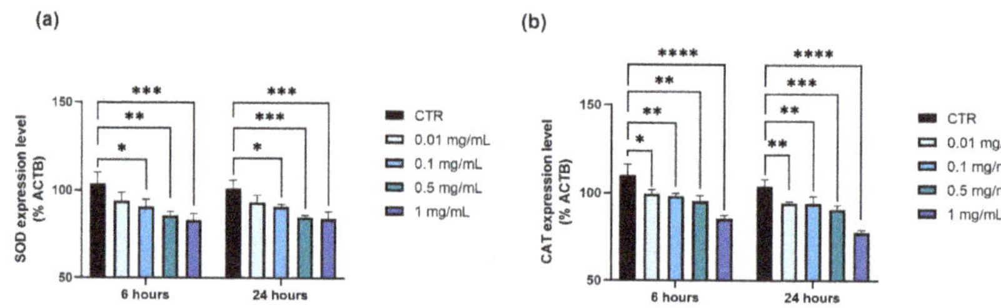

Figure 6. Expression levels of genes involved in oxidative stress in HepG2-OA cells treated with *P. domestica* extract at different concentrations and at different time points. (**a**) Expression levels of superoxide dismutase (SOD) after 6 and 24 h of treatment with *P. domestica* in HepG2-OA cells. (**b**) Expression levels of catalase (CAT) after 6 and 24 h of treatment with *P. domestica* in HepG2-OA cells. Experiments were conducted using RT-qPCR, and results are expressed as percentages representing mean of three separate experiments, each performed in triplicate. Values are normalized against expression levels of housekeeping gene β-actin (ACTB) (ACTB = 100%). * $p < 0.05$; ** $p < 0.01$; *** $p < 0.001$; **** $p < 0.0001$ (Two-Way ANOVA multiple comparison, Dunnett test).

For CAT gene expression, a significant dose-dependent decrease was observed in the HepG2-OA cells, with the most notable reduction at 1 mg/mL after 6 (−22.2%; $p < 0.0001$) and 24 h (−25%; $p < 0.0001$) (Figure 6b).

4. Discussion

MASLD is an escalating global health concern arising from the convergence of multiple pathogenetic mechanisms. Unhealthy dietary habits, a high fructose intake, and a sedentary lifestyle represent important background conditions of MASLD and may exacerbate disease progression [23]. Additionally, visceral obesity [24], T2DM [1], dyslipidemia [25], and arterial hypertension [26] are well-established risk factors promoting MASLD onset and progression, with genetic predispositions, such as PNPLA3 and TM6SF2 [27] polymorphisms, further increasing susceptibility. Notably, MASLD patients face an elevated risk of cardiovascular diseases, including heart disease and stroke, due to overlapping metabolic dysfunctions [28]. Given the chronic nature of the disease and its limited pharmacological options, nutraceutical interventions hold promise for both prevention and management. Exploring the effects of novel, sustainable plant extracts on selected mechanisms relevant to MASLD pathogenesis by using experimental cell-based models of human origin can provide valuable insights before clinical assessment and application. Importantly, the use of a sustainable extract also aligns with the principles of the UN 2030 Agenda for Sustainable Development and the One Health concept.

In this study, we took advantage of a cell-based model of steatotic human hepatocytes (HepG2-OA) to explore the effects of a sustainable extract derived from *Prunus domestica* L. subsp. *syriaca*. Our findings underscore the pathophysiological relevance of targeting lipid dysregulation, glucose imbalance, and oxidative stress in MASLD, highlighting the potential of *P. domestica* extract as an effective nutraceutical approach. Our results demonstrated that treatment with *P. domestica* extract significantly reduced lipid content and downregulated the expression of genes involved in lipid biosynthesis. Additionally, the extract enhanced glucose uptake in a dose-dependent manner in HepG2-OA cells. Furthermore, treatment with *P. domestica* extract effectively reduced ROS production and modulated the expression of genes related to oxidative stress in these cells, reinforcing its potential as a nutraceutical agent in MASLD management.

Importantly, *P. domestica* extract did not affect cell viability, confirming that the selected concentrations were suitable for the experiments. This approach ensured experimental consistency and enhanced the relevance of our findings for future applications.

Lipid accumulation in hepatocytes is a key feature of MASLD, driven by disrupted lipid metabolism and metabolic stress [8]. Notably, *P. domestica* extract reduced both gene expression levels and lipid accumulation in a dose-dependent manner in HepG2-OA cells, highlighting its potential in mitigating this hallmark of MASLD. DGAT1 is a key enzyme in lipid homeostasis, and in MASLD, its overactivity drives excessive lipid production, contributing to hepatic steatosis and to metabolic disturbances like lipotoxicity, oxidative stress, and inflammation [29]. The extract's ability to reduce DGAT1 expression levels is consistent with findings on other polyphenolic compounds [30], such as green tea catechins, which inhibit hepatic lipogenesis by directly targeting lipid synthesis pathways [31]. Additionally, the anthocyanins in *P. domestica*, known for their lipid-lowering properties, likely contribute to DGAT1 inhibition, further reducing lipid buildup in hepatocytes [32]. FASN gene expression, another key enzyme in lipogenesis, was also significantly suppressed by the *P. domestica* extract, aligning with the actions of other polyphenolic compounds such as resveratrol [33] and quercetin [34], which inhibit fatty acid synthesis by downregulating FASN expression and modulating transcription factors like sterol regulatory element-binding protein 1c, SREBP-1c, a critical regulator of lipid metabolism [35]. These findings highlight the potential of *P. domestica* extract, particularly its anthocyanin and catechin content, in addressing lipid dysregulation. By downregulating the genes involved in lipid metabolism and reducing lipid accumulation, the extract targets the mechanisms responsible for excessive hepatic lipid buildup. A limitation of this study is the lack of data on the potential contribution of genes related to lipolysis in the observed lipid content reduction, such as PPARα/γ, CPT1, and SREBP-1c, which play essential roles in lipid oxidation and synthesis. Nevertheless, given the complexity of MASLD pathophysiology, these findings suggest that *P. domestica* extract may be useful for prevention or as part of a combined therapeutic approach. Its lipid-lowering effects, especially when used alongside agents targeting inflammation, fibrosis, or insulin resistance, could provide a more comprehensive strategy for managing the disease.

Impaired glucose metabolism is another hallmark of MASLD [36]. Notably, *P. domestica* extract significantly enhanced glucose uptake in HepG2-OA cells in a dose-dependent manner, with a maximal effect of +39.1% at the highest concentration tested (1 mg/mL). This effect is likely attributable to the extract's flavonoid content, as flavonoids are known to enhance glucose uptake and improve insulin sensitivity [37]. Compounds such as quercetin and anthocyanins, present in *P. domestica*, are particularly effective in improving insulin signaling pathways [38], thereby mitigating insulin resistance, a major driver of MASLD progression. These findings are consistent with research on related compounds like berberine [39] and curcumin [40], which similarly enhance hepatic glucose uptake and insulin sensitivity by modulating pathways such as AMP-activated protein kinase (AMPK) [41] and insulin receptor substrate 1 (IRS-1) [42]. This effect is particularly relevant to MASLD, where the interplay between glucose and lipid dysregulation exacerbates disease severity. Given the liver's central role in maintaining glucose balance, the ability of

P. domestica extract to enhance glucose uptake in HepG2-OA cells suggests its potential to address key metabolic derangements associated with MASLD.

The antioxidant properties of *P. domestica* represent a significant aspect of its protective potential, especially considering the critical role that oxidative stress plays in MASLD progression [43]. The ROS produced in hepatocytes can lead to cellular damage, inflammation, and fibrosis, advancing the condition from simple steatosis to MASH [44]. MASH is more severe as persistent inflammation results in the deposition of extracellular matrix proteins, leading to fibrosis and liver dysfunction [45]. In turn, advanced fibrosis disrupts liver architecture and function, potentially progressing to cirrhosis, liver failure, and an increased risk of liver cancer [46]. In our experimental model, the ROS production increase induced by H_2O_2 treatment in HepG2-OA cells reached a very high extent (+65.5%), possibly recapitulating the elevated oxidative stress characteristic of steatotic liver conditions. The *P. domestica* extract partially but significantly reduced ROS production in a dose-dependent manner, with up to a 22.9% ROS decrease in HepG2-OA cells. The observed antioxidant effects of *P. domestica* are likely attributed to its high anthocyanin content, known to directly neutralize ROS [47] and influence antioxidant enzyme activity in hepatocyte models [48,49]. These effects align with findings from studies on anthocyanin-rich fruits like blueberries and black currants [50]. Additionally, the flavonoids and phenolic acids in *P. domestica* may enhance the body's antioxidant defenses [51] by boosting the activity of endogenous antioxidant enzymes. Our study also demonstrated that *P. domestica* extract modulated the expression of oxidative stress-related genes, specifically downregulating SOD and CAT gene expression in association with reduced oxidative stress. SOD, a key antioxidant enzyme, dismutates superoxide radicals into hydrogen peroxide and oxygen, preventing oxidative damage. This reduction in SOD expression likely reflects a decreased oxidative burden, as lower ROS levels reduce the need for heightened SOD activity [52]. This regulatory effect is consistent with other polyphenolic compounds, such as those from green tea [53] and curcumin [54], which similarly downregulate oxidative stress-related genes as ROS levels decline, thus protecting liver cells from oxidative damage and inflammation. Likewise, CAT, another crucial antioxidant enzyme, decomposes hydrogen peroxide into water and oxygen, preventing oxidative damage. The observed reduction in CAT expression aligns with decreased ROS levels and suggests that lower oxidative stress reduces the need for enhanced CAT activity [55]. This regulatory effect mirrors findings from other studies on polyphenolic compounds, which similarly downregulated oxidative stress-related enzymes following ROS reduction. For instance, salicylic acid treatment was shown to enhance CAT activity and gene expression levels, thereby enhancing antioxidant capacity [56]. Similarly, tart cherry pit extracts modulated CAT gene expression, contributing to their antioxidant effects [57]. By reducing ROS levels and altering the expression of oxidative stress-related genes, *P. domestica* extract may help preserve cellular function and integrity in the context of MASLD. This dual action positions *P. domestica* as a promising treatment agent for the mitigation of oxidative damage and the improvement in metabolic function in in vitro liver disease models at least.

Beyond its biological efficacy, *P. domestica* extract exemplifies the innovative reuse of agro-food waste, aligning with the One Health approach, which underscores the interconnectedness of human, animal, and environmental health [58]. By valorizing agricultural and food processing by-products, this extract promotes a circular economy while minimizing environmental impacts. This sustainability-focused strategy directly supports the United Nations' 2030 Agenda for Sustainable Development, advancing multiple Sustainable Development Goals (SDGs) [59]. It enhances food security by reducing waste and optimizing resource efficiency, contributing to SDG 2 (Zero Hunger) [60]. The health-promoting properties of *P. domestica* extract, including its antioxidant and metabolic benefits, align with SDG 3 (Good Health and Well-being) by aiding in the prevention and management of non-communicable diseases [61]. Additionally, by minimizing food waste and promoting sustainable agricultural practices, *P. domestica* extract advances SDG 12 (Responsible Consumption and Production) while also mitigating environmental impacts such as greenhouse gas emissions, thus supporting SDG 13 (Climate Action) [62].

5. Conclusions

In conclusion, this study highlighted the potential of *P. domestica* extract in positively modulating pathogenic pathways that are hallmarks of MASLD, including lipid metabolism, glucose uptake, and oxidative stress. *P. domestica*'s rich polyphenolic content underscores its promise as an accessible and effective nutraceutical for MASLD management, particularly for patients with limited treatment options.

One limitation of this study is the use of just an in vitro model, which, while providing a cost-effective and reproducible platform for the assessment of metabolic dysfunction related to MASLD, does not fully capture the complexity of liver pathology. Additionally, the direct bioavailability of the *P. domestica* extract to hepatic cells remains uncertain, as the digestion and absorption processes were not considered in this study. Future studies should incorporate bioaccessible fractions obtained through in vitro digestion or relevant metabolites to better understand the extract's physiological relevance. Furthermore, these findings underscore the need for further investigation into additional mechanisms, such as insulin sensitivity, glucose transporter (GLUT) trafficking, and other oxidative stress regulators like Nuclear factor erythroid 2-related factor 2, Nrf2. Moreover, given that MASLD is a chronic condition requiring prolonged intervention, future studies should assess the extract's long-term effects beyond the 48 h time frame used in this study to better evaluate its safety and efficacy.

With the rising prevalence of MASLD and the demand for sustainable treatment solutions, *P. domestica* extract represents a promising addition to nutraceutical-based strategies for liver disease prevention and management, potentially slowing disease progression and improving patient outcomes.

Author Contributions: Conceptualization, L.C. and P.M.; methodology, L.C., C.G., L.D.D. and P.M.; validation, L.C., C.G. and P.M.; investigation, L.C., C.G., M.D., H.U. and F.T.K.; data curation, L.C.; writing—original draft preparation, L.C.; writing—review and editing, L.C., C.G. and P.M.; supervision, P.M.; project administration, P.M.; funding acquisition, P.M. All authors have read and agreed to the published version of the manuscript.

Funding: The work of P.M. is supported in part by the European Union (AtheroNET COST Action-CA21153; HORIZON-MSCA-2021-SE-01-01-MSCA Staff Exchanges 2021 CardioSCOPE 101086397); Italian Space Agency (N. 2023-7-HH.0 CUP F13C23000050005 MicroFunExpo).

Institutional Review Board Statement: Not applicable.

Informed Consent Statement: Not applicable.

Data Availability Statement: The data presented in this study are available on request from the corresponding author.

Acknowledgments: The authors acknowledge the valuable support of Chiara Oliveri, Marco Ruzza, Maddalena Farina, Giorgia Cadamuro, Cristina Cardilli, Margherita Buontempo, Giulia Caputi, Benedetta Pezzini, Francesca Crotti, Alessandro Falcone, Luca Nenzi, Reham Hattab, and Hygerta Berisha.

Conflicts of Interest: The authors declare no conflicts of interest. The funders had no role in the design of the study; in the collection, analyses, or interpretation of data; in the writing of the manuscript; or in the decision to publish the results.

References

1. Chan, W.-K.; Chuah, K.-H.; Rajaram, R.B.; Lim, L.-L.; Ratnasingam, J.; Vethakkan, S.R. Metabolic Dysfunction-Associated Steatotic Liver Disease (MASLD): A State-of-the-Art Review. *J. Obes. Metab. Syndr.* **2023**, *32*, 197–213. [CrossRef]
2. Miao, L.; Targher, G.; Byrne, C.D.; Cao, Y.-Y.; Zheng, M.-H. Current Status and Future Trends of the Global Burden of MASLD. *Trends Endocrinol. Metab.* **2024**, *35*, 697–707. [CrossRef] [PubMed]
3. Forlano, R.; Martinez-Gili, L.; Takis, P.; Miguens-Blanco, J.; Liu, T.; Triantafyllou, E.; Skinner, C.; Loomba, R.; Thursz, M.; Marchesi, J.R.; et al. Disruption of Gut Barrier Integrity and Host–Microbiome Interactions Underlie MASLD Severity in Patients with Type-2 Diabetes Mellitus. *Gut Microbes* **2024**, *16*, 2304157. [CrossRef] [PubMed]
4. Takahashi, Y. Histopathology of Nonalcoholic Fatty Liver Disease/Nonalcoholic Steatohepatitis. *World J. Gastroenterol.* **2014**, *20*, 15539. [CrossRef]
5. Schott, A.-K.; Zipančić, I.; Hernández-Rabaza, V.; Becker-Kojić, Z.A. Human Liver Spheroids from Peripheral Blood for Liver Disease Studies. *J. Vis. Exp.* **2023**, *191*, e64703. [CrossRef] [PubMed]
6. Eynaudi, A.; Díaz-Castro, F.; Bórquez, J.C.; Bravo-Sagua, R.; Parra, V.; Troncoso, R. Differential Effects of Oleic and Palmitic Acids on Lipid Droplet-Mitochondria Interaction in the Hepatic Cell Line HepG2. *Front. Nutr.* **2021**, *8*, 775382. [CrossRef]
7. Wang, S.; Friedman, S.L. Found in Translation—Fibrosis in Metabolic Dysfunction–Associated Steatohepatitis (MASH). *Sci. Transl. Med.* **2023**, *15*, eadi0759. [CrossRef]
8. Schwärzler, J.; Grabherr, F.; Grander, C.; Adolph, T.E.; Tilg, H. The Pathophysiology of MASLD: An Immunometabolic Perspective. *Expert. Rev. Clin. Immunol.* **2024**, *20*, 375–386. [CrossRef]
9. Mattavelli, E.; Olmastroni, E.; Bonofiglio, D.; Catapano, A.L.; Baragetti, A.; Magni, P. Adherence to the Mediterranean Diet: Impact of Geographical Location of the Observations. *Nutrients* **2022**, *14*, 2040. [CrossRef]
10. Machado, M.V. Aerobic Exercise in the Management of Metabolic Dysfunction Associated Fatty Liver Disease. *Diabetes Metab. Syndr. Obes.* **2021**, *14*, 3627–3645. [CrossRef]
11. Rojas, Á.; Lara-Romero, C.; Muñoz-Hernández, R.; Gato, S.; Ampuero, J.; Romero-Gómez, M. Emerging Pharmacological Treatment Options for MAFLD. *Ther. Adv. Endocrinol. Metab.* **2022**, *13*, 204201882211424. [CrossRef]
12. Zhao, M.; Chen, S.; Ji, X.; Shen, X.; You, J.; Liang, X.; Yin, H.; Zhao, L. Current Innovations in Nutraceuticals and Functional Foods for Intervention of Non-Alcoholic Fatty Liver Disease. *Pharmacol. Res.* **2021**, *166*, 105517. [CrossRef] [PubMed]
13. Hefer, M.; Petrovic, A.; Roguljic, L.K.; Kolaric, T.O.; Kizivat, T.; Wu, C.H.; Tabll, A.A.; Smolic, R.; Vcev, A.; Smolic, M. Green Tea Polyphenol (-)-Epicatechin Pretreatment Mitigates Hepatic Steatosis in an In Vitro MASLD Model. *Curr. Issues Mol. Biol.* **2024**, *46*, 8981–8994. [CrossRef] [PubMed]
14. Mijangos-Trejo, A.; Nuño-Lambarri, N.; Barbero-Becerra, V.; Uribe-Esquivel, M.; Vidal-Cevallos, P.; Chávez-Tapia, N. Prebiotics and Probiotics: Therapeutic Tools for Nonalcoholic Fatty Liver Disease. *Int. J. Mol. Sci.* **2023**, *24*, 14918. [CrossRef]
15. Ma, L.; Lu, Q.-Y.; Lim, S.; Han, G.; Boros, L.G.; Desai, M.; Yee, J.K. The Effect of Flavonoids and Topiramate on Glucose Carbon Metabolism in a HepG2 Steatosis Cell Culture Model: A Stable Isotope Study. *Nutrients* **2025**, *17*, 564. [CrossRef]
16. Sokal-Dembowska, A.; Jarmakiewicz-Czaja, S.; Ferenc, K.; Filip, R. Can Nutraceuticals Support the Treatment of MASLD/MASH, and Thus Affect the Process of Liver Fibrosis? *Int. J. Mol. Sci.* **2024**, *25*, 5238. [CrossRef]
17. Ullah, H.; Sommella, E.; Santarcangelo, C.; D'avino, D.; Rossi, A.; Dacrema, M.; Di Minno, A.; Di Matteo, G.; Mannina, L.; Campiglia, P.; et al. Hydroethanolic Extract of *Prunus domestica* L.: Metabolite Profiling and In Vitro Modulation of Molecular Mechanisms Associated to Cardiometabolic Diseases. *Nutrients* **2022**, *14*, 340. [CrossRef]
18. Ullah, H.; De Filippis, A.; Khan, H.; Xiao, J.; Daglia, M. An Overview of the Health Benefits of Prunus Species with Special Reference to Metabolic Syndrome Risk Factors. *Food Chem. Toxicol.* **2020**, *144*, 111574. [CrossRef]
19. Barbera, M. Reuse of Food Waste and Wastewater as a Source of Polyphenolic Compounds to Use as Food Additives. *J. AOAC Int.* **2020**, *103*, 906–914. [CrossRef]
20. Xia, H.; Zhu, X.; Zhang, X.; Jiang, H.; Li, B.; Wang, Z.; Li, D.; Jin, Y. Alpha-Naphthoflavone Attenuates Non-Alcoholic Fatty Liver Disease in Oleic Acid-Treated HepG2 Hepatocytes and in High Fat Diet-Fed Mice. *Biomed. Pharmacother.* **2019**, *118*, 109287. [CrossRef]
21. Atchan Nwakiban, A.P.; Fumagalli, M.; Piazza, S.; Magnavacca, A.; Martinelli, G.; Beretta, G.; Magni, P.; Tchamgoue, A.D.; Agbor, G.A.; Kuiaté, J.-R.; et al. Dietary Cameroonian Plants Exhibit Anti-Inflammatory Activity in Human Gastric Epithelial Cells. *Nutrients* **2020**, *12*, 3787. [CrossRef] [PubMed]

22. Atchan Nwakiban, A.P.; Passarelli, A.; Da Dalt, L.; Olivieri, C.; Demirci, T.N.; Piazza, S.; Sangiovanni, E.; Carpentier-maguire, E.; Martinelli, G.; Shivashankara, S.T.; et al. Cameroonian Spice Extracts Modulate Molecular Mechanisms Relevant to Cardiometabolic Diseases in Sw 872 Human Liposarcoma Cells. *Nutrients* **2021**, *13*, 4271. [CrossRef]
23. Vilar-Gomez, E.; Martinez-Perez, Y.; Calzadilla-Bertot, L.; Torres-Gonzalez, A.; Gra-Oramas, B.; Gonzalez-Fabian, L.; Friedman, S.L.; Diago, M.; Romero-Gomez, M. Weight Loss Through Lifestyle Modification Significantly Reduces Features of Nonalcoholic Steatohepatitis. *Gastroenterology* **2015**, *149*, 367–378.e5. [CrossRef] [PubMed]
24. Huttasch, M.; Roden, M.; Kahl, S. Obesity and MASLD: Is Weight Loss the (Only) Key to Treat Metabolic Liver Disease? *Metabolism* **2024**, *157*, 155937. [CrossRef]
25. Bril, F.; Sninsky, J.J.; Baca, A.M.; Superko, H.R.; Portillo Sanchez, P.; Biernacki, D.; Maximos, M.; Lomonaco, R.; Orsak, B.; Suman, A.; et al. Hepatic Steatosis and Insulin Resistance, But Not Steatohepatitis, Promote Atherogenic Dyslipidemia in NAFLD. *J. Clin. Endocrinol. Metab.* **2016**, *101*, 644–652. [CrossRef] [PubMed]
26. Ji, Y.; Lee, H.; Kaura, S.; Yip, J.; Sun, H.; Guan, L.; Han, W.; Ding, Y. Effect of Bariatric Surgery on Metabolic Diseases and Underlying Mechanisms. *Biomolecules* **2021**, *11*, 1582. [CrossRef]
27. Cherubini, A.; Casirati, E.; Tomasi, M.; Valenti, L. PNPLA3 as a Therapeutic Target for Fatty Liver Disease: The Evidence to Date. *Expert. Opin. Ther. Targets* **2021**, *25*, 1033–1043. [CrossRef]
28. Gutiérrez-Cuevas, J.; Santos, A.; Armendariz-Borunda, J. Pathophysiological Molecular Mechanisms of Obesity: A Link between MAFLD and NASH with Cardiovascular Diseases. *Int. J. Mol. Sci.* **2021**, *22*, 11629. [CrossRef]
29. Longo, M.; Paolini, E.; Di Benedetto, P.; Tomassini, E.; Meroni, M.; Dongiovanni, P. DGAT1 and DGAT2 Inhibitors for Metabolic Dysfunction-Associated Steatotic Liver Disease (MASLD) Management: Benefits for Their Single or Combined Application. *Int. J. Mol. Sci.* **2024**, *25*, 9074. [CrossRef]
30. Nwakiban Atchan, A.P.; Shivashankara, S.T.; Piazza, S.; Tchamgoue, A.D.; Beretta, G.; Dell'Agli, M.; Magni, P.; Agbor, G.A.; Kuiaté, J.-R.; Manjappara, U.V. Polyphenol-Rich Extracts of Xylopia and Aframomum Species Show Metabolic Benefits by Lowering Hepatic Lipid Accumulation in Diet-Induced Obese Mice. *ACS Omega* **2022**, *7*, 11914–11928. [CrossRef]
31. Musial, C.; Kuban-Jankowska, A.; Gorska-Ponikowska, M. Beneficial Properties of Green Tea Catechins. *Int. J. Mol. Sci.* **2020**, *21*, 1744. [CrossRef] [PubMed]
32. Velliquette, R.A.; Grann, K.; Missler, S.R.; Patterson, J.; Hu, C.; Gellenbeck, K.W.; Scholten, J.D.; Randolph, R.K. Identification of a Botanical Inhibitor of Intestinal Diacylglyceride Acyltransferase 1 Activity via in Vitro Screening and a Parallel, Randomized, Blinded, Placebo-Controlled Clinical Trial. *Nutr. Metab.* **2015**, *12*, 27. [CrossRef]
33. Wang, S.; Moustaid-Moussa, N.; Chen, L.; Mo, H.; Shastri, A.; Su, R.; Bapat, P.; Kwun, I.; Shen, C.-L. Novel Insights of Dietary Polyphenols and Obesity. *J. Nutr. Biochem.* **2014**, *25*, 1–18. [CrossRef]
34. Maleki, M.H.; Abdizadeh Javazm, S.; Dastghaib, S.; Panji, A.; Hojjati Far, M.; Mahmoodi, H.; Siri, M.; Shafiee, S.M. The Effect of Quercetin on Adipogenesis, Lipolysis, and Apoptosis in 3T3-L1 Adipocytes: The Role of SIRT1 Pathways. *Obes. Sci. Pract.* **2024**, *10*, e752. [CrossRef]
35. Saleh Al-maamari, J.N.; Rahmadi, M.; Panggono, S.M.; Prameswari, D.A.; Pratiwi, E.D.; Ardianto, C.; Balan, S.S.; Suprapti, B. The Effects of Quercetin on the Expression of SREBP-1c MRNA in High-Fat Diet-Induced NAFLD in Mice. *J. Basic. Clin. Physiol. Pharmacol.* **2021**, *32*, 637–644. [CrossRef] [PubMed]
36. Bansal, S.K.; Bansal, M.B. Pathogenesis of MASLD and MASH—Role of Insulin Resistance and Lipotoxicity. *Aliment. Pharmacol. Ther.* **2024**, *59*, S10–S22. [CrossRef]
37. Gravandi, M.M.; Fakhri, S.; Zarneshan, S.N.; Yarmohammadi, A.; Khan, H. Flavonoids Modulate AMPK/PGC-1α and Interconnected Pathways toward Potential Neuroprotective Activities. *Metab. Brain. Dis.* **2021**, *36*, 1501–1521. [CrossRef]
38. Naz, R.; Saqib, F.; Awadallah, S.; Wahid, M.; Latif, M.F.; Iqbal, I.; Mubarak, M.S. Food Polyphenols and Type II Diabetes Mellitus: Pharmacology and Mechanisms. *Molecules* **2023**, *28*, 3996. [CrossRef]
39. Li, Z.; Wang, Y.; Xu, Q.; Ma, J.; Li, X.; Yan, J.; Tian, Y.; Wen, Y.; Chen, T. Berberine and Health Outcomes: An Umbrella Review. *Phytother. Res.* **2023**, *37*, 2051–2066. [CrossRef]
40. Pivari, F.; Mingione, A.; Brasacchio, C.; Soldati, L. Curcumin and Type 2 Diabetes Mellitus: Prevention and Treatment. *Nutrients* **2019**, *11*, 1837. [CrossRef]
41. Patel, S.S.; Acharya, A.; Ray, R.S.; Agrawal, R.; Raghuwanshi, R.; Jain, P. Cellular and Molecular Mechanisms of Curcumin in Prevention and Treatment of Disease. *Crit. Rev. Food Sci. Nutr.* **2020**, *60*, 887–939. [CrossRef] [PubMed]
42. Maithilikarpagaselvi, N.; Sridhar, M.G.; Swaminathan, R.P.; Zachariah, B. Curcumin Prevents Inflammatory Response, Oxidative Stress and Insulin Resistance in High Fructose Fed Male Wistar Rats: Potential Role of Serine Kinases. *Chem. Biol. Interact.* **2016**, *244*, 187–194. [CrossRef] [PubMed]
43. Li, Y.; Yang, P.; Ye, J.; Xu, Q.; Wu, J.; Wang, Y. Updated Mechanisms of MASLD Pathogenesis. *Lipids Health Dis.* **2024**, *23*, 117. [CrossRef] [PubMed]

44. Guo, X.; Yin, X.; Liu, Z.; Wang, J. Non-Alcoholic Fatty Liver Disease (NAFLD) Pathogenesis and Natural Products for Prevention and Treatment. *Int. J. Mol. Sci.* **2022**, *23*, 15489. [CrossRef]
45. Meyer, M.; Schwärzler, J.; Jukic, A.; Tilg, H. Innate Immunity and MASLD. *Biomolecules* **2024**, *14*, 476. [CrossRef]
46. Berumen, J.; Baglieri, J.; Kisseleva, T.; Mekeel, K. Liver Fibrosis: Pathophysiology and Clinical Implications. *WIREs Mech. Dis.* **2021**, *13*, e1499. [CrossRef]
47. Pérez-Torres, I.; Castrejón-Téllez, V.; Soto, M.E.; Rubio-Ruiz, M.E.; Manzano-Pech, L.; Guarner-Lans, V. Oxidative Stress, Plant Natural Antioxidants, and Obesity. *Int. J. Mol. Sci.* **2021**, *22*, 1786. [CrossRef]
48. Atchan, A.P.N.; Monthe, O.C.; Tchamgoue, A.D.; Singh, Y.; Shivashankara, S.T.; Selvi, M.K.; Agbor, G.A.; Magni, P.; Piazza, S.; Manjappara, U.V.; et al. Anti-Inflammatory, Antioxidant Activities, and Phytochemical Characterization of Edible Plants Exerting Synergistic Effects in Human Gastric Epithelial Cells. *Antioxidants* **2023**, *12*, 591. [CrossRef]
49. de Morais Sousa, M.; de Lima, R.M.T.; de Lima, A.; Reis, A.C.; de Carvalho Melo Cavalcante, A.A.; Sattler, J.A.G.; de Almeida-Muradian, L.B.; de Sousa Lima Neto, J.; dos Reis Moreira-Araujo, R.S.; do Nascimento Nogueira, N. Antioxidant Action and Enzyme Activity Modulation by Bioaccessible Polyphenols from Jambolan (*Syzygium cumini* (L.) Skeels). *Food Chem* **2021**, *363*, 130353. [CrossRef]
50. Cásedas, G.; Les, F.; Gómez-Serranillos, M.P.; Smith, C.; López, V. Anthocyanin Profile, Antioxidant Activity and Enzyme Inhibiting Properties of Blueberry and Cranberry Juices: A Comparative Study. *Food Funct.* **2017**, *8*, 4187–4193. [CrossRef]
51. Hu, Q.; Liu, Z.; Guo, Y.; Lu, S.; Du, H.; Cao, Y. Antioxidant Capacity of Flavonoids from Folium Artemisiae Argyi and the Molecular Mechanism in Caenorhabditis Elegans. *J. Ethnopharmacol.* **2021**, *279*, 114398. [CrossRef] [PubMed]
52. Che, M.; Wang, R.; Li, X.; Wang, H.-Y.; Zheng, X.F.S. Expanding Roles of Superoxide Dismutases in Cell Regulation and Cancer. *Drug Discov. Today* **2016**, *21*, 143–149. [CrossRef] [PubMed]
53. Li, Y.; Chang, S.-C.; Goldstein, B.Y.; Scheider, W.L.; Cai, L.; You, N.-C.Y.; Tarleton, H.P.; Ding, B.; Zhao, J.; Wu, M.; et al. Green Tea Consumption, Inflammation and the Risk of Primary Hepatocellular Carcinoma in a Chinese Population. *Cancer Epidemiol.* **2011**, *35*, 362–368. [CrossRef] [PubMed]
54. Yang, Y.; Liu, Y.; Zhang, A.-L.; Tang, S.-F.; Ming, Q.; Ao, C.-Y.; Liu, Y.; Li, C.-Z.; Yu, C.; Zhao, H.; et al. Curcumin Protects against Manganese-Induced Neurotoxicity in Rat by Regulating Oxidative Stress-Related Gene Expression via H3K27 Acetylation. *Ecotoxicol. Environ. Saf.* **2022**, *236*, 113469. [CrossRef]
55. Quan, X.; Lim, S.-O.; Jung, G. Reactive Oxygen Species Downregulate Catalase Expression via Methylation of a CpG Island in the Oct-1 Promoter. *FEBS Lett.* **2011**, *585*, 3436–3441. [CrossRef]
56. Zhang, X.; Liu, Y.; Zhang, W.; Yang, W.; An, S.; Guo, M.; Chen, G. Salicylic Acid Treatment Ameliorates Postharvest Quality Deterioration in 'France' Prune (*Prunus domestica* L. 'Ximei') Fruit by Modulating the Antioxidant System. *Foods* **2024**, *13*, 2871. [CrossRef]
57. Decot, H.; Sudhakaran, M.; Boismier, E.; Schilmiller, A.; Claucherty, E.; Doseff, A.I.; Aliakbarian, B. Tart Cherry (*Prunus cerasus* L.) Pit Extracts Protect Human Skin Cells against Oxidative Stress: Unlocking Sustainable Uses for Food Industry Byproducts. *Foods* **2023**, *12*, 3748. [CrossRef]
58. Humboldt-Dachroeden, S.; Mantovani, A. Assessing Environmental Factors within the One Health Approach. *Medicina* **2021**, *57*, 240. [CrossRef]
59. Gentili, P.L. Why Is Complexity Science Valuable for Reaching the Goals of the UN 2030 Agenda? *Rend. Lincei Sci. Fis. Nat.* **2021**, *32*, 117–134. [CrossRef]
60. Atukunda, P.; Eide, W.B.; Kardel, K.R.; Iversen, P.O.; Westerberg, A.C. Unlocking the Potential for Achievement of the UN Sustainable Development Goal 2—'Zero Hunger'—In Africa: Targets, Strategies, Synergies and Challenges. *Food Nutr. Res.* **2021**, *65*, 7686. [CrossRef]
61. Manandhar, M.; Hawkes, S.; Buse, K.; Nosrati, E.; Magar, V. Gender, Health and the 2030 Agenda for Sustainable Development. *Bull. World Health Organ.* **2018**, *96*, 644–653. [CrossRef] [PubMed]
62. Raman, R.; Nair, V.K.; Shivdas, A.; Bhukya, R.; Viswanathan, P.K.; Subramaniam, N.; Nedungadi, P. Mapping Sustainability Reporting Research with the UN's Sustainable Development Goal. *Heliyon* **2023**, *9*, e18510. [CrossRef] [PubMed]

nutrients

MDPI

Communication

Genetic Variants and Lifestyle Factors in Androgenetic Alopecia Patients: A Case–Control Study of Single Nucleotide Polymorphisms and Their Contribution to Baldness Risk

Roberto Ambra [1,*], Simona Mastroeni [2], Sonia Manca [1], Thomas J. Mannooranparampil [3], Fabio Virgili [4], Barbara Marzani [5], Daniela Pinto [5] and Cristina Fortes [6]

1 Research Centre for Food and Nutrition, Council for Agricultural Research and Economics (CREA-AN), 00178 Rome, Italy; sonia.manca84@gmail.com

2 National Centre for Disease Prevention and Health Promotion, Italian National Health Institute, 00161 Rome, Italy; simona.mastroeni@iss.it

3 Dermatology Unit, Salus Infirmorum Clinic, 00135 Rome, Italy; tjmannooran@gmail.com

4 Interuniversitary Consortium "National Institute for Bio-Structures and Bio-Systems" (INBB), 00165 Rome, Italy; fvirgili@outlook.it

5 R&D Giuliani S.p.A., 20129 Milan, Italy; bmarzani@giulianipharma.com (B.M.); dpinto@giulianipharma.com (D.P.)

6 Epidemiology Unit, Istituto Dermopatico dell'Immacolata (IDI-IRCCS-FLMM), 00167 Rome, Italy; c.deppermannfortes@idi.it

* Correspondence: roberto.ambra@crea.gov.it

Abstract: Single nucleotide polymorphisms (SNPs) found to be associated with Androgenetic Alopecia (AGA) to date, are characterized by an apparent reduced penetrance into the phenotype suggesting a role of other factors in the etiology of AGA. Objective: We conducted a study to investigate the role of specific allelic variants in AGA controlling for nutritional and lifestyle factors. Methods: Individual patterns of SNPs present in the baldness susceptibility locus at 20p11 (rs1160312 and rs6113491) or close to the androgen receptor (AR) gene in chromosome X (rs1041668) were investigated in 212 male subjects. Information on socio-demographic characteristics, medical history, smoking, and diet was also collected. Logistic regression was used to estimate odds ratios (ORs) and 95% confidence intervals (CIs). Results: After controlling for age, diet, BMI, family history of AGA, and smoking, an increased risk of AGA was found for subjects with [A] alleles for both rs1160312 (OR: 2.97; 95% CI: 1.34–6.62) and rs6113491 (OR: 2.99; 95% CI: 1.37–6.52), and for subjects with the TT genotype for rs1041668 (OR: 4.47; 95% CI: 1.60–12.5). Multivariate logistic regression indicates that diet, familiarity, and BMI, but not smoking, remain statistically significant despite the different SNP genotypes. Conclusions: To our knowledge, this is the first indication that the rs1160312, rs6113491, and rs1041668 polymorphisms are independent risk factors for AGA that can be modulated by diet.

Keywords: androgenetic alopecia; single nucleotide polymorphisms; diet

1. Introduction

Androgenetic Alopecia (AGA) is a sex-limited and age-related dermatological condition that affects around 80% of European men and is characterized by the severe shrinking of hair follicles and eventually by evident hair loss [1]. The proportion of affected males is strongly influenced by race/ethnicity, but shows a worldwide increasing trend [2]. Epidemiological studies have shown that AGA is associated with an increased risk of many chronic diseases, including cardiovascular diseases, diabetes, and prostate cancer [3], suggesting common pathophysiological mechanisms and/or nutritional and environmental factors.

Early studies on twins attributed ≈80% of the phenotypical variance of AGA to additive genetic factors [4]. Accordingly, genome-wide association studies (GWASs) conducted over the subsequent two decades identified more than 350 risk genomic regions and more than 600 independent, common, single nucleotide polymorphisms (SNPs) [5]. However, a recent, large, pedigree-based heritability analysis reduced the contribution of genetics and SNPs to AGA phenotypic variance at 60% and 39%, respectively [6], supporting the role of other factors in the etiology of AGA, including lifestyle and nutritional factors. In fact, hair function and appearance have been reported to rely largely on an adequate and balanced nutritional intake [7], with recent evidence supporting the protective role of the phytochemicals of nutritional plants typical of the Mediterranean diet, naturally rich in polyphenols and antioxidants [8–10].

From this perspective, we conducted a study aimed at investigating the relationships between previously associated SNPs and environmental factors in determining the risk of AGA. For such a purpose, individual patterns of genetic variants strongly associated with AGA located in the baldness susceptibility loci at 20p11 (rs1160312 and rs6113491) [11,12] or in chromosome X between the AR and the ecto-dysplasin A2 receptor (EDA2R) genes (rs1041668) [13] were compared to the individual dietary intake and smoking status of 104 males affected by AGA and 108 controls.

2. Materials and Methods

2.1. Subjects and Food Items

This case–control study was conducted as part of a study that investigated the possible risk factors for the development and the severity of AGA [9,14]. Briefly, males affected by AGA (N = 104) of European ethnicity aged 18 years or more and resident in the Lazio region were drawn from out-patient clinics of the hospital "Istituto Dermopatico dell'Immacolata" (IDI), the reference hospital for dermatological diseases in the Lazio region, between 2011 and 2012. Males not affected by AGA (N = 108) of European ethnicity aged 18 years or older, resident in the Lazio region, were chosen as controls. To avoid bias, both cases and controls were drawn from the same geographic region. A trained dermatologist collected information on socio-demographic and clinical characteristics, including weight and height, the presence of chronic diseases (e.g., diabetes, dyslipidemia, cancer, cerebrovascular, and cardiovascular diseases), family history of AGA, smoking, and dietary habits. The trained dermatologist, with the help of 12 series of figures, observed the subject's head from two angles (side and top) and classified the hair pattern according to the Hamilton baldness scale, as modified by Norwood [15].

Dietary intake was assessed by a validated food-frequency questionnaire [16,17]. The consumption of food groups was defined on a seven-point scale and then combined in two categories according to the frequency distribution among the controls. Food items were grouped on the basis of rough phytochemicals' content. For example, spinach, chicory, and beet leaves formed the "dark leafy green vegetables" (a good source of phenols, lutein, and zeaxanthin) and broccoli, cauliflower, and cabbage formed the "cruciferous vegetables" (good sources of isothiocyanates and indoles). The use of fresh herbs, such as parsley, sage, basil, and rosemary, were categorized as the "number of fresh herbs regularly used". In the latter case, low intake was defined as the regular consumption of two or less fresh herbs, while the regular consumption of three or more herbs was considered a high intake. Smoking status was categorized into two groups (ever-smoker/non-smoker).

Body mass index was calculated as weight in kilograms divided by height in meters squared. Family history was defined as having a first-degree relative affected by AGA.

All participants in the study who filled in the questionnaire were asked to provide a saliva sample. DNA was obtained from 212 subjects. Individual patterns of SNPs located in chromosome 20 (rs1160312 and rs6113491) or in chromosome X between the AR and the ectodysplasin A2 receptor (EDA2R) genes (rs1041668) were investigated in all 212 subjects. The study was approved by the IDI ethical committee and written consent was obtained from all participants.

2.2. SNP Genotyping

DNA was extracted from saliva samples using the Puregene DNA purification kit (DNA Genotek, Kanata, Ontario, Canada), slightly modifying the manufacturer's instructions. Briefly, 500 μL of the saliva sample mixed with the Oragene DNA Stabilizing solution was transferred in a 2 mL reaction tube and incubated for 1 h at 50 °C, with shaking the tube every 5 min. A total of 125 μL of a cell lysis solution and 3 μL of RNase A were added. After incubation for 10 min at RT, 200 μL of a protein precipitation solution was added, and the tubes were centrifuged at 10,000 rpm for 10 min. One volume of isopropanol and 5 μL of glycogen were added, and the tubes were centrifuged at 13,000 rpm for 5 min. The supernatant was discarded, and the pellets washed with 70% ethanol and then centrifuged again at 13,000 rpm for 5 min. Finally, the pellets were resuspended in 50 μL of a DNA hydration solution. Genomic DNA was quantified using a Nanodrop ND-1000 instrument (Agilent technologies, Santa Clara, CA, USA) and diluted to a final concentration of 5 μg/μL.

A Tecan Freedom EVO75 robot was utilized to handle and load genomic DNA (10 ng) and Master mixes in 384-well PCR plates. Genotyping was performed using TaqMan assays specific for every SNP, run on an ABI Prism 7900 HT Sequence Detection system using the TaqMan® Universal PCR Master mix (Applied Biosystems, Foster City, CA, USA). The thermal cycling conditions were: pre-PCR read for the fluorescence background; PCR cycling: 95 °C for 10 min for activating AmpliTaq Gold; 40 cycles at 92 °C for 15 s for denaturing genomic DNA and 1 min at 60 °C for annealing/extension; and finally, a post-PCR read for fluorescence quantification at the end of the run. Standard curves using serial dilutions of known concentrations of genomic DNA were performed to verify the assays' sensitivity, and technical replicates were performed for each sample to assess the consistency of the results. Both the positive controls (known genotypes) and negative controls (no template controls) were included in each run to verify the assays' specificity and detect possible contamination. For each SNP, a raw data table was created, and the major and minor allele frequencies for each sample were subjected to statistical analysis.

2.3. Statistical Analysis

Unconditional logistic regression was used to investigate the association between SNPs and AGA in the baldness susceptibility locus at 20p11 (rs1160312 and rs6113491) or near the AR gene (rs1041668) located in chromosome X. Odds ratios (ORs) and 95% confidence intervals (CIs) for the intermediate- and high-exposure categories were calculated using as reference categories the TC genotype for rs1041668 and the GG and CC homozygotes for rs1160312 and rs6113491, respectively, and pooling the AA and AG genotypes for rs1160312 and the AA and AC ones for rs6113491. Different multivariate logistic regression models controlling for possible confounders were run. We included, in the multivariable models, only variables that were statistically significant in the univariate analysis (p-value < 0.05). The following variables were considered in the same multivariate regression model, to adjust for each other as potential confounders: age, BMI, family history of AGA, smoking, and food items previously shown to be associated with AGA. All analyses were performed using the statistical software package PC-STATA (Stata Statistical Software: Release 15. College Station, TX, USA: StataCorp LLC).

3. Results

Table 1 shows the characteristics of the subjects participating in the study. The mean age of the participants was 28.5 years old for the cases and 38.9 years old for the controls. Out of 104 AGA subjects, 35 (37.5%) had a moderate/severe AGA. Age, BMI, family history of AGA (p-value < 0.001), and smoking ($p = 0.05$) were all associated with AGA. No difference was found for education and the presence of chronic diseases. AGA subjects had a higher frequency of allele A in rs1160312 (76.0% vs. 57.4%) and rs6113491 (75.0% vs. 58.3%) SNPs in comparison to the controls. Also, the TT genotype of rs1041668 was more frequent in AGA subjects than in the controls (91.3% vs. 74.1%).

Table 1. Characteristics and genotypes of the subjects participating in the study.

	Cases (N = 104)		Controls (N = 108)		
	N. [a]	**%**	**N.** [a]	**%**	***p*-Value** [b]
Sex					
male	104	100	108	100	
Age, y					
mean (SD)	28.5 (8.7)		38.9 (12.2)		
median (IQR)	26 (22–33)		38 (29–47)		0.0001 [c]
Educational level					
up to intermediate school	9	8.7	13	12.0	
high school	58	55.8	51	47.2	
degree	37	35.6	44	40.7	0.43
Body mass index (kg/m^2)					
<25	86	82.7	58	53.7	
≥25	18	17.3	50	46.3	<0.0001
Family history of AGA (1st-degree relatives)					
no	43	41.7	82	80.4	
yes	60	58.3	20	19.6	<0.0001
Presence of some illness–condition [d]					
no	43	41.7	48	44.9	
yes	61	59.2	59	55.1	0.61
Ever-smoking					
never	68	65.4	56	51.9	
quit and current	36	34.6	52	48.1	0.05
Norwood–Hamilton scale					
mild	69	66.3	...		
moderate/severe	35	37.5	...		
rs1160312					
GG	25	24.0	44	40.7	
AA	27	26.0	18	16.7	
AG	52	50.0	44	40.7	
00	...		2	1.9	0.02
rs1041668					
TC	9	8.7	27	25.0	
TT	95	91.3	80	74.1	
00	...		1	0.9	0.001
rs6113491					
CC	26	25.0	45	41.7	
AC	52	50.0	44	40.7	
AA	26	25.0	19	17.6	0.03

Abbreviations: SD, standard deviation; IQR, interquartile range. [a]: Totals may vary because of missing values. [b]: χ^2 or Fisher's exact test, where appropriate. [c]: Mann–Whitney U test. [d]: e.g., diabetes, cardio-cerebrovascular disease, cancer, and dyslipidemia.

Table 2 shows the crude and adjusted risk estimates for rs1160312, rs6113491, and rs1041668. After the adjustments for age, BMI, family history of AGA, ever-smoking, and consumption of salad and fresh herbs, an increased risk was found for the TT genotype of rs1041668 near the AR gene locus (OR: 4.47; 95% CI: 1.60–12.5) and for subjects carrying allele A of rs1160312 (OR: 2.97; 95% CI: 1.34–6.62) and rs6113491 (OR: 2.99; 95% CI: 1.37–6.52). In the multivariate models, the consumption of salad, the use of fresh herbs, familiarity, and BMI remained statistically significant, while smoking was no longer statistically significant (in model 2, for those who have quit smoking and current smokers vs. never having smoked, OR: 0.61; 95% CI: 0.30–1.25, OR: 0.58; 95% CI: 0.29–1.17, and OR: 0.60; 95% CI: 0.30–1.20 for rs1160312, rs1041668, and rs6113491, respectively).

Table 2. Association between AGA and rs1160312, rs6113491, and rs1041668 genotypes of the subjects participating in the study.

	Model 0		Model 1		Model 2	
	OR [a]	95%CI	OR [b]	95%CI	OR [c]	95%CI
rs1160312						
GG	1		1		1	
AA AG	2.24	(1.24–4.06)	2.51	(1.20–5.25)	2.97	(1.34–6.62)
rs1041668						
TC	1		1		1	
TT	3.56	(1.58–8.02)	4.44	(1.66–11.9)	4.47	(1.60–12.5)
rs6113491						
CC	1		1		1	
AA AC	2.14	(1.19–3.85)	2.53	(1.22–5.27)	2.99	(1.37–6.52)

[a]: Model 0, crude odds ratio. [b]: Model 1, odds ratio adjusted for age, BMI, family history of AGA, and ever-smoking. [c]: Model 2, odds ratio adjusted for age, BMI, family history of AGA, ever-smoking, and consumption of salad and fresh herbs.

4. Discussion

Our study shows that genetic variants located in the baldness susceptibility loci at 20p11 or in chromosome X between the AR and the ectodysplasin A2 receptor (EDA2R) genes are associated with an increased risk of AGA after controlling for all possible confounders. Our observations confirm the early associations of rs1041668 [13], rs1160312 [11], and rs6113491 [12] SNPs with AGA and subsequent reports [18–22], but also indicate that other factors, i.e., high consumption of foods rich in phytochemicals, BMI, and family history, are independent risk factors for AGA among subjects bearing the variants.

The associations found in our study between AGA and BMI and family history in first-degree relatives are in agreement with a number of studies [23]. The role of smoking in AGA is controversial. Several studies reported an association between smoking and AGA development [14,24–27], while other studies showed no association [9,18,28–30]. In our study, smoking was associated with an increased risk in the univariate analysis, but the effect disappeared in the multivariate analysis after controlling for diet and genetic factors. Similarly, Ellis and coworkers reported that smoking status had little effect on the estimated OR of the SNP rs6152 [31], one of the first chromosome X polymorphisms near the AR locus that has been linked to baldness.

As mentioned in the introduction, AGA is linked to many chronic diseases. In our study, the presence of chronic diseases was not associated with an increased risk of AGA. As aging is a well-known contributor to the risk of chronic diseases, the observed lack of an association may trivially depend on the fact that our AGA subjects were indeed younger than the controls. On the other hand, the inclusion of older non-AGA subjects has the theoretical advantage of avoiding potential false-negative controls, since AGA is an age-dependent condition. Nonetheless, even if the ORs were adjusted for age, a residual confounding of age is not excluded.

After the adjustments for age, BMI, family history of AGA, smoking, salad consumption, and the use of fresh herbs, we found an increased risk for the TT genotype of the rs1041668 SNP present near the AR gene locus that has been associated with AGA, even if the definition of its exact role is still unknown [8]. After the adjustment, we found an increased risk also for subjects carrying the alleles A of rs1160312 and rs6113491 present on chromosome 20. Marcińska and coworkers reported that the two SNPs, rs1160312 and rs6113491, have a strong linkage disequilibrium (94%), even though both were included in their predictive test [19]. Both SNPs are present in intergenic zones, but rs1160312 is present within LINC01432, a non-coding RNA gene that was found differentially expressed in the testes of three out of seven individuals [32], where androgen biosynthesis occurs, suggesting a link between the rs1160312 polymorphism and AGA etiopathogenesis involving differential production or sensitivity to androgen levels through the modulation of LINC01432 gene activity. Further research is required to clarify how rs1160312 contributes to AGA susceptibility, starting for example from the correlation of the SNP genotype with LINC01432 expression in hair follicles.

The effects of familiarity and the protective effect of a high consumption of salad and of the use of fresh herbs remained statistically significant for all three polymorphisms, showing that the etiopathogenesis of AGA has a strong genetic component but is affected by nutrition, and thus confirming its multifactorial nature [33]. Specifically, the observed effects of fresh herb use and salad consumption are in agreement with the results of randomized clinical trials employing phytochemicals either topically [34,35] or simultaneously topically and orally [36]. Phytochemicals have antioxidant, anti-inflammatory, and anti-tumor properties that are considered responsible for the ability of plant food nutrients to prevent chronic diseases [37]. In this respect, Agaoglu et al. recognized the insufficient intake of plant foods as a risk factor for early-onset AGA in young men [26], and Bazmi and coworkers found higher dietary inflammatory index and lower antioxidant index scores in women with AGA [38]. With respect to fresh herbs, among molecules characterized by high bioactivity and included in the abovementioned trials, rosmarinic acid is noteworthy, with its properties well-known for hair health [10]. Further studies are warranted, especially clinical trials with genetic risk screening and controlled diets of at-risk subjects, in order to confirm our findings and eventually set up personalized approaches to AGA management that could include specific dietary modifications and other factors, such as, for example, the gut microbiota that has been recently linked to AGA [39].

Author Contributions: Conceptualization: F.V., C.F., R.A., B.M. and D.P.; methodology: R.A., S.M. (Simona Mastroeni), S.M. (Sonia Manca), T.J.M. and C.F.; investigation: R.A., S.M. (Simona Mastroeni) and T.J.M.; data curation: S.M. (Sonia Manca) and C.F.; writing—original draft preparation: R.A., F.V. and C.F.; writing—review and editing: R.A., S.M. (Sonia Manca), B.M., D.P. and C.F. All authors have read and agreed to the published version of the manuscript.

Funding: This study was supported by the Italian Ministry of Health (Ricerca Corrente 5.1) and by Giuliani S.p.A., Milan, Italy.

Institutional Review Board Statement: This study was conducted in accordance with the Declaration of Helsinki and approved by the Ethics Committee of the Istituto Dermopatico dell'Immacolata (Study EC.295, Prot. n 69/CR/2009, 22 June 2009).

Informed Consent Statement: Informed consent was obtained from all subjects involved in the study.

Data Availability Statement: The data presented in this study are available on request from the corresponding author.

Acknowledgments: We are indebted to Stefano Tabolli for helping us to organize the study and to Sergio Salvi for setting up the Tecan instrument.

Conflicts of Interest: Barbara Marzani and Daniela Pinto are employed by Giuliani S.p.A. The rest of the authors declare no conflict of interest.

References

1. Hamilton, J.B. Patterned Loss of Hair in Man: Types and Incidence. *Ann. N. Y. Acad. Sci.* **1951**, *53*, 708–728. [CrossRef]
2. Ellis, J.A.; Sinclair, R.D. Male Pattern Baldness: Current Treatments, Future Prospects. *Drug Discov. Today* **2008**, *13*, 791–797. [CrossRef]
3. Chen, S.; Xie, X.; Zhang, G.; Zhang, Y. Comorbidities in Androgenetic Alopecia: A Comprehensive Review. *Dermatol. Ther.* **2022**, *12*, 2233. [CrossRef] [PubMed]
4. Nyholt, D.R.; Gillespie, N.A.; Heath, A.C.; Martin, N.G. Genetic Basis of Male Pattern Baldness. *J. Investig. Dermatol.* **2003**, *121*, 1561–1564. [CrossRef] [PubMed]
5. Henne, S.K.; Nöthen, M.M.; Heilmann-Heimbach, S. Male-Pattern Hair Loss: Comprehensive Identification of the Associated Genes as a Basis for Understanding Pathophysiology. *Med. Genet.* **2023**, *35*, 3–14. [CrossRef] [PubMed]
6. Yap, C.X.; Sidorenko, J.; Wu, Y.; Kemper, K.E.; Yang, J.; Wray, N.R.; Robinson, M.R.; Visscher, P.M. Dissection of Genetic Variation and Evidence for Pleiotropy in Male Pattern Baldness. *Nat. Commun.* **2018**, *9*, 5407. [CrossRef] [PubMed]
7. Goldberg, L.J.; Lenzy, Y. Nutrition and Hair. *Clin. Dermatol.* **2010**, *28*, 412–419. [CrossRef] [PubMed]
8. Gokce, N.; Basgoz, N.; Kenanoglu, S.; Akalin, H.; Ozkul, Y.; Ergoren, M.C.; Beccari, T.; Bertelli, M.; Dundar, M. An Overview of the Genetic Aspects of Hair Loss and Its Connection with Nutrition. *J. Prev. Med. Hyg.* **2022**, *63*, E228. [CrossRef] [PubMed]
9. Fortes, C.; Mastroeni, S.; Mannooranparampil, T.; Abeni, D.; Panebianco, A. Mediterranean Diet: Fresh Herbs and Fresh Vegetables Decrease the Risk of Androgenetic Alopecia in Males. *Arch. Dermatol. Res.* **2018**, *310*, 71–76. [CrossRef]
10. Bassino, E.; Gasparri, F.; Munaron, L. Protective Role of Nutritional Plants Containing Flavonoids in Hair Follicle Disruption: A Review. *Int. J. Mol. Sci.* **2020**, *21*, 523. [CrossRef] [PubMed]
11. Richards, J.B.; Yuan, X.; Geller, F.; Waterworth, D.; Bataille, V.; Glass, D.; Song, K.; Waeber, G.; Vollenweider, P.; Aben, K.K.H.; et al. Male-Pattern Baldness Susceptibility Locus at 20p11. *Nat. Genet.* **2008**, *40*, 1282–1284. [CrossRef]
12. Hillmer, A.M.; Brockschmidt, F.F.; Hanneken, S.; Eigelshoven, S.; Steffens, M.; Flaquer, A.; Herms, S.; Becker, T.; Kortüm, A.K.; Nyholt, D.R.; et al. Susceptibility Variants for Male-Pattern Baldness on Chromosome 20p11. *Nat. Genet.* **2008**, *40*, 1279–1281. [CrossRef]
13. Hillmer, A.M.; Hanneken, S.; Ritzmann, S.; Becker, T.; Freudenberg, J.; Brockschmidt, F.F.; Flaquer, A.; Freudenberg-Hua, Y.; Jamra, R.A.; Metzen, C.; et al. Genetic Variation in the Human Androgen Receptor Gene Is the Major Determinant of Common Early-Onset Androgenetic Alopecia. *Am. J. Hum. Genet.* **2005**, *77*, 140–148. [CrossRef] [PubMed]
14. Fortes, C.; Mastroeni, S.; Mannooranparampil, T.J.; Ribuffo, M. The Combination of Overweight and Smoking Increases the Severity of Androgenetic Alopecia. *Int. J. Dermatol.* **2017**, *56*, 862–867. [CrossRef] [PubMed]
15. Norwood, O.T. Male Pattern Baldness: Classification and Incidence. *South. Med. J.* **1975**, *68*, 1359–1365. [CrossRef]
16. Fortes, C.; Mastroeni, S.; Melchi, F.; Pilla, M.A.; Antonelli, G.; Camaioni, D.; Alotto, M.; Pasquini, P. A Protective Effect of the Mediterranean Diet for Cutaneous Melanoma. *Int. J. Epidemiol.* **2008**, *37*, 1018–1029. [CrossRef] [PubMed]
17. Fortes, C.; Forastiere, F.; Farchi, S.; Mallone, S.; Trequattrinni, T.; Anatra, F.; Schmid, G.; Perucci, C.A. The Protective Effect of the Mediterranean Diet on Lung Cancer. *Nutr. Cancer* **2003**, *46*, 30–37. [CrossRef] [PubMed]
18. Lai, C.H.; Chu, N.F.; Chang, C.W.; Wang, S.L.; Yang, H.C.; Chu, C.M.; Chang, C.T.; Lin, M.H.; Chien, W.C.; Su, S.L.; et al. Androgenic Alopecia Is Associated with Less Dietary Soy, Higher Blood Vanadium and Rs1160312 1 Polymorphism in Taiwanese Communities. *PLoS ONE* **2013**, *8*, e79789. [CrossRef]
19. Marcińska, M.; Pośpiech, E.; Abidi, S.; Andersen, J.D.; Van Den Berge, M.; Carracedo, Á.; Eduardoff, M.; Marczakiewicz-Lustig, A.; Morling, N.; Sijen, T.; et al. Evaluation of DNA Variants Associated with Androgenetic Alopecia and Their Potential to Predict Male Pattern Baldness. *PLoS ONE* **2015**, *10*, 012785. [CrossRef] [PubMed]
20. Hagenaars, S.P.; Hill, W.D.; Harris, S.E.; Ritchie, S.J.; Davies, G.; Liewald, D.C.; Gale, C.R.; Porteous, D.J.; Deary, I.J.; Marioni, R.E. Genetic Prediction of Male Pattern Baldness. *PLoS Genet.* **2017**, *13*, 1006594. [CrossRef]
21. Ye, M.; Yang, Z.; Li, M.; Xing, Y.; Zeng, F.; Cheng, B. Association of Eight Single Nucleotide Polymorphisms of Chromosomes 20 and X with Androgenetic Alopecia among Ethnic Han Chinese from Yunnan. *Chin. J. Med. Genet.* **2016**, *33*, 383–387. [CrossRef]
22. Liu, F.; Hamer, M.A.; Heilmann, S.; Herold, C.; Moebus, S.; Hofman, A.; Uitterlinden, A.G.; Nöthen, M.M.; Van Duijn, C.M.; Nijsten, T.E.C.; et al. Prediction of Male-Pattern Baldness from Genotypes. *Eur. J. Hum. Genet.* **2015**, *24*, 895–902. [CrossRef] [PubMed]

23. Qiu, Y.; Zhou, X.; Fu, S.; Luo, S.; Li, Y. Systematic Review and Meta-Analysis of the Association Between Metabolic Syndrome and Androgenetic Alopecia. *Acta Derm. Venereol.* **2022**, *102*, 1012. [CrossRef] [PubMed]
24. Su, L.H.; Chen, T.H.H. Association of Androgenetic Alopecia With Smoking and Its Prevalence Among Asian Men: A Community-Based Survey. *Arch. Dermatol.* **2007**, *143*, 1401–1406. [CrossRef] [PubMed]
25. Salem, A.S.; Ibrahim, H.S.; Abdelaziz, H.H.; Elsaie, M.L. Implications of Cigarette Smoking on Early-Onset Androgenetic Alopecia: A Cross-Sectional Study. *J. Cosmet. Dermatol.* **2021**, *20*, 1318–1324. [CrossRef]
26. Agaoglu, E.; Erdogan, H.K.; Acer, E.; Atay, E.; MetïNtas, S.; Saracoglu, Z.N. Prevalence of Early-Onset Androgenetic Alopecia and Its Relationship with Lifestyle and Dietary Habits. *Ital. J. Dermatol. Venereol.* **2021**, *156*, 675–680. [CrossRef] [PubMed]
27. Mosley, J.G.; Gibbs, A.C.C. Premature Grey Hair and Hair Loss among Smokers: A New Opportunity for Health Education? *BMJ Br. Med. J.* **1996**, *313*, 1616. [CrossRef] [PubMed]
28. Severi, G.; Sinclair, R.; Hopper, J.L.; English, D.R.; McCredie, M.R.E.; Boyle, P.; Giles, G.G. Androgenetic Alopecia in Men Aged 40–69 Years: Prevalence and Risk Factors. *Br. J. Dermatol.* **2003**, *149*, 1207–1213. [CrossRef] [PubMed]
29. Esen Salman, K.; Kucukunal, N.A.; Kivanc Altunay, I.; Aksu Cerman, A. Frequency, Severity and Related Factors of Androgenetic Alopecia in dermatology Outpatient Clinic: Hospital-Based Cross-Sectional Study In. *An. Bras. Dermatol.* **2017**, *92*, 35. [CrossRef]
30. Danesh-Shakiba, M.; Poorolajal, J.; Alirezaei, P. Androgenetic Alopecia: Relationship to Anthropometric Indices, Blood Pressure and Life-Style Habits. *Clin. Cosmet. Investig. Dermatol.* **2020**, *13*, 137. [CrossRef]
31. Ellis, J.A.; Scurrah, K.J.; Cobb, J.E.; Zaloumis, S.G.; Duncan, A.E.; Harrap, S.B. Baldness and the Androgen Receptor: The AR Polyglycine Repeat Polymorphism Does Not Confer Susceptibility to Androgenetic Alopecia. *Hum. Genet.* **2007**, *121*, 451–457. [CrossRef] [PubMed]
32. Fagerberg, L.; Hallstrom, B.M.; Oksvold, P.; Kampf, C.; Djureinovic, D.; Odeberg, J.; Habuka, M.; Tahmasebpoor, S.; Danielsson, A.; Edlund, K.; et al. Analysis of the Human Tissue-Specific Expression by Genome-Wide Integration of Transcriptomics and Antibody-Based Proteomics. *Mol. Cell. Proteom.* **2014**, *13*, 397–406. [CrossRef] [PubMed]
33. Li, Y.; Dong, T.; Wan, S.; Xiong, R.; Jin, S.; Dai, Y.; Guan, C. Application of Multi-Omics Techniques to Androgenetic Alopecia: Current Status and Perspectives. *Comput. Struct. Biotechnol. J.* **2024**, *23*, 2623–2636. [CrossRef]
34. Panahi, Y.; Taghizadeh, M.; Marzony, E.T.; Sahebkar, A. Rosemary Oil vs Minoxidil 2% for the Treatment of Androgenetic Alopecia: A Randomized Comparative Trial. *Skinmed* **2015**, *13*, 15–21. [PubMed]
35. Welzel, J.; Wolff, H.H.; Gehring, W. Reduction of Telogen Rate and Increase of Hair Density in Androgenetic Alopecia by a Cosmetic Product: Results of a Randomized, Prospective, Vehicle-Controlled Double-Blind Study in Men. *J. Cosmet. Dermatol.* **2022**, *21*, 1057–1064. [CrossRef]
36. Feldman, P.R.; Fiebig, K.M.; Piwko, C.; Mints, B.M.; Brown, D.; Cahan, D.J.; Guevara-Aguirre, J. Safety and Efficacy of ALRV5XR in Men with Androgenetic Alopecia: A Randomised, Double-Blinded, Placebo-Controlled Clinical Trial. *EClinicalMedicine* **2021**, *40*, 101124. [CrossRef]
37. Wallace, T.C.; Bailey, R.L.; Blumberg, J.B.; Burton-Freeman, B.; Chen, C.y.O.; Crowe-White, K.M.; Drewnowski, A.; Hooshmand, S.; Johnson, E.; Lewis, R.; et al. Fruits, Vegetables, and Health: A Comprehensive Narrative, Umbrella Review of the Science and Recommendations for Enhanced Public Policy to Improve Intake. *Crit. Rev. Food Sci. Nutr.* **2020**, *60*, 2174–2211. [CrossRef]
38. Bazmi, S.; Sepehrinia, M.; Pourmontaseri, H.; Bazyar, H.; Vahid, F.; Farjam, M.; Dehghan, A.; Hébert, J.R.; Homayounfar, R.; Shakouri, N. Androgenic Alopecia Is Associated with Higher Dietary Inflammatory Index and Lower Antioxidant Index Scores. *Front. Nutr.* **2024**, *11*, 1433962. [CrossRef]
39. Fu, H.; Xu, T.; Zhao, W.; Jiang, L.; Shan, S. Roles of Gut Microbiota in Androgenetic Alopecia: Insights from Mendelian Randomization Analysis. *Front. Microbiol.* **2024**, *15*, 1360445. [CrossRef]

nutrients

MDPI

Article

Microencapsulation of Anthocyanins from *Zea mays* and *Solanum tuberosum*: Impacts on Antioxidant, Antimicrobial, and Cytotoxic Activities

Carlos Barba-Ostria [1,2,*], Yenddy Carrero [3], Jéssica Guamán-Bautista [4], Orestes López [5], Christian Aranda [5], Alexis Debut [6,7] and Linda P. Guamán [8,*]

1 Escuela de Medicina, Colegio de Ciencias de la Salud Quito, Universidad San Francisco de Quito (USFQ), Quito 170901, Ecuador
2 Instituto de Microbiología, Universidad San Francisco de Quito (USFQ), Quito 170901, Ecuador
3 Facultad de Ciencias de la Salud, Universidad Técnica de Ambato, Ambato 180105, Ecuador; yenddycarrero@yahoo.es
4 Facultad de Ciencias de la Hospitalidad, Carrera de Gastronomía, Universidad de Cuenca, Cuenca 010201, Ecuador; jessica.guaman@ucuenca.edu.ec
5 Facultad de Ciencia e Ingeniería en Alimentos, Universidad Técnica de Ambato, Ambato 180207, Ecuador; od.lopez@uta.edu.ec (O.L.); caranda6747@uta.edu.ec (C.A.)
6 Centro de Nanociencia y Nanotecnología, Universidad de Las Fuerzas Armadas ESPE, Sangolquí 171103, Ecuador; apdebut@espe.edu.ec
7 Departamento de Ciencias de la Vida y Agricultura, Universidad de las Fuerzas Armadas ESPE, Sangolquí 171103, Ecuador
8 Facultad de Ciencias de la Salud Eugenio Espejo, Universidad UTE, Centro de Investigación Biomédica (CENBIO), Quito 170527, Ecuador
* Correspondence: cbarbao@usfq.edu.ec (C.B.-O.); linda.guaman@ute.edu.ec (L.P.G.); Tel.: +593-2-2990800 (ext. 2115) (L.P.G.)

Abstract: Objectives: This study investigates the biological activities of microencapsulated anthocyanins extracted from two Andean ancestral edible plants, *Solanum tuberosum*, and *Zea mays*, with a focus on their potential applications in functional foods and therapeutics. The primary objective was to evaluate their antioxidant, antimicrobial, and cytotoxic properties alongside structural and functional analyses of the microencapsulation process. **Methods:** Anthocyanins were extracted and microencapsulated using maltodextrin as a carrier. Fourier-transform infrared spectroscopy (FTIR) and scanning electron microscopy (SEM) were employed to analyze the stability and structure of the microencapsulated particles. The antioxidant, antimicrobial, and cytotoxic activities of the microencapsulated were assessed through established assays. **Results:** *S. tuberosum* exhibited superior antioxidant capacity and potent anticancer activity against HepG2 and THJ29T cell lines, while *Z. mays* demonstrated significant antimicrobial efficacy against multidrug-resistant bacterial strains and biofilm-forming pathogens. Fourier-transform infrared spectroscopy (FTIR) and scanning electron microscopy (SEM) confirmed the stabilization of anthocyanins within a maltodextrin matrix, enhancing their bioavailability and application potential. **Conclusions:** These results highlight the versatility of microencapsulated anthocyanins as bioactive agents for industrial and therapeutic applications. Future studies should explore in vivo validation and synergistic formulations to optimize their efficacy and broaden their use in nutraceutical and pharmaceutical fields.

Keywords: functional foods; natural antimicrobials; biocompounds; antioxidant activity; anthocyanins

1. Introduction

Cancer and infectious diseases represent significant global public health challenges, underscoring the need for research aimed at identifying adjuvants that optimize conventional treatments [1]. In this context, phytocompounds obtained from plant sources, such as roots, stems, leaves, and fruits, have garnered increasing attention. Among these, anthocyanins—pigmented flavonoids—have gained recognition because of their diverse pharmacological and therapeutic properties [2,3].

Anthocyanins are natural pigments widely distributed in fruits, vegetables, and cereals, contributing to the vibrant red, blue, and purple hues of many plants. Prominent sources of anthocyanins include berries (e.g., blueberries, blackberries, and raspberries), grapes, red cabbage, eggplant, and Andean crops such as purple maize (*Zea mays* L.) and purple potato (*Solanum tuberosum* L.) [4,5]. Chemically, anthocyanins belong to the flavonoid class of polyphenols and are characterized by their basic C6-C3-C6 structure, which includes two aromatic rings connected by a three-carbon bridge, forming a heterocyclic flavylium ion. This unique structure allows anthocyanins to exist in multiple chemical forms depending on pH, enabling diverse biological activities [6,7].

Anthocyanins have been linked to numerous health benefits, including anti-inflammatory, antihypertensive, antibacterial, anticancer, and neuroprotective effects, which are mediated by a variety of bioactive mechanisms [8]. Their potent antioxidant properties have also been associated with the prevention and management of diseases such as cancer, metabolic disorders, and cardiovascular conditions [3,9]; however, the application of anthocyanins in functional foods and therapeutic formulations is significantly hindered by their inherent instability. Environmental factors such as pH, temperature, and light exposure contribute to their degradation, thereby limiting their bioavailability and efficacy [10,11].

Several strategies have been developed to address these limitations. Microencapsulation offers a promising solution to these challenges by embedding anthocyanins in protective matrices, which enhance their stability, prolong shelf life, and maintain their functional properties under diverse conditions [12]. Encapsulation protects anthocyanin molecules from harsh conditions in the gastrointestinal tract, allowing them to reach the small intestine intact, where absorption into the bloodstream occurs [13]. Nano- and microencapsulation techniques, such as spray drying, freeze drying, emulsification, gelation, and polyelectrolyte complex formation, have shown promise in overcoming the instability of anthocyanins and enhancing their distribution in functional foods and nutraceuticals [14].

Anthocyanins, as natural pigments, are widely recognized for their antioxidant, anti-inflammatory, anticancer, and antimicrobial properties [15,16]. Found in a variety of plant species, these compounds have attracted significant interest for their role in scavenging free radicals, inhibiting harmful microorganisms, and promoting apoptosis in cancer cells. This makes them promising candidates for developing novel therapeutic agents against chronic and degenerative diseases, including cancer and cardiovascular disorders [3,17].

Two particularly rich sources of anthocyanins are *Zea mays* L. (cultivar INIAP-Racimo de Uva [18]) and *Solanum tuberosum* L. (cultivar INIAP-Yana Shungo [19]), which are cultivated in the Andean region. The anthocyanins in these plants contribute to their distinct pigmentation and have been studied extensively for their bioactive properties [9,20]; however, the content and efficacy of anthocyanins can vary based on genetic and environmental factors, which can influence their antioxidant and antimicrobial activities [21,22].

Despite the growing interest in anthocyanins, their use in functional foods and nutraceuticals remains limited by their inherent instability and poor bioavailability. To address these challenges, microencapsulation techniques have been developed to improve anthocyanin stability and functionality [10,23].

This study aims to investigate the biological activities of microencapsulated anthocyanins extracted from *Z. mays* L. and *S. tuberosum* L., with a focus on their antioxidant, antimicrobial, and cytotoxic properties. The goal is to evaluate the potential of these encapsulated pigments, particularly regarding their effectiveness against pathogenic bacteria and cancer cells. Through this research, we seek to contribute to the growing body of knowledge on the health benefits of anthocyanins and explore their potential applications in both the food and pharmaceutical industries.

2. Materials and Methods

2.1. Chemicals and Reagents

All reagents and chemicals used in this study were of analytical grade unless otherwise specified. A 100 ppm chlorine solution, sourced from local suppliers, was used for disinfection. Ethanol (96%) and distilled and deionized water were also locally sourced as laboratory-grade reagents.

Hydrochloric acid (1.5 mol/L), Folin–Ciocalteu reagent, and sodium carbonate (7.5%) were purchased from Sigma-Aldrich (Merck, Darmstadt, Hesse, Germany) for extract preparation and analysis. Standards such as gallic acid, catechin, cyanidin-3-glucoside (C3G, reference compound), Trolox (reference antioxidant), and 2,2-diphenyl-1-picrylhydrazyl (DPPH, analytical grade) were also obtained from Sigma-Aldrich. Maltodextrin (10–20 DE) was used as a carrier agent for microencapsulation. Dimethyl sulfoxide (DMSO) and Trypan Blue (TB, analytical grade) were sourced from the same supplier.

Cell culture media and supplements, including Dulbecco's Modified Eagle Medium (DMEM), fetal bovine serum (FBS), L-glutamine, penicillin (10,000 U/mL), and streptomycin (10,000 μg/mL), were obtained from Gibco™ (Thermo Fisher Scientific, Waltham, MA, USA). The MTT reagent (3-(4,5-dimethylthiazol-2-yl)-2,5-diphenyl tetrazolium bromide) was provided by Thermo Fisher Scientific (Waltham, MA, USA).

Antibodies for apoptosis assays, including Bax (6A7), Bcl-2 (7), and caspase-8 (8CSP03), were sourced from Santa Cruz Biotechnology, Inc. (Dallas, TX, USA). Additional reagents, such as fluorescein isothiocyanate (FITC)-conjugated secondary antibody, IgG control conjugated with phycoerythrin (PE), and Aqueous Mounting Medium, were also obtained from Santa Cruz Biotechnology, Inc.

All reagents were prepared following standard laboratory protocols and utilized according to the manufacturer's guidelines to ensure accuracy and reproducibility.

2.2. Plant Material

Z. mays L. and *S. tuberosum* were obtained from a local market in Ambato, Ecuador. Specifically, the cultivars used were *Zea mays* L. (cultivar INIAP-Racimo de Uva, [18]) and *Solanum tuberosum* L. (INIAP-Yana Shungo, [19]). The samples were washed, disinfected with a 100-ppm chlorine solution, and then freeze-dried, ground, and finally stored at −20 °C. The freeze-drying process lasted a total of 72 h. Afterward, the dried samples were ground into a fine powder using an electric laboratory blender (between 100 μm and 500 μm), followed by sieving with a N35 (500 μm) sieve. Anthocyanins were extracted from the corn grains of *Zea mays* L. and the underground portions (tubers) of *Solanum tuberosum* L. The samples were then stored at −20 °C until use in the experiments for this study.

2.3. Anthocyanin Extraction

Ethanolic extracts were prepared according to Perez et al. (2021) with some modifications: The powder material was mixed with twenty times the volume of 96% ethanol:1.5 mol/L HCl (85:15 v/v). This blend was added to a stirrer tank to extract anthocyanins and extracted for 60 min at 70 °C [24].

The solid part was separated from the blend by using an Andreas Hettich GmbH & Co., Ltd. (Tuttlingen, Germany) Rotine 380 centrifuge. The extract was transferred to a 500 mL balloon with continuous stirring and was applied by a rotary evaporator in a water bath to 70 °C for 2 h under a vacuum to remove the solvent.

2.4. Determination of Total Polyphenol Content (TPC) and Anthocyanin Content

The total polyphenol content (TPC) and anthocyanin content of microencapsulated anthocyanins extracted from *S. tuberosum* L. and *Z. mays* L. were carried out using the Folin–Ciocalteu reagent with catechin as the standard [25].

The TPC was measured using the Folin–Ciocalteu method. A 0.5 mL aliquot of the extract was mixed with 2.5 mL of 10% Folin–Ciocalteu reagent and incubated for 5 min at room temperature. Then, 2 mL of 7.5% sodium carbonate solution was added, and the mixture was incubated in the dark for 30 min. The absorbance was measured at 760 nm using a Thermo Scientific (Waltham, MA, USA) Genesys 10S UV-Vis spectrophotometer. Gallic acid was used as a standard, and TPC was expressed in mg of gallic acid equivalents (GAE) per kg of fresh weight of fruit.

The anthocyanin content was determined by the pH differential method [26]. Extracts were diluted in buffers at pH 1.0 and pH 4.5, and the absorbance was measured at 510 nm and 700 nm, respectively, using a Thermo Scientific (Waltham, MA, USA) Genesys 10S UV-Vis spectrophotometer. The anthocyanin content was calculated using the formula:

$$\text{Anthocyanin content (mg C3G/100 g)} = \frac{(\text{A510} - \text{A700}) \times \text{MW} \times \text{DF} \times 1000}{\varepsilon \times \text{L}}$$

where A is the absorbance, MW is the molecular weight of cyanidin-3-glucoside (449.2 g/mol), DF is the dilution factor, ε is the molar absorptivity (26,900 L/mol·cm), and L is the path length (1 cm). The results were expressed in mg of cyanidin-3-glucoside (C3G) per 100 g of fresh weight of fruit.

All measurements were performed in triplicate, and the results were expressed as mean ± standard deviation (SD). Statistical analysis was performed using a *t*-test to determine significant differences between the two extracts ($p < 0.001$).

2.5. Microencapsulation

Microencapsulation Process

The microencapsulation of anthocyanins was performed using maltodextrin (10–20 DE) as the carrier agent. Anthocyanin extracts with a total solids content of 27% (equivalent to 20 g of anthocyanins) were prepared at a 20:80 anthocyanins-to-maltodextrin ratio. For each extract, 280 mL of distilled water was mixed with the anthocyanin solution and combined with maltodextrin. The mixtures were homogenized separately for *S. tuberosum* L. and *Z. mays* L. extracts using an IKA mixer (RH Digital, Staufen, Baden-Württemberg, Germany).

The microencapsulation process for each extract was conducted independently using a laboratory-scale mini spray dryer Büchi B-290 (Flawil, St. Gallen, Switzerland). The solutions were fed into the spray dryer under controlled conditions: an inlet air temperature of 150 ± 2 °C, an outlet air temperature of 90 ± 2 °C, an internal pressure of -50 mbar, an atomizing air flow of 400–600 L/h, and a drying air flow rate of 60 m^3/h [27].

During the spray drying process, each anthocyanin solution was atomized within the drying chamber, forming solid microspheres encapsulated in maltodextrin-based polymers [28]. The resulting microspheres for both extracts were collected in separate collection flasks and stored in HDPE-aluminum bags at a controlled temperature of 15–25 °C.

2.6. Characterization by FTIR

Fourier transform infrared (FTIR) spectroscopy was employed to identify the functional groups in the microcapsules. The spectra were obtained using a JASCO FTIR 4100 spectrometer (Tokyo, Japan) with the ATR method, covering a wave number range of 4000–500 cm^{-1} at a resolution of 4 cm^{-1} across 36 scans.

2.7. Morphological Characterization by Scanning Electron Microscope (SEM)

Each sample was mounted on a stub for electron microscopy with conductive double-sided carbon tape. The samples were coated with a ~20 nm layer of conductive gold (99.99% purity) for 60 s using a Quorum Q150R ES sputtering evaporator (Lewes, East Sussex, UK). Micrographs were captured using a TESCAN MIRA 3 Scanning Electron Microscope (SEM) with the Secondary Electron (SE) detector (Brno, South Moravia, Czech Republic).

The images were analyzed using the Fiji biological-image analysis platform (version 2.9.0) [29]. Area data were extracted from the images using Fiji, and the diameter of each sphere was calculated using the following formula:

$$D = \frac{2\sqrt{A}}{\pi}$$

where D is the diameter, and A is the area obtained from Fiji.

2.8. Antioxidant Capacity

The antioxidant activity of the microencapsulated anthocyanins extracted from *Z. mays* L. and *S. tuberosum* L. was assessed using the DPPH (2,2-diphenyl-1-picrylhydrazyl) radical scavenging assay. The assay was conducted following a modified protocol of Brand-Williams et al. (1995) [30]. A mass of 100 mg of each microencapsulated powder was dissolved in 10 mL of methanol and sonicated for 30 min at room temperature. The solutions were then centrifuged at 4000 rpm for 10 min, and the supernatants were collected for further analysis.

A 0.2 mM DPPH solution was prepared in methanol. For the assay, 100 µL of the DPPH solution was mixed with 100 µL of the microencapsulated in a Corning 96-well microplate (Corning, NY, USA) at concentrations ranging from 10 to 500 µg/mL. The mixtures were incubated in the dark at room temperature for 30 min to allow the reaction to occur. After the incubation period, the absorbance was measured at 517 nm using a Cytation 5 microplate reader. The DPPH radical scavenging activity was calculated for each concentration of the extract using the following formula:

$$\%\text{DPPH scavenging} = 100 \times \frac{A_{solvent} - A_{sample}}{A_{solvent}}$$

where the absorbance of the solvent is the absorbance of the DPPH solution without any extract, and the absorbance of the sample is the absorbance of the DPPH solution with the plant extract after incubation.

The DPPH scavenging activity for each concentration was expressed as a percentage. The concentration that resulted in the highest % DPPH scavenging activity was identified, and a dose–response curve was generated to visualize the antioxidant capacity of the extracts. All experiments were conducted in triplicate, and the results were presented as mean ± standard deviation (SD). To calculate IC_{50} for *S. tuberosum* and *Z. mays*, a cubic polynomial was fitted to DPPH inhibition data. The polynomial equations were derived using the least squares method to minimize error and ensure a smooth trend. IC_{50} was determined by solving the polynomial equation for the concentration corresponding to 50% DPPH inhibition using numerical root-finding methods. The fit's accuracy was validated by high R^2 values (0.995).

Trolox, a water-soluble vitamin E analog, was used as a reference antioxidant to validate the assay. A standard curve of Trolox was prepared in the range of 10 to 200 µM, and results for the extracts were compared to the standard to ensure the accuracy and reliability of the assay.

2.9. Antimicrobial Activity by Well Diffusion Agar

Antibacterial activity assessment was conducted using the agar-well diffusion method [31]. Five bacterial strains were selected for the antimicrobial evaluation of Gram-positives: *Staphylococcus aureus*, *Listeria monocytogenes*, and *Bacillus cereus*, and Gram-negatives: *Pseudomonas aeruginosa* and *Escherichia coli*. All bacterial strains were obtained from a standard microbial culture collection. The bacteria were cultured in Mueller–Hinton broth (MHB) and incubated overnight at 37 °C. The bacterial suspensions were adjusted to a concentration of 1×10^8 CFU/mL (corresponding to 0.5 McFarland standard) using sterile saline solution.

A mass of 100 mg of each microencapsulated powder was dissolved in 10 mL of sterile distilled water. The solutions were sonicated for 30 min at room temperature to ensure complete dissolution and then filtered through a 0.22 μm membrane filter to remove any particulate matter. The resulting filtrates were used as the stock solutions for the antimicrobial assay.

Mueller–Hinton agar (MHA) plates were prepared and inoculated with 100 μL of the bacterial suspension. Wells of 6 mm in diameter were punched into the agar, and 50 μL of each extract solution was dispensed into the wells. Gentamicin, a broad-spectrum antibiotic, was used as a positive control at a 500 μg/mL concentration.

Plates were incubated at 37 °C for 24 h. The diameters of the inhibition zones around each well were measured in millimeters. The measurements were taken at three different points around each well, and the average diameter was calculated. Sterile distilled water was used as a negative control to ensure that no contamination or intrinsic antibacterial activity was present in the solvents used for extract preparation. Gentamicin, a broad-spectrum antibiotic, was used as a positive control at a 500 μg/mL concentration. All experiments were conducted in triplicate to ensure reproducibility and reliability of these data. The results were expressed as the mean inhibition zone diameter (mm) ± standard deviation (SD) for each bacterial strain tested. Differences in inhibition zones between the extracts from *S. tuberosum* and *Z. mays* were analyzed to assess their relative efficacy against each bacterial strain.

2.10. Cell Culture

HeLa cells (ATCC® CCL-2™) were obtained from frozen (−196 °C) cells suspended in a freezing medium consisting of 90% fetal bovine serum (FBS) and 10% Dimethyl Sulfoxide (DMSO). Following thawing, cells were cultivated in a 75 cm^3 flask (Thermo Fisher Scientific, Waltham, MA, USA) containing Dulbecco's Modified Eagle Medium (DMEM Gibco™, Waltham, MA, USA) with 10% FBS, 1% L-glutamine, penicillin (10,000 U/mL), and streptomycin (10,000 μg/mL) at 37 °C, 5% CO_2, and humid atmosphere for 24 h.

2.11. MTT Assay

The number of living cells was determined using the MTT (3-(4,5-dimethylthiazol-2-yl)-2,5-diphenyl tetrazole bromide) metabolic reduction assay according to manufacturer's instructions (Thermo Fisher, Waltham, MA, USA).

Trypan Blue (TB) exclusion was used to assess the viability of the cells once confluence was greater than 80% (TB: Sigma-Aldrich 200-786-7). The cellular monolayer in DMEM (1%) was disaggregated using a sterile syringe. A volume of 30 μL of this cellular suspension reacted with 30 μL of TB. Viable cells (TB-negative) were visualized by an optical microscope (AmScope, Irvine, CA, USA) at a 40× magnification.

To determine the degree of proliferation and living cell proportion, Hela cells were seeded in 96-well plates at 10×10^3 cells/well and incubated at 37 °C and 5% CO_2 for 24 h to allow their adhesion. Afterward, cells were treated with microencapsulated anthocyanins at 267.05 mg/100 g and 168.5 mg/100 g concentrations (serial dilutions: 10^{-1} to 10^{-11} mg/mL) for 24 h, the medium was discarded, and 100 μL of MTT reagent in FBS and the phenol-free medium was added. After incubation for 4 h at 37 °C to allow the formazan formation, 100 μL of sodium dodecyl sulfate (1 mg/mL in 0.01 mol/L HCl) was added to dissolve the formazan crystals [32]. Plates were read using a Victor X3 spectrophotometer (Perkin Elmer, Waltham, MA, USA) at 570 nm. The IC_{50} values were obtained through no lineal regression analysis using GraphPad Prism 7.0 Software (GraphPad Software Inc., San Diego, CA, USA).

2.12. Determination of the Expression of Apoptosis-Associated Molecules

HeLa cells (ATCC®CCL-2™) were seeded on sterile coverslips and placed on six-well plates at a concentration of 50×10^4 cells/well in the conditioned medium at 37 °C and 5% CO_2 for 48 h to allow cell adhesion. The microencapsulated anthocyanins were then added to each well at the IC_{50} value determined from the MTT assay, and the plates were incubated for an additional 24 h. After washing three times (PBS), cells were fixed with a solution of 4% paraformaldehyde in PBS for 15 min. Permeabilization was carried out using 1 mL of permeability buffer (20 mM glycine, 0.5x Triton 100x) for 15 min.

Cells were incubated with primary antibodies against Bax (6A7), Bcl-2 (7), or caspase-8 (8CSP03) (Santa Cruz Biotechnology, Inc., USA) at a 1:500 dilution. The localization of Bax and Bcl-2 was determined using a fluorescein isothiocyanate (FITC)-conjugated secondary antibody (m-IgGκ BP-FITC, Santa Cruz Biotechnology, Inc., USA). IgG control was performed with mouse kappa conjugated to phycoerythrin (PE) (m-IgGκ BP-PE, Santa Cruz Biotechnology, Inc., USA). Cultures were incubated at 37 °C for 30 min in a humidified chamber. After washing with PBS, coverslips were mounted with Aqueous Mounting Medium (Santa Cruz Biotechnology, Inc., USA) and analyzed using a Leica DMi8 fluorescence microscope (Leica microsystems, Wetzlar, Hesse, Germany) at 630× magnification with GFP (500–550 nm), DAPI (358–461 nm), and Texas Red (595–615 nm) filters. Images were captured using the Leica Application Suite (LAS) X software version 5.2.0 (Leica Microsystems, Wetzlar, Germany). Fluorescence intensity was quantified by determining the ratio of total pixels to the pixels in areas considered positive.

2.13. Calculation of Apoptotic Index

The apoptotic index (AI) was calculated to assess the balance between pro-apoptotic and anti-apoptotic proteins [33,34] in HeLa cells treated with microencapsulated anthocyanins from *Z. mays* L. and *S. tuberosum* L. The expression levels of the pro-apoptotic markers Bax and Caspase-8, along with the anti-apoptotic marker Bcl-2, were quantified by counting the number of positive cells. The AI was calculated using the following formula:

$$AI = \frac{\text{Bax}(\text{mean positive cells}) + \text{Caspase} - 8(\text{mean positive cells})}{\text{Bcl} - 2(\text{mean positive cells})}$$

For both control and treated groups, the mean number of positive cells for Bax, Caspase-8, and Bcl-2 was obtained from multiple fields. Standard deviations were calculated using error propagation formulas to account for variability.

2.14. Statistical Analysis

All experiments were performed in triplicate at least three times. The results were expressed as mean ± standard deviation (SD). Differences between groups were detected using *t*-tests performed using GraphPad Prism software (version 7.04, GraphPad Software Inc., San Diego, CA, USA). Statistical significance was considered at $p < 0.05$.

3. Results and Discussion

3.1. Total Polyphenol Content (TPC) and Anthocyanin Content

The total polyphenol content (TPC) and anthocyanin content of the microencapsulated anthocyanins from *S. tuberosum* L. and *Z. mays* L. were evaluated. The results are summarized in Table 1.

Table 1. Polyphenol and anthocyanin content of *S. tuberosum* L. and *Z. mays* L.

Parameter	*S. tuberosum*	*Z. mays*
TPC (mg of gallic acid equivalents (GAE) per kg of fresh weight (fw))	554 * ± 25.16	494 * ± 24.03
Anthocyanin content (mg C3G/100 g)	71.40	63.5

TPC: Total polyphenols content. * The asterisk (*) indicates that the difference between samples is statistically significant ($p < 0.001$).

The TPC of the *S. tuberosum* extract was 554 ± 25.16 mg GAE/kg fresh weight, significantly higher ($p < 0.001$) compared to the *Z. mays* extract, which showed a TPC of

494 ± 24.03 mg GAE/kg fresh weight. These findings indicate that *S. tuberosum* has a greater total polyphenol content, suggesting a potentially higher antioxidant capacity. This finding aligns with the known variation in TPC across different potato cultivars and genotypes, which is influenced by factors such as genetic differences, environmental conditions, and the specific parts of the plant analyzed [35]. For example, studies on Slovak potato varieties have reported TPC values ranging from 795.05 mg/kg dry matter (DM) in the Victoria variety to 1238.42 mg/kg DM in the Laura variety, highlighting the significant influence of varietal differences and growing localities on TPC [36].

The anthocyanin content was also higher in *S. tuberosum* (71.40 mg C3G/100 g) compared to *Z. mays* (63.5 mg C3G/100 g). This result suggests that *S. tuberosum* is a richer source of anthocyanins, which may contribute to its superior antioxidant properties. Previous studies have demonstrated significant variation in anthocyanin content among different potato cultivars and related species, ranging from 2 to 40 mg/100 g of fresh weight in red-fleshed potatoes [37]. A study on Peruvian purple potatoes reported anthocyanin content as high as 75.71 mg/100 g under specific extraction conditions [38], which aligns closely with our findings for *S. tuberosum*. These variations are influenced by genetic factors, such as the presence of genes related to the flavonoid-anthocyanin biosynthetic pathway, including those at the D, P, and R loci, which govern anthocyanin accumulation [39].

3.2. Fourier Transform Infrared Spectroscopy (FTIR) Analysis

Fourier Transform Infrared (FTIR) spectroscopy was employed to analyze the structural changes in anthocyanins extracted from *Z. mays* L. and *S. tuberosum* L. in both non-microencapsulated and microencapsulated forms. The encapsulation was performed using maltodextrin as a matrix through spray drying. The FTIR spectra provide insights into the functional groups present and how they interact with the encapsulation matrix, helping to understand the effects of microencapsulation on the molecular structure of anthocyanins. A summary of the main results is shown in Table 2 for *Z. mays* and Table 3 for *S. tuberosum*. The FTIR spectra images for *Z. mays* and *S. tuberosum* are also included in Supplementary Figures S1 and S2, respectively.

Table 2. Summary of FTIR Comparative Visual Analysis of *Z. mays* L. Comparative visual analysis of FTIR spectra of non-microencapsulated and microencapsulated anthocyanins from *Z. mays* L.

Wavenumber (cm^{-1})	Functional Group	Non-Microencapsulated (Qualitative Intensity)	Microencapsulated (Qualitative Intensity)
3200–3600	O-H stretching (hydroxyl)	High	Medium
2800–3000	C-H stretching (alkanes)	Medium	Low
1700–1750	C=O stretching (carbonyl)	High	Low
1500–1600	C=C stretching (aromatic rings)	Medium	Low
1000–1300	C-O, C-O-C stretching (ethers, glycosidic bonds)	Medium	Low
1027	C-O-C stretching (polysaccharides, matrix interactions)	-	Medium
840–760	New peaks (maltodextrin matrix vibrations)	-	Medium

Table 3. Summary of FTIR Comparative Visual Analysis of *S. tuberosum* L. Comparative visual analysis of FTIR spectra of non-microencapsulated and microencapsulated anthocyanins from *S. tuberosum* L.

Wavenumber (cm^{-1})	Functional Group	Non-Microencapsulated (Qualitative Intensity)	Microencapsulated (Qualitative Intensity)
3200–3600	O-H stretching (hydroxyl)	High	Medium
2800–3000	C-H stretching (alkanes)	Low	Medium
1700–1750	C=O stretching (carbonyl)	High	Low
1500–1600	C=C stretching (aromatic rings)	Medium	Low
1000–1300	C-O, C-O-C stretching (ethers, glycosidic bonds)	Medium	Low
1027	C-O-C stretching (polysaccharides, matrix interactions)	-	Medium
840–760	New peaks (maltodextrin matrix vibrations)	-	Medium

3.2.1. O-H Stretching (3200–3600 cm^{-1})

The O-H stretching region is critical for understanding the presence of hydroxyl groups, which are abundant in anthocyanins. In both *Z. mays* L. and *S. tuberosum* L., the non-microencapsulated anthocyanins exhibited a high-intensity peak in this region (Tables 2 and 3), indicating free hydroxyl groups. Upon microencapsulation, this intensity reduced to a medium level, suggesting that the hydroxyl groups are involved in hydrogen bonding with the maltodextrin matrix. This result supports the hypothesis that microencapsulation leads to the shielding of functional groups, reducing their availability for interaction. The similar reduction in intensity for both species indicates that the maltodextrin matrix interacts similarly with the anthocyanins' hydroxyl groups, limiting their free vibration.

3.2.2. C-H Stretching (2800–3000 cm^{-1})

C-H stretching, representative of aliphatic bonds in anthocyanins, showed varying behavior between the two species. In *Z. mays* L., both the non-microencapsulated and microencapsulated forms exhibited medium intensity (Table 2), indicating that microencapsulation had minimal impact on the availability of aliphatic C-H bonds; however, in *S. tuberosum* L., the non-microencapsulated form displayed a low intensity, which increased to a medium level after microencapsulation (Table 3). This increase may suggest that microencapsulation alters the conformation of anthocyanins in *S. tuberosum* L., possibly due to a reorganization of aliphatic groups during the encapsulation process.

3.2.3. C=O Stretching (1700–1750 cm^{-1})

The carbonyl group (C=O) is crucial for the stability of anthocyanins, and FTIR data revealed notable differences before and after encapsulation. In both species, the non-microencapsulated anthocyanins exhibited high intensity in the C=O stretching region (Tables 2 and 3), confirming the presence of carbonyl groups typical of anthocyanins; however, upon encapsulation, the intensity dropped to a low level. This result suggests that the carbonyl groups are involved in strong interactions with the maltodextrin matrix, likely through hydrogen bonding or dipole-dipole interactions, which effectively shield the carbonyl groups from detection in the FTIR spectrum.

3.2.4. C=C Stretching (1500–1600 cm^{-1})

The C=C stretching region, associated with aromatic rings, showed medium intensity in the non-microencapsulated forms of both species (Tables 2 and 3); however, the intensity dropped to a low level after microencapsulation. This change indicates that the encapsulation process affects the vibration of aromatic rings in the anthocyanins, likely due to the protective effects of maltodextrin, which limits their free movement.

3.2.5. C-O and C-O-C Stretching (1000–1300 cm^{-1})

In both species, the C-O and C-O-C stretching regions, corresponding to glycosidic bonds, exhibited medium intensity in the non-microencapsulated anthocyanins (Tables 2 and 3). After encapsulation, the intensity was reduced to a low level, reflecting the interaction of anthocyanins' glycosidic bonds with the maltodextrin matrix. The reduced intensity indicates that encapsulation decreases the exposure of these bonds to the environment, which could be beneficial in protecting anthocyanins from degradation.

New peaks observed in the 840–760 cm^{-1} region in both microencapsulated forms (Tables 2 and 3) are attributable to maltodextrin matrix vibrations. The absence of these peaks in the non-microencapsulated forms confirms the presence of the matrix and its encapsulating role. These peaks demonstrate the successful encapsulation of anthocyanins within the maltodextrin matrix.

Overall, the FTIR spectra reveal that microencapsulation using maltodextrin significantly alters the molecular environment of anthocyanins in both *Z. mays* L. and *S. tuberosum* L. The reduced intensity of key functional groups such as O-H, C=O, and C=C stretching after encapsulation suggests strong interactions with the matrix, providing protection to the anthocyanins. The instability of anthocyanins has long been recognized as a major limitation for their use in food and pharmaceutical industries, as factors such as pH, temperature, and light can rapidly degrade their structure, reducing their bioactivity. In this study, microencapsulation with maltodextrin was employed as an innovative approach to mitigate these challenges. The FTIR analysis confirmed the successful interaction of anthocyanins with the encapsulation matrix, providing a protective barrier against environmental stressors. Furthermore, the enhanced antioxidant activity observed in the microencapsulated anthocyanins supports the hypothesis that encapsulation not only preserves their stability but also optimizes their functional potential.

In addition to spray-drying microencapsulation with maltodextrin, other methods have been explored to enhance the stability of anthocyanins, each with unique advantages and disadvantages. Encapsulation using liposomes offers excellent protection because of their bilayer structure, which can shield anthocyanins from environmental factors; however, the high cost and complexity of liposome preparation limit their scalability for industrial applications [40,41]. Another approach involves the use of protein-based carriers, such as casein or gelatin, which provide a natural and biocompatible matrix for anthocyanin stabilization. While effective, protein-based methods often face challenges related to allergenicity and sensitivity to temperature and pH during processing [41]. Freeze-drying, another common technique, can preserve anthocyanin stability well, but its high energy demand and long processing time make it less cost-effective compared to spray-drying [42].

Spray-drying with maltodextrin, as utilized in this study, offers a balance of cost-efficiency, scalability, and protection. The interaction between maltodextrin and anthocyanins, as evidenced by FTIR analysis, suggests that this method provides robust encapsulation while maintaining bioactivity. Nevertheless, it is worth noting that spray-drying microencapsulation may result in particle size heterogeneity, as observed in *S. tuberosum*. By addressing these comparative aspects, our study demonstrates the practicality of spray-drying microencapsulation as a viable method for enhancing anthocyanin stability in functional food and nutraceutical applications.

3.3. Morphological Analysis by Scanning Electron Microscope (SEM)

Scanning electron microscopy (SEM) was utilized to assess the morphology and surface characteristics of microencapsulated anthocyanins from *S. tuberosum* L. (*S. tuberosum*) and *Z. mays* L. (*Z. mays*), both encapsulated using maltodextrin via spray drying. Distinct differences in particle morphology were observed between the two samples.

For *S. tuberosum*, the SEM image (Figure 1) reveals a heterogeneous mixture of spherical and irregularly shaped particles, with significant variation in particle size. Larger particles are clearly visible alongside smaller, irregular fragments, and the presence of agglomerates suggests potential challenges in the spray drying process, such as inconsistent atomization or uneven drying conditions. While the particle surfaces appear generally smooth, occasional unevenness further indicates variability in the encapsulation process.

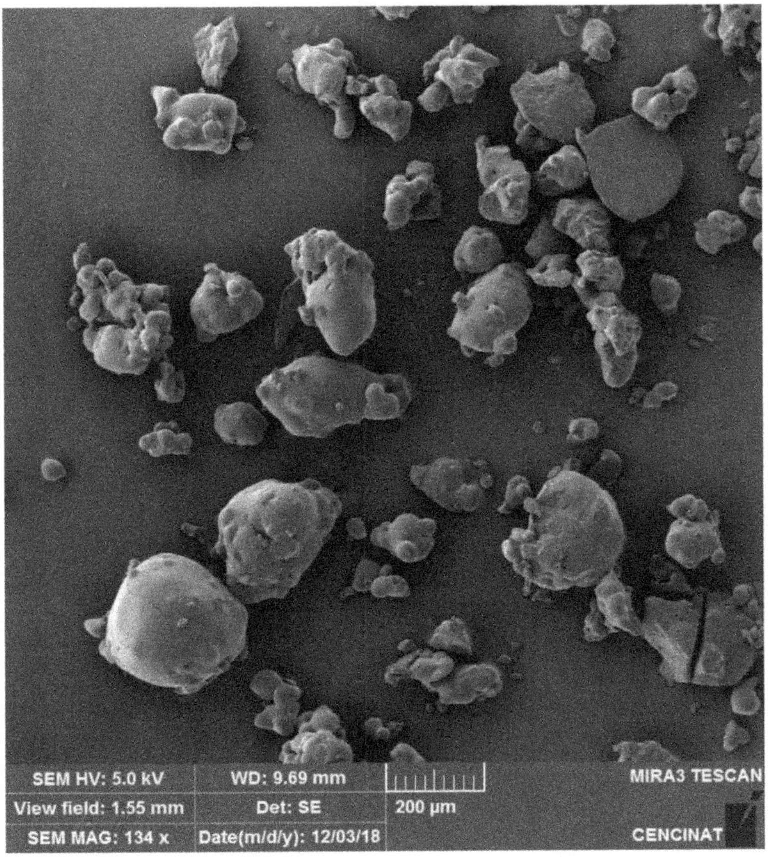

Figure 1. SEM image of *S. tuberosum* L. microencapsulated particles prepared by spray drying, captured with a TESCAN MIRA 3 SEM at 134× magnification and a 200 μm scale bar.

In contrast, the SEM analysis of *Z. mays* (Figure 2) shows a more uniform morphology, still, some degree of agglomeration and clustering is still present. The particle surfaces of *Z. mays* appear more textured than those of *S. tuberosum*, possibly because of differences in drying temperature or the interaction between anthocyanins and the encapsulating matrix. Nevertheless, the overall morphology suggests a more controlled encapsulation process, making *Z. mays* better suited for applications requiring fine particle dispersibility and rapid dissolution [43].

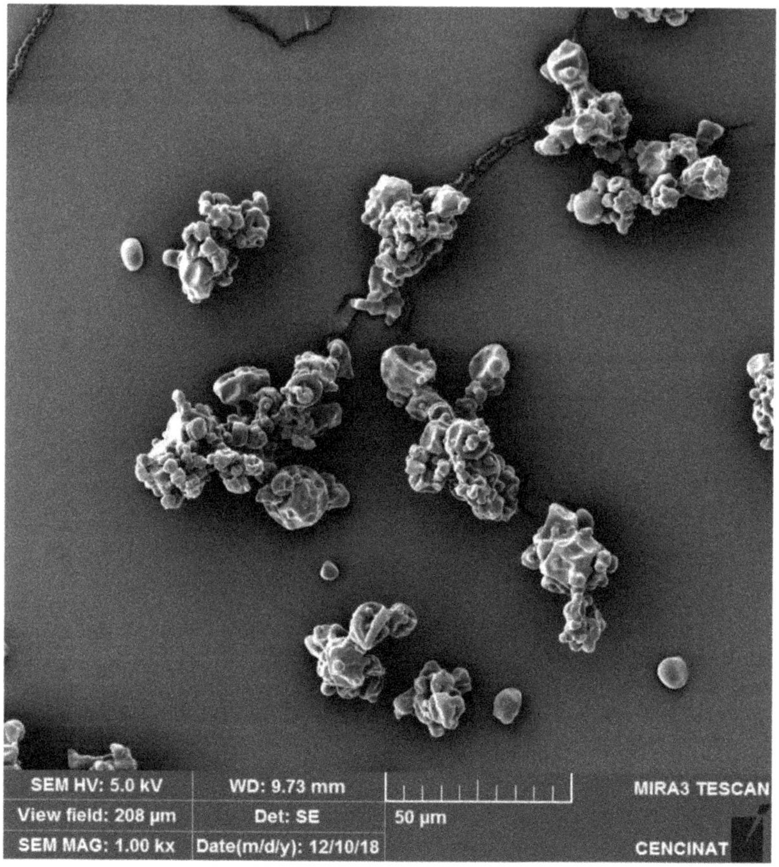

Figure 2. SEM image of *Z. mays* L. microencapsulated particles prepared by spray drying, captured with a TESCAN MIRA 3 SEM at 1000× magnification and a 50 μm scale bar.

Particle size distribution (PSD) analysis underscores the differences between the two samples and offers valuable information for potential applications. The PSD of *S. tuberosum* (Figure 3) shows a broad distribution, with the most frequent particle size ranging between 80 and 100 μm. The mean particle size is approximately 100–150 μm, with 80% of particles smaller than 200 μm; however, the presence of particles larger than 500 μm indicates variability in the spray drying process. These larger particles suggest that *S. tuberosum* anthocyanins could be ideal for applications requiring controlled or sustained release, such as in food formulations where prolonged release of active compounds is advantageous [44]. This size distribution may also be advantageous in nutraceutical products, where larger particles provide stability and support a sustained release mechanism [45].

On the other hand, the PSD of *Z. mays* (Figure 4) shows a much finer distribution, with the majority of particles ranging between 1 and 2 μm. Approximately 80% of the particles are smaller than 3 μm, making *Z. mays* suitable for applications requiring rapid dissolution or quick dispersion. The fine particle distribution enhances the surface area-to-volume ratio, facilitating faster release of encapsulated anthocyanins. This property makes *Z. mays* particularly valuable in functional beverages, pharmaceuticals, or cosmetics, where immediate bioavailability is essential [46].

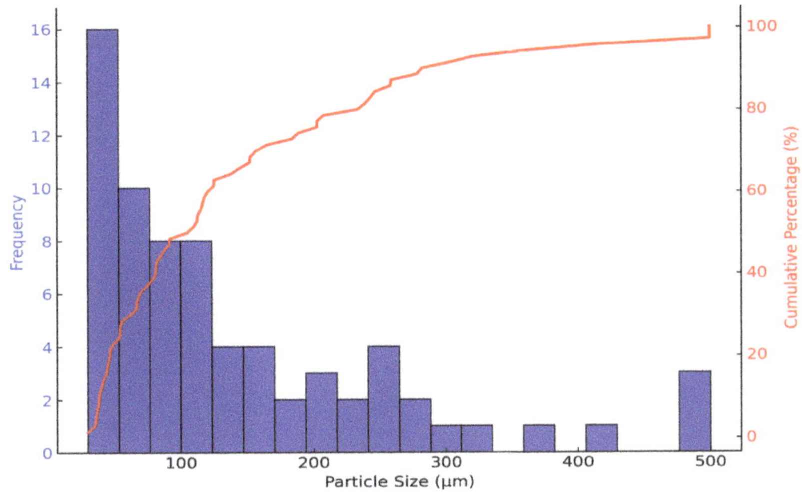

Figure 3. Particle size distribution analysis of *S. tuberosum* L. microencapsulated spheres. Particle size distribution and cumulative distribution curve of *S. tuberosum* L microencapsulated spheres, measured using FIJI software (version 2.9.0).

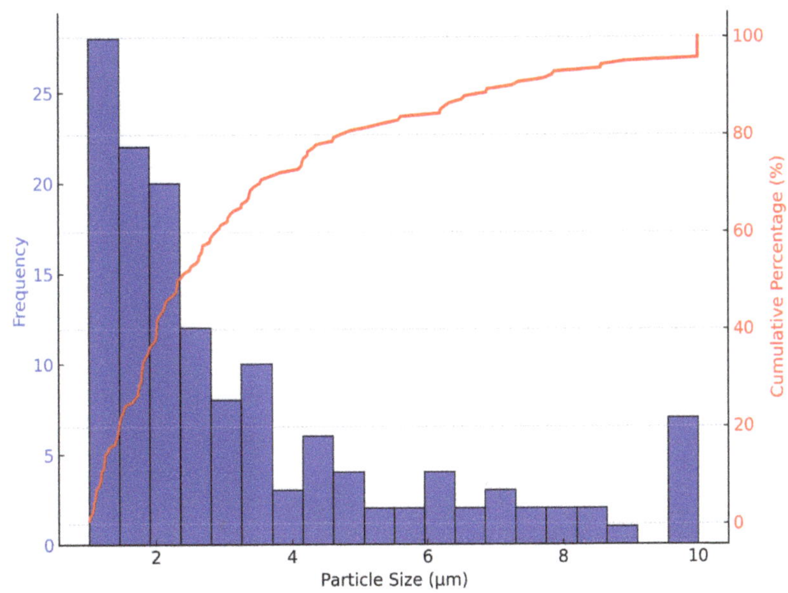

Figure 4. Particle size distribution analysis of *Z. mays* L. microencapsulated spheres. Particle size distribution and cumulative distribution curve of *Z. mays* microencapsulated spheres were measured using FIJI software (version 2.9.0).

The significant differences in particle size and morphology between the microencapsulated anthocyanins from *S. tuberosum* and *Z. mays* have direct implications for their respective applications. In food and nutraceutical formulations, particle size and morphology not only influence the release kinetics of the active compounds but also their stability and interactions with other formulation components [47].

The larger, more heterogeneous particles observed in *S. tuberosum* (Figures 1 and 3) suggest that this sample is better suited for applications requiring sustained or controlled release. Functional snacks, powdered supplements, or nutraceutical capsules could benefit from the slower dissolution rates associated with larger particles, offering prolonged antioxidant activity or extended color stability potentially enhancing shelf life [48].

In contrast, the finer particle size distribution observed in *Z. mays* (Figures 2 and 4) makes it ideal for applications requiring rapid dissolution. Functional beverages, instant powders, and pharmaceutical formulations would benefit from the quick release of active anthocyanins, enhancing bioavailability and providing immediate physiological effects. Additionally, the smaller particle size of *Z. mays* anthocyanins improves sensory qualities in food products, contributing to smoother textures and more uniform color dispersion, which are critical in beverages, dairy products, and cosmetics [49].

These morphological differences underscore the importance of optimizing spray drying parameters to tailor encapsulated anthocyanins for specific applications. For *S. tuberosum*, minimizing agglomeration and achieving a narrower particle size distribution could enhance its performance in applications requiring more uniform release. For *Z. mays*, the relatively fine and uniform particles suggest an optimized spray drying process, though further refinement could reduce agglomeration and improve particle stability [50].

3.4. DPPH Radical Scavenging Activity

The antioxidant activity of microencapsulated anthocyanins from *Z. mays* and *S. tuberosum* was assessed using the 2,2-diphenyl-1-picrylhydrazyl (DPPH) radical scavenging assay, with results expressed as % DPPH inhibition. While both extracts demonstrated notable antioxidant activity, significant differences in their efficacy were evident.

As shown in Figure 5 and Table S1, anthocyanins from *S. tuberosum* exhibited superior antioxidant potential, achieving a maximum DPPH inhibition of 65% at 500 µg/mL, compared to 52% for *Z. mays* at the same concentration. The steeper slope of the dose–response curve for *S. tuberosum* reflects more efficient free radical scavenging activity, whereas *Z. mays* displayed a more gradual increase in % DPPH inhibition.

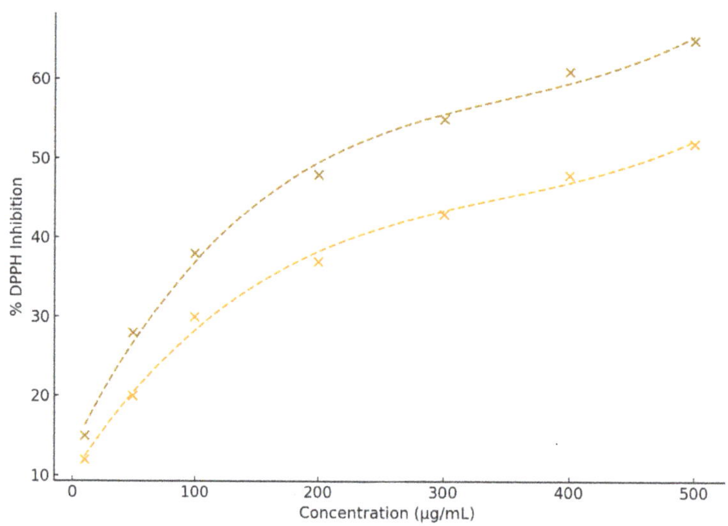

Figure 5. Antioxidant activity (% DPPH inhibition) of microencapsulated anthocyanins from *S. tuberosum* L. and *Z. mays* L. The plot illustrates the relationship between anthocyanin concentration and % DPPH inhibition. Data points represent the mean % DPPH inhibition, with *S. tuberosum* depicted as dark goldenrod cross and *Z. mays* as orange cross. Cubic polynomial fits (dashed lines).

The calculated IC_{50} values further support these observations, with *S. tuberosum* reaching 50% DPPH inhibition at 205.84 µg/mL, significantly lower than the 463.62 µg/mL required for *Z. mays*. Cubic polynomial fitting (R^2 = 0.995) provided an accurate representation of these trends. These findings align with previous research, which highlights the superior radical scavenging efficiency of cyanidin-based anthocyanins, predominant in *S. tuberosum*, compared to other anthocyanin types [51,52]. This emphasizes the potential of *S. tuberosum* as a valuable natural source of antioxidants.

3.5. Antimicrobial Activity

The antimicrobial activity of microencapsulated anthocyanins extracted from *S. tuberosum* L. and *Z. mays* L. was evaluated using a well-based diffusion assay against five bacterial strains: *Staphylococcus aureus* subsp. *aureus* Rosenbach ATCC 25923, *Listeria monocytogenes* ATCC 19115, *Pseudomonas aeruginosa* ATCC 10145, *Bacillus cereus* ATCC 10876, and *Escherichia coli* ATCC 25922. The results, expressed as the inhibition zone diameter in millimeters (mm), are summarized in Figure 6 (*S. tuberosum* L.) and Figure 7 (*Z. mays* L.).

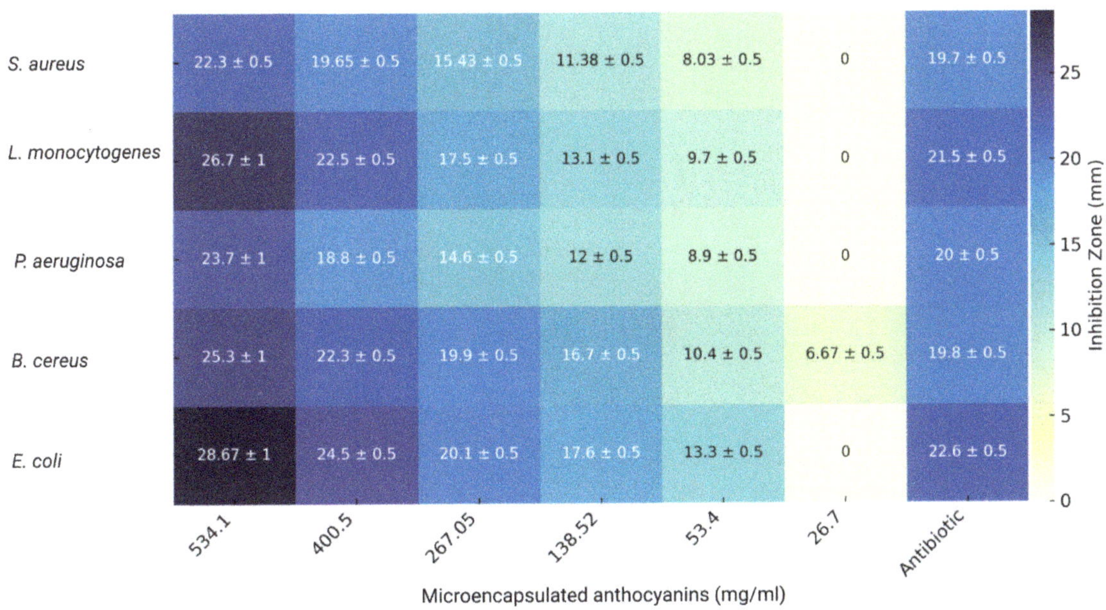

Figure 6. Antimicrobial activity of microencapsulated *S. tuberosum* anthocyanin extract against different bacterial strains. Heatmap showing the inhibition zones (in mm) with standard deviations for *S. aureus*, *L. monocytogenes*, *P. aeruginosa*, *B. cereus*, and *E. coli* at various concentrations (534.1 to 26.7 mg/mL) of the microencapsulated *S. tuberosum* extract. Antibiotic (gentamicin) was used at the standard concentration.

The Minimum Inhibitory Concentration (MIC) was determined based on the lowest concentration of the extract that completely inhibited bacterial growth. Gentamicin served as the control antibiotic. The results showed that both extracts had notable antimicrobial properties, though their efficacy varied by bacterial strain and extract concentration.

The antimicrobial activity of microencapsulated anthocyanin extracts from *S. tuberosum* was tested at concentrations ranging from 26.7 mg/mL to 534.1 mg/mL (Figure 6). The extract exhibited strong inhibitory effects, especially against *B. cereus*, which showed an inhibition zone of 25.3 ± 1 mm at 534.1 mg/mL. *E. coli* also displayed a notable inhibition zone of 28.67 ± 1 mm, indicating that the *S. tuberosum* anthocyanin extract was highly effective against this Gram-negative bacterium; however, *P. aeruginosa* exhibited a smaller inhibition zone of 23.7 ± 1 mm under the same concentration, indicating moderate susceptibility.

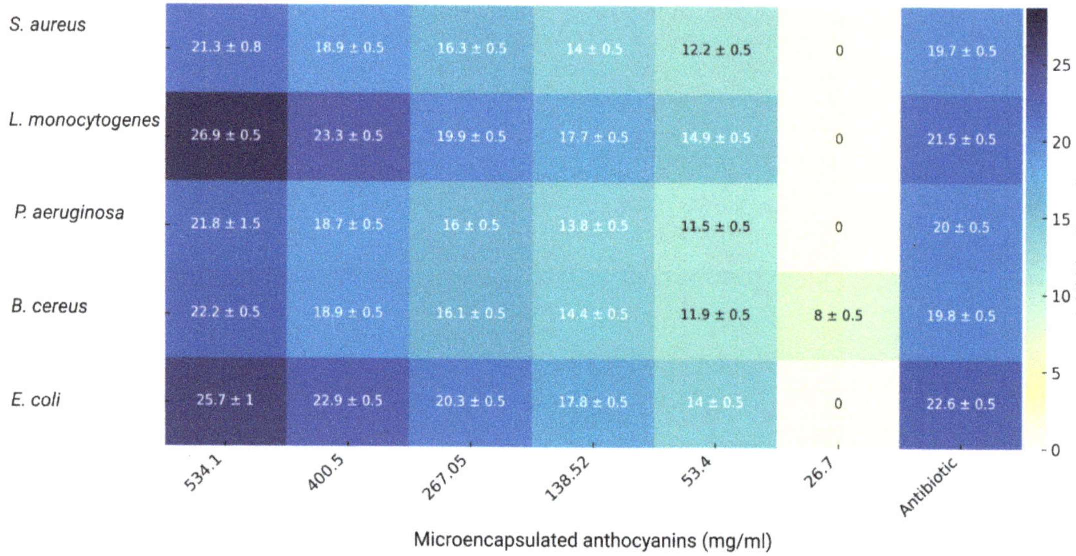

Figure 7. Antimicrobial activity of microencapsulated *Z. mays* anthocyanin extracts against different bacterial strains. Heatmap showing the inhibition zones (in mm) with standard deviations for *S. aureus*, *L. monocytogenes*, *P. aeruginosa*, *B. cereus*, and *E. coli* at various concentrations (534.1 to 26.7 mg/mL) of the microencapsulated *S. tuberosum* extract. Antibiotic (gentamicin) was used at the standard concentration.

At lower concentrations, the antimicrobial efficacy of the *S. tuberosum* extract decreased considerably. For example, at 138.52 mg/mL, inhibition zones were significantly smaller, with *S. aureus* showing an inhibition zone of 11.38 ± 0.5 mm and *P. aeruginosa* at 12.0 ± 0.5 mm. At the lowest concentration of 26.7 mg/mL, no inhibition zones were observed for most bacterial strains, indicating that higher concentrations are necessary for effective bacterial inhibition. These findings suggest that the microencapsulation of *S. tuberosum* anthocyanins enhances their stability, allowing for sustained antimicrobial activity, but higher doses are critical for optimal efficacy, which is consistent with previous research [53,54].

The antimicrobial activity of the *Z. mays* extract was assessed across various bacterial strains (Figure 7). Similar to *S. tuberosum*, the microencapsulated anthocyanins from *Z. mays* demonstrated broad-spectrum inhibitory effects. *L. monocytogenes* exhibited an inhibition zone of 26.7 ± 1 mm at 534.1 mg/mL, indicating high susceptibility, while *B. cereus* showed an inhibition zone of 25.7 ± 1 mm at the same concentration. These findings align with previous research highlighting the efficacy of anthocyanins, particularly against Gram-positive bacteria such as *B. cereus* and *L. monocytogenes* [4,55].

As with *S. tuberosum*, lower concentrations of *Z. mays* extract resulted in reduced antimicrobial activity. At 138.52 mg/mL, the inhibition zone for *B. cereus* decreased to 16.7 ± 0.5 mm, while for *P. aeruginosa*, it was recorded at 12.0 ± 0.5 mm. At the lowest concentration of 26.7 mg/mL, no inhibition was observed for *S. aureus*, *L. monocytogenes*, or *P. aeruginosa*. Gentamicin, used as the antibiotic control, produced higher inhibition zones at lower concentrations. For instance, it showed an inhibition zone of 19.7 ± 0.5 mm against *S. aureus* and 22.6 ± 0.5 mm against *E. coli*. While the anthocyanin extracts were effective, gentamicin proved more potent at lower concentrations.

To quantify the antimicrobial potency of the microencapsulated extracts, MIC values were determined from these disk diffusion data by identifying the lowest concentration of the extract that completely inhibited bacterial growth (Table 4). The MIC values revealed that both *Z. mays* and *S. tuberosum* extracts had similar minimal inhibitory concentrations for most bacterial strains. The MIC for *S. aureus* and *L. monocytogenes* was 53.4 mg/mL for both extracts, while *B. cereus* had a lower MIC of 26.7 mg/mL for both extracts, indicating a higher susceptibility to anthocyanins.

Table 4. MIC of Microencapsulated anthocyanin extracts.

Bacterial Strain	MIC (mg/mL)	
	S. tuberosum	*Z. mays*
S. aureus	53.4	53.4
L. monocytogenes	53.4	53.4
P. aeruginosa	53.4	53.4
B. cereus	26.7	26.7
E. coli	53.4	53.4

MIC data confirmed that Gram-positive bacteria, such as *B. cereus* and *L. monocytogenes*, were generally more susceptible to anthocyanin extracts than Gram-negative bacteria [56], such as *P. aeruginosa*. This trend aligns with the inhibition zone results and the existing literature, which suggests that the simpler cell wall structure of Gram-positive bacteria makes them more vulnerable to phenolic compounds such as anthocyanins [57,58]. In contrast, the outer membrane of Gram-negative bacteria tends to present greater resistance to damage caused by these molecules.

The results from this study indicate that microencapsulated anthocyanin extracts from both *S. tuberosum* and *Z. mays* exhibit significant antimicrobial activity against a range of bacterial strains in agreement with prior research [59].

Future studies should focus on improving the antimicrobial efficacy of anthocyanin extracts by developing synergistic formulations or optimizing their delivery mechanisms. Additionally, exploring the mode of action of these extracts on bacterial cell walls could provide valuable insights into how anthocyanins can be made more effective. Given the global concern over antibiotic resistance, plant-based antimicrobials such as anthocyanins represent a promising avenue for addressing this pressing issue.

3.6. Cytotoxic Activity and Induction of Apoptosis

The cytotoxic effects of microencapsulated anthocyanin extracts from *Z. mays* L. and *S. tuberosum* L. on HeLa cells were evaluated using the MTT assay. Serial dilutions, ranging from 0.1 mg/mL to 1×10^{-11} mg/mL, were applied to the cells for 24 h, after which cell viability was measured spectrophotometrically. Dose–response curves were generated, and IC_{50} values were determined for both extracts, as shown in Figure 8 (Dose–response curves of the cytotoxic effects of *Z. mays* and *S. tuberosum* microencapsulated anthocyanin extracts on HeLa cells).

For *Z. mays*, the dose–response curve showed a gradual decrease in cell viability with increasing concentration. At lower concentrations (0.0039–0.0625 mg/mL), cell viability remained near 100%, but at 0.125 mg/mL, a reduction to 90% was observed. Further increases in concentration led to more marked reductions, with 60% viability at 0.25 mg/mL, 20% at 0.5 mg/mL, and complete cell death at 1 mg/mL. The IC_{50} value for *Z. mays* was calculated at 0.275 mg/mL (95% confidence interval: 0.227–0.322 mg/mL), with a slope (k) of -7.32, indicating a gradual decline in viability across the concentration range.

In contrast, *S. tuberosum* exhibited a much steeper decline in viability. At lower concentrations (1×10^{-11}–1×10^{-7} mg/mL), viability remained above 90%, but a sharp drop occurred at 1×10^{-5} mg/mL, reducing viability to 85%. This steep decline continued, with 60% viability at 1×10^{-4} mg/mL and 10% at 1×10^{-3} mg/mL, leading to 0% viability at 1×10^{-2} mg/mL. The IC_{50} value for *S. tuberosum* was significantly lower, at 0.070 mg/mL

(95% CI: 0.061–0.079 mg/mL), with a much steeper slope of −41.83. These results indicate a concentration-dependent cytotoxic effect for both extracts, with *S. tuberosum* showing greater potency at lower concentrations compared to *Z. mays* (Figure 8).

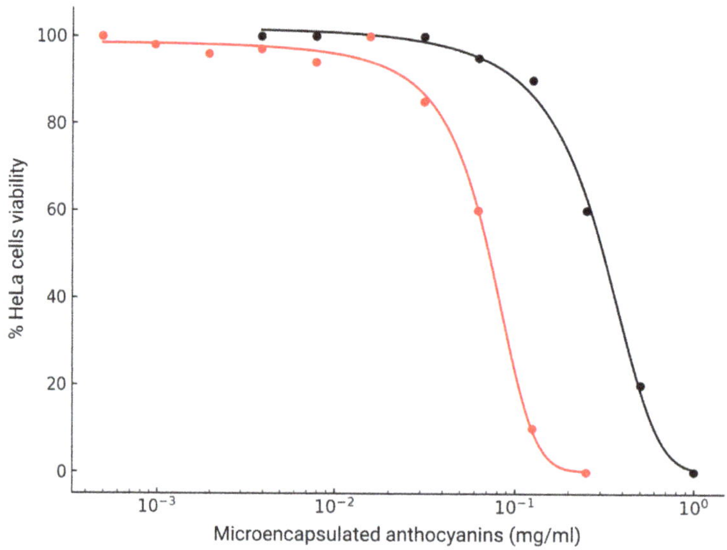

Figure 8. Dose–response curves of the cytotoxic effects of *Z. mays* and *S. tuberosum* L. The *X*-axis (log scale) represents the concentration of anthocyanin extract in mg/mL, while the *Y*-axis shows the percentage of viable cells. Data points for *Z. mays* are depicted as black circles, with the fitted sigmoid curve shown as a solid black line. Red circles denote data points for *S. tuberosum*, with the corresponding fitted curve represented by a red line.

The comparison of IC_{50} values highlights the greater potency of *S. tuberosum*, which achieved similar cytotoxic effects at significantly lower concentrations than *Z. mays*. The IC_{50} for *S. tuberosum* (0.070 mg/mL) was markedly lower than that of *Z. mays* (0.275 mg/mL). The increased potency observed in *S. tuberosum* L. may be attributable to its higher total polyphenol content (TPC) and elevated anthocyanin levels (Table 1). The greater cytotoxicity exhibited by *S. tuberosum* in HeLa cells, as indicated by its lower IC_{50} value, is likely a direct result of its enriched polyphenol and anthocyanin concentrations. These compounds are well-established for their cytotoxic properties across various cancer cell lines, including HeLa cells [60–63], and their presence reinforces the potential of *S. tuberosum* as a potent source of bioactive molecules for cancer therapy.

Further differences were apparent in the slopes of the dose–response curves, with *Z. mays* exhibiting a slope of −7.32 and *S. tuberosum* showing a much steeper slope of −41.83. The steeper slope for *S. tuberosum* reflects a more rapid and pronounced reduction in cell viability over a narrow concentration range, suggesting a highly efficacious cytotoxic mechanism. This sharper response could be attributable to the higher total polyphenol content (TPC) and anthocyanin levels in *S. tuberosum*, which are likely driving more potent bioactive effects (Table 1). The steep slope associated with *S. tuberosum* suggests a sharp therapeutic window, where small variations in concentration around the IC_{50} could lead to substantial biological effects.

The differences in potency and slope between the two extracts may be attributable to their distinct anthocyanin compositions. *Z. mays* is known to be rich in cyanidin-based anthocyanins, which have shown moderate cytotoxicity in various cancer models. In contrast, *S. tuberosum* may contain delphinidin or petunidin derivatives, which could account for its stronger cytotoxic effects [61]. Differences in anthocyanin structure, including glycosylation and acylation, play a critical role in determining their bioactivity [64].

Additionally, the observed differences in cytotoxicity may stem from factors such as solubility, stability, and bioavailability of the anthocyanins in each extract. Anthocyanins are sensitive to environmental factors such as pH and temperature [65,66], which can affect their stability and efficacy. It is possible that *S. tuberosum* anthocyanins are more stable or more readily absorbed by cells, leading to their more potent cytotoxic effects. Conversely, *Z. mays* anthocyanins may degrade more rapidly, resulting in a slower and less pronounced reduction in cell viability.

To investigate whether apoptosis was the primary mechanism behind the cytotoxic effects observed with both microencapsulated anthocyanins, the apoptotic index (AI) was analyzed by measuring the expression of pro-apoptotic markers Bax and Caspase-8 relative to the anti-apoptotic marker Bcl-2. The AI provided a measure of the balance between cell death promotion and inhibition (Table S2). For *Z. mays* L., the control group showed an AI of 2.32 (±1.02), while treatment with the microencapsulated anthocyanins resulted in a slightly higher AI of 2.47 (±0.95). Although this increase indicates a modest rise in pro-apoptotic activity, the marginal difference, and overlapping standard deviations suggest that apoptosis is not the primary mechanism underlying the cytotoxic effects of *Z. mays* L. anthocyanins. While apoptosis likely contributes, these data imply that *Z. mays* L.'s cytotoxicity results from the interplay of multiple pathways.

Treatment with *S. tuberosum* L. anthocyanins increased the AI to 2.60 (±0.90), suggesting a stronger apoptotic response compared to *Z. mays* L. Nonetheless, the cytotoxic effects observed in previous studies likely involve additional mechanisms beyond apoptosis. The relatively high standard deviations in AI, coupled with the pronounced reduction in cell viability (Table S2), point to other processes—such as oxidative stress or mitochondrial dysfunction—as critical contributors to *S. tuberosum* L. anti-tumor effects.

These findings indicate that while both *Z. mays* L. and *S. tuberosum* L. anthocyanin extracts induce apoptosis in HeLa cells, apoptosis is unlikely to be the sole driver of their cytotoxic effects. Anthocyanins exhibit a range of biological activities that contribute to their antitumoral effects, including inhibition of cell proliferation, suppression of angiogenesis, and modulation of signaling pathways. These multifaceted actions suggest that while apoptosis is a significant mechanism, it is not the major pathway through which anthocyanins exert their anticancer effects [67,68].

Further investigation into the molecular pathways affected by these anthocyanin extracts is warranted to elucidate their cytotoxic mechanisms fully. Exploring the interplay between apoptosis and other processes—such as autophagy, necrosis, or cell cycle disruption—will be crucial in optimizing anthocyanin-based therapeutic strategies for cancer treatment.

4. Conclusions

This study provides comprehensive insights into the biological potential of microencapsulated anthocyanins derived from *S. tuberosum* and *Z. mays*, emphasizing their relevance as sources of bioactive compounds with therapeutic and functional food applications. The superior antioxidant activity of *S. tuberosum*, coupled with its strong cytotoxic effects against HepG2 and THJ29T cancer cell lines, highlights its promise as a natural therapeutic agent for oxidative stress-related diseases and cancer. On the other hand, *Z. mays* demonstrated notable antimicrobial activity against clinically relevant multidrug-resistant bacterial strains and biofilm-forming pathogens, addressing critical global health challenges such as antimicrobial resistance. The use of microencapsulation significantly improved the stability and bioavailability of anthocyanins, as evidenced by FTIR and SEM analyses, providing a robust platform for enhancing their functional properties. These findings reinforce the value of ancestral Andean edible plants as untapped reservoirs of bioactive molecules, paving the way for their integration into modern nutraceuticals and pharmaceutical formulations. Future studies should prioritize in vivo validations, detailed mechanistic investigations, and the development of optimized formulations to maximize their therapeutic potential and applicability in diverse fields, including healthcare and food sciences.

Supplementary Materials: The following supporting information can be downloaded at: https://www.mdpi.com/article/10.3390/nu16234078/s1, Figure S1: FTIR Spectral Curves of Anthocyanins from *Solanum tuberosum* L.; Figure S2: FTIR Spectral Curves of Anthocyanins from *Zea mays* L.; Table S1. Antioxidant activity of the microencapsulated anthocyanins from *Zea mays* L.; Table S2. Apoptosis index (AI) of HeLa cells treated with microencapsulated anthocyanins of *Zea mays* L. and *S. tuberosum* L.

Author Contributions: Conceptualization, C.B.-O. and L.P.G.; methodology, C.B.-O., Y.C., J.G.-B., O.L., C.A. and L.P.G.; formal analysis, C.B.-O., Y.C., J.G.-B., O.L., C.A., A.D. and L.P.G.; investigation, C.B.-O., Y.C., J.G.-B., O.L., C.A., A.D. and L.P.G.; writing—original draft preparation, C.B.-O., Y.C., J.G.-B., O.L., C.A., A.D. and L.P.G.; writing—review and editing, C.B.-O., Y.C., J.G.-B., O.L., C.A., A.D. and L.P.G.; supervision, C.B.-O. and L.P.G.; project administration, C.B.-O. and L.P.G.; funding acquisition, C.B.-O. and L.P.G. All authors have read and agreed to the published version of the manuscript.

Funding: This research received no external funding.

Institutional Review Board Statement: Not applicable.

Informed Consent Statement: Not applicable.

Data Availability Statement: The original contributions presented in the study are included in the article/Supplementary Materials, further inquiries can be directed to the corresponding author.

Conflicts of Interest: The authors declare no conflicts of interest.

References

1. Marchini, S.; D'Incalci, M.; Broggini, M. New molecules and strategies in the field of anticancer agents. *Curr. Med. Chem. Anticancer. Agents* **2004**, *4*, 247–262. [CrossRef] [PubMed]
2. Gonçalves, A.C.; Nunes, A.R.; Falcão, A.; Alves, G.; Silva, L.R. Dietary effects of anthocyanins in human health: A comprehensive review. *Pharmaceuticals* **2021**, *14*, 690. [CrossRef] [PubMed]
3. Liu, J.; Zhou, H.; Song, L.; Yang, Z.; Qiu, M.; Wang, J.; Shi, S. Anthocyanins: Promising Natural Products with Diverse Pharmacological Activities. *Molecules* **2021**, *26*, 3807. [CrossRef] [PubMed]
4. Barba-Ostria, C.; Carrera-Pacheco, S.E.; Gonzalez-Pastor, R.; Zuñiga, J.; Mayorga-Ramos, A.; Tejera, E.; Guamán, L. Exploring the Multifaceted Biological Activities of Anthocyanins Isolated from Two Andean Berries. *Foods* **2024**, *13*, 2625. [CrossRef] [PubMed]
5. Pappalardo, I.; Convertini, P.; Infantino, V. Anthocyanins. In *Natural Molecules in Neuroprotection and Neurotoxicity*; Elsevier: Amsterdam, The Netherlands, 2024; pp. 1221–1239, ISBN 9780443237638.
6. Sangeeta, S.; Rai, S.; Bisht, S.; Nazim, M. Chemical Properties of Anthocyanins Sourced from Different Subtropical Fruits. In *Anthocyanins in Subtropical Fruits: Chemical Properties, Processing, and Health Benefits*; CRC Press: New York, NY, USA, 2023; pp. 33–58. ISBN 9781003242598.
7. Guo, Y.; Zhang, H.; Shao, S.; Sun, S.; Yang, D.; Lv, S. Anthocyanin: A review of plant sources, extraction, stability, content determination and modifications. *Int. J. Food Sci. Technol.* **2022**, *57*, 7573–7591. [CrossRef]
8. Teixeira, M.; Tao, W.; Fernandes, A.; Faria, A.; Ferreira, I.M.P.L.V.O.; He, J.; de Freitas, V.; Mateus, N.; Oliveira, H. Anthocyanin-rich edible flowers, current understanding of a potential new trend in dietary patterns. *Trends Food Sci. Technol.* **2023**, *138*, 708–725. [CrossRef]
9. Oancea, S.; Oprean, L. Anthocyanins, from Biosynthesis in Plants to Human Health Benefits. 2011. Available online: https://saiapm.ulbsibiu.ro/cercetare/ACTA_E/AUCFT_2011_I_3_16.pdf (accessed on 12 October 2024).
10. Herrera-Balandrano, D.D.; Chai, Z.; Beta, T.; Feng, J.; Huang, W. Blueberry anthocyanins: An updated review on approaches to enhancing their bioavailability. *Trends Food Sci. Technol.* **2021**, *118*, 808–821. [CrossRef]
11. Oancea, S. A review of the current knowledge of thermal stability of anthocyanins and approaches to their stabilization to heat. *Antioxidants* **2021**, *10*, 1337. [CrossRef]
12. Wu, X.; Yan, X.; Zhang, J.; Wu, X.; Zhang, Q.; Zhang, B. Intelligent films based on dual-modified starch and microencapsulated Aronia melanocarpa anthocyanins: Functionality, stability and application. *Int. J. Biol. Macromol.* **2024**, *275*, 134076. [CrossRef]
13. Rocha, F.; de Paula Rezende, J.; Maciel Dos Santos Dias, M.; Rodrigues Arruda Pinto, V.; César Stringheta, P.; Clarissa Dos Santos Pires, A.; Cristina Teixeira Ribeiro Vidigal, M. Complexation of anthocyanins, betalains and carotenoids with biopolymers: An approach to complexation techniques and evaluation of binding parameters. *Food Res. Int.* **2023**, *163*, 112277. [CrossRef]

14. Machado, M.H.; Almeida, A.d.R.; Maciel, M.V.d.O.B.; Vitorino, V.B.; Bazzo, G.C.; da Rosa, C.G.; Sganzerla, W.G.; Mendes, C.; Barreto, P.L.M. Microencapsulation by spray drying of red cabbage anthocyanin rich extract for the production of a natural food colorant. *Biocatal. Agric. Biotechnol.* **2022**, *39*, 102287. [CrossRef]
15. Cappellini, F.; Marinelli, A.; Toccaceli, M.; Tonelli, C.; Petroni, K. Anthocyanins: From mechanisms of regulation in plants to health benefits in foods. *Front. Plant Sci.* **2021**, *12*, 748049. [CrossRef] [PubMed]
16. Burton-Freeman, B.; Sandhu, A.; Edirisinghe, I. Anthocyanins. In *Nutraceuticals*; Elsevier: Amsterdam, The Netherlands, 2016; pp. 489–500, ISBN 9780128021477.
17. Ockermann, P.; Headley, L.; Lizio, R.; Hansmann, J. A review of the properties of anthocyanins and their influence on factors affecting cardiometabolic and cognitive health. *Nutrients* **2021**, *13*, 2831. [CrossRef] [PubMed]
18. Yánez, G.C.; Zambrano Mendoza, J.L.; Caicedo, M.; Heredia, J.; Sangoquiza Caiza, C.A.; Villacrés, E.; Racines Jaramillo, M.R.; Caballero, D. *Ficha Técnica de la Variedad de Maíz Negro INIAP-199 "Racimo de Uva"*; INIAP, Estación Experimental Santa Catalina, Programa de Maíz; INIAP: Quito, Ecuador, 2016.
19. Monteros, J.C.; Yumisaca Jiménez, S.F.; Tello Torres, C.M.; Montesdeoca, L.; Reinoso, R.I.A.; Garófalo, J.; Carrera, E.; Andrade-Piedra, J.; Cuesta Subía, H.X. INIAP-Yana Shungo: Variedad Para Consumo en Fresco y Procesado. Boletín Plegable INAP. 2011. Available online: https://repositorioslatinoamericanos.uchile.cl/handle/2250/8270208 (accessed on 19 October 2024).
20. Reyes, L.F.; Miller, J.C.; Cisneros-Zevallos, L. Antioxidant capacity, anthocyanins and total phenolics in purple-and red-fleshed potato (*Solanum tuberosum* L.) genotypes. *Am. J. Pot Res.* **2005**, *82*, 271–277. [CrossRef]
21. Ponder, A.; Hallmann, E.; Kwolek, M.; Średnicka-Tober, D.; Kazimierczak, R. Genetic Differentiation in Anthocyanin Content among Berry Fruits. *Curr, ISsues Mol. Biol.* **2021**, *43*, 36–51. [CrossRef]
22. Connor, A.M.; Finn, C.E.; McGhie, T.K.; Alspach, P.A. Genetic and Environmental Variation in Anthocyanins and their Relationship to Antioxidant Activity in Blackberry and Hybridberry Cultivars. *J. Am. Soc. Hort. Sci.* **2005**, *130*, 680–687. [CrossRef]
23. Salarbashi, D.; Bazeli, J.; Fahmideh Rad, E. An update on the new achievements in the nanocapsulation of anthocyanins. *Nanomed. J.* **2020**, *7*, 87–97.
24. Pérez, B.P.; Endara, A.B.; Garrido, J.A.; Ramírez Cárdenas, L.d.L.Á. Extraction of anthocyanins from Mortiño (*Vaccinium floribundum*) and determination of their antioxidant capacity. *Rev. Fac. Nac. Agron. Medellín* **2021**, *74*, 9453–9460. [CrossRef]
25. Singleton, V.L.; Orthofer, R.; Lamuela-Raventós, R.M. [14] Analysis of total phenols and other oxidation substrates and antioxidants by means of folin-ciocalteu reagent. In *Oxidants and Antioxidants Part A*; Methods in Enzymology; Elsevier: Amsterdam, The Netherlands, 1999; Volume 299, pp. 152–178, ISBN 9780121822002.
26. Wrolstad, R.E.; Durst, R.W.; Lee, J. Tracking color and pigment changes in anthocyanin products. *Trends Food Sci. Technol.* **2005**, *16*, 423–428. [CrossRef]
27. Righi da Rosa, J.; Nunes, G.L.; Motta, M.H.; Fortes, J.P.; Cezimbra Weis, G.C.; Rychecki Hecktheuer, L.H.; Muller, E.I.; Ragagnin de Menezes, C.; Severo da Rosa, C. Microencapsulation of anthocyanin compounds extracted from blueberry (*Vaccinium* spp.) by spray drying: Characterization, stability and simulated gastrointestinal conditions. *Food Hydrocoll.* **2019**, *89*, 742–748. [CrossRef]
28. Laokuldilok, T.; Kanha, N. Microencapsulation of Black Glutinous Rice Anthocyanins Using Maltodextrins Produced from Broken Rice Fraction as Wall Material by Spray Drying and Freeze Drying. *J. Food Process. Preserv.* **2017**, *41*, e12877. [CrossRef]
29. Schindelin, J.; Arganda-Carreras, I.; Frise, E.; Kaynig, V.; Longair, M.; Pietzsch, T.; Preibisch, S.; Rueden, C.; Saalfeld, S.; Schmid, B.; et al. Fiji: An open-source platform for biological-image analysis. *Nat. Methods* **2012**, *9*, 676–682. [CrossRef] [PubMed]
30. Brand-Williams, W.; Cuvelier, M.E.; Berset, C. Use of a free radical method to evaluate antioxidant activity. *LWT Food Sci. Technol.* **1995**, *28*, 25–30. [CrossRef]
31. Cutler, R.R.; Wilson, P. Antibacterial activity of a new, stable, aqueous extract of allicin against methicillin-resistant Staphylococcus aureus. *Br. J. Biomed. Sci.* **2004**, *61*, 71–74. [CrossRef] [PubMed]
32. Barone, D.; Cito, L.; Tommonaro, G.; Abate, A.A.; Penon, D.; De Prisco, R.; Penon, A.; Forte, I.M.; Benedetti, E.; Cimini, A.; et al. Antitumoral potential, antioxidant activity and carotenoid content of two Southern Italy tomato cultivars extracts: San Marzano and Corbarino. *J. Cell. Physiol.* **2018**, *233*, 1266–1277. [CrossRef]
33. Gao, C.; Wang, A.-Y. Significance of increased apoptosis and Bax expression in human small intestinal adenocarcinoma. *J. Histochem. Cytochem.* **2009**, *57*, 1139–1148. [CrossRef]
34. Vaskivuo, T.E.; Stenbäck, F.; Tapanainen, J.S. Apoptosis and apoptosis-related factors Bcl-2, Bax, tumor necrosis factor-alpha, and NF-kappaB in human endometrial hyperplasia and carcinoma. *Cancer* **2002**, *95*, 1463–1471. [CrossRef]
35. Čeryová, N. Monitoring of Selected Heavy Metals and Bioactive Compounds in Potato (*Solanum tuberosum* L.) Tubers. *Agrobiodivers. Improv. Nutr. Health Life Qual.* **2022**, *6*, 213–219. [CrossRef]
36. Volnová, B.; Musilová, J.; Kopernická, M.; Kavalcová, P.; Harangozo, Ľ.; Medvecký, M. The content of total polyphenols in different varieties of Solanum tuberosum grow in Spiš area. *Potravinarstvo Slovak. J. Food Sci.* **2016**, *10*, 72–77. [CrossRef]
37. Rodriguez-Saona, L.E.; Giusti, M.M.; Wrolstad, R.E. Anthocyanin pigment composition of red-fleshed potatoes. *J. Food Sci.* **1998**, *63*, 458–465. [CrossRef]
38. Neciosup-Puican, A.A.; Barreda, E.F.; Quinayá, C.P. Stability and content of anthocyanins in Peruvian purple potato INIA 328—Kulli Papa. *LWT* **2024**, *199*, 116125. [CrossRef]

39. Riveros-Loaiza, L.M.; Benhur-Cardona, N.; Lopez-Kleine, L.; Soto-Sedano, J.C.; Pinzón, A.M.; Mosquera-Vásquez, T.; Roda, F. Uncovering anthocyanin diversity in potato landraces (*Solanum tuberosum* L. Phureja) using RNA-seq. *PLoS ONE* **2022**, *17*, e0273982. [CrossRef] [PubMed]
40. Sun, Y.; Chi, J.; Ye, X.; Wang, S.; Liang, J.; Yue, P.; Xiao, H.; Gao, X. Nanoliposomes as delivery system for anthocyanins: Physicochemical characterization, cellular uptake, and antioxidant properties. *LWT* **2021**, *139*, 110554. [CrossRef]
41. Wang, N.; Li, X.-J.; Wang, L.; Li, B.; Tian, J.-L. Design of a liposome casein hydrogel as an efficient front-end homeostatic anthocyanin loading system. *Int. J. Biol. Macromol.* **2024**, *278*, 134928. [CrossRef]
42. Aldiyeva, A.B.; Khamitova, D.D. Influence of freeze-drying parameters on the content of polyphenols and anthocyanins in strawberries. *J. Almaty Technol. Univ.* **2023**, *1*, 52–56. [CrossRef]
43. Mohammadalinejhad, S.; Kurek, M.A. Microencapsulation of anthocyanins—Critical review of techniques and wall materials. *Appl. Sci.* **2021**, *11*, 3936. [CrossRef]
44. Gulin-Sarfraz, T.; Kalantzopoulos, G.N.; Haugen, J.-E.; Axelsson, L.; Raanaas Kolstad, H.; Sarfraz, J. Controlled Release of Volatile Antimicrobial Compounds from Mesoporous Silica Nanocarriers for Active Food Packaging Applications. *Int. J. Mol. Sci.* **2022**, *23*, 7032. [CrossRef]
45. Fangueiro, J.F.; Souto, E.B.; Silva, A.M. Encapsulation of nutraceuticals in novel delivery systems. In *Nutraceuticals*; Elsevier: Amsterdam, The Netherlands, 2016; pp. 305–342, ISBN 9780128043059.
46. Alemzadeh, I.; Hajiabbas, M.; Pakzad, H.; Dehkordi, S.S.; Vossoughi, A. Encapsulation of food components and bioactive ingredients and targeted release. *Int. J. Eng.* **2020**, *33*, 1–11. [CrossRef]
47. Patil, S.; Chaudhari, B.; Acharya, M. Emerging Nano-Formulation Strategies for Nutraceutical Delivery. *Adv. Food Process. Technol.* **2023**, *4*, 127. [CrossRef]
48. Boggia, R.; Zunin, P.; Turrini, F. Functional foods and food supplements. *Appl. Sci.* **2020**, *10*, 8538. [CrossRef]
49. Chen, T.; Zhang, M.; Bhandari, B.; Yang, Z. Micronization and nanosizing of particles for an enhanced quality of food: A review. *Crit. Rev. Food Sci. Nutr.* **2018**, *58*, 993–1001. [CrossRef] [PubMed]
50. Catalkaya, G.; Guldiken, B.; Capanoglu, E. Encapsulation of anthocyanin-rich extract from black chokeberry (*Aronia melanocarpa*) pomace by spray drying using different coating materials. *Food Funct.* **2022**, *13*, 11579–11591. [CrossRef] [PubMed]
51. Takahata, Y.; Kai, Y.; Tanaka, M.; Nakayama, H.; Yoshinaga, M. Enlargement of the variances in amount and composition of anthocyanin pigments in sweetpotato storage roots and their effect on the differences in DPPH radical-scavenging activity. *Sci. Hortic.* **2011**, *127*, 469–474. [CrossRef]
52. Frestasya, L.; Pangsibidang, R.C.A. Purple sweet potato antioxidants for oxidative stress caused by intense physical exercise. *Pharm. Educ.* **2024**, *24*, 128–133. [CrossRef]
53. Shi, Y.; Chen, X.; Gao, Q.; Zou, Y.; Xing, D.; Chen, R.; He, X.; Li, Q. Preparation and chemical properties of microencapsulation developed with mulberry anthocyanins and silk fibroin. *Ind. Crops Prod.* **2024**, *212*, 118383. [CrossRef]
54. Baysal, E.; Kazan, A. Microencapsulation of black carrot anthocyanins for enhanced thermal stability. *J. Innov. Sci. Eng.* **2024**, *8*, 92–102. [CrossRef]
55. Yuan, G.; Xia, X.; Guan, Y.; Yi, H.; Lai, S.; Sun, Y.; Cao, S. The antimicrobial quantitative relationship and mechanism of plant flavonoids to gram-positive bacteria. *Res. Sq.* **2022**, *15*, 1190. [CrossRef]
56. Tallam, A.K.; Sahithi, A.; Nuli, M.V. Evaluation of antibacterial property of anthyocyanin extracted from brassica oleracea against gram positive and gram negative bacteria by using erythromycin as a standard drug. *Int. J. Indig. Herb. Drug.* **2023**. [CrossRef]
57. Álvarez-Martínez, F.J.; Barrajón-Catalán, E.; Encinar, J.A.; Rodríguez-Díaz, J.C.; Micol, V. Antimicrobial Capacity of Plant Polyphenols against Gram-positive Bacteria: A Comprehensive Review. *Curr. Med. Chem.* **2020**, *27*, 2576–2606. [CrossRef]
58. Bouarab-Chibane, L.; Forquet, V.; Lantéri, P.; Clément, Y.; Léonard-Akkari, L.; Oulahal, N.; Degraeve, P.; Bordes, C. Antibacterial Properties of Polyphenols: Characterization and QSAR (Quantitative Structure-Activity Relationship) Models. *Front. Microbiol.* **2019**, *10*, 829. [CrossRef]
59. Zhao, X.; Zhang, C.; Guigas, C.; Ma, Y.; Corrales, M.; Tauscher, B.; Hu, X. Composition, antimicrobial activity, and antiproliferative capacity of anthocyanin extracts of purple corn (*Zea mays* L.) from China. *Eur. Food Res. Technol.* **2009**, *228*, 759–765. [CrossRef]
60. Pan, F.; Liu, Y.; Liu, J.; Wang, E. Stability of blueberry anthocyanin, anthocyanidin and pyranoanthocyanidin pigments and their inhibitory effects and mechanisms in human cervical cancer HeLa cells. *RSC Adv.* **2019**, *9*, 10842–10853. [CrossRef] [PubMed]
61. Lazzè, M.C.; Savio, M.; Pizzala, R.; Cazzalini, O.; Perucca, P.; Scovassi, A.I.; Stivala, L.A.; Bianchi, L. Anthocyanins induce cell cycle perturbations and apoptosis in different human cell lines. *Carcinogenesis* **2004**, *25*, 1427–1433. [CrossRef] [PubMed]
62. Navarro, M.; Arnaez, E.; Moreira, I.; Quesada, S.; Azofeifa, G.; Wilhelm, K.; Vargas, F.; Chen, P. Polyphenolic Characterization, Antioxidant, and Cytotoxic Activities of Mangifera indica Cultivars from Costa Rica. *Foods* **2019**, *8*, 384. [CrossRef]
63. Wang, L.; Li, X.; Wang, B. The cytotoxicity activity of Hohenbuehelia serotina polyphenols on HeLa cells via induction of cell apoptosis and cell cycle arrest. *Food Chem. Toxicol.* **2019**, *124*, 239–248. [CrossRef]
64. Koss-Mikołajczyk, I.; Bartoszek, A. Relationship between Chemical Structure and Biological Activity Evaluated In Vitro for Six Anthocyanidins Most Commonly Occurring in Edible Plants. *Molecules* **2023**, *28*, 6156. [CrossRef]
65. Janseerat; Kolekar, M.; Reddy, C.S.; Sharma, S.; Roy, S. Anthocyanin-Based Natural Color Induced Intelligent Food Packaging Sensor: A Review. *Curr. Food Sci. Technol. Rep.* **2024**, *2*, 157–167. [CrossRef]

66. Koop, B.L.; Soares, L.S.; Cesca, K.; Souza, V.G.L.; Valencia, G.A.; Monteiro, A.R. Enhancing the stability of anthocyanins extracts through adsorption into nanoclays—Development of a smart biohybrid sensor for intelligent food packaging or as natural food additive/preservative. *Food Bioprod. Process.* **2024**, *147*, 315–326. [CrossRef]
67. Selvamuthukumaran, M. Natural Anthocyanins from Subtropical Fruits for Cancer Prevention. In *Anthocyanins in Subtropical Fruits: Chemical Properties, Processing, and Health Benefits*; CRC Press: New York, NY, USA, 2023; pp. 97–103, ISBN 9781003242598.
68. Kim, M.J.; Paramanantham, A.; Lee, W.S.; Yun, J.W.; Chang, S.H.; Kim, D.C.; Park, H.S.; Choi, Y.H.; Kim, G.S.; Ryu, C.H.; et al. Anthocyanins Derived from Vitis coignetiae Pulliat Contributes Anti-Cancer Effects by Suppressing NF-κB Pathways in Hep3B Human Hepatocellular Carcinoma Cells and In Vivo. *Molecules* **2020**, *25*, 5445. [CrossRef]

nutrients

MDPI

Article

Diet Biofunctionality in Modulating Cardiovascular Parameters in Obese Patients After Bioenteric Intragastric Balloon Bariatric Surgery

Edyta Barbara Balejko [1,*] and Jarosław Lichota [2]

[1] Department of Commodity Sciences, Quality Assessment, Process Engineering and Human Nutrition, Faculty of Food Sciences and Fisheries, West Pomeranian University of Technology in Szczecin, 70-310 Szczecin, Poland

[2] Unii Lubelskiej 1, Department of General, Minimally Invasive and Gastroenterological Surgery, Independent Public Clinical Hospital No. 1 of Pomeranian Medical University in Szczecin, 71-252 Szczecin, Poland

* Correspondence: edyta.balejko@zut.edu.pl

Abstract: Background/Objectives: Adiposopathy is the cause of many secondary disorders in the function and structure of many organs and systems in the body. In the progression of obesity and the increasing dysfunction of anti-inflammatory me-diators, chronic inflammation occurs. This may be accompanied by the development of metabolic complications. Methods: A diet with highly bioactive properties was formulated, and an element of diet therapy was introduced as a key component to support treatment in obese patients following bariatric surgery. Patients underwent a BIB (Bioenteric Intragastric Balloon) procedure. As obesity is a risk factor for cardiovascular diseases, this study aimed to regulate cardiovascular factors in adiposopathy. Anti-inflammatory dietary components with modulating properties were included, with increased bioflavonoids, vitamins A, E, C, folic acid, and synbiotics, and altered fatty acid composition. Results: The results showed satisfactory effects on fat reduction and the regulation of isoprostanes, plasminogen, angiotensin, prostacyclin, triglycerides, blood pressure, and blood rheology parameters. Cardiovascular co-morbidities are common in obesity. This is due to the endocrine function of adipocytes. As such, we decided to investigate the possibility of using bioactive dietary components as an adjunct to the safety of reducing prothrombotic parameters in obese patients after BIB surgery. This study hypothesised that the enrichment of the recommended diet after bariatric surgery with the addition of n-3 EFAs, bioflavonoids, vitamins, and synbiotics might result in comparable or greater fat mass loss in the subjects. In addition, the use of a functional diet might show a beneficial modifying effect on antihyperglycemic parameter values. We then compared the results to those obtained among patients fed a reducing, standard diet. Conclusions: Using a functional diet, a significant reduction in visceral fat was achieved. A decrease in VFA was shown to reduce whole-blood viscosity. Furthermore, this study showed a significant effect of bioactive components on pro-thrombotic parameters in obese patients.

Keywords: obesity; bariatric; dietotherapy; isoprostanes; plasminogen activator inhitor-1; angitensin; prostacyclins; triglycerides; hypertension; blood rheology

1. Introduction

The development of civilisation has greatly contributed to the extension of human life. At the same time, modern lifestyles have exacerbated the problem of obesity to epidemic proportions. Visceral fat dysfunction results from inflammation, oxidative stress, hypoxia, and mitochondrial dysfunction. The increased chemotaxis of immune cells into adipose tissue leads to the development of a chronic inflammatory process. With obesity come dysfunctions in blood volume and flow, systolic cardiac output, minute volume, cardiac hypertrophy, hypertension, and haemorheological properties. Due to interdependent metabolic disturbances, vascular wall damage, thrombus formation, and atherosclerotic plaques occur [1]. Most adipokines from visceral adipose tissue are pro-inflammatory. Adiposopathy is the cause of many secondary disorders in the function and structure of many organs and systems in the body. Adipokines entering the circulation exert effects on the function of the vascular walls of circulation and heart muscles. Atherosclerotic plaques in obese patients contain more lipids, are brittle, and easily rupture [2]. In the progression of obesity and the increasing dysfunction of anti-inflammatory mediators, chronic inflammation occurs. This may be accompanied by the development of metabolic complications. This fact explains the association of co-morbidities such as diabetes with an increased risk of inflammatory diseases, hypertension, and atherosclerosis. The exceptional incidence of cardiovascular complications prompts the search for support for therapeutic management. The functional properties of nutrients offer opportunities for the natural modulation of concentrations of factors that cause metabolic disorders [3–5]. Current diet therapy is based on designer foods that meet specific needs of the body. Long-term reduction diets very often lead to deficiencies. Therefore, this paper proposes a greater supply of bioactive natural ingredients such as bioflavonoids, fatty acids, and probiotics, with the expectation of significantly better treatment effects. A diet with functional characteristics offers the possibility of prevention and effective care. Therefore, the enrichment of weight-loss diets with functional food components may be appropriate.

For obese patients with BMI values ≥ 35 kg/m^2, experiencing no effects in terms of weight reduction by conservative methods, bariatric surgery and procedures are used [6–8]. An intragastric balloon is the least invasive bariatric procedure. The aim of this study was to modify the recommended standard reduction diet after bariatric surgery to achieve the regulation of isoprostanes, plasminogen, angiotensin, prostacyclin, triglycerides, blood pressure, and blood rheological parameters. The regulation of the concentrations of these parameters was expected to increase the health safety of patients. The diet was modified, increasing the proportion of natural regulatory bioactive compounds.

2. Material and Methods

2.1. Study Group

This study was conducted at the Sonomed Medical Centre in Szczecin. Sixty obese female patients were observed after balloon insertion into the stomach using the Bioenteric Intragastric Balloon (BIB) method. All patients were diagnosed with hypertension. The follow-up time was 1 year. Measurements were carried out immediately before the bariatric surgery and at the end of the follow-up period. Ethical approval was obtained from the Bioethics Committee of the Regional Chamber of Physicians in Szczecin on 6 May 2015 (OIL-Sz/Mf/KB/452/06/05/2015).

A body composition analysis was performed, using a body composition analyser, by the bioimpedance analysis (BIA) method. The IOI 353 analyser was CEO 123 certified and complied with the MDD 93/42/EEC medical device directive. The mean age of the women was 40.0. The mean BMI was 37.2 ± 3.5 kg/m^2. All patients had a history of numerous unsuccessful attempts at weight reduction by conservative methods, i.e., diet. The patients were under the care of a dietician and a psychologist.

Division of the Study Group and Dietary Characteristics

Patients were divided into the following groups (20 each):

Group I—control, not following dietary recommendations;
Group II—following dietary recommendations developed by American specialists from the University of Nevada School of Medicine;
Group III—using proprietary modifications of the US recommendations.

The diet increased the proportion of bioflavonoids, *n*-3 EFAs, and vitamins A, E, and C. Thus, 20 mL of flaxseed oil was introduced into the daily diet of patients in Group III as the main source of *n*-3 EFAs. The patients added the selected oil to soups after cooking, without heat treatment, or as an addition to salads or hummus. Dietary ingredients were selected to increase the anti-inflammatory effect. In addition, patients in this group took a synbiotic every other month. A chemical analysis of the antioxidant properties of the proprietary diet was performed: the antioxidant capacity TEAC (Trolox Equivalent Antioxidant Capacity) was determined according to Re et al. [9], the FRAP (Ferric Reducing Antioxidant Power) capacity was established according to Benzie and Strain [10], and the total polyphenol content was measured according to Cheung et al. [11]. In addition, fatty acid composition and content were assessed, and a sensory evaluation of the proposed diet was carried out [4]. It was assumed that an appropriate combination of bioactive components would confer antioxidant properties to the diet. Groups I and II had similar proportions of macronutrients. The protein content of the diet was 80–85 g/day, whereas that of total carbohydrates was 70 g/day and total fat 42 g/day. The caloric value of the diets at month 1 was about 400 kcal, at month 3 about 600–800 kcal, and at month 5–12 about 1200 kcal.

Patients in Group III supplemented their diet with the addition of 20 mL of flaxseed oil and smoothies (twice a day) high in antioxidants and probiotics. They also took probiotics once a day every other month.

A 5-point sensory analysis was carried out according to PN-ISO 4121:1998 [12] for unrefined Budwig flaxseed oil ('LenVitol' Olfarm Sp.z.o.o, Pietrzykowice), evening primrose oil ('Wiesiołek' Olfarm Sp.z.o.o., Pietrzykowice), and Icelandic cod-liver oil ('LYSIHF' Reykjavik, Iceland). The discriminants assessed during the evaluation were colour, taste, and odour. The evaluation was carried out at the sensory laboratory of the West Pomeranian University of Technology in Szczecin. The sensory profile analysis of taste and colour was carried out according to PN-ISO 11036:1999 [13], PN-ISO 6658:1998 [14], and PN-ISO 6564:1999 [15]. Sensory evaluation was carried out by a team of 10 assessors trained in oil quality analysis.

The following rating scale was used:

- 5 points—very good;
- 4 points—good;
- 3 points—satisfactory;
- 2 points—barely satisfactory;
- 1 point—unsatisfactory.

The sensory scores were calculated based on the average of the determinants analysed (Table 1).

Table 1. Sensory analysis of oils.

Oil	Discriminants				
	Appearance	Colour	Taste	Smell	Total Score
Linseed oil	4.50	4.20	1.80	2.80	3.33
Evening primrose oil	4.00	4.00	1.25	1.80	2.76
Icelandic cod-liver oil	3.80	4.00	1.00	1.00	2.45

Based on the analyses, the following composition of fatty acids was determined in the diets of patients from Group III: SFA 26.95%, MUFA 44.98%, *n*-3 PUFA 9.87%, *n*-6 PUFA 18.20, (*n*-6)/(*n*-3) PUFA 1.84, and fat content 8.4%.

Moreover, in food ratios, the composition of fatty acids was determined (Table 2) according to AOAC 2004, (Aa 9-86). The methyl esters of fatty acids were analysed with gas chromatography (AOAC 991.39) using gas chromatography–mass spectrometry (GC-MS). The conditions of the analysis were the following: column SP^{TM}-2560, 100× 0.25 cm^3/min, split 1:50, injector temperature of 220 °C, oven temperature initially at 140 °C, then temperature growth from 140 °C to 240 °C/4 min, reaching a final temperature of 240 °C/10 min.

Table 2. Fatty acid composition analysis.

Systematic Name of Fatty Acid	Lipid Number	Fatty Acid Content [%]	SD
Tetradecanoic	C14:0	2.862	0.09
Pentadecanoic	C15:0	0.163	0.02
Hexadecanoic	C16:0 C16:1	19.986 4.339	0.15 0.11
Octadecanoic	C18:0 C18:1	3.94 38.156	0.09 0.21
Octadecadienoic	C18:2 *n*-6 C18:3 *n*-3	15.63 6.65	0.18 0.12
Octatetraenoic	C18:4 *n*-3	0.777	0.02
Docosanoic	C22:1	2.382	0.08
Eikosatetraenoic	C20:4 *n*-6 C20:4 *n*-3	2.571 0.10	0.03 0.01
Eikosapentaenoic Tetracosanoic Docosapentaenoic Docosahexaenoic	C20:5 *n*-3 C24:1 C22:5 *n*-3 C22:6 *n*-3	1.10 0.101 0.20 1.05	0.04 0.01 0.03 0.07
	SFA MUFA *n*-3 PUFA *n*-6 PUFA (*n*-6)/(*n*-3) PUFA Fat content	26.95 44.98 9.87 18.20 1.84 8.4	 0.16

The cocktails, which were the basis of the diet, contained many more bioactive compounds than the meals of the standard diet. The smoothies were based on vegetables and fruits such as pomegranate, raspberry, currant, orange, apple, spinach, kale, parsley, ginger, beetroot, and pumpkin, and flaxseed was also added. The daily intake of antioxidant components, depending on the type of smoothie consumed, was 5479–8414 µMTE/day in terms of antioxidant capacity (TEAC), 1642–4896 µM TE/day for the reducing capacity, and 1.2–2.2 g catechin equivalents/day for the total polyphenol content [4].

2.2. Immunoenzymatic Assays

An immunoenzymatic ELISA technique was used to determine serum prostacyclin, angiotensin, plasminogen, and isoprostane. Absorbance was read at 450 nm ± 2 nm using an ELx808 multichannel ELISA reader (BIO-TEK Instruments, Inc., Winooski, VT, USA). The KC Junior for the Windows calculator programme from BIO-TEK Instruments, Inc., USA, was used to develop calibration curves and calculate the concentration values of the test parameters. The following commercial kits were used for this study:

- Prostacyclin (catalogue no. 515211, Cayman Chemical Company, Ann Arbor, MI, USA), with a method accuracy of ±1% ± 0.010 absorbance and a measurement range of 1.6–1000 pg/mL;
- Angiotensin (catalogue no. E0797h, EIAab Science Co., Wuhan, China), with a method accuracy of ±1% ± 0.010 absorbance and a measurement range of 15.6–1000 pg/mL;
- Plasminogen (catalogue no. E0532h, EIAab Science Co, Wuhan, China), with a method accuracy of ±1% ± 0.010 absorbance and a measurement range of 0.156–10 ng/mL;
- Isoprostane (catalogue no. 516351, Cayman Chemical Company, Ann Arbor, MI, USA), with a method accuracy of ±1% ± 0.010 absorbance and a measurement range of 0.8–500 pg/mL.

2.3. Blood Rheological Measurements

Rheological tests were performed using an AR2000 ex rotational rheometer from TA Instruments (New Castle, DE, USA). The tests were carried out on whole blood at 32 °C using the plate-to-plate method with a diameter of 40 mm, at a constant shear rate of 1 [1/s], to determine apparent viscosity η.

2.4. Measurement of Triglyceride Levels and Blood Pressure

In all patient groups, serum triglyceride concentrations were determined in the collected blood. TG determination was performed using a colourimetric method. These tests were performed before the start of treatment and after the weight loss process. Analyses were performed in accredited diagnostic laboratories. Blood pressure was also measured in accordance with the current recommendations of the Polish Society of Hypertension.

2.5. Statistical Analysis

Statistica 13 from Statsoft was used for the calculations. To demonstrate statistically significant differences in concentrations between groups, the non-parametric Wilcoxon paired-rank order test, a non-parametric alternative to Student's *t*-test for dependent samples, was used.

3. Results

All patients had a history of multiple unsuccessful attempts at weight loss with conservative methods, including dieting. The standard diet used in Group II followed the recommendations of the Polish Society for the Treatment of Obesity regarding the nutrition of people after bariatric surgery [16]. The diet for Group III was antioxidant and anti-inflammatory [4]. At the baseline after treatment, the caloric value of all diets at month 1 was about 400 kcal, while, at month 3, it was about 600–800 kcal and, at months 5–12, about 1200 kcal. A diet of about 1000 kcal had the following values: protein, 80–85 g/day; total carbohydrates, 70 g/day; and total fat, 42 g/day. The *n*-6/*n*-3 value was 1.84. The diet of Group III contained two meals with high antioxidant potential [4]. The caloric value of the diets at month 1 was about 400 kcal, at month 3 about 600–800 kcal, and at months 5–12 about 1200 kcal. Patients in Group III took a synbiotic once a day, every other month. The total number of colony-forming units (CFUs) was 1 × 109 CFUs.

All measurements were performed in duplicate, at the beginning and at the end of the observation period. Using bioelectrical impedance measurements, the effects of fat reduction were compared.

Patients adhering to a diet rich in bioflavonoids, vitamins, minerals, *n*-3 fatty acids, and synbiotics achieved the highest weight reduction from an average of 98.5 kg to 70.0 kg, compared to Group II, from 95.0 kg to 80.0 kg, and Group I, from 89.5 kg to 83.4 kg. Group III achieved the highest reduction in body fat mass and visceral fat area, with the lowest loss of muscle mass and BMI (Table 3, Figure 1). The effects of the body composition analysis in Group III are shown in Table 1 and Figure 1. Statistically significant differences were found between Groups I and II, I and III, and II and III, at $p < 0.05$.

Table 3. Analysis of body composition by bioelectrical impedance ($\bar{x} \pm SD$).

	Fat Mass [kg]		Visceral Fat Area [cm^2]		Muscle Tissue Mass [kg]	
	Before	After	Before	After	Before	After
Gr.1	39.5 ± 3.2	36.6 ± 1.2	140 ± 22.5	132 ± 16.3	40.4 ± 2.0	37.2 ± 1.8
Gr.2	40.2 ± 2.5	31.1 ± 2	149.5 ± 25.7	124.5 ± 12.3	45.3 ± 1.6	39.5 ± 2.2
Gr.3	42.4 ± 1.2	20.1 ± 1.5	139.8 ± 19.9	95.8 ± 8.3	46.1 ± 3.1	39.9 ± 2.0

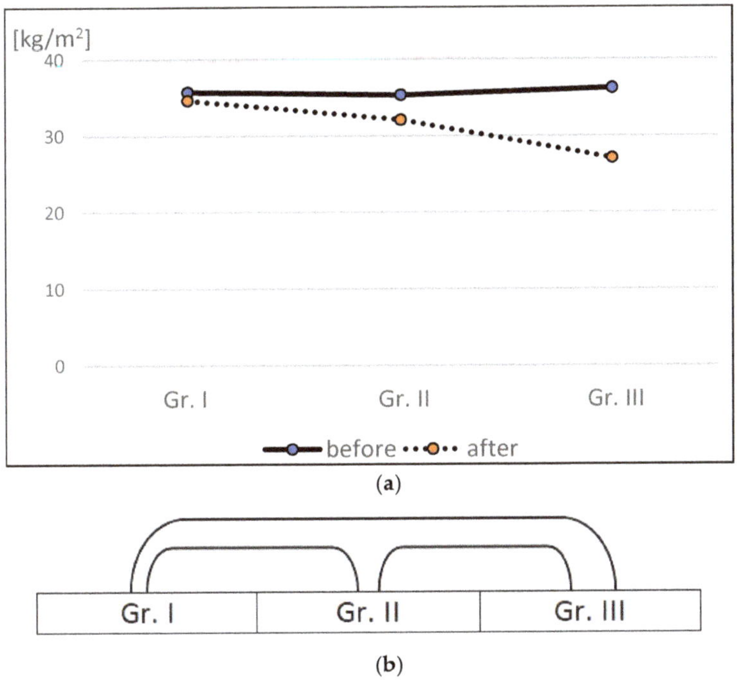

Figure 1. (**a**) BMI values of patients in three groups before and after BIB surgery and weight loss diets. (**b**) Incidence of statistically significant differences between the obtained BMI values of patients in the three groups after BIB surgery and weight loss diets.

In Group II, the blood pressure values before surgery were 149 ± 10/91 ± 6 mmHg and decreased to 139 ± 10/87 ± 2 mmHg after surgery. In Group III, the pressure values before surgery were 143 ± 10/85 ± 5 mmHg and decreased to 130 ± 10/80 ± 3 mmHg after surgery. The changes in systolic and diastolic blood pressure values in Group II, obtained after the diet-assisted BIB procedure, can be considered high but normal. The systolic and diastolic blood pressure values in Group II after the diet-assisted BIB procedure can be considered high but below the threshold for hypertension. The mean systolic and diastolic blood pressures of the patients before and after the treatment are shown in Figures 2 and 3.

According to the standards of the Polish Society of Cardiology, normal triglyceride levels are 35–150 mg/dL (Polish Society of Lipidology 2016) [17]. The triglyceride levels in patients in Group I, before BIB, were 165 mg/dL and, after the procedure, 150 mg/dL. In Group II patients, following international dietary recommendations, the triglyceride levels before BIB were 172 mg/dL and, after the procedure, 120 mg/dL. In Group III, in patients following the authors' diet, the triglyceride level before BIB was 165 mg/dL and, after the procedure, 90 mg/dL (Figure 4). Statistically significant differences were found between Groups I and II, I and III, and II and III, at $p < 0.05$.

A non-parametric Wilcoxon paired-rank order test was used, with an assumption of $p < 0.05$, for the results of triglyceride concentrations, comparing data before weight loss to data after treatment. Group I showed no statistically significant differences. Groups II and III showed statistically significant differences in triglyceride concentrations.

Isoprostane concentrations were determined by immunoenzymatic assay, using the ELISA method, and the mean values obtained are shown in Table 4. Lower values of isoprostane levels were obtained in patients on the experimental diet. The determination of isoprostanes provides a reliable and sensitive indicator of the lipid peroxidation metabolism in vivo, allowing the estimation of the contribution of free radicals to the pathophysiology of many diseases. The results obtained may be a marker of reduced free radical processes in the body associated with the pathogenesis of many metabolic diseases associated with obesity.

Using Wilcoxon's non-parametric paired-rank order test, statistically significant differences were shown between Groups I and II, I and III, and II and III (Figure 5) at $p < 0.05$. There was a significant indication of differences between the results obtained for Groups II and III. It can therefore be assumed that antioxidant components taken systematically significantly inhibit free radical reactions.

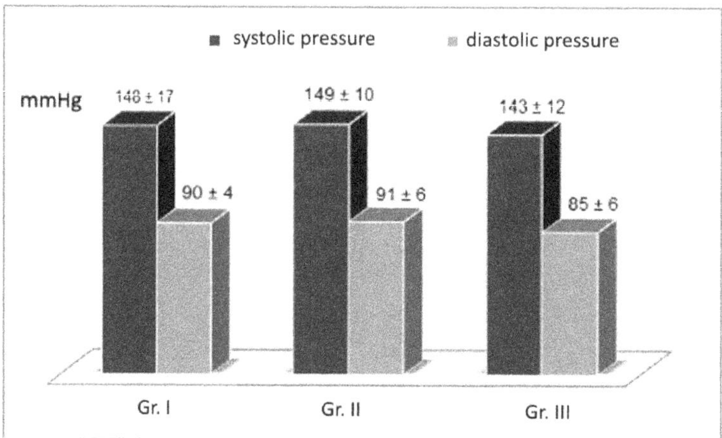

Figure 2. Blood pressure values of patients in the three groups before BIB treatment. Group I—control; Group II—receiving the standard diet; and Group III—receiving the modified diet.

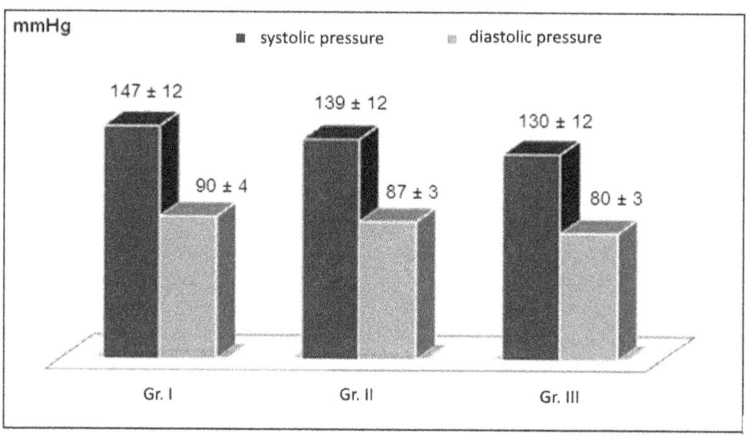

Figure 3. Blood pressure values of patients in the three groups after the BIB procedure and weight loss diets.

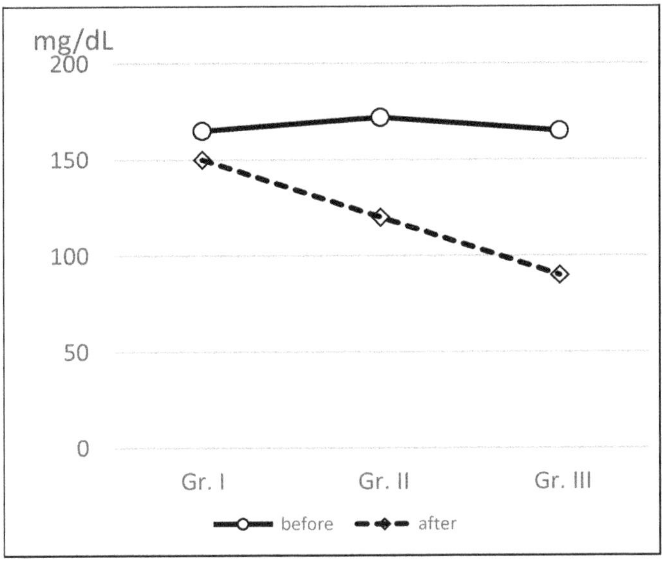

(**a**)

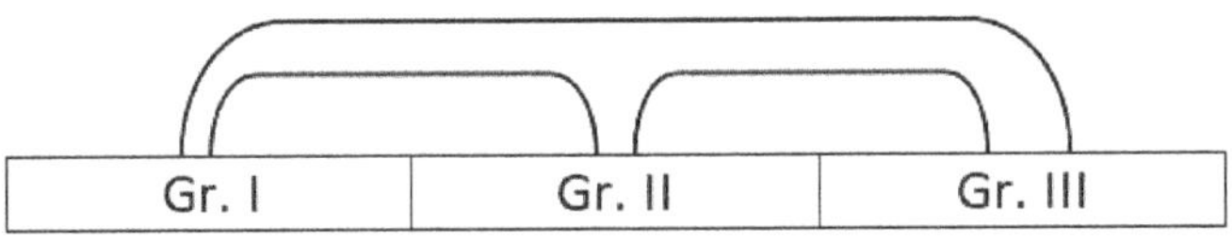

(**b**)

Figure 4. (**a**) Mean triglyceride levels of patients in the three groups before and after BIB surgery and weight loss diets. (**b**) Incidence of statistically significant differences between the achieved triglyceride levels of patients in the three groups after BIB surgery and weight loss diets.

Table 4. Mean values of serum isoprostane levels [pg/mL] in patients in the three groups before and after the BIB procedure and the weight loss diet.

Group I		Group II		Group III	
Before BIB ($\bar{x} \pm$ SD)	**After BIB ($\bar{x} \pm$ SD)**	**Before BIB ($\bar{x} \pm$ SD)**	**After BIB ($\bar{x} \pm$ SD)**	**Before BIB ($\bar{x} \pm$ SD)**	**After BIB ($\bar{x} \pm$ SD)**
145.8 ± 16.8	148.3 ± 21.1	137.4 ± 20.5	110 ± 20.8	143.3 ± 23.8	94.3 ± 23.2

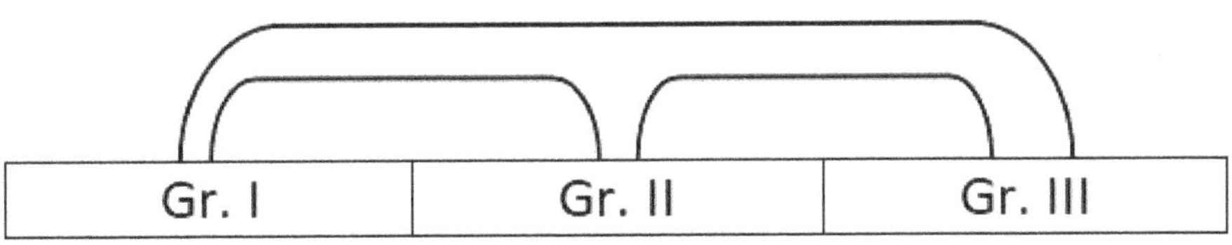

Figure 5. To assess the occurrence of statistically significant differences between the obtained concentrations of isoprostanes, prostacyclins, plasminogen, and angiotensinogen in patients in the three groups after BIB surgery and the weight loss diets.

Prostacyclin concentrations were determined with an immunoenzymatic assay, using the ELISA method. The mean values obtained are shown in Table 5. In our study, after one year of follow-up, we found higher values of serum prostacyclin in patients from Groups II and III treated with a diet after the BIB procedure. For Group III patients receiving a modified diet, the effect was better because the support was a diet with functional characteristics. The components of the diet that had been modified with functional foods could positively influence the results regarding prostacyclin concentrations in comparisons between Group II and Group III patients. Using Wilcoxon's non-parametric paired-rank order test, statistically significant differences were shown between Groups I and II, I and III, and II and III at $p < 0.05$, after the patients had completed their weight loss (Figure 5). There was a statistically significant increase in prostacyclin levels in patients who had reduced their body weight. Excess body fat in obesity highly correlates with the development of atherosclerosis. The components of the diet that had been modified with functional foods may have favourably influenced the results of PGI2 concentrations in comparisons between Groups II and III.

Table 5. Mean prostacyclin levels [pg/mL] in the serum of patients in the three groups before and after BIB surgery and relevant weight loss diets.

Group I		Group II		Group III	
Before BIB ($\bar{x} \pm$ SD)	**After BIB ($\bar{x} \pm$ SD)**	**Before BIB ($\bar{x} \pm$ SD)**	**After BIB ($\bar{x} \pm$ SD)**	**Before BIB ($\bar{x} \pm$ SD)**	**After BIB ($\bar{x} \pm$ SD)**
9.51 ± 1.09	9.84 ± 1.31	9.39 ± 1.22	16.93 ± 1.66	8.58 ± 1.39	21.81 ± 1.37

Plasminogen concentrations were determined by immunoenzymatic assay, using the ELISA method. The mean values obtained are shown in Table 6. In the case of Group I, the effect of a small but unfavourable increase in plasminogen was demonstrated. There were decreases in the values of serum plasminogen concentrations in Group II and Group III patients treated with a diet after BIB treatment. The effect was stronger in Group III patients receiving a modified diet. The components of the modified diet containing functional foods may have favourably influenced the results regarding plasminogen concentrations in comparisons between Group II and III patients. Using Wilcoxon's non-parametric paired-rank order test, statistically significant differences were shown between Groups I and II, Groups I and III, and Groups II and III at $p < 0.05$, after the patients had completed their weight loss (Figure 5).

Table 6. Mean plasminogen levels [ng/mL] in the serum of patients in the three groups before and after BIB surgery and relevant weight loss diets.

Group I		Group II		Group III	
Before BIB ($\bar{x} \pm$ SD)	**After BIB ($\bar{x} \pm$ SD)**	**Before BIB ($\bar{x} \pm$ SD)**	**After BIB ($\bar{x} \pm$ SD)**	**Before BIB ($\bar{x} \pm$ SD)**	**After BIB ($\bar{x} \pm$ SD)**
20.03 ± 0.6	20.59 ± 0.91	19.26 ± 0.53	12.13 ± 0.53	19.29 ± 0.59	9.57 ± 0.59

Angiotensinogen concentrations were determined by immunoenzymatic assay, using the ELISA method. The mean values obtained are shown in Table 7. In all patients in Group III, there were decreases in angiotensinogen concentrations after one year of follow-up. The significant decreases in the values obtained in Groups II and III were due to the reduction diet. In Group III, the strongest reduction effects were seen after a diet rich in antioxidants. The results of the comparison of statistically significant differences between the groups are shown in Figure 5.

Since the concentrations of isoprostanes, prostacyclins, plasminogen, and angiotensinogen in all the groups studied showed statistically significant differences, they are presented jointly and graphically in 5. As is well known, excess body fat in obesity promotes the development of atherosclerosis. The components of the diet modified with functional foods may have favourably modified the concentrations of the parameters studied in comparisons between Groups II and III.

Table 7. Mean values of angiotensinogen [pg/mL] in the serum levels of patients in the three groups before and after BIB surgery and relevant weight loss diets.

Group I		Group II		Group III	
Before BIB ($\bar{x} \pm$ SD)	**After BIB ($\bar{x} \pm$ SD)**	**Before BIB ($\bar{x} \pm$ SD)**	**After BIB ($\bar{x} \pm$ SD)**	**Before BIB ($\bar{x} \pm$ SD)**	**After BIB ($\bar{x} \pm$ SD)**
4.16 ± 0.41	3.71 ± 0.48	3.57 ± 0.68	2.88 ± 0.25	3.39 ± 0.41	2.34 ± 0.37

In the absence of significant changes in Group I, Table 8 compares the results of the final concentrations of the studied parameters for Groups II and III only.

Table 8. Comparison of parameter concentrations for Groups II and III after 12 months of observation ($p < 0.05$).

Parameter	II gr (*n*-20)	III gr (*n*-20)
BMI [kg/m^2]	32.07 ± 5.82	27.07 ± 4.86
VFA [cm^2]	124.5 ± 12.3	95.8 ± 8.3
Blood pressure [mmHg]	139 ± 12/87 ± 3	130 ± 12/80 ± 3
TG [mg/dL]	120 ± 9.23	90 ± 6.78
Isoprostanes [pg/mL]	110 ± 20.88	94.32 ± 23.27
Plasminogenes [ng/mL]	12.13 ± 0.53	9.57 ± 0.59
Angiotensines [pg/mL]	2.88 ± 0.26	2.34 ± 0.37
Prostacyclines [pg/mL]	16.93 ± 1.66	21.81 ± 1.37

Among the haemorheological properties used in the diagnosis of cardiovascular disease, the outstanding parameter is blood viscosity. The viscosity value is mainly influenced by the morphotic elements of the blood and its properties, in addition to changes in temperature and blood flow velocity [18].

As VFA (visceral fat area) values depend on the structure of one's diet, an attempt was made to demonstrate the dependence of viscosity on this parameter (Figure 6). In all patients, lower whole-blood apparent viscosity values were found as the VFA values decreased.

The results are illustrated in the graph below.

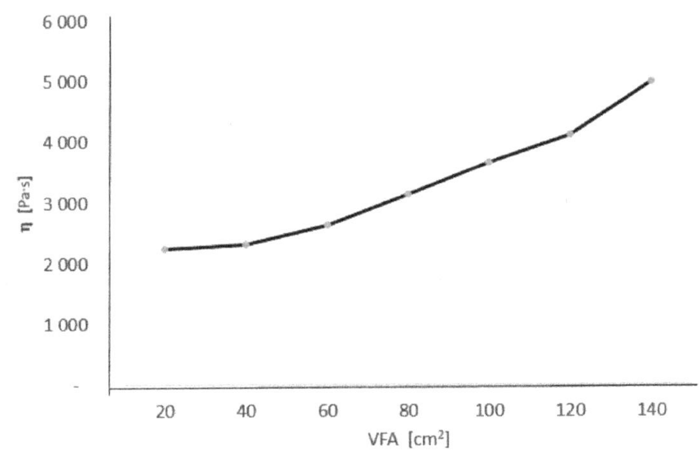

Figure 6. Dependence of blood viscosity on VFA for women (*n*-60).

4. Discussion

We hypothesised that natural biofunctional food ingredients would show potential to modulate many metabolic responses. By creating a diet enriched with bioactive ingredients, a higher reduction in visceral adipose tissue and the regulation of procoagulant parameters were expected. Unfortunately, not all patients showed willingness to cooperate. Patients who did not follow the dietary recommendations formed the control group. The most effective average weight loss was observed in Group III patients following the authors' diet, rich in bioflavonoids, vitamins, minerals, *n*-3 acids, and synbiotics. There was a reduction in visceral fat in Group II and a stronger reduction in Group III. Patients in Group I, with no diet, did not achieve weight loss. Visceral fat highly correlates with vascular problems [19]. Group III, whose patients received *n*-3/*n*-6 fatty acids in the ratio (*n*-6)/(*n*-3) PUFA = 1.84, showed statistically significant differences in the triglyceride concentrations after the diet period.

As shown in our study, normalisation of blood pressure occurred in the group following the authors' dietary recommendations. Compared to the control group, statistically significant differences were obtained in Group II and Group III. Despite the application of BIB, persistently high systolic and diastolic blood pressure values were indicated in patients who did not follow the dietary recommendations and did not reduce their body weight (Group I). It can be stated that dietary intervention is necessary. Appropriate dietary components not only support a reduction in adipose tissue but also regulate blood pressure values in patients [20,21]. The development of obesity is accompanied by increased inflammatory activation in adipose tissue.

Increased levels of inflammatory markers are found in obese patients [22,23]. Analyses of isoprostanes are used to monitor oxidative stress levels and eliminate disease factors such as arteriosclerosis, insulin-dependent diabetes, hypercholesterolaemia, obesity, neurodegenerative diseases, asthma, or pneumonia [24–27]. Chronic platelet activation, that is, the increased synthesis of pro-aggregating isoprostanes as a result of increased oxidative stress, has been observed in obese individuals [28,29]. Weight loss decreased the synthesis of pro-aggregating isoprostanes. 8-iso-PGF2α has been shown to stimulate smooth-muscle contraction in the blood vessel wall of the brain, heart, and kidneys. Under conditions of oxidative stress, 8-iso-PGF2α may increase the risk of embolic complications in patients with cardiovascular disease, including ischaemic stroke or myocardial infarction [30]. Numerous studies have shown significantly higher isoprostane concentrations in obese individuals compared to control groups with normal BMI values. A positive correlation with waist circumference and visceral fatness has been shown [31,32]. Obesity is accompanied by oxidative stress. Metabolic diseases exacerbate lipid peroxidation, increasing isoprostane concentrations. It is known that some dietary components, such as vitamins, plant pigments, bioflavonoids, tannins, fatty acids, and other compounds belonging to the phytamine group, are bioactive compounds which were intentionally increased in our diet. A significant decrease in serum isprostane levels was observed in patients with inflammatory diseases who received higher doses of anthocyanins, derived from berries, strawberries, currants, and blueberries, through their diet [33–35]. Oxidative stress is characterised by a lack of capacity of the body's natural antioxidant defence mechanisms. Therefore, the structure of the designed diet with antioxidant features was not random. In the group of patients receiving the author's diet, enriched with flavonoids, vitamins, and *n*-3 fatty acids, the obtained values of blood isoprostane concentrations were the lowest compared to the results of serum isoprostane concentrations before balloon implantation and weight loss surgery. When comparing the isoprostane concentrations before and after balloon removal, statistically significant differences were obtained between Groups I and II, I and III, and II and III. No changes in isoprostane concentrations after the follow-up period were seen in the control group of patients not adhering to dietary recommendations. In Group II, the isoprostane concentrations decreased, but this was strongest in Group III.

The favourable *n*-6/*n*-3 EFA ratio was 4:1. Arachidonic acid metabolism leads to the formation of prostacyclin PGI2. It is used in the prevention of atherosclerosis. It exhibits anticoagulant effects, dilates arteries, prevents platelet aggregation, and dissolves preformed thrombi. In addition, its immunomodulatory and anti-inflammatory properties have also been discovered [36]. Visceral obesity promotes thrombus formation and induces endothelial dysfunction. Obese patients show an impaired protective response to nitric oxide and prostacyclin [37]. In obese patients, there is a reduced ability of prostacyclins to activate cAMP synthesis and prevent platelet aggregation [38]. A high correlation between the presence of hypertension and low serum prostacyclin levels has been indicated [39]. In our study, in Group III patients, there was a significant reduction in visceral adipose tissue, an improvement in blood pressure values and TG levels, and elevated prostacyclin levels compared to the results obtained in Group II and I patients. The improvement in test parameters may indicate a reduction in the patients' risk of atherosclerosis. Analysing the results of the obtained prostacyclin concentrations, statistically significant differences were indicated between Groups I and II, I and III, and, significantly, II and III.

The endocrine–enzymatic system, AAR (renin–angiotensin–aldosterone), is responsible for the regulation of blood pressure and water–electrolyte balance. It acts systemically in the bloodstream and locally, e.g., in blood vessel walls or the myocardium [40]. Clinical trials targeting angiotensinogen in the treatment of hypertension and heart failure are ongoing. Higher levels of angiotensinogen correlate strongly with the incidence of obesity and hypertension, especially in women [41,42]. As adipocytes are a local source of angiotensinogen synthesis [43], their concentration as angiotensin prohormones was determined in our study. Increased adipose tissue contributes to the systemic up-regulation of the AAR system. This promotes inflammation, lipogenesis, and reactive oxygen species production and impairs insulin signalling. The increase in blood concentrations of AAR components mediated by adipocytes is the link between hypertension and inflammation in obesity. This is an example of a vicious circle. In our own observation, initially, in the presence of obesity, all patients had high levels of angiotensinogen. After BIB and a diet based on natural regulating ingredients, a significant decrease in the angiotensin prohormone was found. An association of high-sugar and high-fat diets with the components of the AAR has been established [44]. In contrast, regulating the proportion of polyunsaturated acids (PUFAs) in one's diet positively regulates blood pressure. Gamma linolenic acid attenuates the development of hypertension. It lowers the plasma aldosterone levels and decreases the density and affinity of AT1 in the adrenal glands [45]. A diet rich in omega-3, compared to a diet poor in this acid, reduces hypertension through the modulation of the RAS [46]. Group III, in which patients received n-3/n-6 fatty acids at a ratio of (n-6)/(n-3) PUFA = 1.84, showed beneficial changes in angiotensinogen regulation.

The potential involvement of the overproduction of plasminogen activator inhibitor type 1 in the pathogenesis of increased prothrombotic activity in obese individuals has been analysed. It has been shown that the adipocytes of an obese person produce 2-fold more PAI-1 than in a lean person. PAI-1 is also identified with the development of atherosclerosis and coronary thrombosis accompanying atherosclerotic plaque rupture [47]. PAI-1 is considered an acute-phase protein. Its regulation is influenced by pro-inflammatory factors (IL-1, TNFα) but also angiotensin II and IV [48,49]. Elevated levels of PAI-1 have been shown to highly correlate with coronary artery disease and myocardial infarction [50,51]. In our study, patients receiving a diet rich in antioxidant compounds showed the lowest plasminogen concentrations.

Haemorheological properties are used in the diagnosis of cardiovascular diseases. A prominent parameter is blood viscosity. The viscosity value is mainly influenced by the morphotic elements of the blood and its properties, in addition to changes in temperature and blood flow velocity [18].

Severe haemorheological disorders are diagnosed in the presence of obesity. Obese patients show increased viscosity values and decreased rheological values for blood flow velocity, especially through the capillaries. This results in increased peripheral resistance and, thus, the need for haemodynamic adaptation.

This study showed that, after a diet rich in antioxidants, the surface area of visceral fat decreases, which had a direct effect on the decrease in blood viscosity. Adipocytes are connected to capillaries. Their excess forces the synthesis of newly formed vessels. This leads to an increase in the vascular bed area. Vascular reactivity is altered. Under typical stimuli, they do not contract or contract insufficiently [2]. This results in higher systolic blood pressure values, increased left ventricular contractile force, overload, and hypertrophy. The higher the BMI values, the higher the circulating blood volume in the body. At the same time, the haematocrit index highly correlates with increased body fat [2]. Due to impaired blood flow through adipose tissue, a weaker organ blood flow is observed [52]. The increase in venous pressure probably depends on the slower outflow of blood from the large veins and the right half of the heart. Oxygen's concentration in venous blood is markedly reduced [52]. In our study, the dependence of blood viscosity on the visceral fat area (VFA) was indicated. A decrease in the VFA values was obtained, thereby lowering the apparent blood viscosity values, regulating the prothrombotic parameters, and improving the haemorheological properties of the patients' blood.

The study shows that the BIB procedure, followed by dietary support, is an effective method of weight reduction. By modifying the diet, enriching it with natural bioactive ingredients, significantly better fat reduction results and favourable values for cardiovascular parameters were achieved.

5. Conclusions

At the beginning of follow-up, obese patients showed unfavourable values for triglycerides, blood pressure, and prothrombotic indices. Using a functional diet, a significant reduction in visceral fat was achieved. A decrease in VFA was shown to reduce whole-blood viscosity. Furthermore, this study showed a significant effect of bioactive components on prothrombotic parameters in obese patients. The improvement in the parameters analysed may indicate a reduction in the risk of atherosclerosis in these patients.

Author Contributions: Methodology, E.B.B.; Validation, E.B.B.; Formal analysis, E.B.B.; Investigation, E.B.B.; Resources, E.B.B. and J.L.; Data curation, E.B.B.; Writing—original draft, E.B.B.; Writing—review & editing, E.B.B.; Project administration, J.L. All authors have read and agreed to the published version of the manuscript.

Funding: This research received no external funding.

Institutional Review Board Statement: This research project received the approval of the Bioethics Committee of the Regional Chamber of Physicians in Szczecin on 6 May 2015 (consent no. OIL-Sz/Mf/KB/452/06/05/2015).

Informed Consent Statement: Written informed consent was obtained from the patient(s) for participation in the study and publication.

Data Availability Statement: The original contributions presented in this study are included in the article. Further inquiries can be directed to the corresponding author.

Conflicts of Interest: The authors of this paper report no conflicts of interest.

References

1. Alcala, M.; Calderon-Dominguez, M.; Bustos, E.; Ramos, P.; Casals, N.; Serra, D.; Viana, M.; Herrero, L. Increased inflammation, oxidative stress and mitochondrial respiration in brown adipose tissue from obese mice. *Sci. Rep.* **2017**, *7*, 16082. [CrossRef]
2. Czech, A.; Bernas, M.; Tatoń, J. Cardiovascular symptoms of overweight and obesity. *Endokrynol. Otyłość I Zaburzenia Przemiany Materii.* **2007**, *3*, 85–94.
3. Balejko, E.; Bogacka, A.; Pawlus, J.; Lichota, J. Effects of Bioactive Dietary Components on Changes in Lipid and Liver Parameters in Women after Bariatric Surgery and Procedures. *Nutrients* **2024**, *16*, 1379. [CrossRef]
4. Balejko, E.; Balejko, J.; Plust, D. Assessment of the Effect of Dietary Modifications and Bioenteric Intragastric Balloon Treatment on the Changes of Some Morphological and Biochemical Parameters in Obese Patients. *Ann. Nutr. Metab.* **2018**, *73*, 290–301. [CrossRef] [PubMed]

5. Yue, T.; Sheng, Q.; Luo, Y.; Xiao, Z.; Wang, Y.; Song, W.; Yan, M.; Niu, H.; Zang, T.; Li, N. Biflavonoids and Oligomeric Flavonoids from Food. In *Handbook of Dietary Phytochemicals*; Xiao, J., Sarker, S., Asakawa, Y., Eds.; Springer: Singapore, 2020; ISBN 978-981-13-1745-3. [CrossRef]
6. Fernandez, A.Z.; Demaria, E.J.; Tichansky, D.S.; Kellum, J.M.; Wolfe, L.G.; Meador, J.; Sugerman, H.J. Multivariate analysis of risk factors for death following gastric bypass for treatment of morbid obesity. *Ann. Surg.* **2004**, *239*, 698–703. [CrossRef]
7. Sjostrom, L.; Narbro, K.; Sjostrom, C.D.; Karason, K.; Larsson, B.; Wedel, H.; Lystig, T.; Sullivan, M.; Bouchard, C.; Carlsson, B.; et al. Swedish obese subjects study. Effects of bariatric surgery on mortality in swedish obese study. *Engl. J. Med.* **2007**, *8*, 741–752. [CrossRef] [PubMed]
8. Gulinac, M.; Miteya, D.G.; Petshevska-Sekulovska, M.; Novakov, I.P.; Svetozar, A.; Peruhova, M.; Snegarova, V.; Kabakchieva, P.; Assyoy, Y.; Vasiley, G.; et al. Long-term effectiveness, outcomes and complications of bariatric surgery. *World J. Clin. Cases* **2023**, *6*, 4504–4512. [CrossRef]
9. Re, R.; Pellegrini, N.; Proteggente, A.; Pannal, A.A.; Yang, M.; Rice-Evans, C. Antioxidant activity applying an improved ABTS radical cation decolorization assay. *Free Rad. Biol. Med.* **1999**, *26*, 1231–1237. [CrossRef]
10. Benzie, I.F.F.; Strain, J.J. The ferric reducing ability of plasma FRAP as a measure of antioxidant power: The FRAP assay. *Anal. Bioch.* **1996**, *239*, 70–76. [CrossRef]
11. Cheung, L.M.; Cheung, P.C.K.; Ooi, V.E.C. Antioxidant activity and total phenolics of edible mushroom extracts. *Food Chem.* **2003**, *81*, 249–255. [CrossRef]
12. *PN-ISO 4121:1998*; Sensory Analysis—Methodology—Evaluation of Food Products by Methods Using Scales. Polish Committee for Standardisation: Warsaw, Polish, 1998.
13. *PN-ISO 11036:1999*; Sensor Analysis—Methodology—Texture Profile. Polish Committee for Standardisation: Warsaw, Polish, 1999.
14. *PN-ISO 6658:1998*; Sensory Analysis—Methodology—General Guidance. Polish Committee for Standardisation: Warsaw, Polish, 1998.
15. *PN-ISO 6564:1999*; Sensory Analysis—Methodology—Flavour Profile Methods. Polish Committee for Standardisation: Warsaw, Polish, 1999.
16. Bąk Sosnowska, M.; Białkowska, M.; Bogdanski, P.; Chomiuk, T.; Gałązka Sobotka, M.; Holecki, M.; Jarosińska, A.; Jezierska, M.; Kamiński, P.; Kłoda, K.; et al. Clinical recommendations for the management of patients with obesity 2022—The position of the Polish Society for the Treatment of Obesity. *Med. Prakt.* **2022**, *5*, 1–87.
17. Banach, M.; Jankowski, P.; Jóźwiak, J.; Cybulska, B.; Windak, A.; Guzik, T.; Mamcarz, A.; Broncel, M.; Tomasik, T. *PTL/KLRwP/PTK Guidelines for the Management of Lipid Disorders for Family Physicians*; Polish Society of Lipidology: Poznań, Poland, 2016.
18. Pryzwan, T.; Dolibog, P.; Kierszniok, K.; Pietrzyk, B. Blood rheological properties and methods of their measurement. *Ann. Acad. Med. Siles.* **2024**, *78*, 1–10. [CrossRef]
19. Claria, J.; Lopez-Vicario, C.; Rius, B.; Titos, E. Pro-resolving actions of SPM in adipose tissue biology. *Mol. Asp. Med.* **2017**, *58*, 83–92. [CrossRef] [PubMed]
20. Savica, V.; Bellinghieri, G.; Kopple, J. The Effect of Nutrition on Blood Pressure. *Annu. Rev. Nutr.* **2010**, *30*, 365–401. [CrossRef] [PubMed]
21. Kucharska, A.; Gajewska, D.; Kiedrowski, M.; Sińska, B.; Juszczyk, G.; Czerw, A.; Augustynowicz, A.; Bobiński, K.; Deptała, A.; Niegowska, J. The impact of individualised nutritional therapy according to DASH diet on blood pressure, body mass, and selected biochemical parameters in overweight/obese patients with primary arterial hypertension: A prospective randomised study. *Kardiol. Polska.* **2018**, *1*, 158–165. [CrossRef]
22. German, A.J.; Ryan, V.H.; German, A.C.; Wood, I.S.; Trayhurn, P. Obesity, its associated disorders and the role of inflammatory adipokines in companion animals. *Vet. J.* **2010**, *185*, 4–9. [CrossRef]
23. Skinner, A.C.; Steiner, M.J.; Henderson, F.W.; Perrin, E.M. Multiple markers of inflammation and weight status: Cross-sectional analyses throughout childhood. *Pediatrics* **2010**, *125*, e801–e809. [CrossRef]
24. Morrow, J.D.; Minton, T.A.; Badr, K.F.; Roberts, L.J. Evidence that the F2-isoprostane, 8-epi-prostaglandin F2 alpha, is formed in vivo. *Biochim. Biophyts. Acta* **1994**, *1210*, 244–248. [CrossRef]
25. Souvignet, C.; Cracowski, J.L.; Stanke-Labesque, F.; Bessard, G. Are Isoprostans a Clinical Marker for Antioxidant Drug Investigation. *Fundam. Clin. Pharmacol.* **2000**, *14*, 1–10. [CrossRef]
26. Erve, J.; Kadiiska, B.; London, J.; Mason, P. Classifying oxidative stress by F_2-isoprostane levels across human diseases: A meta-analysis. *Redox Biol.* **2017**, *12*, 582–599. [CrossRef]
27. Erve, J. Strategies to decrease oxidative stress biomarker levels in human medical conditions: A meta-analysis on 8-iso-prostaglandin $F_{2\alpha}$. *Redox Biol.* **2018**, *17*, 282–296.
28. Davi, G.; Guagnano, M.; Ciabattoni, G. Platelet activation in obese women: Role of inflammation and oxidant stress. *JAMA* **2002**, *288*, 2008–2014. [CrossRef] [PubMed]
29. Davi, G.; Patrono, C. Platelet activation and atherotrombosis. *N. Engl. J. Med.* **2007**, *357*, 2482–2494. [CrossRef]
30. Patrignani, P. Aspirin insensitive eicosanoid biosynthesis in cardiovascular disease. *Thromb. Res.* **2003**, *110*, 281–286. [CrossRef]
31. Dennis, B.; Ergul, A.; Gower, B.; Allison, J.; Davis, C. Oxidative stress and cardiovascular risk in overweight children in an exercise intervention program. *Child. Obes.* **2013**, *9*, 15–21. [CrossRef]

32. Kaikkonen, J.; Vilppo, T.; Asikainen, J.; Voutilainen, S.; Kurl, S.; Salonen, J. Fatty acids as determinants of in-vivo lipid peroxidation: The EFFGE study in Eastern Finnish hypertensive and non-hypertensive subjects. *Ann. Med.* **2013**, *5*, 455–464. [CrossRef] [PubMed]
33. Khan, F.; Ray, S.; Craigie, A.; Kennedy, G.; Hill, A.; Barton, K.; Broughton, J.; Belch, J. Lowering of oxidative stress improves endothelial function in healthy subjects with habitually low intake of fruit and vegetables: A randomized controlled trial of antioxidant- and polyphenol-rich blackcurrant juice. *Free Radic. Biol. Med.* **2014**, *72*, 232–237. [CrossRef] [PubMed]
34. Alvarez-Suarez, J.; Giampieri, F.; Tulipani, S.; Casoli, T.; Stefano, G.; González-Paramás, A.; Santos-Buelga, C.; Busco, F.; Quiles, J.; Cordero, M.; et al. One-month strawberry-rich anthocyanin supplementation ameliorates cardiovascular risk, oxidative stress markers and platelet activation in humans. *J. Nutr. Biochem.* **2014**, *25*, 289–294. [CrossRef]
35. McAnulty, S.; Nieman, D.; Dumke, C.; Shooter, L.; Henson, D.; Utter, A.; Milne, G.; McAnulty, S.R. Effect of blueberry ingestion on natural killer cell counts, oxidative stress, and inflammation prior to and after 2.5 h of running. *Appl. Physiol. Nutr. Metab.* **2011**, *36*, 976–984. [CrossRef]
36. Mitchell, J.; Kirkby, N. Eicosanoids, prostacyclin and cyclooxygenase in the cardiovascular system. *BJP* **2018**, *176*, 1038–1050. [CrossRef]
37. Grundy, S.M. Obesity, metabolic syndrome, and coronary atherosclerosis. *Circulation* **2002**, *105*, 2696–2698. [CrossRef] [PubMed]
38. Russo, I.; Traversa, M.; Bonomo, K.; De Salve, A.; Matiello, L.; Del Mese, P.; Doronzo, G.; Cavalot, F.; Trovati, M.; Anfossi, G. In centralo, weight loss restores platelet sensitivity to nitric oxide and prostacyclin. *Obesity* **2010**, *18*, 788–797. [CrossRef] [PubMed]
39. Yuriy, V.; Marushko, Y.; Tatiana, V.; Hyschak, T. Endothelium dependent factors of vasoconstriction (thromboxane B and vasodilation (6-prostaglandin F1α in children with primary arterial hypertension. *Puls Uczelni.* **2015**, *3*, 3–6. [CrossRef]
40. Ferrario, C.; Martell, N.; Yunis, C.; Flack, J.; Chappell, M.; Brosnihan, K.; Dean, R.; Fernandez, A.; Novikov, S.; Pinillas, C.; et al. Characterization of angiotensin-(1-7) in the urine of normal and essential hypertensive subjects. *Am. J. Hypertens* **1998**, *11*, 137–146. [CrossRef]
41. Umemura, S.; Nyui, N.; Tamura, K.; Hibi, K.; Yamaguchi, S.; Nakamaru, M.; Ishigami, T.; Yabana, M.; Kihara, M.; Inoue, S.; et al. Plasma angiotensinogen concentrations in obese patients. *Clin. Trial.* **1997**, *10*, 629–633. [CrossRef]
42. Trainor, P.; Brambatti, M.; Carlisle, S.; Mullick, A.; Shah, S.; Kahlon, T.; Otero Mostacero, D.; Mousavi, H.; Morgan, E.; Tami, Y.; et al. Blood Levels of Angiotensinogen and Hypertension in the Multi-Ethnic Study of Atherosclerosis. *J. Am. Coll. Cardiol.* **2023**, *81*, 1248–1259. [CrossRef] [PubMed]
43. Van Harmelen, M.; Ariapart, P.; Hoffstedt, J.; Lundkvist, I.; Bringman, S.; Arner, P. Increased Adipose Angiotensinogen Gene Expression in Human Obesity. *Obesity* **2000**, *4*, 337–341. [CrossRef]
44. Frigolet, M.; Torres, N.; Tovar, A. The renin–angiotensin system in adipose tissue and its metabolic consequences during obesity. *J. Nutr. Biochem.* **2013**, *24*, 2003–2015. [CrossRef]
45. Engler, M.; Engle, M.B.; Erickson, S.; Paul, S. Dietary gamma-linolenic acid lowers blood pressure and alters aortic reactivity and cholesterol metabolism in hypertension. *J. Hypertens.* **1992**, *10*, 1197–1204. [CrossRef]
46. Engler, M.; Schambelan, M.; Engle, R.M.; Ball, D.; Goodfriend, T. Effects of dietary gamma-linolenic acid on blood pressure and adrenal angiotensin receptors in hypertensive rats. *Proc. Soc. Exp. Bio Med.* **1998**, *218*, 234–237. [CrossRef]
47. Mertens, I.; Van der Planken, M.; Corthouts, B. Visceral fat is a determinant of PAI-1 activity in diabetic and non-diabetic overweight and obese women. *Horm. Metab. Res.* **2001**, *33*, 602–660. [CrossRef] [PubMed]
48. Araki, S.; Dobashi, K.; Kubo, K.; Yamamoto, Y.; Asayama, K.; Shirahata, A. N-acetylcysteine attenuates TNF-alpha induced changes in secretion of interleukin-6, plasminogen activator inhibitor-1 and adiponectin from 3T3- -L1 adipocytes. *Life Sci.* **2006**, *79*, 2405–2412. [CrossRef] [PubMed]
49. Eren, M.; Painter, C.; Gleaves, L. Tissue- and agonist-specific regulation of human and murine plasminogen activator inhibitor-1 promoters in transgenic mice. *J. Thromb. Haemost.* **2003**, *1*, 2389–2396. [CrossRef]
50. Collet, J.; Montalescot, G.; Vicaut, E. Acute release of plasminogen activator inhibitor-1 in ST-segment elevation myocardial infarction predicts mortality. *Circulation* **2003**, *108*, 391–394. [CrossRef]
51. Song, C.; Burgess, S.; Eicher, J.; O'Donnell, C.; Johnson, A. Causal Effect of Plasminogen Activator Inhibitor Type 1 on Coronary Heart Disease. *J. Am. Heart Assoc.* **2017**, *6*, 6. [CrossRef]
52. Collis, T.; Devereux, R.B.; Roman, M.J. Relations of stroke volume and cardiac output to body composition: The Strong Heart Study. *Circulation* **2001**, *103*, 820–825. [CrossRef]

nutrients

MDPI

Article

Cannabidiol Enhances Mitochondrial Metabolism and Antioxidant Defenses in Human Intestinal Epithelial Caco-2 Cells

Alejandro Bravo Iniguez [1], Qi Sun [1], Qiaorong Cui [1], Min Du [2] and Mei-Jun Zhu [1,*]

[1] School of Food Science, Washington State University, Pullman, WA 99164, USA; a.bravoiniguez@wsu.edu (A.B.I.); qi.sun6@wsu.edu (Q.S.); qiaorong.cui@wsu.edu (Q.C.)
[2] Department of Animal Sciences, Washington State University, Pullman, WA 99164, USA; min.du@wsu.edu
* Correspondence: meijun.zhu@wsu.edu; Fax: +(509)-335-4815

Abstract: Background: The reintroduction of hemp production has resulted in increased consumption of cannabidiol (CBD) products, particularly CBD oil, yet their effects on intestinal health are not fully understood. Proper mitochondrial function and antioxidant defenses are vital for maintaining the intestinal epithelial barrier. AMP-activated protein kinase (AMPK) and peroxisome proliferator-activated receptor gamma coactivator (PGC)1α are key mediators of mitochondrial metabolism. Methods & Results: Using Caco-2 cells, we found that CBD oil promoted AMPK phosphorylation, upregulated differentiation markers, and enhanced PGC1α/SIRT3 mitochondrial signaling. CBD oil reduced reactive oxygen species production and increased antioxidant enzymes. Moreover, CBD oil also increased levels of citrate, malate, and succinate—key metabolites of the tricarboxylic acid cycle—alongside upregulation of pyruvate dehydrogenase and isocitrate dehydrogenase 1. Similarly, pure CBD induced metabolic and antioxidant signaling. Conclusions: CBD enhances mitochondrial metabolic activity and antioxidant defense in Caco-2 cells, making it a promising candidate for treating intestinal dysfunction.

Keywords: AMPK; antioxidant activity; cannabidiol; intestinal epithelium; mitochondria

1. Introduction

The intestinal epithelium is a self-renewing, tightly regulated barrier essential for nutrient absorption, tissue protection, and the coordination of immune responses [1]. Dysregulation of the epithelium, such as impaired barrier function, is characteristic of gut diseases such as inflammatory bowel disease (IBD) [2]. The intestinal epithelium is constantly renewed, depending on the proliferation and differentiation of stem cells residing in crypts. Extensive oxidative metabolic transition and mitochondrial biogenesis occur during epithelial differentiation [3]. Proper cellular energetics, orchestrated by functional mitochondria, are vital for epithelial health. Mice with enhanced intestinal oxidative phosphorylation and ATP production develop less severe colitis than their peers [4]. In humans, patients with colitis exhibit decreased levels of mitochondrial respiratory chain complexes compared to healthy counterparts [5].

Mitochondria are major producers of free radicals, and their dysfunction results in increased oxidative damage that contributes to the progression of pathological intestinal conditions [6]. The inability of the body to balance the production of free radicals, such as reactive oxygen species (ROS), with appropriate defense mechanisms results in damaging oxidative stress, which plays a role in the pathology of numerous conditions including IBD [7]. Managing ROS is an intricate process vital for maintaining redox homeostasis. The body employs various defenses to control levels of oxidative stress, including antioxidative enzymes, whose levels can be influenced by lifestyle factors and aging [8]. Patients with gastrointestinal diseases exhibit both elevated levels of ROS and decreased activity of antioxidative enzymes [9]. Inhibition of these mediators increases ROS levels and promotes inflammasome activation [10]. Thus, it is important to identify strategies to maintain adequate antioxidative activity.

NF-E2-related factor 2 (NRF2) is an important transcription factor that regulates the expression of antioxidant genes and controls ROS levels in the intestines [11]. NRF2 is regulated by Kelch-like ECH-associated protein 1 (KEAP1), and it binds to the antioxidant response element (ARE) to promote the expression of enzymes such as NAD(P)H quinone dehydrogenase 1 (NQO1) and heme oxygenase 1 (HO-1) [12]. In the canonical pathway of NRF2 activation, oxidative stress decreases the ability of KEAP1 to sequester NRF2, allowing NRF2 to translocate to the nucleus and activate ARE-driven gene expression [13]. Alternatively, the scaffold protein p62 plays a role in the noncanonical activation of NRF2 by disrupting the interaction between KEAP1 and NRF2 [14,15]. Several upstream pathways regulate NRF2/HO-1, including phosphoinositide 3-kinase (PI3K)/AKT [16], p38 mitogen-activated protein kinase (MAPK) [17], and AMP-activated protein kinase (AMPK) [18]. AMPK also regulates intestinal differentiation and barrier function through the activation of caudal type homeobox 2 (CDX2) [19], illustrating the interconnection between metabolic and antioxidant pathways, which is essential for maintaining intestinal homeostasis.

Cannabidiol (CBD) is a non-psychoactive cannabinoid found in cannabis that can reach the gut depending on the method of delivery [20,21]. In the human colorectal carcinoma cell line Caco-2, CBD reduces ROS production and improves transepithelial resistance upon exposure to H_2O_2 or H_2O_2/Fe^{2+} [22,23]. We previously demonstrated that mice with dextran sodium sulfate (DSS)-induced colitis that received 200 mg kg^{-1} CBD in their diet for 5 weeks showed reduced inflammation, associated with increased phosphorylation and activation of AMPK [24].

Several studies showed the effects of CBD in improving mitochondrial energetics. Hippocampal neurons treated with 5 μM CBD exhibit greater mitochondrial respiration compared to untreated neurons [25]. In mice, intraperitoneal injections of CBD ameliorate the negative effects of doxorubicin on mitochondrial biogenesis in the myocardium [26]. The effect of CBD on intestinal mitochondrial energetics and signaling remains to be elucidated. This study used human epithelial Caco-2 cells to investigate the effects of CBD on the antioxidant and metabolic activities of colon cells. We hypothesized that CBD treatment upregulates the phosphorylation of AMPK in Caco-2 cells, which is accompanied by enhanced mitochondrial energetics and the upregulation of antioxidant enzymes.

2. Materials and Methods

2.1. Cannabidiol

A commercial full-spectrum CBD hemp oil was purchased directly from the manufacturer (Nutra Pure LLC, Vancouver, WA, USA). As per the test results provided by the producer, analysis by a published method [27] determined the CBD content in the oil to be 18.3 mg/mL, while other cannabinoids were below the limit of quantification. A CBD stock solution (10 mM) was prepared by diluting the oil in dimethylsulfoxide (DMSO) (VWR, Radnor, PA, USA). Additionally, cannabidiol (≥98%) was purchased from Cayman Chemical (Ann Arbor, MI, USA) and dissolved in DMSO to prepare a stock solution at 10 mM. All CBD stock solutions were stored at −20 °C.

2.2. Cell Line

Caco-2 cells were obtained from the American Type Culture Collection (Manassas, VA, USA). The cells were routinely cultured in Dulbecco's modified Eagle medium (DMEM) (Sigma; St. Louis, MO, USA) supplemented with 10% fetal bovine serum (Sigma), 100 units/mL of penicillin G, and 100 μg/mL of streptomycin (Sigma) at 37 °C with 5% CO_2. Cells were seeded into 12-well plates for analyses unless stated otherwise. Following overnight incubation, cells were treated with or without 10μM CBD for 1, 2, or 4 days.

2.3. Intracellular Reactive Oxygen Species (ROS) Measurement

Levels of intracellular ROS were evaluated as previously described [28]. In brief, Caco-2 cells were seeded into 96-well plates and cultured in complete DMEM overnight, followed by incubation with media containing the cell-permeable fluorescent probe, 2,7-dichlorofluorescein diacetate (H_2DCFDA) (MilliporeSigma, Burlington, MA, USA), for 45 min. After replacing the media, the cells were treated with or without CBD and with or without H_2O_2 for 24 h. Fluorescence was measured using a BioTek Synergy H1 microplate reader (Agilent Technologies, Palo Alto, CA, USA) with an excitation wavelength of 485 nm and an emission wavelength of 530 nm. The fluorescence of H_2DCFDAobtained from the plate reader was reported in arbitrary units and normalized to the values of the untreated controls.

2.4. Immunoblotting

Proteins were extracted from Caco-2 cells, separated by SDS-PAGE gels, and transferred onto nitrocellulose membrane as described previously [29,30]. Antibodies against acetyl-CoA carboxylase (ACC), AMPK, CDX2, catalase, HO-1, isocitrate dehydrogenase 1 (IDH1), p62, p-ACC, p-AMPK, pyruvate dehydrogenase (PDH), sirtuin3 (SIRT3), and superoxide dismutase (SOD)2 were purchased from Cell Signaling Technology (Danvers, MA, USA). The antibody for claudin-2 was purchased from Thermo Fisher Scientific (Waltham, MA, USA), while the antibody for proliferator-activated receptor gamma coactivator 1 alpha (PGC1α) was obtained from ProteinTech (Rosemont, IL, USA). The antibody for SOD1 was purchased from Santa Cruz Biotechnology (Dallas, TX, USA). Horseradish peroxidase-coupled anti-rabbit or anti-mouse IgGs were used for visualization by chemiluminescence. Band density quantification was normalized to the signal of β-tubulin. Data are presented as relative to the control group.

2.5. Quantitative Reverse Transcription PCR (qRT-PCR) Analysis

Total mRNA was extracted from Caco-2 cells or animal tissue using Trizol Reagent (Thermo Fisher) per the manufacturer's instructions. Reverse transcription was completed using an iScript™ kit (Bio-Rad, Hercules, CA, USA). The produced cDNA served as templates for qRT-PCR analysis, using SYBR Green Master Mix (Bio-Rad) and a CFX96™ Real-Time PCR Detection System (Bio-Rad). The primers used for qRT-PCR are listed in Supplementary Materials Table S1, with 18S serving as the housekeeping gene.

2.6. Tricarboxylic Acid Cycle Metabolite Analysis by GC-MS

Caco-2 cells were treated with or without CBD for 2 days. Following the treatment period, the cells were collected and processed for analysis using an Agilent 7890B gas chromatography system equipped with a 5977A single-quadrupole mass spectrometer and a 7693 autosampler system (Agilent Technologies), following previously established procedures [31]. The column utilized was an HP-5 ms column (30 m $\times$ 250 μM i.d., 0.25 μM film thickness; Agilent Technologies). Ribitol, purchased from Sigma, served as the internal standard. Citrate and malate standards were purchased from Sigma. The succinate standard was purchased from ThermoFisher Scientific. The relative abundances of metabolites were determined by calculating the area ratios of the target peaks to the ribitol (internal standard) peaks.

2.7. Statistical Analysis

Statistical analysis was performed as previously described using GraphPad Prism 7 [31]. The data are presented relative to the control group as mean $\pm$ SEM (standard error of the mean). Treatments were compared using either a two-tailed Student's t-test or one-way ANOVA. Significance was determined using a p-value ≤ 0.05.

3. Results

3.1. CBD Oil Induces Phosphorylation of AMPK and Upregulates Downstream Targets

Incubation with CBD oil increased the phosphorylation of AMPK compared to controls (Figure 1A). CBD oil treatment also enhanced the phosphorylation of ACC, a downstream target of AMPK (Figure 1A). Moreover, at both the protein and mRNA levels, CBD oil exhibited a promotive effect on CDX2, another downstream target of AMPK and the key transcription factor governing epithelial differentiation (Figure 1B,C). Additionally, exposure to CBD oil decreased the protein level of claudin-2 and increased the mRNA level of zonula occludens-1 (*ZO-1*), indicating positive effects on epithelial differentiation and barrier function (Figure 1B,C).

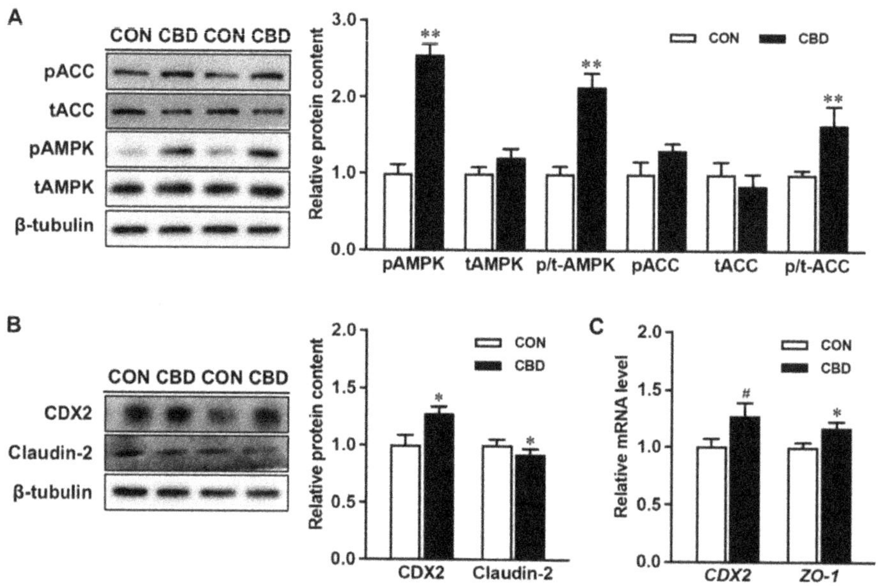

Figure 1. Cannabidiol oil induces AMP-activated protein kinase (AMPK) phosphorylation and upregulates downstream targets overseeing epithelial differentiation and barrier function. (**A**) Protein contents of p-AMPK, t-AMPK, p- acetyl-CoA carboxylase (ACC), and t-ACC. (**B**) The protein content of caudal type homeobox 2 (CDX2) and claudin-2. (**C**) mRNA expression of *CDX2* and zonula occludens-1 (*ZO-1*). CON: untreated Caco-2 cells; CBD: Caco-2 cells treated with 10 μM cannabidiol (CBD) oil. Mean ± SEM, $n = 4$, #: $p \leq 0.10$; *: $p \leq 0.05$; **: $p \leq 0.01$.

3.2. CBD Oil Treatment Promotes Mitochondrial Energetics

CBD oil treatment increased protein contents of the transcription factor Peroxisome proliferator-activated receptor gamma coactivator 1 alpha (PGC1α) and the deacetylase enzyme, Sirtuin 3 (SIRT3) (Figure 2A). Treatment with CBD oil also upregulated the mRNA expression of the mitochondrially encoded NADH-ubiquinone oxidoreductase core subunit 1 (*mtND1*), *mtND4*, and cytochrome b (*CYTB*) (Figure 2B). Additionally, CBD oil promoted oxidative phosphorylation in Caco-2 cells. GC-MS analysis of key tricarboxylic acid (TCA) cycle metabolites revealed elevated contents of citrate, malate, and succinate in CBD-treated cells (Figure 3A). This effect was accompanied by increased protein contents of isocitrate dehydrogenase 1 (IDH1), an enzyme in the TCA cycle responsible for the conversion of isocitrate to alpha-ketoglutarate (αKG), and pyruvate dehydrogenase (PDH), the enzyme responsible for directing pyruvate to oxidative phosphorylation (Figure 3B).

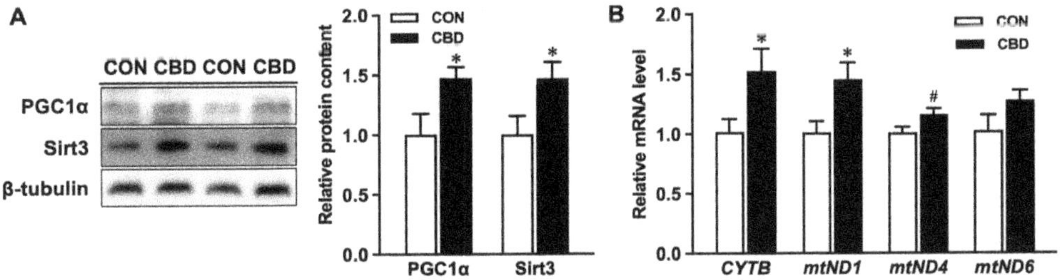

Figure 2. Cannabidiol oil enhances mitochondrial signaling and activity. (**A**) Protein contents of Peroxisome proliferator-activated receptor gamma coactivator 1 alpha (PGC1α) and sirtuin 3 (SIRT3). (**B**) mRNA expression of cytochrome b (*CYTB*), mitochondrially encoded NADH-ubiquinone oxidoreductase core subunit 1 (*mtND1*), *mtND4*, and *mtND6*. CON: untreated Caco-2 cells; CBD: Caco-2 cells treated with 10 µM cannabidiol (CBD) oil. Mean ± SEM, $n = 4$, #: $p \leq 0.10$; *: $p \leq 0.05$.

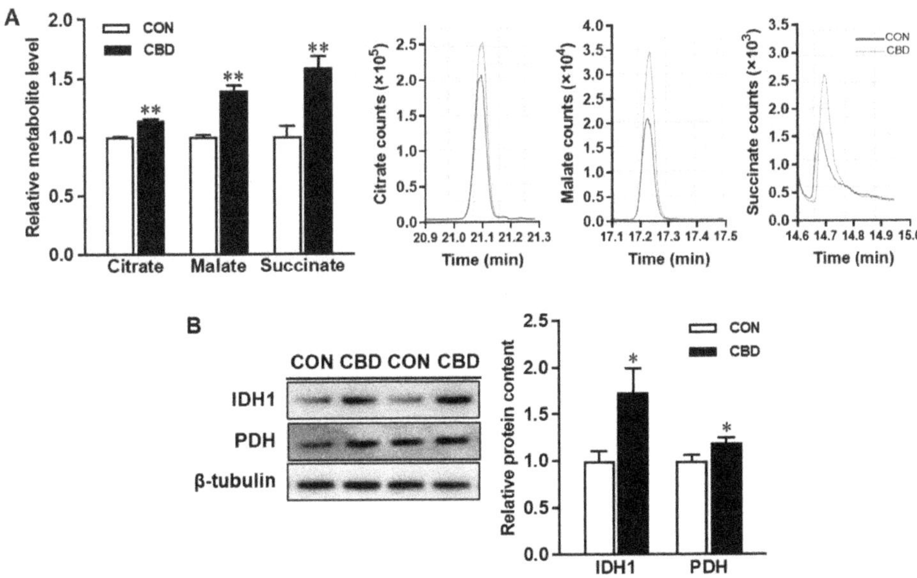

Figure 3. Cannabidiol oil alters tricarboxylic acid (TCA) cycle activity and metabolite levels. (**A**) Levels of TCA cycle metabolites obtained from gas chromatography/mass spectrometry and representative peaks for citrate, malate, and succinate. (**B**) Protein contents of isocitrate dehydrogenase 1 (IDH1) and pyruvate dehydrogenase (PDH). CON: untreated Caco-2 cells; CBD: Caco-2 cells treated with 10 µM cannabidiol (CBD) oil. Mean ± SEM, $n = 3$–4, *: $p \leq 0.05$; **: $p \leq 0.01$.

3.3. CBD Oil Suppresses ROS Formation and Upregulates Antioxidants

Treating Caco-2 cells with 10 µM CBD oil lowered levels of ROS with or without the H_2O_2 challenge (Figure 4A). CBD oil also induced the expression of the antioxidant enzyme, HO-1 (Figure 4B). Moreover, the protein contents of catalase SOD1, and to a lesser extent SOD2, were increased (Figure 4B). At the mRNA level, CBD oil upregulated heme oxygenase 1 gene (*HMOX1*) and *SOD2* expression (Figure 4C).

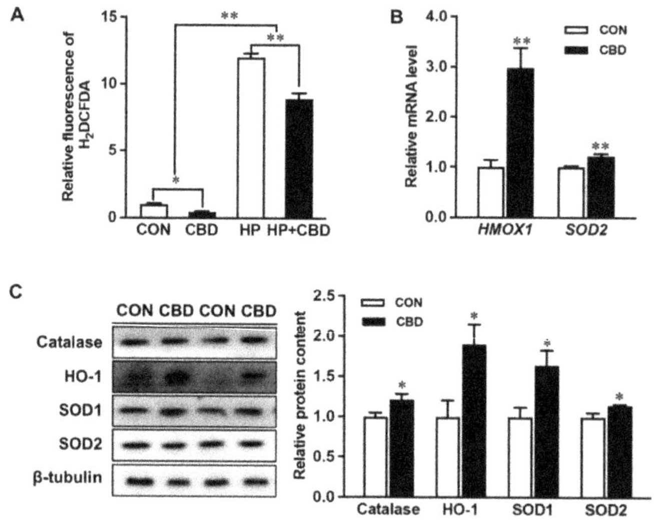

Figure 4. Cannabidiol oil mitigates reactive oxygen species (ROS) production and enhances antioxidant expression. (**A**) ROS production measured with H2DCFDA. (**B**) mRNA expression of heme oxygenase 1 gene (*HMOX1*) and superoxide dismutase 2 (*SOD2*). (**C**) Protein contents of catalase, heme oxygenase 1 (HO-1), SOD1, and SOD2. CON: untreated Caco-2 cells; CBD: Caco-2 cells treated with 10 μM cannabidiol (CBD) oil. Mean ± SEM, $n = 4$, *: $p \leq 0.05$; **: $p \leq 0.01$.

3.4. Exposure to CBD Oil Upregulates NRF2 Signaling Pathway

Consistent with the upregulation of HO-1 protein and mRNA (*HMOX1*) levels in CBD oil-treated cells, the mRNA expression of *NRF2* was also elevated (Figure 5A). Accordingly, the mRNA level of *NQO1*, a target gene of NRF2 encoding the detoxification enzyme, was increased in CBD oil-treated cells. The content of p62 was also upregulated in CBD oil-treated cells (Figure 5B).

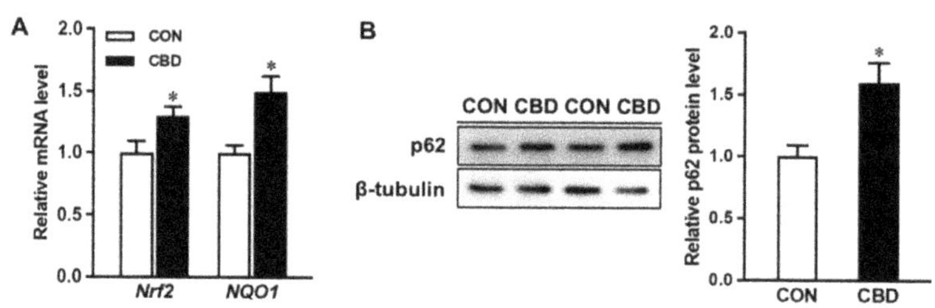

Figure 5. Cannabidiol oil targets NF-E2-related factor 2 (NRF2) signaling. (**A**) mRNA expression of *Nrf2* and NAD(P)H quinone dehydrogenase 1 (*NQO1*). (**B**) Protein content of p62. CON: untreated Caco-2 cells; CBD: Caco-2 cells treated with 10 μM cannabidiol (CBD) oil. Mean ± SEM, $n = 4$, *: $p \leq 0.05$.

3.5. Pure CBD Promotes Signaling Pathways Similarly to CBD Oil

While CBD is the major constituent in commercial CBD oils, it is common for them to contain other cannabinoids at much smaller levels. To confirm that CBD exerts positive effects on AMPK and related signaling, Caco-2 cells were further treated with 10 μM pure CBD compound. Consistently, pure CBD increased phosphorylation of AMPK and upregulated SIRT3 (Figure 6A). Pure CBD exerted beneficial effects on antioxidant signaling, elevating protein levels of HO-1 and catalase (Figure 6B), as well as the mRNA expression of

NQO1 and *SOD2* (Figure 6C). Together these findings show that CBD targets mitochondrial and antioxidant signaling to improve intestinal epithelial health.

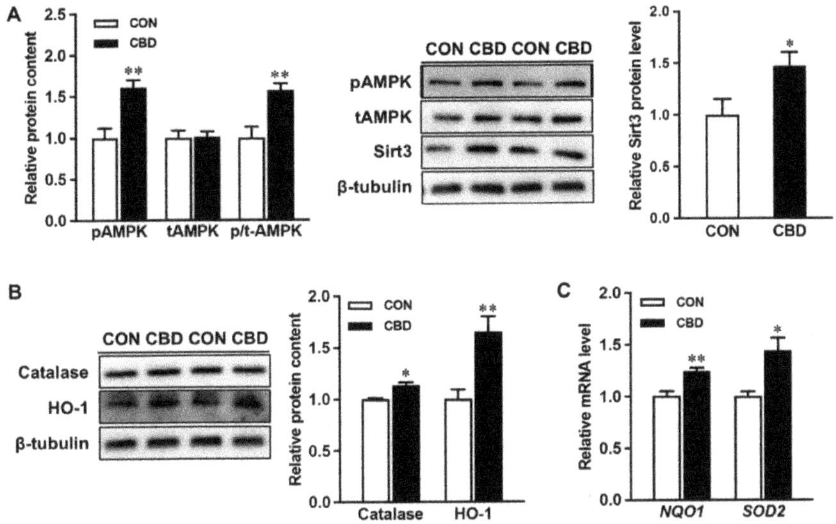

Figure 6. Pure cannabidiol induces phosphorylation of AMPK and upregulates both mitochondrial and antioxidant signaling. (**A**) Protein contents of p- AMP-activated protein kinase (AMPK), t-AMPK, and sirtuin3 (SIRT3). (**B**) Protein contents of catalase and heme oxygenase 1 (HO-1). (**C**) mRNA expression of NAD(P)H quinone dehydrogenase 1 (*NQO1*) and superoxide dismutase 2 (*SOD2*). CON: untreated Caco-2 cells; CBD: Caco-2 cells treated with 10 μM cannabidiol (CBD). Mean ± SEM, $n = 4$, *: $p \leq 0.05$; **: $p \leq 0.01$.

4. Discussion

The average daily intake of CBD among adults who regularly consume CBD-containing products is 50.3 ± 40.7 mg [32]. CBD exhibits poor bioavailability, hampered by its low water solubility [33], and approximately one-third of orally ingested CBD is excreted in the feces [34]. Pharmacokinetic studies with humans have largely focused on serum levels following oral intake. After ingesting an oral capsule containing 10 mg CBD, the maximum concentration measured in serum was 2.47 ng/mL (7.85 nM) [35]. In a different study, a higher oral dose of 200 mg CBD resulted in a maximum serum concentration of 148 ng/mL (470.63 nM) [36]. Multiple factors affect the oral absorption of CBD, including the presence of lipids, which enhances CBD absorption [35,37]. Following oral delivery in rats, CBD levels detected in intestinal lymph far exceeded serum levels, being 250-fold greater [37], suggesting the importance of understanding its effects on gut epithelial health. If the same holds following oral intake in humans, micromolar levels of CBD may be obtainable in the intestines.

Among CBD product consumers, drops are the most commonly used type of product [38]. In this experiment, we employed commercially available CBD oil to best reflect exposure to the average consumers. This CBD oil utilized hempseed oil as a carrier, which contains essential fatty acids and bioactive tocopherols [39]. To account for this, we also utilized pure CBD in the present study. Given that concentration and dosage instructions differ between CBD products, the use of a single treatment condition is a limitation of the present study.

The present study employed the Caco-2 cell line to model the intestinal epithelium of the colon. The cultured cells mimic epithelial differentiation upon achieving confluence which dictated our choice of treatment times [19]. In Caco-2 cell monolayers, 10 μM CBD treatment potentiated the recovery of transepithelial resistance following a challenge with ethylenediaminetetraacetic acid [40]. CBD treatment also resulted in elevated mRNA expression of *ZO-1* [40]. In the present study, CBD oil treatment similarly increased the mRNA expression of *ZO-1*. In agreement with our previous observations in mice with DSS-induced colitis, CBD oil and pure CBD increased the phosphorylation of AMPK in Caco-2 cells. AMPK, a regulator of energy homeostasis, plays a key role in the homeostasis of the intestinal epithelium [19,41]. Considering that AMPK activation upregulates differentiation transcription factor CDX2 at both the mRNA and protein levels [42], the ability of both CBD to activate AMPK and upregulate its downstream targets holds promise as a means to strengthen intestinal epithelial barrier function.

Proper differentiation relies on mitochondrial function, characterized by increased oxidative phosphorylation and mitochondrial biogenesis as epithelial cells differentiate and migrate away from the crypts [43,44]. In intestinal epithelial cells, the proinflammatory signal, tumor necrosis factor-alpha (TNF-α) induces mitochondrial dysfunction, reducing oxygen consumption and mitochondrial membrane potential [45]. It also decreases the expression of alkaline phosphatase, a marker for intestinal epithelial differentiation [46]. CBD oil treatment upregulated the protein contents of PGC1α and SIRT3, a deacetylase controlling mitochondrial quantity, metabolism, and antioxidant activity [47,48].

Furthermore, CBD oil upregulated the TCA cycle enzyme IDH1, responsible for synthesizing α-ketoglutarate, a vital cofactor for epigenetic modifications that is required for the proper differentiation of epithelial cells [49,50]. PDH was also increased in CBD-treated cells. Impairment of the PDH in cancer cells favors greater glycolysis at the expense of mitochondrial oxidation [51]. Changes to TCA cycle enzyme protein levels were accompanied by changes in metabolite levels. CBD treatment increased the intracellular content of citrate, malate, and succinate in Caco-2 cells. In pigs, succinate increased epithelial tight junction protein content [52]. Together, our findings suggest that CBD enhances mitochondrial metabolic function in colon epithelial cells, which may contribute to its beneficial effects.

CBD oil treatment ameliorated ROS production in Caco-2 cells both in the presence or absence of H_2O_2. This effect was accompanied by the upregulation of antioxidant enzymes including HO-1. Similar observations of NRF2 and HO-1 induction have been reported in keratinocytes [53] and endothelial cells [54] treated with 1 and 6 μM CBD, respectively. The scaffold protein p62 can facilitate the degradation of KEAP1, impeding its interactions with NRF2 [55], and also participates in a positive feedback loop with NRF2 [56]. We observed the upregulation of p62 in CBD oil-treated Caco-2 cells. Given its role in regulating the expression of important antioxidants and detoxification enzymes, proper NRF2 expression is crucial for intestinal health. Mice deficient in NRF2 showed increased susceptibility to colitis induced by DSS [57]. Conversely, the activation of NRF2 and the upregulation of its antioxidant signaling pathways in mice mitigated DSS-induced disease severity [58]. In DSS-induced colitis, HO-1 is negatively regulated by transcription factor BTB domain and CNC homology 1 (BACH1), and mice deficient in BACH1 display elevated levels of colonic HO-1 and decreased disease activity [59]. Co-treatment with ZnPP, an inhibitor of HO-1, negated the beneficial effects of BACH1 deficiency on disease activity [59]. Promoting proper expression of HO-1 and other antioxidant defenses through phytochemicals such as CBD may serve as an approach for combatting intestinal dysfunction.

5. Conclusions

As the burden generated by IBD persists, multiple prevention and treatment strategies are needed. The beneficial effects of plant-derived bioactive compounds, such as resveratrol, which ameliorate disease activity of IBD in experimental animal models of colitis, are partially through the promotion of antioxidant activity [60]. Our findings showcase the ability of CBD to combat oxidative stress in colonic epithelial cells, shedding light on potential mechanisms behind these effects such as induction of NRF2/HO-1 signaling. Additionally, our study reveals that CBD treatment impacts mitochondrial energetics and related signaling, inducing the phosphorylation of AMPK and the upregulation of PGC1α and SIRT3. Given that the maintenance of the intestinal epithelium is an energy-demanding process reliant on intricate regulation of mitochondrial activity, our findings help understand the potential of CBD to safeguard against intestinal epithelial dysregulation.

Supplementary Materials: The following supporting information can be downloaded at: https://www.mdpi.com/article/10.3390/nu16223843/s1, Table S1: Lists the primer sets used for quantitative RT-qPCR. References [61–63] are cited in Supplementary Materials.

Author Contributions: Conceptualization, A.B.I. and M.-J.Z.; methodology, A.B.I., Q.S., Q.C. and M.-J.Z.; validation, M.-J.Z.; formal analysis, A.B.I.; writing—original draft preparation, A.B.I.; writing—review and editing, M.D. and M.-J.Z.; visualization, A.B.I. and M.-J.Z.; supervision, M.-J.Z.; project administration, M.-J.Z.; funding acquisition, M.-J.Z. All authors have read and agreed to the published version of the manuscript.

Funding: This research was funded by the United States Department of Agriculture-National Institute of Food and Agriculture (USDA-NIFA) (2018-67017-27517), the Washington State University Agricultural Research Center Emerging Research Issues Competitive Grant, and the Washington State University Dedicated Marijuana Account (DMAc) Grant.

Institutional Review Board Statement: Not applicable.

Informed Consent Statement: Not applicable.

Data Availability Statement: The data presented in this study are available upon request.

Conflicts of Interest: The authors declare no conflicts of interest.

References

1. Martini, E.; Krug, S.M.; Siegmund, B.; Neurath, M.F.; Becker, C. Mend your fences: The epithelial barrier and its relationship with mucosal immunity in inflammatory bowel disease. *Cell Mol. Gastroenterol. Hepatol.* **2017**, *4*, 33–46. [CrossRef] [PubMed]
2. Zeissig, S.; Burgel, N.; Gunzel, D.; Richter, J.; Mankertz, J.; Wahnschaffe, U.; Kroesen, A.J.; Zeitz, M.; Fromm, M.; Schulzke, J.D. Changes in expression and distribution of claudin 2, 5 and 8 lead to discontinuous tight junctions and barrier dysfunction in active Crohn's disease. *Gut* **2007**, *56*, 61–72. [CrossRef] [PubMed]
3. Rodríguez-Colman, M.J.; Schewe, M.; Meerlo, M.; Stigter, E.; Gerrits, J.; Pras-Raves, M.; Sacchetti, A.; Hornsveld, M.; Oost, K.C.; Snippert, H.J.; et al. Interplay between metabolic identities in the intestinal crypt supports stem cell function. *Nature* **2017**, *543*, 424–427. [CrossRef]
4. Bär, F.; Bochmann, W.; Widok, A.; von Medem, K.; Pagel, R.; Hirose, M.; Yu, X.; Kalies, K.; König, P.; Böhm, R.; et al. Mitochondrial gene polymorphisms that protect mice from colitis. *Gastroenterology* **2013**, *145*, 1055–1063. [CrossRef]
5. Sifroni, K.G.; Damiani, C.R.; Stoffel, C.; Cardoso, M.R.; Ferreira, G.K.; Jeremias, I.C.; Rezin, G.T.; Scaini, G.; Schuck, P.F.; Dal-Pizzol, F.; et al. Mitochondrial respiratory chain in the colonic mucosal of patients with ulcerative colitis. *Mol. Cell Biochem.* **2010**, *342*, 111–115. [CrossRef] [PubMed]
6. Beltrán, B.; Nos, P.; Dasí, F.; Iborra, M.; Bastida, G.; Martínez, M.; O'Connor, J.E.; Sáez, G.; Moret, I.; Ponce, J. Mitochondrial dysfunction, persistent oxidative damage, and catalase inhibition in immune cells of naïve and treated Crohn's disease. *Inflamm. Bowel Dis.* **2010**, *16*, 76–86. [CrossRef] [PubMed]
7. Vona, R.; Pallotta, L.; Cappelletti, M.; Severi, C.; Matarrese, P. The impact of oxidative stress in human pathology: Focus on gastrointestinal disorders. *Antioxidants* **2021**, *10*, 201. [CrossRef]
8. Bouzid, M.A.; Filaire, E.; Matran, R.; Robin, S.; Fabre, C. Lifelong voluntary exercise modulates age-related changes in oxidative stress. *Int. J. Sports Med.* **2018**, *39*, 21–28. [CrossRef] [PubMed]
9. Jiménez, P.; Piazuelo, E.; Sánchez, M.T.; Ortego, J.; Soteras, F.; Lanas, A. Free radicals and antioxidant systems in reflux esophagitis and Barrett's esophagus. *World J. Gastroenterol.* **2005**, *11*, 2697–2703. [CrossRef]
10. Chen, Z.; Zhong, H.; Wei, J.; Lin, S.; Zong, Z.; Gong, F.; Huang, X.; Sun, J.; Li, P.; Lin, H.; et al. Inhibition of Nrf2/HO-1 signaling leads to increased activation of the NLRP3 inflammasome in osteoarthritis. *Arthritis Res. Ther.* **2019**, *21*, 300. [CrossRef]
11. Hochmuth, C.E.; Biteau, B.; Bohmann, D.; Jasper, H. Redox regulation by Keap1 and Nrf2 controls intestinal stem cell proliferation in Drosophila. *Cell Stem Cell* **2011**, *8*, 188–199. [CrossRef] [PubMed]
12. Sun, Z.; Zhang, S.; Chan, J.Y.; Zhang, D.D. Keap1 controls postinduction repression of the Nrf2-mediated antioxidant response by escorting nuclear export of Nrf2. *Mol. Cell Biol.* **2007**, *27*, 6334–6349. [CrossRef] [PubMed]
13. Silva-Islas, C.A.; Maldonado, P.D. Canonical and non-canonical mechanisms of Nrf2 activation. *Pharmacol. Res.* **2018**, *134*, 92–99. [CrossRef] [PubMed]

14. Komatsu, M.; Kurokawa, H.; Waguri, S.; Taguchi, K.; Kobayashi, A.; Ichimura, Y.; Sou, Y.S.; Ueno, I.; Sakamoto, A.; Tong, K.I.; et al. The selective autophagy substrate p62 activates the stress responsive transcription factor Nrf2 through inactivation of Keap1. *Nat. Cell Biol.* **2010**, *12*, 213–223. [CrossRef]
15. Lau, A.; Wang, X.J.; Zhao, F.; Villeneuve, N.F.; Wu, T.; Jiang, T.; Sun, Z.; White, E.; Zhang, D.D. A noncanonical mechanism of Nrf2 activation by autophagy deficiency: Direct interaction between Keap1 and p62. *Mol. Cell Biol.* **2010**, *30*, 3275–3285. [CrossRef]
16. Xu, L.; He, S.; Yin, P.; Li, D.; Mei, C.; Yu, X.; Shi, Y.; Jiang, L.; Liu, F. Punicalagin induces Nrf2 translocation and HO-1 expression via PI3K/Akt, protecting rat intestinal epithelial cells from oxidative stress. *Int. J. Hyperth.* **2016**, *32*, 465–473. [CrossRef]
17. Hsu, J.T.; Kan, W.H.; Hsieh, C.H.; Choudhry, M.A.; Schwacha, M.G.; Bland, K.I.; Chaudry, I.H. Mechanism of estrogen-mediated intestinal protection following trauma-hemorrhage: p38 MAPK-dependent upregulation of HO-1. *Am. J. Physiol. Regul. Integr. Comp. Physiol.* **2008**, *294*, R1825–R1831. [CrossRef]
18. Liu, X.M.; Peyton, K.J.; Shebib, A.R.; Wang, H.; Korthuis, R.J.; Durante, W. Activation of AMPK stimulates heme oxygenase-1 gene expression and human endothelial cell survival. *Am. J. Physiol. Heart Circ. Physiol.* **2011**, *300*, H84–H93. [CrossRef]
19. Sun, X.; Yang, Q.; Rogers, C.J.; Du, M.; Zhu, M.J. AMPK improves gut epithelial differentiation and barrier function via regulating Cdx2 expression. *Cell Death Differ.* **2017**, *24*, 819–831. [CrossRef]
20. Birnbaum, A.K.; Karanam, A.; Marino, S.E.; Barkley, C.M.; Remmel, R.P.; Roslawski, M.; Gramling-Aden, M.; Leppik, I.E. Food effect on pharmacokinetics of cannabidiol oral capsules in adult patients with refractory epilepsy. *Epilepsia* **2019**, *60*, 1586–1592. [CrossRef]
21. Lucas, C.J.; Galettis, P.; Schneider, J. The pharmacokinetics and the pharmacodynamics of cannabinoids. *Br. J. Clin. Pharmacol.* **2018**, *84*, 2477–2482. [CrossRef] [PubMed]
22. Cocetta, V.; Governa, P.; Borgonetti, V.; Tinazzi, M.; Peron, G.; Catanzaro, D.; Berretta, M.; Biagi, M.; Manetti, F.; Dall'Acqua, S.; et al. Cannabidiol isolated from *Cannabis sativa* L. protects intestinal barrier from in vitro inflammation and oxidative stress. *Front. Pharmacol.* **2021**, *12*, 641210. [CrossRef] [PubMed]
23. Borrelli, F.; Aviello, G.; Romano, B.; Orlando, P.; Capasso, R.; Maiello, F.; Guadagno, F.; Petrosino, S.; Capasso, F.; Di Marzo, V.; et al. Cannabidiol, a safe and non-psychotropic ingredient of the marijuana plant Cannabis sativa, is protective in a murine model of colitis. *J. Mol. Med.* **2009**, *87*, 1111–1121. [CrossRef] [PubMed]
24. Sun, Q.; Bravo Iniguez, A.; Tian, Q.; Du, M.; Zhu, M.J. Dietary cannabidiol activates PKA/AMPK signaling and attenuates chronic inflammation and leaky gut in DSS-induced colitis mice. *Mol. Nutr. Food Res.* **2024**, *68*, e2300446. [CrossRef]
25. Sun, S.; Hu, F.; Wu, J.; Zhang, S. Cannabidiol attenuates OGD/R-induced damage by enhancing mitochondrial bioenergetics and modulating glucose metabolism via pentose-phosphate pathway in hippocampal neurons. *Redox Biol.* **2017**, *11*, 577–585. [CrossRef]
26. Hao, E.; Mukhopadhyay, P.; Cao, Z.; Erdélyi, K.; Holovac, E.; Liaudet, L.; Lee, W.S.; Haskó, G.; Mechoulam, R.; Pacher, P. Cannabidiol protects against doxorubicin-induced cardiomyopathy by modulating mitochondrial function and biogenesis. *Mol. Med.* **2015**, *21*, 38–45. [CrossRef]
27. Giese, M.W.; Lewis, M.A.; Giese, L.; Smith, K.M. Method for the analysis of cannabinoids and terpenes in cannabis. *J. AOAC Int.* **2015**, *98*, 1503–1522. [CrossRef]
28. Xue, Y.; Zhang, S.; Du, M.; Zhu, M.-J. Dandelion extract suppresses reactive oxidative species and inflammasome in intestinal epithelial cells. *J. Funct. Foods* **2017**, *29*, 10–18. [CrossRef]
29. Xue, Y.; Zhang, H.; Wang, H.; Hu, J.; Du, M.; Zhu, M.-J. Host inflammatory response inhibits Escherichia coli O157: H7 adhesion to gut epithelium through augmentation of mucin expression. *Infect. Immun.* **2014**, *82*, 1921–1930. [CrossRef]
30. Zhu, M.J.; Du, M.; Hess, B.W.; Means, W.J.; Nathanielsz, P.W.; Ford, S.P. Maternal nutrient restriction upregulates growth signaling pathways in the cotyledonary artery of cow placentomes. *Placenta* **2007**, *28*, 361–368. [CrossRef]
31. Sun, Q.; Bravo Iniguez, A.; Tian, Q.; Du, M.; Zhu, M.-J. PGC-1α in mediating mitochondrial biogenesis and intestinal epithelial differentiation promoted by purple potato extract. *J. Funct. Foods* **2022**, *98*, 105291. [CrossRef]
32. Kaufmann, R.; Aqua, K.; Lombardo, J.; Lee, M. Observed impact of long-term consumption of oral cannabidiol on liver function in healthy adults. *Cannabis Cannabinoid Res.* **2023**, *8*, 148–154. [CrossRef] [PubMed]
33. Perucca, E.; Bialer, M. Critical aspects affecting cannabidiol oral bioavailability and metabolic elimination, and related clinical implications. *CNS Drugs* **2020**, *34*, 795–800. [CrossRef]
34. Wall, M.E.; Perez-Reyes, M. The metabolism of delta 9-tetrahydrocannabinol and related cannabinoids in man. *J. Clin. Pharmacol.* **1981**, *21*, 178S–189S. [CrossRef]
35. Millar, S.A.; Stone, N.L.; Yates, A.S.; O'Sullivan, S.E. A systematic review on the pharmacokinetics of cannabidiol in humans. *Front. Pharmacol.* **2018**, *9*, 1365. [CrossRef]
36. Taylor, L.; Crockett, J.; Tayo, B.; Morrison, G. A phase 1, open-label, parallel-group, single-dose trial of the pharmacokinetics and safety of cannabidiol (CBD) in subjects with mild to severe hepatic impairment. *J. Clin. Pharmacol.* **2019**, *59*, 1110–1119. [CrossRef]
37. Zgair, A.; Lee, J.B.; Wong, J.C.M.; Taha, D.A.; Aram, J.; Di Virgilio, D.; McArthur, J.W.; Cheng, Y.K.; Hennig, I.M.; Barrett, D.A.; et al. Oral administration of cannabis with lipids leads to high levels of cannabinoids in the intestinal lymphatic system and prominent immunomodulation. *Sci. Rep.* **2017**, *7*, 14542. [CrossRef] [PubMed]

38. Goodman, S.; Wadsworth, E.; Schauer, G.; Hammond, D. Use and perceptions of cannabidiol products in Canada and in the United States. *Cannabis Cannabinoid Res.* **2022**, *7*, 355–364. [CrossRef]
39. Alonso-Esteban, J.I.; González Fernández, M.; Fabrikov, D.; Sánchez-Mata, M.; Torija-Isasa, E.; Guil-Guerrero, J. Fatty acids and minor functional compounds of hemp (*Cannabis sativa* L.) seeds and other Cannabaceae species. *J. Food Compos. Anal.* **2022**, *115*, 104962. [CrossRef]
40. Alhamoruni, A.; Lee, A.C.; Wright, K.L.; Larvin, M.; O'Sullivan, S.E. Pharmacological effects of cannabinoids on the Caco-2 cell culture model of intestinal permeability. *J. Pharmacol. Exp. Ther.* **2010**, *335*, 92–102. [CrossRef]
41. Olivier, S.; Diounou, H.; Pochard, C.; Frechin, L.; Durieu, E.; Foretz, M.; Neunlist, M.; Rolli-Derkinderen, M.; Viollet, B. Intestinal epithelial AMPK deficiency causes delayed colonic epithelial repair in DSS-induced colitis. *Cells* **2022**, *11*, 590. [CrossRef] [PubMed]
42. Sun, X.; Du, M.; Navarre, D.A.; Zhu, M.-J. Purple potato extract promotes intestinal epithelial differentiation and barrier function by activating AMP-activated protein kinase. *Mol. Nutr. Food Res.* **2018**, *62*, 1700536. [CrossRef] [PubMed]
43. Stringari, C.; Edwards, R.A.; Pate, K.T.; Waterman, M.L.; Donovan, P.J.; Gratton, E. Metabolic trajectory of cellular differentiation in small intestine by Phasor Fluorescence Lifetime Microscopy of NADH. *Sci. Rep.* **2012**, *2*, 568. [CrossRef]
44. D'Errico, I.; Salvatore, L.; Murzilli, S.; Lo Sasso, G.; Latorre, D.; Martelli, N.; Egorova, A.V.; Polishuck, R.; Madeyski-Bengtson, K.; Lelliott, C.; et al. Peroxisome proliferator-activated receptor-gamma coactivator 1-alpha (PGC1alpha) is a metabolic regulator of intestinal epithelial cell fate. *Proc. Natl. Acad. Sci. USA* **2011**, *108*, 6603–6608. [CrossRef] [PubMed]
45. Baregamian, N.; Song, J.; Bailey, C.E.; Papaconstantinou, J.; Evers, B.M.; Chung, D.H. Tumor necrosis factor-alpha and apoptosis signal-regulating kinase 1 control reactive oxygen species release, mitochondrial autophagy, and c-Jun N-terminal kinase/p38 phosphorylation during necrotizing enterocolitis. *Oxid. Med. Cell Longev.* **2009**, *2*, 297–306. [CrossRef] [PubMed]
46. Malo, M.S.; Biswas, S.; Abedrapo, M.A.; Yeh, L.; Chen, A.; Hodin, R.A. The pro-inflammatory cytokines, IL-1beta and TNF-alpha, inhibit intestinal alkaline phosphatase gene expression. *DNA Cell Biol.* **2006**, *25*, 684–695. [CrossRef]
47. Torrens-Mas, M.; Hernández-López, R.; Pons, D.G.; Roca, P.; Oliver, J.; Sastre-Serra, J. Sirtuin 3 silencing impairs mitochondrial biogenesis and metabolism in colon cancer cells. *Am. J. Physiol. Cell Physiol.* **2019**, *317*, C398–C404. [CrossRef]
48. Zhao, C.; Sakaguchi, T.; Fujita, K.; Ito, H.; Nishida, N.; Nagatomo, A.; Tanaka-Azuma, Y.; Katakura, Y. Pomegranate-derived polyphenols reduce reactive oxygen species production via SIRT3-mediated SOD2 activation. *Oxid. Med. Cell Longev.* **2016**, *2016*, 2927131. [CrossRef]
49. Tran, T.Q.; Hanse, E.A.; Habowski, A.N.; Li, H.; Gabra, M.B.I.; Yang, Y.; Lowman, X.H.; Ooi, A.M.; Liao, S.Y.; Edwards, R.A.; et al. α-Ketoglutarate attenuates Wnt signaling and drives differentiation in colorectal cancer. *Nat. Cancer* **2020**, *1*, 345–358. [CrossRef]
50. Tian, Q.; Iniguez, A.B.; Sun, Q.; Wang, H.; Du, M.; Zhu, M.J. Dietary alpha-ketoglutarate promotes epithelial metabolic transition and protects against DSS-induced colitis. *Mol. Nutr. Food Res.* **2021**, *65*, e2000936. [CrossRef]
51. McFate, T.; Mohyeldin, A.; Lu, H.; Thakar, J.; Henriques, J.; Halim, N.D.; Wu, H.; Schell, M.J.; Tsang, T.M.; Teahan, O.; et al. Pyruvate dehydrogenase complex activity controls metabolic and malignant phenotype in cancer cells. *J. Biol. Chem.* **2008**, *283*, 22700–22708. [CrossRef] [PubMed]
52. Li, X.; Mao, M.; Zhang, Y.; Yu, K.; Zhu, W. Succinate modulates intestinal barrier function and inflammation response in pigs. *Biomolecules* **2019**, *9*, 486. [CrossRef] [PubMed]
53. Jastrząb, A.; Gęgotek, A.; Skrzydlewska, E. Cannabidiol regulates the expression of keratinocyte proteins involved in the inflammation process through transcriptional regulation. *Cells* **2019**, *8*, 827. [CrossRef] [PubMed]
54. Böckmann, S.; Hinz, B. Cannabidiol promotes endothelial cell survival by Heme Oxygenase-1-mediated autophagy. *Cells* **2020**, *9*, 1703. [CrossRef] [PubMed]
55. Copple, I.M.; Lister, A.; Obeng, A.D.; Kitteringham, N.R.; Jenkins, R.E.; Layfield, R.; Foster, B.J.; Goldring, C.E.; Park, B.K. Physical and functional interaction of sequestosome 1 with Keap1 regulates the Keap1-Nrf2 cell defense pathway. *J. Biol. Chem.* **2010**, *285*, 16782–16788. [CrossRef]
56. Jain, A.; Lamark, T.; Sjøttem, E.; Larsen, K.B.; Awuh, J.A.; Øvervatn, A.; McMahon, M.; Hayes, J.D.; Johansen, T. p62/SQSTM1 is a target gene for transcription factor NRF2 and creates a positive feedback loop by inducing antioxidant response element-driven gene transcription. *J. Biol. Chem.* **2010**, *285*, 22576–22591. [CrossRef]
57. Khor, T.O.; Huang, M.T.; Kwon, K.H.; Chan, J.Y.; Reddy, B.S.; Kong, A.N. Nrf2-deficient mice have an increased susceptibility to dextran sulfate sodium-induced colitis. *Cancer Res.* **2006**, *66*, 11580–11584. [CrossRef]
58. Zhang, Y.; Yan, T.; Sun, D.; Xie, C.; Wang, T.; Liu, X.; Wang, J.; Wang, Q.; Luo, Y.; Wang, P.; et al. Rutaecarpine inhibits KEAP1-NRF2 interaction to activate NRF2 and ameliorate dextran sulfate sodium-induced colitis. *Free Radic. Biol. Med.* **2020**, *148*, 33–41. [CrossRef]
59. Takagi, T.; Naito, Y.; Mizushima, K.; Hirai, Y.; Harusato, A.; Okayama, T.; Katada, K.; Kamada, K.; Uchiyama, K.; Handa, O.; et al. Heme oxygenase-1 prevents murine intestinal inflammation. *J. Clin. Biochem. Nutr.* **2018**, *63*, 169–174. [CrossRef]
60. Yao, J.; Wang, J.Y.; Liu, L.; Li, Y.X.; Xun, A.Y.; Zeng, W.S.; Jia, C.H.; Wei, X.X.; Feng, J.L.; Zhao, L.; et al. Anti-oxidant effects of resveratrol on mice with DSS-induced ulcerative colitis. *Arch. Med. Res.* **2010**, *41*, 288–294. [CrossRef]
61. Spandidos, A.; Wang, X.; Wang, H.; Seed, B. PrimerBank: A resource of human and mouse PCR primer pairs for gene expression detection and quantification. *Nucleic Acids Res.* **2010**, *38*, D792–D799. [CrossRef] [PubMed]

62. Xue, Y.; Du, M.; Zhu, M.-J. Quercetin suppresses NLRP3 inflammasome activation in epithelial cells triggered by Escherichia coli O157:H7. *Free Radic. Biol. Med.* **2017**, *108*, 760–769. [CrossRef] [PubMed]
63. Xue, Y.; Du, M.; Zhu, M.-J. Raspberry extract prevents NLRP3 inflammasome activation in gut epithelial cells induced by pathogenic Escherichia coli. *J. Funct. Foods* **2019**, *56*, 224–231. [CrossRef]

nutrients

MDPI

Article

The Influence of Maceration and Flavoring on the Composition and Health-Promoting Properties of Roasted Coffee

Joanna Grzelczyk [1,*], Grażyna Budryn [1], Krzysztof Kołodziejczyk [2] and Joanna Ziętala [1]

1 Institute of Food Technology and Analysis, Faculty of Biotechnology and Food Sciences, Lodz University of Technology, 90-537 Lodz, Poland; grazyna.budryn@p.lodz.pl (G.B.); 237523@edu.p.lodz.pl (J.Z.)

2 Department of Sugar Industry and Food Safety Management, Faculty of Biotechnology and Food Sciences, Lodz University of Technology, 90-537 Lodz, Poland; krzysztof.kolodziejczyk@p.lodz.pl

* Correspondence: joanna.grzelczyk@p.lodz.pl

Abstract: Over the years, many methods of refining green beans have been developed, including maceration aimed at enriching the coffee aroma and improving the overall quality. This study aimed to evaluate the influence of different methods of maceration (fruit and wine) and the addition of food flavors to coffee beans on antioxidant activity, caffeine, phenolic and organic acid content, as well as health-promoting properties. This research showed that the use of the maceration in melon and apple fruit pulp (100 g of fruit pulp per 100 g of green coffee, incubated for 24 h, coffee roasting at 230 °C, control trial roasted coffee) ensured the highest polyphenol (hydroxycinnamic acids and their esters—chlorogenic acids) content (in melon pulp—13.56 g/100 g d.b. (dry bean); in apple pulp—13.22 g/100 g d.b., $p < 0.05$ (one-way ANOVA)) and antioxidant activity. Melon (92.11%, IC50 = 3.80 mg/mL extract) and apple (84.55%, IC50 = 4.14 mg/mL) showed the highest α-amylase (enzyme concentration 10 μmol/mL) inhibition activity (0.5 mg/mL for both fruits). The addition of food flavors reduced the total content of chlorogenic acids to the range of 4.64 to 6.48 g/100 g d.b. and increased the content of acrylamide and 5-HMF, which positively correlated with a low antioxidant potential compared to the macerated samples and the control. Studies have shown that coffee macerated in the pulp of melon and apple fruit, due to its great potential to inhibit α-amylase in vivo, may have a preventive effect on type II diabetes. This study complements the current knowledge on the potential health-promoting properties of coffee flavored using different methods; further research should include more advanced models for testing these health-promoting properties. Statistical analysis was based on the determination of the average values of six measurements and their standard deviation, as well as on the one-way ANOVA (analysis of variation) and the Pearson correlation coefficient, using Statistic 10.0 software. The significance was defined at $p \leq 0.05$.

Keywords: antioxidant activity; phenolic acids; organic acids; coffee flavoring

1. Introduction

Due to the increasing interest of consumers in flavored coffee products, many methods and practices used by producers have been developed in this regard. Coffee flavoring initially involved the addition of artificial coffee aromas or natural coffee oil, the purpose of which was to enrich the typical coffee aroma. The next practice was using aromas with quite different food fragrance notes [1].

Traditional methods that naturally improve coffee aroma include, for example, roasting coffee at different temperatures, using various techniques for drying green coffee beans, and mixing several types of coffee [1–4]. Recent years have brought progress in food technology, and modernized production methods allow for the development of more ecological, healthy, and tasty products [2,3]. Consumers expect to buy coffee beans of the highest quality and content of health-promoting compounds [2,3]. Roasted coffee reveals one of the most complex aromas (about 1000 different compounds), like roasted cocoa or wine, although formed by different groups of volatiles. Therefore, one of the most common flavored coffees is that with chocolate aroma. On the other hand, the aroma of wine can enrich coffee beans with fruity characteristics, making them milder in taste [4]. Individual volatile compounds (i.e., pyrazines, aldehydes, ketones) are responsible for specific aroma aromas [5–8]. The sugar content in green coffee has a positive effect on the aromatic properties, causing the formation of furans and pyrroles with a caramel aroma. In turn, lactic and acetic acids add a fruity and winey aroma to coffee, as do the presence of alcohols and alpha-damascene [9–11]. Hydroxycinnamic acids and their esters are chemical compounds that ensure antioxidant properties in coffee. Another critical component of coffee beans is dietary fiber, which intensifies intestinal peristalsis. In green coffee beans, it is cellulose and hemicellulose, which are found in larger amounts in Arabica species compared to the content in Robusta. In roasted beans, the fiber fraction also includes Maillard reaction products. Arabica contains up to 3% more lipids than Robusta. The lipids contribute to the aroma of roasted beans by forming some ketones and aldehydes. The lipids contained in coffee consist of include sterols and tocopherols next to the most abundant triacylglycerols [12].

Coffee accompanies the consumer every day. It is consumed most often due to its energy effect. Other reasons include drinking coffee, which is popular in company at meetings or at work. A smaller proportion of consumers still consume coffee due to its health-promoting qualities. If the consumer decides to drink coffee for health reasons, they have expectations regarding its health claims. The process of flavoring coffee can enrich coffee with valuable ingredients, such as vitamins, or micro- and macro-elements, and include supplying health claims on the packaging [13,14]. On the other hand, for coffee connoisseurs, the highest quality of coffee is important while maintaining taste sensations. Therefore, consumers expect useful information such as the procedure for appropriate preparation of coffee depending on the species, the species and place of coffee bush cultivation, the date of coffee bean harvesting, and methods of pre-treatment [15]. An especially important aspect for today's consumer is whether coffee is grown ethically [16].

One of the most frequently chosen coffees by consumers is old brew. Thanks to this method, the coffee has a unique flavor, and the coffee is characterized by a sweet, floral, and fruity taste. The noticeable bitterness and acidity are low. Consumers are increasingly trying flavored coffees. This is due to aroma marketing. Companies create coffee aromas that we associate with pleasant moments or peace. They use a subconscious technique to "program" our decisions. Only a true coffee connoisseur can appreciate the natural note of coffee [17].

Demanding consumers often look for new products and do not become permanently attached to even the best ones. In the field of coffee brands, many flavored coffees have appeared, giving the opportunity to try new flavors. The most natural improvement in aroma can be achieved by influencing the composition of the beans before roasting [18]. Mechanical drying of green beans after removing the coffee cherry pulp, compared to natural drying, reduces the level of desirable aromatic compounds after roasting. Wetting the beans before roasting or steaming during the process improves the aroma [19–21]. Therefore, one of the methods used in this study was maceration of coffee beans before roasting. The fruit pulp contains high water content, which moisturizes the coffee beans, and together with solutes, this gives it a new, distinctive aroma. After extracting the beans from the fruit and before drying, it is beneficial to leave the beans in high humidity, where the germination can begin triggering the activity of different hydrolases. As a result, sugars, amino acids, and fatty acids are released, which are more reactive during drying and roasting than their precursors [22–25]. Using this method allows for obtaining coffee beans with lower acidity while maintaining high-quality green coffee beans. Therefore, dry-processed coffee was purchased for this research, so that the maceration would improve the properties of the beans.

Nowadays, many advanced methods are used to improve the aroma of coffee beans, including addition of volatile ingredients or their precursors depending on the stage of processing [26]. Initially, it involved enrichment with natural or artificial oils containing characteristic coffee aromas, enhancing the typical coffee smell. This practice continues to present day and applies to instant coffee. Later, the solutions that involved adding other aromas, such as vanilla, nut, chocolate, rum, cherry, and several others were developed [27]. However, coffee connoisseurs look for natural and more healthy solutions than flavoring by adding artificial substances. This has resulted in the emergence of other trends in improving the aroma of coffee and, at the same time, its health-promoting properties. These methods include removing harmful compounds and introducing aroma along with health-promoting substances, as well as maceration or fermentation using various methods [28–31]. The additional steps in processing coffee beans contribute to a higher final product price, making naturally flavored coffees a niche product so far.

For the fermentation of green coffee in fruit, and optionally also in extracted green beans, naturally inhibited coffee bush strains are used. By using microflora naturally adapted to the fermentation of the raw material, advanced fermentation can be achieved to obtain products such as coffee wine or coffee kumiss [32–34].

The content of caffeine, phenolic compounds and other highly bioactive substances may be changed because of natural favoring, which may influence the health-promoting properties of coffee extracts [35–39]. Evaluating the health-promoting properties of naturally flavored coffees may have the beneficial effect of increasing their consumption. Despite previous studies on coffee bean maceration in various media, there is no information in the literature on its effect on the level of hydroxycinnamic acids and their esters, of which coffee is an especially important source in the diet. Previous studies concerned volatile compounds and microbiological safety. Therefore, the novelty of this study is the assessment of the effect of coffee bean flavoring using different methods on the composition of polyphenolic compounds in the final product. The aim of this research was to assess the impact of coffee flavoring vs. maceration in different fruit pulps on properties of coffee extracts. It involved determination of the profile of phenolic and aliphatic acids, as well as antioxidant and α-amylase inhibitory properties.

2. Materials and Methods

2.1. Chemicals and Materials

HPLC- and UHPLC-grade water, formic acid, acetonitrile, methanol, hydroxy-2,5,7,8-tetramethylchroman-2-carboxylic acid (Trolox) (≥97%), 2,4,6-tri(2-pyridyl)-s-triazine (TPTZ, ≥98%), sodium acetate (≥99%), ferric chloride hexahydrate (≥97%), ferrozine (≥97%), 2,2-diphenyl-1-picrylhydrazyl (DPPH, ≥95%), disodium ethylenediaminetetraacetate dihydrate (EDTA, ACS reagent, 99.0–101.0%), and ammonium acetate (≥97%) were purchased from Merck (Darmstadt, Germany). Acrylamide (≥99%), 5-hydroxymethylfurfural (HMF, ≥99%), 5-caffeoylquinic acid (≥99%), lactic acid (≥98%), citric acid (≥98%), malic acid (≥99%), acetic 3,4-dicaffeoylquinic acid (≥98%), ferulic acid (FA, ≥98%), 5-Feruloylquinic acid (5FQ, ≥98%), 4-Feruloylquinic acid (4FQ, ≥98%), 3-Feruloylquinic acid (3FQ, ≥98%), α-amylase from human saliva, and caffeic acid (CA, ≥98%) were purchased from Sigma Aldrich (St. Louis, MO, USA); 3-caffeoylqunic acid (≥99%), 4-caffeoylqunic acid (≥99%), 3,5-dicaffeoylquinic acid (≥99%), and 4,5-dicaffeoylquinic acid (≥99%) were purchased from Phyto Lab (Vestenbergsgreuth, Germany). Ultrapure water (resistivity, 18.2 MΩ cm) was obtained from a Millipore Milli-Q Plus purification system (Bedford, MA, USA). Green Arabica, Brazil Cerrado variety (high-quality harvest, Brazil, Santos region) was purchased from Bero Polska (Gdynia, Poland). The coffee beans came from the 2018 harvest and were subjected to natural dry processing (drying in the sun and warm air). The fruits, food flavorings, and red wine were purchased from a local store.

2.2. Flavoring and Maceration of Coffee Beans

2.2.1. Maceration in Wine

A quantity of 100 g green coffee was roasted at 230 °C for 12 min until the coffee beans were dark in color [40]. Obtaining a dark color (second crack) of the coffee ends the roasting process. The coffee beans were air-cooled. Freshly roasted coffee was cooled to 24 °C and poured with 200 mL of wine into a vessel, mixed, and closed. During maceration in wine, the coffee beans must be completely submerged to ensure that the coffee beans are evenly macerated; 200 mL was enough to immerse 100 g of green coffee beans. The maceration was carried out at a temperature of 4 °C for 12 h, with mixing of the coffee beans after 4 and 8 h. Then, the coffee beans were separated from the wine using a strainer. The procedure was repeated twice. A new portion of the same wine was used after 12 h to avoid the aftertaste of oxidized tannins. Maceration was carried out for a total of 24 h. Three parallel replicates were made from the same bottle of wine. The coffee beans were left on filter paper to evaporate the alcohol, and then the beans were dried at a temperature of 50 °C to ensure 95% solids content. Carlo Rossi (Bols Sp. z o.o., Oborniki, Poland), a sweet red wine (0.75 L, 9%) type with a floral and fruity aroma, was selected for analysis. The high sugar content in wine can cause reduced acidity in coffee. The wine was purchased at the supermarket. The bottles were selected from the same batch. For one-day fermentation, two new portions of wine from one bottle were used. According to the literature, wine fermentation can last longer than 2 days. For example, in the JP2017060455A patent, fermentation was carried out for 48 h and with the same pair of wine.

2.2.2. Maceration in Fruit Pulps

Ripe, undamaged fruits were selected for analysis. The ripeness of the fruit was assessed organoleptically, by color and aroma. The amount of fruit to be macerated and the maceration time were selected experimentally, based on a preliminary study in which color and taste were assessed after various maceration times. Fresh apples, quince, melon, strawberry, raspberry, cherry, and grapefruit were washed and cut; 100 g of fruit, crushed using a kitchen grater and a mixer, was mixed with 100 g of green coffee beans. Coffee beans with fruit pulp were closed in a jar and placed in the refrigerator (4 °C) for 24 h. All variants were thoroughly mixed and placed in the refrigerator for a specified amount of time to carry out the maceration process. Then, the coffee beans were separated from the fruit under running water and dried for one day at a temperature of 50 °C to achieve 95% of solids. Next, 100 g of macerated green coffee was roasted at 230 °C for 12 min until the coffee beans were dark in color. The coffee beans were air-cooled. Figure 1 shows examples of coffee beans after maceration and drying.

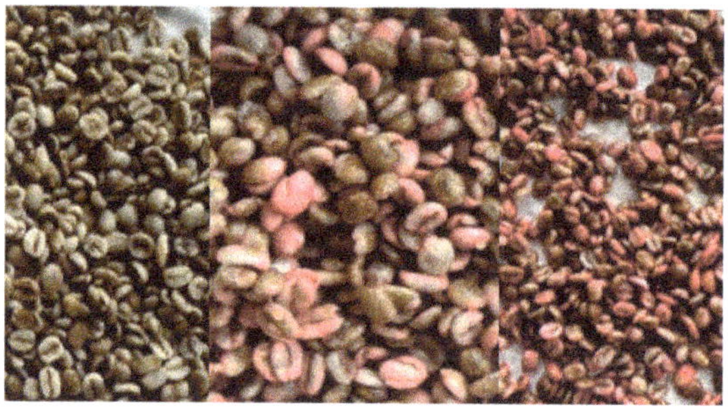

Figure 1. From the left: coffee macerated in melon, raspberry, strawberry.

2.2.3. Flavoring with Aroma Oils

A quantity of 100 g green coffee beans was roasted at 230 °C for 12 min until the beans were dark in color [40]. The coffee beans were air-cooled. Freshly roasted coffee beans were mixed with 0.2 mL food flavoring in a coating machine. The operation was repeated for each flavor (mango, raspberry, grapefruit, strawberry, cherry, and vanilla).

2.2.4. Preparation of Coffee Extracts

Coffee samples were ground in portions in a cast iron grinder (ground to a size range from 480 to 680 µm (Fiamma, MCF C)). Coffee infusion used for the analyses was prepared by placing 7 g of ground beans on filter paper (weight: 60 g/m^2) on a funnel and pouring 100 mL of water at 95 °C.

2.3. Analysis of Phenolic and Organic Acid, Caffeine, HMF, and Acrylamide (UHPLC-ESI-MS)

Hydroxycinnamic, phenolic, and organic acids; caffeine; HMF; and acrylamide were determined in extracts. The analysis was carried out according to the method developed in the previous work [40]. In short: The mobile phase consisted of solvent A—water/formic acid (99.9:0.1, *v*/*v*); solvent B—acetonitrile/formic acid (99.9:0.1, *v*/*v*). A flow rate of 0.2 mL/min and injection volume of 2 µL was used. The calibration curves were constructed for a standard compound using six different concentration levels in a range of 0.01–1.0 mg/mL. Instrument control, data acquisition, and evaluation were carried out with LabSolutions 5.60 SP2, Chromatography Data System, and Postrun Analysis (LabSolutions 5.60 SP2) software, respectively. The mass spectrometric conditions were as follows: capillary voltage of 4500 V, drying gas temperature of 250 °C, drying gas flow of 15 L/min, and nebulizing gas pressure of 1 bar; the capillary temperature was 350 °C, and nitrogen was used as nebulizer. Full-scan mass spectra were acquired over a mass range from *m*/*z* 50 to 2000 in negative ion mode [40]. Figure 2 shows example HPLC chromatogram.

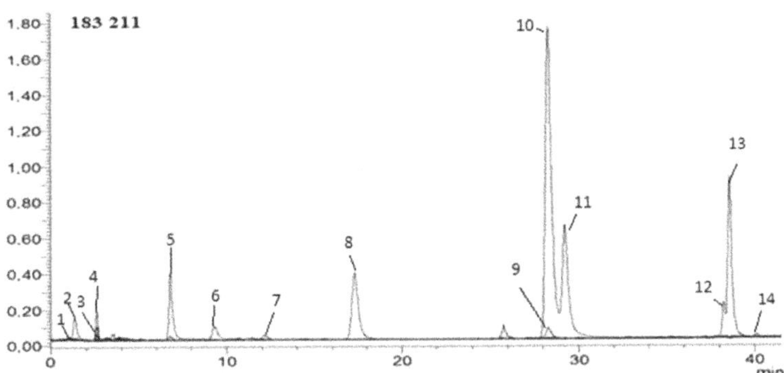

Figure 2. Example HPLC chromatogram of hydroxycinnamic acids, HMF, acrylamide, and caffeine in negative ion mode. 1—5-hydroxymethylfurfural; 2—acrylamide; 3—3-*O*-feruloylquinic acid; 4—4-*O*-feruloylquinic acid; 5—5-*O*-feruloylquinic acid; 6—ferulic acid; 7—caffeic acid; 8—4-*O*-caffeoylquinic acid; 9—3-*O*-caffeoylquinic acid; 10—caffeine; 11—5-*O*-caffeoylquinic acid; 12—3,4-di-*O*-caffeoylquinic acid; 13—3,5-di-O-caffeoylquinic acid; 14—4,5-di-*O*-caffeoylquinic acid.

Determination of the Content of Organic Acids: Lactic, Citric, Malic, and Acetic

The analysis was performed as above, with modifications. The mobile phases were eluent A, water/formic acid (99.9/0.1, *v*/*v*) and eluent B, methanol/formic acid (99.9/0.1, *v*/*v*). The flow rate was 0.3 mL/min, and the gradient was as follows: 0–1.30 min, 0–20% B; 1.31–3.00 min, 20–55% B; 3.01–6.00 min, 55–100% B; 6.01–7.00 min, 100–0% B. The ESI source was operated in positive ion mode and the column was thermostated at 35 °C. Full-scan MS and target MS2 spectral data were obtained from *m*/*z* 50 to 2000. Figure 3 shows example HPLC chromatogram.

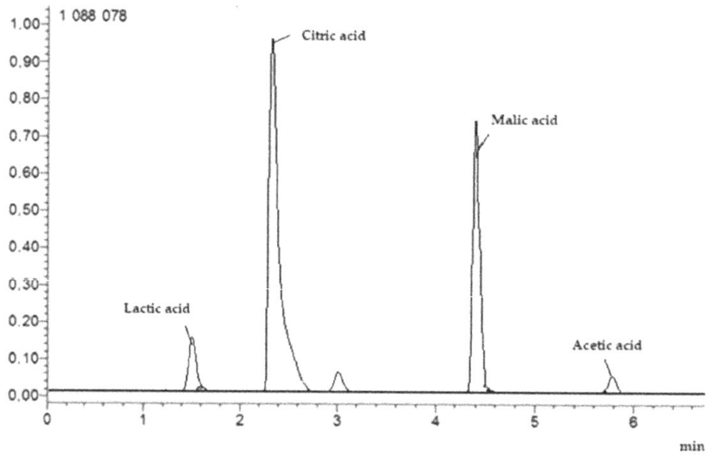

Figure 3. Example HPLC chromatogram of organic acids: lactic, citric, malic, and acetic.

2.4. *Total Antioxidant Capacity Test*

The total antioxidant capacity of the coffee was measured using spectrophotometric (Shimadzu, Kyoto, Japan); 0.2 g of ground coffee was extracted with 20 mL of methanol (70%) in ambient temperature for 30 min and filtered through filter paper. The filtrate was used for analyses. The antioxidant capacity was determined using the measurements of DPPH$^{\bullet}$ scavenging (0.1 mL of coffee extracts was added to 3.9 mL methanol and 1 mL DPPH; absorbance was measured at a wavelength of 517 nm) and of ferric reducing antioxidant power (FRAP) (1 mL of extracts was mixed with 4 mL of FRAP; absorbance was measured at a wavelength of 593 nm). The calibration was based on a reagent test without coffee extract. The DPPH$^{\bullet}$ and FRAP reducing activities were expressed as AC% = [(Acontrol − Asample)/Acontrol] × 100. The FRAP and DPPH were expressed in µmol TE/g [41,42].

2.5. *α-Amylase Inhibitory Assay*

The α-amylase inhibitory activity (AAI) was determined according to the method of Oboh [43]. α-Amylase from human saliva (A103) was dissolved in sodium phosphate buffer (pH 6.9; 20 mM) (1:9 *v*/*v*). Then, 500 µL of buffer and 500 µL of coffee extract prepared according to Section 2.5 were taken. The solution was mixed and incubated (25 °C). After 10 min, 500 µL of starch solution (1%) was added and the incubation was repeated under the same conditions. After 10 min, the incubation was stopped by adding 1.0 mL of dinitrosalicylic acid (DNSA) (5 min in boiling water bath). Then, the sample was cooled to room temperature and 10 mL of distilled water was added. Next, the absorbance was measured at 540 nm. The results were expressed as AAI inhibition (%) = [(Acontrol − Asample)/Acontrol] × 100.

2.6. *Statistical Analysis*

Statistical analysis was based on the determination of the average values of six measurements and their standard deviation, as well as on the one-way ANOVA (analysis of variance) and the Pearson correlation coefficient, using Statistic 10.0 software. The significance was defined at $p \leq 0.05$.

3. Results and Discussion

3.1. *Content of the Hydroxycinnamic and Organic Acid, Caffeine, HMF, and Acrylamide*

The health-promoting properties of coffee extracts depend on the content of belonging to phenolic acids hydroxycinnamic acids (HCAs), in particular chlorogenic acid

(CHAs). Different methods of refining coffee beans may change the content of HCAs [44,45]. Tables 1 and 2 show the concentration of HCAs and caffeine in coffee extracts prepared from beans macerated in fruit pulps or in wine before roasting or with the addition of food flavors after roasting.

Table 1. Concentration of hydroxycinnamic and caffeine in extracts from coffee macerated in fruit pulps and roasted. CA—caffeic acid; FA—ferulic acid; 3-FQA—3-*O*-Feruloylquinic acid; 4-FQA—4-*O*-Feruloylquinic acid; 5-FQA—5-*O*-Feruloylquinic acid; 3-CQA—3-*O*-Caffeoylquinic acid; 4-CQA—4-*O*-Caffeoylquinic acid; 5-CQA—5-*O*-Caffeoylquinic acid; 3,5-diCQA—3,5-*O*-Dicaffeoylquinic acid; 4,5-diCQA—4,5-*O*-Dicaffeoylquinic acid; 3,4-diCQA—3,4-*O*-Dicaffeoylquinic acid; TCA—total chlorogenic acids.

Compound (g/100 g d.b.)	Control	Melon	Strawberry	Apples	Quince	Raspberry	Cherry	Grapefruit
CA	0.13 ± 0.01^{a}	0.08 ± 0.00^{b}	$0.12 \pm 0.01^{a,c}$	0.06 ± 0.00^{b}	0.05 ± 0.00^{b}	$0.12 \pm 0.00^{a,c}$	0.10 ± 0.00^{a}	0.07 ± 0.00^{b}
FA	0.36 ± 0.03^{a}	0.21 ± 0.00^{b}	0.35 ± 0.00^{a}	0.26 ± 0.00^{b}	0.28 ± 0.00^{b}	0.36 ± 0.01^{a}	0.22 ± 0.00^{b}	0.21 ± 0.01^{b}
3-FQA	0.09 ± 0.02^{a}	0.31 ± 0.00^{b}	0.11 ± 0.00^{a}	0.37 ± 0.01^{c}	0.39 ± 0.01^{c}	0.10 ± 0.00^{a}	0.31 ± 0.01^{b}	0.28 ± 0.01^{d}
5-FQA	0.33 ± 0.01^{a}	0.82 ± 0.02^{b}	0.35 ± 0.00^{a}	1.10 ± 0.02^{c}	1.15 ± 0.02^{c}	0.48 ± 0.01^{d}	0.88 ± 0.02^{b}	0.95 ± 0.01^{e}
4-FQA	0.09 ± 0.00^{a}	0.40 ± 0.00^{c}	0.09 ± 0.00^{a}	0.45 ± 0.00^{c}	0.43 ± 0.00^{c}	0.11 ± 0.00^{a}	0.42 ± 0.00^{c}	0.42 ± 0.00^{c}
3-CQA	0.38 ± 0.01^{a}	1.82 ± 0.01^{b}	0.43 ± 0.01^{c}	1.38 ± 0.01^{d}	1.41 ± 0.01^{d}	0.73 ± 0.03^{e}	1.96 ± 0.04^{b}	1.20 ± 0.02^{d}
5-CQA	4.25 ± 0.03^{a}	5.71 ± 0.03^{c}	4.02 ± 0.01^{a}	4.35 ± 0.61^{b}	4.33 ± 0.61^{b}	4.15 ± 0.02^{a}	3.18 ± 0.15^{c}	2.88 ± 0.03^{d}
4-CQA	0.38 ± 0.02^{a}	1.79 ± 0.02^{b}	0.36 ± 0.01^{a}	1.98 ± 0.06^{b}	2.01 ± 0.06^{c}	0.44 ± 0.01^{d}	1.51 ± 0.05^{e}	1.63 ± 0.01^{e}
3,5-diCQA	0.49 ± 0.02^{a}	1.34 ± 0.01^{c}	0.46 ± 0.01^{a}	1.39 ± 0.07^{c}	0.92 ± 0.07^{b}	0.45 ± 0.01^{a}	1.17 ± 0.01^{c}	1.95 ± 0.02^{d}
4,5-diCQA	0.04 ± 0.00^{a}	0.21 ± 0.01^{b}	0.03 ± 0.01^{a}	0.32 ± 0.00^{c}	0.35 ± 0.00^{c}	0.02 ± 0.00^{a}	$0.22 \pm 0.01^{b,d}$	$0.22 \pm 0.00^{d,b}$
3,4-diCQA	0.11 ± 0.00^{a}	0.87 ± 0.01^{b}	0.10 ± 0.00^{a}	1.56 ± 0.03^{c}	1.58 ± 0.03^{c}	0.31 ± 0.01^{d}	0.83 ± 0.01^{b}	0.92 ± 0.01^{b}
TCA	6.50 ± 0.09^{a}	13.56 ± 0.05^{c}	6.42 ± 0.03^{a}	13.22 ± 0.45^{c}	12.72 ± 0.45^{b}	7.27 ± 0.09^{d}	10.80 ± 0.29^{e}	10.73 ± 0.15^{e}
Caffeine	3.51 ± 0.03^{a}	3.50 ± 0.01^{a}	3.49 ± 0.02^{a}	3.51 ± 0.01^{a}	3.51 ± 0.03^{a}	3.50 ± 0.02^{a}	3.50 ± 0.02^{a}	3.52 ± 0.01^{a}

Values are expressed as mean value ± SD; $n = 6$; values with the same superscript letter ($^{a–e}$) along the same row are not significantly different ($p > 0.05$).

Table 2. Concentration of hydroxycinnamic and caffeine in in extracts from coffee macerated in red wine and roasted or flavored with aroma oils after roasting. CA—caffeic acid; FA—ferulic acid; 3-FQA—3-*O*-Feruloylquinic acid; 4-FQA—4-*O*-Feruloylquinic acid; 5-FQA—5-*O*-Feruloylquinic acid; 3-CQA—3-*O*-Caffeoylquinic acid; 4-CQA—4-*O*-Caffeoylquinic acid; 5-CQA—5-*O*-Caffeoylquinic acid; 3,5-diCQA—3,5-*O*-Dicaffeoylquinic acid; 4,5-diCQA—4,5-*O*-Dicaffeoylquinic acid; 3,4-diCQA—3,4-*O*-Dicaffeoylquinic acid; TCA—total chlorogenic acids.

Compound (g/100 g d.b.)	Mango	Raspberry	Strawberry	Cherry	Grapefruit	Vanilla	Red Wine
CA	0.08 ± 0.00^{b}	0.09 ± 0.00^{b}	0.07 ± 0.00^{b}	0.06 ± 0.00^{c}	0.08 ± 0.00^{b}	0.06 ± 0.00^{c}	0.12 ± 0.00^{a}
FA	0.12 ± 0.01^{b}	0.23 ± 0.01^{d}	0.19 ± 0.00^{a}	0.17 ± 0.01^{c}	0.23 ± 0.01^{d}	0.17 ± 0.00^{c}	0.35 ± 0.02^{a}
3-FQA	0.21 ± 0.01^{d}	0.33 ± 0.01^{c}	0.26 ± 0.01^{d}	0.13 ± 0.01^{b}	0.32 ± 0.03^{c}	0.23 ± 0.01^{d}	0.11 ± 0.00^{a}
5-FQA	0.15 ± 0.02^{b}	0.25 ± 0.02^{c}	0.29 ± 0.01^{d}	0.20 ± 0.01^{c}	0.26 ± 0.02^{c}	0.70 ± 0.02^{e}	0.37 ± 0.01^{a}
4-FQA	0.19 ± 0.02^{b}	0.40 ± 0.01^{c}	0.32 ± 0.00^{d}	0.29 ± 0.00^{e}	0.20 ± 0.02^{b}	0.29 ± 0.03^{e}	0.09 ± 0.00^{a}
3-CQA	0.47 ± 0.03^{c}	0.06 ± 0.02^{b}	0.63 ± 0.01^{d}	0.46 ± 0.02^{c}	0.50 ± 0.16^{e}	0.46 ± 0.03^{c}	0.43 ± 0.01^{c}
5-CQA	2.39 ± 0.05^{b}	2.79 ± 0.09^{b}	3.80 ± 0.03^{c}	3.38 ± 0.02^{c}	3.65 ± 0.13^{c}	2.38 ± 0.01^{b}	5.02 ± 0.02^{d}
4-CQA	0.26 ± 0.05^{b}	0.51 ± 0.05^{c}	0.15 ± 0.03^{d}	0.61 ± 0.00^{e}	0.34 ± 0.03^{a}	0.91 ± 0.01^{f}	0.36 ± 0.01^{a}
3,5-diCQA	0.14 ± 0.02^{a}	0.33 ± 0.03^{c}	0.29 ± 0.03^{d}	0.15 ± 0.01^{a}	0.28 ± 0.02^{f}	0.15 ± 0.02^{a}	0.46 ± 0.02^{f}
4,5-diCQA	0.16 ± 0.02^{b}	0.21 ± 0.02^{c}	0.22 ± 0.02^{c}	0.20 ± 0.00^{c}	0.26 ± 0.01^{c}	0.19 ± 0.01^{b}	0.03 ± 0.00^{a}
3,4-diCQA	0.13 ± 0.01^{a}	0.20 ± 0.02^{d}	0.27 ± 0.01^{d}	0.75 ± 0.02^{b}	0.30 ± 0.05^{c}	0.92 ± 0.03^{d}	0.10 ± 0.00^{a}
TCA	4.64 ± 0.15^{b}	5.29 ± 0.10^{c}	6.28 ± 0.03^{a}	6.48 ± 0.09^{a}	6.41 ± 0.03^{d}	6.44 ± 0.15^{a}	7.44 ± 0.15^{d}
Caffeine	3.50 ± 0.01^{a}	3.50 ± 0.02^{a}	3.49 ± 0.01^{a}	3.41 ± 0.02^{a}	3.50 ± 0.04^{a}	3.50 ± 0.02^{a}	3.51 ± 0.00^{a}

Values are expressed as mean value ± SD; $n = 6$; values with the same superscript letter ($^{a–f}$) along the same row are not significantly different ($p > 0.05$).

The content of HCAs ranged from 4.64 to 13.56 g/100 g d.b. for mango food flavor and melon pulp, respectively. The control sample (dark roasted coffee) showed an HCA content of 6.50 g/100 g d.b. The coffee bean maceration in fruit pulps resulted in an increase in the content of HCAs compared to the control ($p < 0.05$), in the following order: melon

(13.56 g/100 g d.b.) > apples (13.22 g/100 g d.b.) > quinice (12.72 g/100 g d.b.) > cherry (10.80 g/100 g d.b.) >grapefruit (10.73 g/100 g d.b.) > raspberry (7.27 g/100 g d.b.). Maceration of coffee beans in strawberry pulp resulted in a statistically insignificant ($p > 0.05$) decrease in HCA content (Table 1). The reduction in HCAs in coffee beans may be due to the fact that strawberries are a rich source of flavonoids and hydroxybenzoic acids but not hydroxycinnamic acids [40]. Maceration in fruit pulps of raspberry, strawberry, cherry, and grapefruit resulted in a decrease of 5-*O*-caffeoylquinic acid concentration after roasting, which may be the result of partial transacylation of this isomer during thermal processing [46].

The most beneficial fruits used for coffee maceration in terms of HCA content increase were melon and apples. In both cases, the HCA concentration was approximately twice as high as in the control coffee extract ($p < 0.05$). The maceration resulted in an increase in the concentration of the isomers of ferulic acid esters with quinic acid (3-, 4-, and 5-O-feruloylquinic acids) and of caffeic acid esters (3- and 4-O-caffeoylquinic acids). However, the 5-O-caffeoylquinic acid isomer significantly increased its concentration only after maceration of coffee beans with melon, by approx. 30%. Dimtsas et al. showed that melon extracts contain 5-CQA acid at a level from 0.51 to 76.96 mg/100 g d.b and 3-CQA from 2.08 to 37.06 mg/100 g d.b. [47]. Melon is a rich source of polyphenols that prevent neurodegenerative diseases and diabetes. It exhibits antioxidant and anti-inflammatory properties. Additionally, it contains vitamins C and E. The main phenolic compounds in melon are chlorogenic acid (3-caffeoylquinic acid), neochlorogenic acid (5-caffeoylquinic acid), and 3-hydroxybenzoic acid. Therefore, during the maceration process, the mango pulp enriched the coffee with valuable HCAs (Table 1) [47–49].

Melon and apple have a high content of ascorbic acid. Ascorbic acid can protect coffee beans from the oxidation process during roasting and consequently yield higher amounts of HCA. Apples contain pectolytic enzymes that could cause an increase in chlorogenic acids as well because of the release from links with pectic substances. [47–49].

Caffeic and ferulic acids in roasted coffee were degraded compared to the control. The reduction may result from a high roasting temperature. For example, the thermostability of caffeic acid is up to 223 °C [50]. However, the acids may be additionally formed as a result of the esters' bond hydrolysis, which is more likely at lower pH in the presence of fruit pulp substances. The feruloylquinic acids accounted for from 5 to 13% of the total chlorogenic acids. The decrease in determined trans-ferulic acid may also be the result of an increase in the content of ferulic acid cis-isomer [51].

The use of maceration in wine increased the HCA content by 0.94 g/100 g d.b. compared to the control sample (Table 2). However, the concentration achieved was not higher than in the case of fruit maceration. This may be related to the use of sweet wine, which could cause chlorogenic acid binding to the proteinaceous material and the formation of Maillard reaction products. In the case of wine-macerated coffee, an increase in 5-O-caffeoylquinic acid (Table 2) was also observed. Regarding polyphenols, coffee contains hydroxycinnamic acids and their esters, which account for about 10% of green beans and 3% of roasted coffee, and a cup of coffee contains 20–650 mg of these polyphenols. The wine is rich in flavan-3-ols, tannins, hydroxycinnamic and benzoic acids, anthocyanins, proanthocyanidins, and stilbenes, which include resveratrol, present in an amount of 3.5 mg/L [52]. Because of the rich and complex composition of wine, during coffee roasting after wine maturation, additional derivatives with unique sensory and health-promoting properties are formed [53]. Moderate drinking of wine and regular consumption of coffee improve cognitive effects in elderly people, inactivate cholinesterases, and provide neurotransmitters [54]. Polyphenols also show anticancer, cardioprotective, hepatoprotective, and immune system-stimulating properties, as well as anti-obesity and antidiabetic activities [55,56]. Phenolic compounds contained in coffee and wine have a beneficial effect on the gastrointestinal microbiota, which is reflected in the reduction in inflammatory and allergic reactions. The mechanism of action of polyphenols from both sources is different, and for this reason, it may be desirable to combine polyphenols from both sources in the diet, achieved with a specific product [57].

Enhancing the aroma of roasted coffee with the addition of food flavor contributed to reducing the content of HCAs. The mango food flavor reduced the HCA content by 1.86 g/100 g d.b., and by 1.21 g/100 g d.b. in the case of the raspberry flavor. However, the addition of strawberry, cherry, vanilla, and grapefruit food flavors had only a slight effect on the HCA reduction (Table 2). The differences resulted from the aroma carrier used. Strawberry, cherry, grapefruit, and vanilla flavors were dissolved in alcohol. However, mango and raspberry were dissolved in oils. Aromatic compounds in food flavors are dissolved in media such as ethyl alcohol, triacetin, propylene glycol, water, and vegetable oils. When adding flavor to hot coffee beans, the moisture content of the coffee beans may increase, which in turn could increase the acrylamide content [58]. On the other hand, food flavors can accelerate the oxidation process of roasted coffee beans, reducing the concentration of chlorogenic acids and lowering the overall quality of the brew [59].

Control coffee extracts, the extracts from beans roasted after maceration, and roasted bean extracts after the addition of aroma oils contained similar, statistically insignificant caffeine contents, amounting to about 3.5 g/100 g d.b. ($p > 0.05$). This was due to the fact that caffeine is a thermostable compound, and on the other hand, fruit pulps or aroma oils are not a source of alkaloids. Caffeine degrades at a temperature exceeding 235 °C [50]. Caffeine is an adenosine receptor inhibitor and has neuronal detoxification activity, influencing the release of glutamine and increasing the intracellular level of cyclic adenosine-3′,5′-monophosphate (cAMP). Caffeine is an antioxidant; in addition to inhibiting the action of adenosine, it helps to inhibit the activity of lipid peroxidase by degrading free radicals. Caffeine also has the ability to inhibit monoamine oxidase B, protecting and increasing the bioavailability of dopamine in the brain. Increasing dopamine concentration improves cognitive functions [60,61].

Maillard reaction products are an important group of coffee ingredients. Compounds from this group are attributed to quite different in vivo activities, ranging from anti-inflammatory and antioxidant activities to carcinogenic and mutagenic potential. HMF and acrylamide are examples of the second group. Table 3 shows the concentration of HMF and acrylamide in extracts from coffee macerated in fruit pulps or red wine as well as those flavored with aroma oils.

Table 3. Concentration of HMF and acrylamide in extracts from coffee macerated in fruit pulps, red wine, or flavored with aroma oils.

Coffee Handling Method	5-Hydroxymethylfurfural (mg/100 g d.b.)	Acrylamide (μg/100 g d.b.)
Control	0.33 ± 0.01^{a}	4.89 ± 0.06^{a}
	Maceration	
Melon	0.44 ± 0.02^{b}	4.90 ± 0.03^{a}
Strawberry	0.30 ± 0.01^{a}	4.91 ± 0.02^{a}
Apples	0.55 ± 0.03^{c}	4.98 ± 0.09^{a}
Quince	0.31 ± 0.01^{a}	5.01 ± 0.03^{b}
Raspberry	0.38 ± 0.02^{a}	4.95 ± 0.02^{a}
Cherry	0.35 ± 0.02^{a}	4.91 ± 0.04^{a}
Grapefruit	0.41 ± 0.03^{b}	4.90 ± 0.01^{a}
Red vine	0.35 ± 0.02^{a}	4.91 ± 0.01^{a}
	Food flavors	
Mango	1.34 ± 0.01^{d}	6.95 ± 0.06^{a}
Raspberry	1.22 ± 0.01^{d}	6.33 ± 0.09^{c}
Strawberry	1.05 ± 0.02^{d}	7.22 ± 0.11^{d}
Cherry	0.95 ± 0.03^{c}	5.51 ± 0.02^{b}
Grapefruit	0.98 ± 0.04^{c}	5.18 ± 0.04^{b}
Vanilla	0.68 ± 0.03^{e}	4.93 ± 0.01^{a}

Values are expressed as mean value ± SD; $n = 6$. Values with the same superscript letter ($^{a-e}$) along the same row are not significantly different ($p > 0.05$).

The HMF content in the extract from the control coffee was 0.33 mg/100 g d.b. (Table 3). The content of HMF in extracts after aromatization and maceration ranged from 0.30 to 1.34 mg/100 g for strawberry pulp and mango food flavor, respectively (Table 3). The maceration contributed to more intense formation of HMF using pulps obtained from melon, apple, raspberry, cherry, and grapefruit. As the fruits ripen, the sugar content increases, in particular sucrose, fructose, and galactosyl sucrose. Melon contains approximately 8 g/100 g; raspberry—4.42 g/100 g; cherry—5.95 g/100 g; grapefruit—7 g/100 g; apple—12.9 g/100 g of simple sugars. The higher the content of sugars, especially fructose, in the product, the higher the HMF content, which is consistent with our research. [62–66]. Most likely, some of the juice from the fruit was absorbed into the bean. A key issue in coffee research is the roasting process and its determining effect on the presence of biologically active phytochemicals. In this context, attention is mainly paid to the role of polyphenols, such as hydroxycinnamic acids and their esters with quinic acid, called chlorogenic acids, trigonelline, and Maillard reaction products (MRP) [67]. Thermal degradation of coffee bean components in the roasting process reduces the content of polyphenolic compounds and the formation of melanoidins, partly related to polyphenols, but also low molecular weight Maillard reaction products, such as acrylamide and 5-hydroxymethylfurfural, which reduce the antioxidant activity of coffee and have potential carcinogenic effects [67]. Already at a roasting temperature of 120–140 °C, an endothermic maximum can be observed; the coffee beans begin to swell, changing their structure. There are also processes of non-enzymatic bean browning, which contribute to the formation of acrylamide because of the reaction of the carboxyl group of reducing sugars with the amino group [68]. When coffee beans reach a temperature of approximately 160 °C, a characteristic crack appears, caused by a simultaneous loss of mass with the formation of gases and an increase in the volume of the bean [68]. At this stage of the coffee roasting process, changes in chemical composition occur, the degradation process of polyphenolic compounds begins, and a number of non-volatile organic compounds are transformed into volatile aroma components [68]. Pyrolysis of polysaccharides and sugars found in coffee beans takes place, producing volatile compounds, aliphatic carbonyls, alcohols, and diketones. At a temperature of 180–190 °C, the characteristic aroma, flavor, and color of light, medium, or dark roasted coffee are created. The reactions occurring in the grain at this temperature are exothermic, causing a rapid increase in grain temperature, leading to the degradation of proteins, chlorogenic acids, trigonelline, and carbohydrates [69]. Carbohydrates are degraded under the influence of aliphatic acids into smaller compounds, such as glycolic or lactic acid. As a result of non-enzymatic browning, because of the degradation of carbohydrates and chlorogenic acid, color-producing compounds such as melanoidins are formed [70,71]. The final stage of roasting coffee until it obtains a dark color is achieved at a bean temperature of 190 to 250 °C. The bean changes its structure, becomes highly porous, carbon dioxide is released, and new aromatic compounds and MRPs are formed, which partially combine with polyphenols [70,71].

Only strawberry and quince slightly reduced the content of HMF. This compound is formed because of the Maillard reaction or caramelization of sugars found in coffee beans [70]. At the same time, the formation of HMF is favored by a pH closer to neutral; therefore, sour strawberries and quince could limit its formation. Food flavors caused higher HMF content in coffee extracts than in the case of maceration because they contributed to increased non-enzymatic browning after adding them to coffee directly after roasting.

Acrylamide content in extracts from coffee macerated with fruit pulps or in wine was statistically at the same level ($p > 0.05$). However, the use of food flavors resulted in an increase in acrylamide to the range of 4.93–7.22 µg/100 g d.b. This may be related to the second possible mechanism of acrylamide formation from oxidized lipids.

Acrylamide consumed in high concentrations is a potentially carcinogenic substance, the permissible daily dose of acrylamide for a person weighing 70 kg amounts 140 µg. It can be noted that drinking coffee in quantities of 2–3 cups per day does not exceed the daily safe dose of acrylamide; however, this substance can be administrated additionally with other foods constituting the daily diet. It is known that consuming green coffee reduces the risk of acrylamide accumulation in the human body [72,73].

Our research confirmed that the addition of artificial flavors negatively affects the quality of the coffee infusion and its health-promoting properties. Food flavors contain partially natural plant and fruit extracts that contain simple sugars. This results in increased HMF and acrylamide. This is due to a reduction in the content of hydroxycinnamic acids and their esters in coffee extracts and the formation of a higher quantity of harmful compounds such as acrylamide. The content of some Maillard reaction products like HMF and acrylamide in coffee should be minimized, taking into account their anti-nutritional characteristics [74].

3.2. Concentration of Organic Acids

Roasted coffee beans subjected to the maceration in fruit pulps were richer in organic acids, except for apple fruit pulp. Apple pulp decreased organic acids by 0.02 g/100 g d.b. compared to the control sample. This is caused by a reduction in acetic acid and malic acid. Apples are a rich source of malic acid. However, the organic compound did not pass into the bean in sufficient quantity to compensate for the degradation of the compounds during coffee roasting [75]. Malic acid degrades at temperatures above 140 °C. A similar tendency of malic acid can be seen in raspberries and red wine. However, the content of malic acid increased in strawberries, melon, quince, cherries, and grapefruit. This may be related to the higher acidity in the fruit. Their concentrations increased from 0.87 to maximally 1.05 g/100 g d.b. in coffee macerated with melon pulp (Table 4). The contents of acetic and lactic acids increased in most variants. Enriching coffee beans with fruit pulp and wine resulted in an increase in the citric acid content in the beans, which at the same time had a protective effect on the citric acid present in the beans themselves. Citric acid degrades in the range of 177–501 °C, which makes it a stable compound [76]. A similar tendency was observed for lactic acid, which degrades only at a temperature of 185 °C [77].

Table 4. Concentration of organic acids in extracts from coffee macerated in fruit pulps, red wine, or flavored with aroma oils.

Coffee Handling Method	Acetic Acid (mg/100 g d.b.)	Lactic Acid (mg/100 g d.b.)	Malic Acid (g/100 g d.b.)	Citric Acid (g/100 g d.b.)	Total Organic Acids (g/100 g d.b.)
Control	0.72 ± 0.02^{a}	3.23 ± 0.01^{a}	0.25 ± 0.02^{a}	0.61 ± 0.01^{a}	0.87 ± 0.03^{a}
			Maceration		
Melon	1.24 ± 0.01^{b}	4.16 ± 0.12^{b}	0.29 ± 0.04^{b}	0.71 ± 0.05^{b}	1.05 ± 0.05^{b}
Strawberry	1.44 ± 0.01^{c}	7.05 ± 0.05^{c}	0.29 ± 0.01^{b}	0.65 ± 0.07^{c}	0.95 ± 0.09^{c}
Apples	0.22 ± 0.01^{d}	3.71 ± 0.11^{d}	0.20 ± 0.03^{c}	0.65 ± 0.02^{c}	0.85 ± 0.05^{a}
Quince	0.63 ± 0.00^{e}	4.89 ± 0.03^{e}	0.28 ± 0.02^{b}	0.66 ± 0.01^{c}	0.94 ± 0.03^{c}
Raspberry	1.22 ± 0.01^{b}	4.72 ± 0.10^{e}	0.23 ± 0.04^{a}	0.65 ± 0.02^{c}	0.89 ± 0.04^{a}
Cherry	1.59 ± 0.02^{c}	4.66 ± 0.05^{e}	0.27 ± 0.02^{b}	0.63 ± 0.05^{a}	0.91 ± 0.02^{c}
Grapefruit	1.61 ± 0.02^{c}	3.73 ± 0.09^{d}	0.26 ± 0.03^{a}	0.65 ± 0.04^{c}	0.93 ± 0.02^{c}
Red vine	1.13 ± 0.06^{b}	3.76 ± 0.09^{d}	0.23 ± 0.03^{c}	0.76 ± 0.02^{b}	0.99 ± 0.09^{c}
			Food flavors		
Mango	0.04 ± 0.00^{f}	0.01 ± 0.00^{f}	0.27 ± 0.01^{b}	0.46 ± 0.02^{d}	0.73 ± 0.02^{d}
Raspberry	0.05 ± 0.01^{f}	0.01 ± 0.00^{f}	0.23 ± 0.02^{c}	0.55 ± 0.02^{e}	0.78 ± 0.03^{d}
Strawberry	0.19 ± 0.01^{g}	0.01 ± 0.00^{f}	0.20 ± 0.02^{d}	0.58 ± 0.03^{e}	0.78 ± 0.03^{d}
Cherry	0.16 ± 0.01^{g}	0.01 ± 0.00^{f}	0.21 ± 0.05^{d}	0.58 ± 0.08^{e}	0.79 ± 0.02^{d}
Grapefruit	0.22 ± 0.01^{h}	0.01 ± 0.00^{f}	0.16 ± 0.03^{e}	0.57 ± 0.02^{e}	0.73 ± 0.03^{d}
Vanilla	0.02 ± 0.00^{f}	0.01 ± 0.00^{f}	0.21 ± 0.02^{d}	$0.59 \pm 0.0 1^{e}$	0.80 ± 0.03^{e}

Values are expressed as mean value ± SD; $n = 6$. Values with the same superscript letter ($^{a-h}$) along the same row are not significantly different ($p > 0.05$).

The addition of food flavors contributed to reducing the content of organic acids by 0.07–0.14 g/100 g d.b., respectively, for vanilla and mango/grapefruit aroma oils (Table 4).

In the case of food aromas, the total content of organic acids decreased compared to the control sample. This may be due to the fact that coffee beans are sprinkled with food flavors right after roasting. A sticky layer is formed on the beans, which extends the cooling time of the beans. The consequence of this is the formation of a higher content of HMF and acrylamide, at the expense of acetic acid. Individual volatile compounds or groups of them are responsible for specific aroma characteristics. Lactic acid of low volatility and acetic acid result in a fruity and winey aroma in coffee [5–8,78]. In our study, coffee extracts after maceration with fruit pulps or red wine showed increased contents of lactic and acetic acids, which may give them fruitier aroma. Additionally, maceration with fruits may also result in the formation of an increased amount of furans and pyrroles, softening the taste of coffee [79,80]. This might result not only from absorption of phytochemicals from a pulp, because aromatic improvement was also observed after soaking green beans in water, followed by drying and roasting, which increased the content of free polyphenols and amino acids because of proteolysis [79,80].

3.3. Antioxidant Potential

Figure 4 shows antioxidant properties of coffee extracts prepared from coffee beans after maceration determined by DPPH and FRAP methods. Both methods showed a high positive correlation of the results, amounting to $r = 0.98$. Coffee methanolic extracts form the beans that had been pretreated by maceration with fruit pulps before roasting had increased antioxidant potential compared to the control ($p < 0.05$). Fruits such as melon (FRAP—416.77 µmol TE/g; DPPH—418.33 µmol TE/g), apple (FRAP—395.02 µmol TE/g; DPPH—418.22 µmol TE/g), and quince (FRAP—366.15 µmol TE/g; DPPH—368.12 µmol TE/g) showed the highest potential to increase the antioxidant activity in coffee. However, maceration in wine or the addition of food flavors such as cherry, strawberry, grapefruit, and vanilla resulted in similar antioxidant properties to the control coffee extract. In turn, mango and raspberry aroma reduced antioxidant properties. Melon has a high antioxidant potential because it is a source of vitamin C and A, β-carotene, and phytoene, with a total polyphenol content of 40–80 mg/100 g [80]. Maceration with the participation of hydrolytic enzymes releases sugars, amino acids, and polyphenols, which undergo non-enzymatic browning during roasting, so macerated coffees darken faster and show higher antioxidant activity after roasting. In addition to producing dark dyes, coffee fermentation contributes to enriching the aroma with a number of desirable compounds from the pyrazine, alcohol, aldehyde, ketone, phenol, furan, pyrrole, and other groups [81–83]. In fermented coffees, the content of organic acids such as malic and lactic increases, which give the infusions a pleasant acidity [84]. Maceration in strawberry pulp showed low antioxidant potential, which is related to the low content of chlorogenic acids. A better maceration effect could have been achieved with seasonal strawberries.

In turn, food flavors did not significantly increase the antioxidant potential of coffee extracts. In the case of mango aroma, there was a decrease in antioxidant activity, which was related to the decrease in HCA concentrations (Table 2). In food flavors, mango and cherry had the lowest value, which may be supplemented with more artificial additives to obtain the desired aroma. Some of the ingredients of food aromas with unsaturated bonds may create radicals with pro-oxidant action. The main antioxidant substances in coffee are chlorogenic acid and their volatile degradation products, caffeine, melanoidins, and trigonelline. It should be taken into account that coffee extracts are a rich source of antioxidants that are helpful in the prevention of, among others, Alzheimer's and Parkinson's diseases, type 2 diabetes, and metabolic orders [62,63].

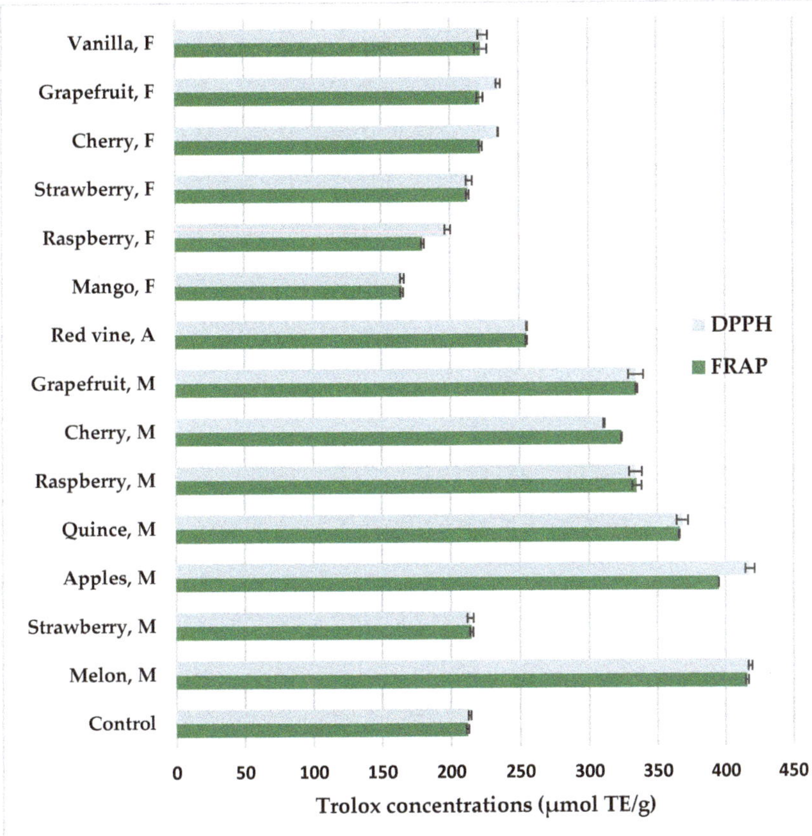

Figure 4. Antioxidant properties of methanolic extracts from flavored coffee, determined by DPPH and FRAP methods. Control—coffee without additives; M—maceration in fruit pulps; F—food flavors; A—maceration in red wine. Values are expressed as mean value ± SD.

3.4. *α-Amylase Inhibitory Activity*

α-Amylase is the main enzyme responsible for the decomposition of α-glucans by hydrolytic catalysis, making them bioavailable and potentially bioabsorbable. The use of α-amylase inhibitors is an essential element in the prevention of diabetes [43]. Coffee extracts subjected to various aromatization methods showed properties of over 50% inhibition of the enzyme (Table 5, Figures 5 and 6). The inhibitory activity almost linearly increased with increasing concentrations of coffee extract in the tested range. The method of coffee bean maceration with fruit pulps of melon (92.11%, IC_{50} = 3.80 mg/mL), apple (84.55%, IC_{50} = 4.14 mg/mL), and red wine (88.33% IC_{50} = 3.96 mg/mL) showed the highest enzyme inhibition activity (α-amylase 0.5 mg/mL, 10 μmol/mL). However, the aromatization method with the addition of aroma oils from mango and raspberry showed enzyme inhibition activity lower than in the control sample.

Table 5. IC_{50} values of α- amylase inhibitory activity of coffee extract form flavored beans.

				IC_{50} (mg/mL) *			
				Maceration			
Control	Melon	Strawberry	Apples	Quince	Raspberry	Cherry	Grapefruit
4.47 ± 0.05 [a]	3.80 ± 0.15 [b]	4.79 ± 0.09 [a]	4.14 ± 0.03 [a]	4.36 ± 0.29 [a]	5.73 ± 0.15 [c]	4.37 ± 0.18 [a]	4.40 ± 0.07 [a]
		Food flavors				Maceration	
Mango	Raspberry	Strawberry	Cherry	Grapefruit	Vanilla	Red wine	
6.72 ± 0.34 [d]	6.50 ± 0.09 [d]	6.56 ± 0.02 [d]	6.46 ± 0.10 [d]	5.62 ± 0.13 [c]	5.47 ± 0.05 [c]	3.96 ± 0.35 [b]	

Values are expressed as mean value ± SD; $n = 6$. Values with the same letter [a–d] along the same column are not significantly different ($p > 0.05$). * IC_{50}—the half-maximal inhibitory concentration values for α-amylase by water-extracted coffee.

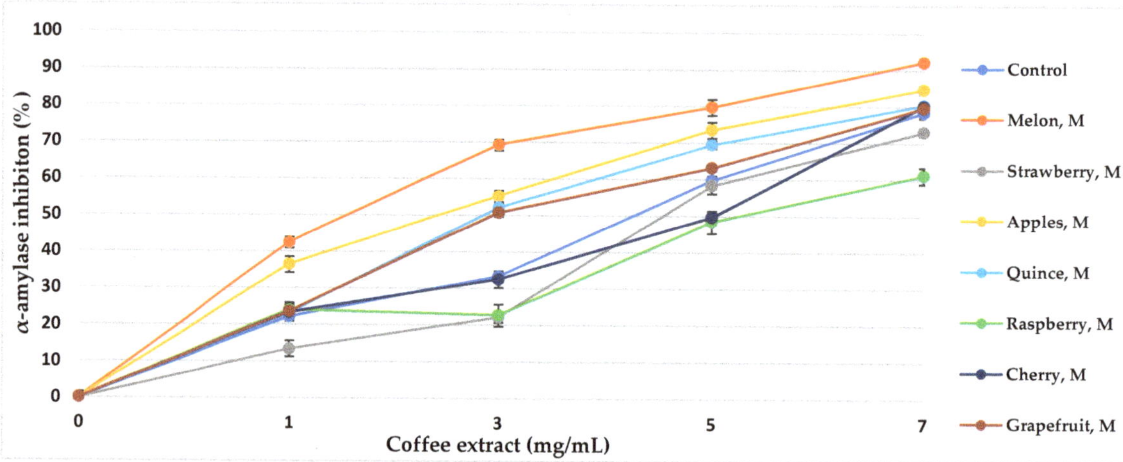

Figure 5. α-Amylase inhibitory activity of coffee extracts. Control—coffee without additives; M—maceration.

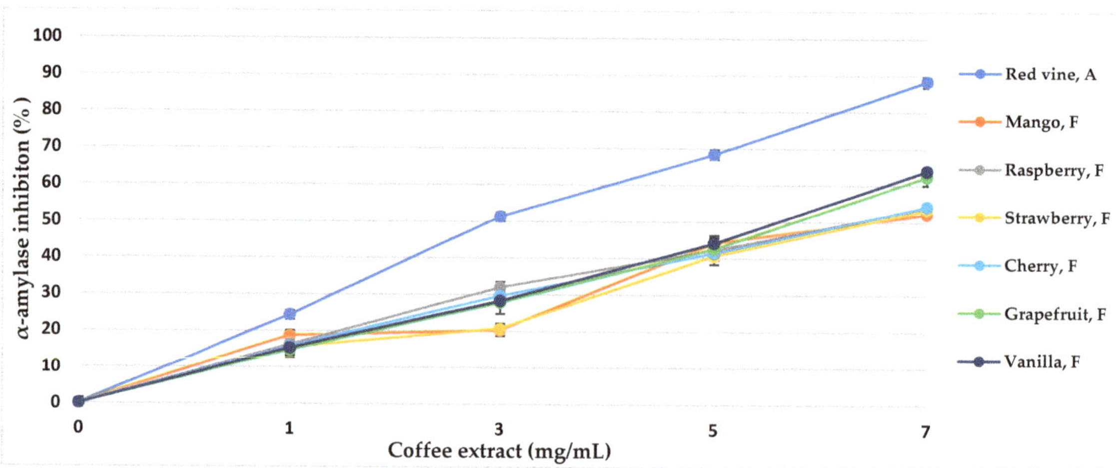

Figure 6. α-Amylase inhibitory activity of coffee extracts. Control—coffee without additives; F—food flavor; A—maceration in red wine.

Thanks to the maceration of coffee with fruits and wine, the activity of α-amylase inhibition increased, while the addition of food flavors generally decreased the mentioned inhibitory properties in coffee extracts. Sun et al. [85] showed that coffee treated with ultrasound before roasting increases the inhibitory effect towards α-amylase, and the compounds responsible for the activity bind the enzyme in a competitive manner. 5-*O*-Caffeoylquinic acid (5-CQA) and 3,5-*O*-dicaffeoylquinic acid (3,5-diCQA) were identified as the main coffee ligands linking the active site of α-amylase [85]. In our study, a similar relationship was observed. The extract of roasted coffee obtained after maceration in melon fruit pulp contained 5-CQA in relatively high amounts, at 5.76 g/100 g d.b., and at 1.34 g/100 g d.b. for 3,5-diCQA; the IC_{50} of the enzyme inhibition amounted to 3.80 mg/mL, and maceration in wine resulted in concentrations of 5.02 g/100 g d.b. and 0.46 g/100 g d.b., respectively, with IC_{50} = 3.96 mg/mL, comparing to other coffee aromatization methods and a control coffee. It can be noticed that maceration with fruit pulps not only increased the content of hydroxycinnamic acids and their esters in roasted coffee but also resulted in high alpha-amylase inhibition activity and antioxidant potential. However, food flavors showed low enzyme inhibition activity, which correlates with the low content of chlorophyll acids. Additionally, artificial flavors contain toxic substances and increased the content of acrylamide and HMF in the coffee extract, which resulted in lower antioxidant activity.

4. Conclusions

This study showed that the content of phenolic compounds and organic acids in coffee extracts depended on the coffee flavoring method. It was found that maceration of green coffee beans with mango, apple, and red wine is the best way to flavor coffee in terms of health-promoting properties. Maceration had a positive effect on the protection of beans against the degradation of phenolic compounds. Roasted coffee with added food flavors had the lowest content of polyphenols and organic acids, which resulted in a deterioration in quality. The obtained results suggest a beneficial effect of using fruit pulps or wine for green bean maceration on antioxidant and α-amylase-inhibiting activity. The results of this study will be used in future research on an innovative method of coffee bean refining, optimizing maceration conditions using wastes from the food industry, the aim of which is not only to improve the taste but also to have a beneficial effect on the health-promoting properties of coffee beans, evaluated in complex in vitro and in vivo models.

Author Contributions: Conceptualization, J.G.; methodology, J.G.; formal analysis, J.G., J.Z., G.B. and K.K.; data curation, J.G., G.B. and K.K.; writing—original draft preparation, J.G.; writing—review and editing, G.B. and K.K.; visualization, J.G. and J.Z.; supervision, J.G.; funding acquisition, J.G. and G.B. All authors have read and agreed to the published version of the manuscript.

Funding: This research received no external funding.

Institutional Review Board Statement: Not applicable.

Informed Consent Statement: Not applicable.

Data Availability Statement: The data presented in this study are available on request from the corresponding author due to he data are part of an ongoing study.

Conflicts of Interest: The authors declare no conflicts of interest.

References

1. Pszczola, D.E. Beverage Flavors 'Spill Over' Into Foods. Food Technology Magazine. pp. 1–31. Available online: https://www.ift.org/news-and-publications/food-technology-magazine/issues/2009/february/columns/ingredients (accessed on 1 August 2024).
2. F 1ebrianto, N.A.; Zhu, F. Coffee bean processing: Emerging methods and their effects on chemical, biological and sensory properties. *Food Chem.* **2023**, *412*, 135489. [CrossRef] [PubMed]
3. Mahmud, M.M.C.; Shellie, R.A.; Keast, R. Unravelling the relationship between aroma compounds and consumer acceptance: Coffee as an example. *Compr. Rev. Food Sci. Food Saf.* **2020**, *19*, 2380–2420. [CrossRef] [PubMed]

4. Fujioka, K.; Tomizawa, Y.; Shimizu, N.; Manome, Y. Description of coffee aroma with the electronic nose which learned wine aromas, Le nez du vin. In Proceedings of the of the 1st International Electronic Conference on Sensors and Applications, Sciforum Electronic Conference Series, online, 1–16 June 2014. [CrossRef]
5. Vezzulli, F.; Lambri, M.; Bertuzzi, T. Volatile compounds in green and roasted arabica specialty coffee: Discrimination of origins, post-harvesting processes, and roasting level. *Foods* **2023**, *12*, 489. [CrossRef] [PubMed]
6. Barea-Ramos, J.D.; Cascos, G.; Mesías, M.; Lozano, J.; Martín-Vertedor, D. Evaluation of the olfactory quality of roasted coffee beans using a digital nose. *Sensors* **2022**, *22*, 8654. [CrossRef]
7. Zhao, L.; Wang, Y.; Wang, D.; He, Z.; Gong, J.; Tan, C. Effects of different probiotics on the volatile components of fermented coffee were analyzed based on headspace-gas chromatography-ion mobility spectrometry. *Foods* **2023**, *12*, 2015. [CrossRef]
8. Shen, X.; Zi, C.; Yang, Y.; Wang, Q.; Zhang, Z.; Shao, J.; Zhao, P.; Liu, K.; Li, X.; Fan, J. Effects of different primary processing methods on the flavor of coffea arabica beans by metabolomics. *Fermentation* **2023**, *9*, 717. [CrossRef]
9. Partida-Sedas, J.G.; Muñoz Ferreiro, M.N.; Vázquez-Odériz, L.; Romero-Rodríguez, M.Á.; Pérez-Portilla, E. Influence of the postharvest processing of the "Garnica" coffee variety on the sensory characteristics and overall acceptance of the beverage. *J. Sens. Stud.* **2019**, *34*, e12502. [CrossRef]
10. Wang, C.; Sun, J.; Lassabliere, B.; Yu, B.; Liu, S.Q. Coffee flavour modification through controlled fermentation of green coffee beans by Saccharomyces cerevisiae and Pichia kluyveri: Part II. Mixed cultures with or without lactic acid bacteria. *Food Res. Int.* **2020**, *136*, 109452. [CrossRef]
11. Bastian, F.; Hutabarat, O.S.; Dirpan, A.; Nainu, F.; Harapan, H.; Emran, T.B.; Simal-Gandara, J. From plantation to cup: Changes in bioactive compounds during coffee processing. *Foods* **2021**, *10*, 2827. [CrossRef]
12. Macheiner, L.; Schmidt, A.; Schreiner, M.; Mayer, H.K. Green coffee infusion as a source of caffeine and chlorogenic acid. *J. Food Compos. Anal.* **2019**, *84*, 103307. [CrossRef]
13. Marques, D.S.; Memento, G.S.; Salgado, A.L.; Freire, A.P. Quality Coffee Information Needs and Implications for Information Systems: A Study with Coffee Consumers. In Proceedings of the 20th Brazilian Symposium on Information Systems, Juiz de Fora, Brazil, 20–23 May 2014. [CrossRef]
14. Mili, S.; Ferro-Soto, C. Precursors and outcomes of satisfaction of fair trade coffee consumers. *Eur. J. Manag. Bus. Econ.* **2024**, *33*, 195–211. [CrossRef]
15. Samoggia, A.; Riedel, B. Consumers' Perceptions of Coffee Health Benefits and Motives for Coffee Consumption and Purchasing. *Nutrients* **2019**, *11*, 653. [CrossRef] [PubMed]
16. Bercík, J.; Gálová, J.; Pavelka, A. *The Use of Consumer Neuroscience in Aroma Marketing*; BRIIL: Leiden, The Netherlands, 2021. [CrossRef]
17. Yang, A.; Zhang, Z.; Jiangm, K.; Xu, K.; Meng, F.; Wu, W.; Li, Z.; Wang, B. Study on ultrasound-assisted extraction of cold brew coffee using physicochemical, flavor, and sensory evaluation. *Food Biosci.* **2024**, *61*, 104455. [CrossRef]
18. Lee, L.W.; Cheong, M.W.; Curran, P.; Yu, B.; Liu, S.Q. Coffee fermentation and flavor—An intricate and delicate relationship. *Food Chem.* **2015**, *185*, 182–191. [CrossRef] [PubMed]
19. Seninde, D.R.; Chambers, E. Coffee flavor: A review. *Beverages* **2020**, *6*, 44. [CrossRef]
20. Schenker, S.; Heinemann, C.; Huber, M.; Pompizzi, R.; Perren, R.; Escher, R. Impact of roasting conditions on the formation of aroma compounds in coffee beans. *J. Food Sci.* **2002**, *67*, 60–66. [CrossRef]
21. Baggenstoss, J.; Poisson, L.; Kaegi, R.; Perren, R.; Escher, F. Coffee roasting and aroma formation: Application of different time-temperature conditions. *J. Agric. Food Chem.* **2008**, *56*, 5836–5846. [CrossRef]
22. Erlacher, W.A.; Amaral, J.F.; Amaral, J.A.; Christo, B.F.; Ferreira, D.S.; Tatagiba, S.D.; Rocha, B.C.; Tomaz, M.A.; Rodrigues, W.N.; Partelli, F.L. Effect of indole-3-acetic acid on growth, physiology and nutritional status of young arabica coffee plants. *Coffee Sci.* **2023**, *17*, 172050. [CrossRef]
23. da Costa, D.S.; Albuquerque, T.G.; Costa, H.S.; Bragotto, A.P.A. Thermal contaminants in coffee induced by roasting: A review. *Int. J. Environ. Res. Public Health* **2023**, *20*, 5586. [CrossRef]
24. Cao, X.; Wu, H.; Viejo, C.G.; Dunshea, F.R.; Suleria, H.A.R. Effects of postharvest processing on aroma formation in roasted coffee—A review. *Int. J. Food Sci. Technol.* **2023**, *58*, 1007–1027. [CrossRef]
25. Di Stefano, V.; Buzzanca, C.; Ruvutuso, F.; Scuderi, D.; Palazzolo, E.; Gugliuzza, G.; Tinebra, I.; Farina, V. Chemical composition and anti-radical properties of coffee cherry cultivated in Mediterranean climate. *Food Biosci.* **2023**, *56*, 103349. [CrossRef]
26. Pua, A.; Goh, R.M.V.; Huang, Y.; Tang, V.C.Y.; Ee, K.H.; Cornuz, M.; Liu, S.Q.; Lassabliere, B.; Yu, B. Recent advances in analytical strategies for coffee volatile studies: Opportunities and challenges. *Food Chem.* **2022**, *388*, 132971. [CrossRef] [PubMed]
27. Zhang, S.J.; De Bruyn, F.; Pothakos, V.; Contreras, G.F.; Cai, Z.; Moccand, C.; Weckx, S.; De Vuyst, L. Influence of various processing parameters on the microbial community dynamics, metabolomic profiles, and cup quality during wet coffee processing. *Front. Microbiol.* **2019**, *10*, 2621. [CrossRef] [PubMed]
28. Rahma, S.K.; Sarofa, U.; Anggreini, R.A. The effect of the proportion of ginger and spices extracts and the addition of sugar on the physicochemical properties of instant spiced coffee. *Asian J. Appl. Res. Community Dev. Empower.* **2024**, *8*, 37–43. [CrossRef]
29. Wan, L.; Wang, H.; Mo, X.; Wang, Y.; Song, L.; Liu, L.; Liang, W. Applying HS-SPME-GC-MS combined with PTR-TOF-MS to analyze the volatile compounds in coffee husks of Coffea arabica with different primary processing treatments in Yunnan. *LWT* **2024**, *191*, 115675. [CrossRef]

30. Maligan, J.M.; Kosasih, S.U.; Nurcholis, M.; Sriherfyna, F.H. Effect of fermentation time and roasting temperature on the characteristics of wine coffee arabica semeru. *J. Pangan Agroindustri* **2024**, *12*, 31–42. [CrossRef]
31. Abubakar, Y.; Hasni, D.; Baihaqi, A.; Rasdiansyah, R.; Sumardi, S. Consumer preferences on arabica coffee bag with cinnamon flavors from different roasting degrees. *AIP Conf. Proc.* **2024**, *3082*, 040047. [CrossRef]
32. Zhang, S.J.; De Bruyn, F.; Pothakos, V.; Torres, J.; Falconi, C.; Moccand, C.; Weckx, S.; De Vuyst, L. Following coffee production from cherries to cup: Microbiological and metabolomic analysis of wet processing of Coffea Arabica. *Appl. Environ. Microbiol.* **2019**, *85*, e02635-18. [CrossRef]
33. Elhalis, H.; Cox, J.; Frank, D.; Zhao, J. The crucial role of yeasts in the wet fermentation of coffee beans and quality. *Int. J. Food Microbiol.* **2020**, *333*, 108796. [CrossRef]
34. Bressani, A.P.P.; Martinez, S.J.; Sarmento, A.B.I.; Borém, F.M.; Schwan, R.F. Influence of yeast inoculation on the quality of fermented coffee (*Coffea arabica* var. Mundo Novo) processed by natural and pulped natural processes. *Int. J. Food Microbiol.* **2021**, *343*, 109107. [CrossRef]
35. Zofia, N.-Ł.; Aleksandra, Z.; Tomasz, B.; Martyna, Z.-D.; Magdalena, Z.; Zofia, H.-B.; Tomasz, W. Effect of fermentation time on antioxidant and anti-ageing properties of green coffee kombucha ferments. *Molecules* **2020**, *25*, 5394. [CrossRef] [PubMed]
36. Liu, J.; Fu, B.; Liu, S.; Qu, H.; Luo, H.; Yuan, W. Study on the wine brewing technology of coffee pulp grown in Yunnan province. *Sci. Technol. Food Ind.* **2017**, *10*, 194–199. [CrossRef]
37. Muzykiewicz-Szymańska, A.; Nowak, A.; Wira, D.; Klimowicz, A. The Effect of brewing process parameters on antioxidant activity and caffeine content in infusions of roasted and unroasted arabica coffee beans originated from different countries. *Molecules* **2021**, *26*, 3681. [CrossRef]
38. Stanek, N.; Zarębska, M.; Biłos, Ł.; Barabosz, K.; Nowakowska-Bogdan, E.; Semeniuk, I.; Błaszkiewicz, J.; Kulesza, R.; Matejuk, R.; Szkutnik, K. Influence of coffee brewing methods on the chromatographic and spectroscopic profiles, antioxidant, and sensory properties. *Sci. Rep.* **2021**, *11*, 21377. [CrossRef] [PubMed]
39. Portela, C.D.S.; Almeida, I.F.; Reis, T.A.D.D.; Hickmann, B.R.B.; Benassi, M.T. Effects of brewing conditions and coffee species on the physicochemical characteristics, preference, and dynamics of sensory attributes perception in cold brews. *Food Res. Int.* **2022**, *151*, 110860. [CrossRef]
40. Grzelczyk, J.; Szwajgier, D.; Baranowska-Wójcik, E.; Budryn, G.; Zakłos-Szyda, M.; Sosnowska, B. Bioaccessibility of coffee bean hydroxycinnamic acids during in vitro digestion influenced by the degree of roasting and activity of intestinal probiotic bacteria, and their activity in Caco-2 and HT29 cells. *Food Chem.* **2022**, *392*, 133328. [CrossRef]
41. Wolska, J.; Janda, K.; Jakubczyk, K.; Szymkowiak, M.; Chlubek, D.; Gutowska, I. Levels of antioxidant activity and fluoride content in coffee infusions of Arabica, Robusta, and green coffee beans in according to their brewing methods. *Biol. Trace Elem. Res.* **2017**, *179*, 327–333. [CrossRef]
42. Yashin, A.; Yashin, Y.; Wang, J.Y.; Nemzer, B. Antioxidant and antiradical activity of coffee. *Antioxidants* **2013**, *2*, 230–245. [CrossRef]
43. Oboh, G.; Akinyemi, A.J.; Ademiluyi, A.O. Inhibition of α-amylase and α-glucosidase activities by ethanolic extract of *Telfairia occidentalis* (fluted pumpkin) leaf. *Asian Pac. J. Trop. Biomed.* **2012**, *2*, 733–738. [CrossRef]
44. Kim, Y.K.; Lim, J.-M.; Kim, Y.J.; Kim, W. Alterations in pH of coffee bean extract and properties of chlorogenic acid based on the roasting degree. *Foods* **2024**, *13*, 1757. [CrossRef]
45. Mättä-Riihinen, K.R.; Kamal-Eldin, A.; Törrönen, A.R. Identification and quantification of phenolic compounds in berries of *Fragaria* and *Rubus* Sp. (Family *Rosaceae*). *J. Agric. Food Chem.* **2004**, *52*, 6178–6187. [CrossRef]
46. Dawidowicz, A.L.; Typek, R. Thermal transformation of trans-5-O-caffeoylquinic acid (trans-5-CQA) in alcoholic solutions. *Food Chem.* **2015**, *167*, 52–60. [CrossRef] [PubMed]
47. Gong, L.; Feng, D.; Wang, T.; Ren, Y.; Liu, Y.; Wang, J. Inhibitors of α-amylase and α-glucosidase: Potential linkage for whole cereal foods on prevention of hyperglycemia. *Food Sci. Nutr.* **2020**, *8*, 6320–6337. [CrossRef] [PubMed]
48. Dimtsas, V.; Douma, A.; Soukia, D.; Chatzimitakos, T.; Athanasiadis, V.; Kotsou, K.; Bozinou, E.; Lalas, S.I. Exploring varied (green) extraction methods to optimize galia melon peel antioxidant potential. *Separations* **2024**, *11*, 135. [CrossRef]
49. Gómez-García, R.; Campos, D.A.; Aguilar, C.N.; Madureira, A.R.; Pintad, M. Valorization of melon fruit (*Cucumis melo* L.) by-products: Phytochemical and biofunctional properties with emphasis on current trends and advances. *Trends Food Sci. Technol.* **2020**, *99*, 507–519. [CrossRef]
50. Mihalev, K.; Schieber, A.; Mollov, P.; Carle, R. Effect of mash maceration on the polyphenolic content and visual quality attributes of cloudy apple juice. *J. Agric. Food Chem.* **2004**, *52*, 7306–7310. [CrossRef] [PubMed]
51. Mehaya, F.M.; Mohammad, A.A. Thermostability of bioactive compounds during roasting process of coffee beans. *Heliyon* **2020**, *6*, e05508. [CrossRef]
52. Ludwig, I.A.; Bravo, J.; De Peña, M.P.; Cid, C. Effect of sugar addition (torrefacto) during roasting process on antioxidant capacity and phenolics of coffee. *LWT Food Sci. Technol.* **2013**, *51*, 553–559. [CrossRef]
53. Ohishi, T.; Fukutomi, R.; Shoji, Y.; Goto, S.; Isemura, M. The beneficial effects of principal polyphenols from green tea, coffee, wine, and curry on obesity. *Molecules* **2021**, *26*, 453. [CrossRef]
54. Garrido, J.; Borges, F. Wine and grape polyphenols—A chemical perspective. *Food Res. Int.* **2013**, *54*, 1844–1858. [CrossRef]
55. Haller, S.; Montandon, M.-L.; Rodriguez, C.; Herrmann, F.R.; Giannakopoulos, P. Impact of coffee, wine, and chocolate consumption on cognitive outcome and MRI parameters in old age. *Nutrients* **2018**, *10*, 1391. [CrossRef] [PubMed]

56. Nguyen, T.; Kuchera, M.; Smoot, K.; Diako, C.; Vixie, B.; Ross, C.F. Consumer acceptance of a polyphenolic coffee beverage. *J. Food Sci.* **2016**, *81*, S2817–S2823. [CrossRef] [PubMed]
57. Cao, H.; Ou, J.; Chen, L.; Zhang, Y.; Szkudelski, T.; Delmas, D.; Daglia, M.; Xiao, J. Dietary polyphenols and type 2 diabetes: Human Study and Clinical Trial. *Crit. Rev. Food Sci. Nutr.* **2019**, *59*, 3371–3379. [CrossRef] [PubMed]
58. Budryn, G.; Nebesny, E.; Oracz, J. Correlation between the stability of chlorogenic acids, antioxidant activity and acrylamide content in coffee beans roasted in different conditions. *Int. J. Food Prop.* **2015**, *18*, 290–302. [CrossRef]
59. Zanin, R.C.; Smrke, S.; Kurazawa, L.E.; Yamashita, F.; Yeretzian, C. Modulation of aroma release of instant coffees through microparticles of roasted coffee oil. *Food Chem.* **2021**, *341*, 128193. [CrossRef]
60. Hong, C.T.; Chan, L.; Bai, C.-H. The Effect of caffeine on the risk and progression of Parkinson's disease: A meta-analysis. *Nutrients* **2020**, *12*, 1860. [CrossRef]
61. Schepici, G.; Silvestro, S.; Bramanti, P.; Mazzon, E. Caffeine: An overview of its beneficial effects in experimental models and clinical trials of Parkinson's disease. *Int. J. Mol. Sci.* **2020**, *21*, 4766. [CrossRef] [PubMed]
62. Singh, J.; Metrani, R.; Jayaprakasha, G.K.; Crosby, K.M.; Jifon, J.L.; Ravishankar, S.; Brierley, P.; Leskovar, D.L.; Turini, T.A.; Schultheis, J.; et al. Profiling carotenoid and sugar contents in unique Cucumis melo L. cultigens harvested from different climatic regions of the United States. *J. Food Compos. Anal.* **2022**, *106*, 104306. [CrossRef]
63. Aprea, E.; Charles, M.; Endrizzi, I.; Laura Corollaro, M.; Betta, E.; Biasioli, F.; Gasperi, F. Sweet taste in apple: The role of sorbitol, individual sugars, organic acids and volatile compounds. *Sci. Rep.* **2017**, *7*, 44950. [CrossRef]
64. Ross, K.; Siow, Y.; Brown, D.; Isaak, C.; Fukumoto, L.; Godfrey, D. Characterization of Water Extractable Crude Polysaccharides from Cherry, Raspberry, and Ginseng Berry Fruits: Chemical Composition and Bioactivity. *Int. J. Food Prop.* **2015**, *18*, 670–689. [CrossRef]
65. Faienza, M.F.; Corbo, F.; Carocci, A.; Catalano, A.; Clodoveo, M.L.; Grano, M.; Wang, D.Q.; D'Amato, G.; Muraglia, M.; Franchini, C.; et al. Novel insights in health-promoting properties of sweet cherries. *J. Funct. Foods.* **2020**, *69*, 103945. [CrossRef] [PubMed]
66. Weingart, E.; Tschirner, S.; Teevs, L.; Prüße, U. Conversion of Fructose to HMF in a Continuous Fixed Bed Reactor with Outstanding Selectivity. *Molecules* **2018**, *23*, 1802. [CrossRef] [PubMed]
67. Tsegay, G.; Redi-Abshiro, M.; Chandravanshi, B.S.; Ele, E.; Mohammed, A.M.; Mamo, H. Efect of altitude of cofee plants on the composition of fatty acids of green coffee beans. *BMC Chem.* **2020**, *14*, 36. [CrossRef]
68. Schouten, M.A.; Tappi, S.; Romani, S. Acrylamide in coffee: Formation and possible mitigation strategies—A review. *Crit. Rev. Food Sci. Nutr.* **2020**, *60*, 3807–3821. [CrossRef]
69. de Melo Pereira, G.V.; de Carvalho Neto, D.P.; Júnior, A.I.; Vásquez, Z.S.; Medeiros, A.B.; Vandenberghe, L.P.; Soccol, C.R. Exploring the impacts of postharvest processing on the aroma formation of coffee beans—A review. *Food Chem.* **2019**, *272*, 441–452. [CrossRef]
70. Hamzalıoğlu, A.; Gökmen, V. 5-Hydroxymethylfurfural accumulation plays a critical role on acrylamide formation in coffee during roasting as confirmed by multiresponse kinetic modeling. *Food Chem.* **2020**, *318*, 126467. [CrossRef] [PubMed]
71. Münchow, M.; Alstrup, J.; Steen, I.; Giacalone, D. Roasting conditions and coffee flavor: A multi-study empirical investigation. *Beverages* **2020**, *6*, 29. [CrossRef]
72. Rattanarat, P.; Chindapan, N.; Sakamon, D. Comparative evaluation of acrylamide and polycyclic aromatic hydrocarbons contents in Robusta coffee beans roasted by warm air and superheated steam. *Food Chem.* **2021**, *341*, 128266. [CrossRef]
73. Oikawa, N.; Wakabayashi, M.; Ota, H. Processing Method of Coffee Bean, Roasting Method of Coffee Bean, and Method for increasing Amino Acid in Coffee Bean. U.S. Patent 11/664,218, 18 September 2008.
74. Sturm, K.; Hudina, M.; Solar, A.; Marn, M.V.; Stampar, F. Fruit Quality of Different 'Gala' Clones. *Europ. J. Hort. Sci.* **2003**, *68*, 169–175.
75. Marques, C.; Sotiles, R.A.; Farias, F.O.; Oliveira, G.; Mitterer-Daltoe, M.L.; Masson, M.L. Full physicochemical characterization of malic acid: Emphasis in the potential as food ingredient and application in pectin gels. *Arab. J. Chem.* **2020**, *13*, 9118–9129. [CrossRef]
76. Wiecinska, P. Thermal degradation of organic additives used in colloidal shaping of ceramics investigated by the coupled DTA/TG/MS analysis. *J. Therm. Anal. Calorim.* **2016**, *123*, 1419–1430. [CrossRef]
77. Komesu, A.; Martinez, P.F.M.; Lunelli, B.H.; Oliveira, J.; Maciel, M.R.W.; Fiho, R.M. Study of Lactic Acid Thermal Behavior Using Thermoanalytical Techniques. *J. Chem.* **2017**, *2017*, 4149592. [CrossRef]
78. Cuervo, A.; Hevia, A.; López, P.; Suárez, A.; Diaz, C.; Sánchez, B.; Margolles, A.; González, S. Phenolic compounds from red wine and coffee are associated with specific intestinal microorganisms in allergic subjects. *Food Funct.* **2016**, *7*, 104–109. [CrossRef]
79. Zulfiqar, H.; Hussain, A.I.; Ali, Q.; Rathore, H.A.; Ahmed, I. Phenolic profile, nutritional potential and biological activities of wildly grown accessions of Cucumis melo var. Agrestis. *J. King Saud Univ. Sci.* **2024**, *36*, 10332. [CrossRef]
80. Haile, M.; Bae, H.M.; Kang, W.H. Comparison of the Antioxidant Activities and Volatile Compounds of Coffee Beans Obtained Using Digestive Bio-Processing (Elephant Dung Coffee) and Commonly Known Processing Methods. *Antioxidants* **2020**, *9*, 408. [CrossRef] [PubMed]
81. Zeb, A. Phenolic Profile and antioxidant activity of melon (*Cucumis melo* L.) seeds from Pakistan. *Foods* **2016**, *5*, 67. [CrossRef] [PubMed]
82. Fetsch, V.T.; Kalschne, D.L.; Canan, C.; Flores, É.L.M.; Viegas, M.C.; Peiter, G.C.; Zara, R.F.; Amaral, J.S.; Corso, M.P. Coffee extract as a natural antioxidant in fresh pork sausage—A model approach. *Foods* **2024**, *13*, 1409. [CrossRef]

83. Freitas, V.V.; Borges, L.L.R.; Vidigal, M.C.T.R.; das Santos, M.H.; Stringheta, P.C. Coffee: A comprehensive overview of origin, market, and the quality process. *Trends Food Sci. Technol.* **2024**, *146*, 104411. [CrossRef]
84. Yeager, S.E.; Batali, M.E.; Guinard, J.E.; Ristenpart, W.D. Acids in coffee: A review of sensory measurements and meta-analysis of chemical composition. *Crit. Rev. Food Sci. Nutr.* **2021**, *63*, 1010–1036. [CrossRef]
85. Sun, Y.; Cao, Q.; Huang, Y.; Lu, T.; Ma, H.; Chen, X. Mechanistic study on the inhibition of α-amylase and α-glucosidase using the extract of ultrasound-treated coffee leaves. *J. Sci. Food Agric.* **2024**, *104*, 63–74. [CrossRef]

nutrients

MDPI

Article

Beneficial Effects of Ginger Extract on Eye Fatigue and Shoulder Stiffness: A Randomized, Double-Blind, and Placebo-Controlled Parallel Study

Fumiko Higashikawa [1,*], Yuta Nakaniida [2,3], Hongyang Li [4], Lian Liang [4], Keishi Kanno [5], Keiko Ogawa-Ochiai [4] and Yoshiaki Kiuchi [2]

1 Medical Center for Translational and Clinical Research, Hiroshima University Hospital, 1-2-3 Kasumi, Minami-ku, Hiroshima 734-8551, Japan
2 Department of Ophthalmology and Visual Science, Graduate School of Biomedical and Health Sciences, Hiroshima University, 1-2-3 Kasumi, Minami-ku, Hiroshima 734-8551, Japan; d224004@hiroshima-u.ac.jp (Y.N.); ykiuchi@hiroshima-u.ac.jp (Y.K.)
3 Department of Ophthalmology, Saneikai Tsukazaki Hospital, 68-1 Aboshi Waku, Himeji 671-1227, Japan
4 Kampo Clinical Center, Hiroshima University Hospital, 1-2-3 Kasumi, Minami-ku, Hiroshima 734-8551, Japan; hoyalee328@yahoo.co.jp (H.L.); lianglian96@gmail.com (L.L.); ikkandoo@gmail.com (K.O.-O.)
5 Department of General Internal Medicine, Hiroshima University Hospital, 1-2-3 Kasumi, Minami-ku, Hiroshima 734-8551, Japan; kkanno@hiroshima-u.ac.jp
* Correspondence: fumiko@hiroshima-u.ac.jp; Tel.: +81-(82)-257-1909

Abstract: This study aimed to assess ginger extract's impact on ocular and peripheral blood flow and its potential to alleviate eye fatigue and shoulder stiffness. This study included 100 healthy individuals aged 20–73 years with eye fatigue and shoulder stiffness. Participants were randomly assigned to receive either placebo capsules or ginger extract capsules daily for eight weeks. Ocular blood flow, peripheral blood flow, eye fatigue (visual analog scale [VAS]), shoulder stiffness (VAS), body warmth (VAS), and shoulder muscle stiffness were assessed at weeks 0, 4, and 8, respectively. No improvement in ocular blood flow was observed under the study conditions. Conversely, peripheral blood flow in deep areas was enhanced in females ($p = 0.033$). Subgroup analysis by age ($\geq$51 or <51 years) revealed that ginger's effect on enhancing peripheral blood flow in deep vessels was restricted in females under 51 ($p = 0.017$). Similarly, subjective complaints of eye fatigue and shoulder stiffness were improved by ginger consumption in females under 51. Body warmth was favorably changed significantly in males $\geq$51 years due to ginger consumption. The muscle stiffness showed no statistically significant changes. In conclusion, ginger consumption reduces eye fatigue and shoulder stiffness by enhancing peripheral blood flow in relatively young females.

Keywords: ginger; ocular blood flow; peripheral blood flow; eye fatigue; shoulder stiffness

1. Introduction

For centuries, ginger (*Zingiber officinale*) has been widely used as a spice for cooking and as a medicinal herb worldwide. The main active components of ginger are gingerols, shogaols, and zingerones, which are pungent compounds. These components show anti-inflammatory and anti-oxidative activities, as confirmed in in vitro and in vivo animal models and in cancer patients [1–3]. Several systematic reviews have shown that consuming ginger can alleviate nausea and vomiting during pregnancy [4–10] and improve metabolic syndrome [4,10–17] and pain [4,18–22]. Nevertheless, further research is needed to elucidate the differences among clinical trial conditions, including ginger form, dosage, consumption period, and evaluation outcomes.

Ginger is also a staple ingredient in traditional Japanese cuisine and is believed to offer various health benefits, such as improvements to thermogenetic function and blood flow acceleration. Despite the many studies concerning ginger's effects, there is limited scientific evidence to support the claims of improved blood flow, still less in the eyes, or warming of the body, which are long-held beliefs in Japan. Consequently, additional research is necessary to explore the possibility of ginger enhancing blood flow and promoting body warmth.

In recent years, there has been a significant increase in the use of visual display terminals (VDTs), such as computers, smartphones, tablets, and video games, owing to rapid advancements in IT. Prolonged exposure to VDTs has been associated with a variety of health issues, most notably VDT Syndrome. This condition is characterized by symptoms such as dry eyes, eye fatigue, and stiffness of the neck and shoulders. The prevalence of dry eye disease in VDT users ranges from 26% to 70% [23,24]. This condition has become a pressing social issue that must be addressed because it negatively impacts an individual's quality of life [24,25]. Studies have associated low ocular blood flow with eye diseases such as glaucoma and myopia [26–28]. These findings suggest that improving ocular blood flow may be an effective strategy for preventing or treating eye diseases since proper blood flow to the eye is crucial for providing sufficient oxygen and nutrients to the optic nerve.

Hence, we conducted a randomized, double-blind, placebo-controlled clinical study in individuals with symptoms similar to VDT syndrome to explore whether consuming ginger could enhance both peripheral and ocular blood flow, leading to improvements in shoulder stiffness and eye fatigue. Our evaluation not only assessed ocular and peripheral blood flow, but also recorded self-reported conditions, such as eye fatigue, shoulder stiffness, and body warmth. It also measured shoulder muscle stiffness.

2. Materials and Methods

2.1. Materials

The ginger extract powder capsule weighed 250 mg and consisted of 100 mg of ginger extract powder E (2 mg of 6-shogaol, 0.5 mg of 6-gingerol; Ikeda Tohka Industries Co., Ltd., Hiroshima, Japan), 147 mg of dextrin, and 3 mg of calcium stearate. The placebo capsule contained the same constituents as the ginger capsule, except for the ginger powder, which was substituted for 100 mg of dextrin. The capsules were provided by Ikeda Food Research Co., Ltd. (Hiroshima, Japan).

2.2. Subjects

Participants were recruited via advertisements. The inclusion criteria were healthy individuals between the ages of 20 and 75 who experienced both eye fatigue and shoulder stiffness. Excluded from this study were subjects with eye symptoms requiring immediate treatment, patients taking medication or dietary supplements that might impact the study results, including those intended to alleviate eye fatigue, shoulder stiffness, or affect blood flow, patients who participated in another clinical trial within the past three months, or were pregnant or nursing.

2.3. Study Design

This randomized, double-blind, placebo-controlled, parallel clinical study was conducted at Hiroshima University Hospital from August to December 2021. One hundred study participants meeting the inclusion and exclusion criteria determined by the principal investigator were randomly assigned to either the ginger or placebo group at a 1:1 allocation ratio. The assignment table was generated using a computer with a randomization program. The subjects were stratified by sex and allocated using the block randomization method with a block size of 4. The investigator responsible for allocation was not involved in assessing the study results. The principal investigator, physicians, and clinical staff were blinded to the randomization assignment.

The participants were instructed to take one capsule of either ginger extract or a placebo daily for 8 weeks. Clinical examinations were conducted every four weeks.

The subjects were instructed as follows: (1) to maintain their usual lifestyle, including food consumption, especially ginger in dishes, and exercise; (2) to keep a daily record of their compliance with capsule intake, health conditions, medications, and dietary supplements; (3) to record their diet, including beverages and alcohol, for three consecutive days prior to each clinical visit; (4) not to take the experimental capsules before, but rather after, the clinical examination on the day of the scheduled clinical visits; (5) not to start taking new dietary supplements; and (6) not to donate blood during the study period.

In this study, we measured the change in blood flow in the macular and optic disc areas using a Laser Speckle Flowgraphy System, LSFG-NAVI (Softcare Ltd., Fukuoka, Japan), as the primary outcome. Secondary outcomes included changes in peripheral blood flow, eye fatigue (VAS), shoulder stiffness (VAS), body warmth (VAS), and shoulder muscle stiffness. The participants' compliance rates were evaluated based on their records. Any negative effects that occurred during the study were recorded in a questionnaire at the clinical visit, in the subjects' diaries, and assessed using the Common Terminology Criteria for Adverse Events (CTCAE) v5.0.

This clinical trial was registered in the University Hospital Medical Information Network Clinical Trials Registry (UMIN-CTR, www.umin.ac.jp) as UMIN000044983.

2.4. Ocular Blood Flow

Real-time changes in blood flow were detected using LSFG-NAVI. Specifically, this system allows the calculation of ocular blood flow in a particular area of interest. This system measures blood flow using the Mean Blur Rate (MBR), a relative value and not an exact measure of blood flow speed. This study measured ocular blood flow in the macular and optic disc areas. Blood flow in the optic disc was determined by subtracting the MBR of the tissue area (MT) from that of the vascular area (MV). The average of the three measurements was used for each analysis. Data from the right eye were used for all analyses.

2.5. Peripheral Blood Flow

O2C ("Oxygen-to-see", LEA Medizintechnik, Giessen, Germany) is a device that allows non-invasive measurement of tissue oxygenation and microcirculation [29,30]. The present study measured blood flow and flow velocity at depths of 2 mm (cutaneous tissue) and 8 mm (subcutaneous tissue) using O2C. The data were collected as previously described [30]. Briefly, an O2C probe was placed in the middle of the dorsal aspect of the right forearm. After the patient sat for 10 min, the microcirculation was measured continuously for 3 min. The data were obtained as an average of three minutes of measurement. The measuring room was set at a comfortable temperature.

2.6. Visual Analog Scales (VAS)

Visual analog scales (VAS) were used to assess the level of subjective symptoms related to eye fatigue, shoulder stiffness, and body warmth. Participants were asked to mark their symptoms on a 100 mm line, ranging from 0 to 100. The VAS indicators were as follows: for eye fatigue, 0 represented "no eye fatigue at all" and 100 represented "the most severe eye fatigue imaginable"; for shoulder stiffness, 0 represented "no shoulder stiffness at all" and 100 represented "the most extreme shoulder stiffness imaginable"; for body warmth, 0 represented "the worst feeling of coldness" and 100 represented "the best feeling of warmth".

2.7. Shoulder Muscle Stiffness

The firmness of the shoulder muscles in the depression midway between the acromion and cervical spine (Jianjing, GB21) was measured using a muscle hardness meter (TDM-NA1; Sato Shouji Inc., Kanagawa, Japan).

2.8. Statistical Analysis

We determined a sample size of 100, assuming a 10% difference between groups in outcome changes, with a standard deviation of 15%, 85% power, and 5% alpha error, because there was no reference to ginger's effect on ocular blood flow to calculate the sample size. We assessed the data as FAS, including all cases in the final analyses, according to the intention-to-treat principle (Figure 1). The multiple imputation method was repeated 20 times to handle missing data.

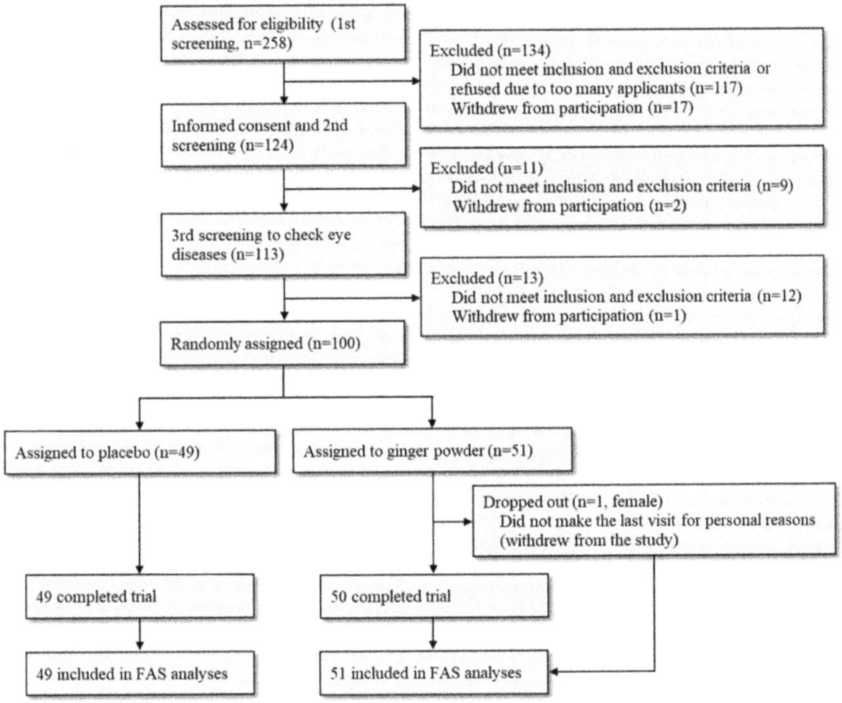

Figure 1. Summary of the subject flow.

We compared changes in each outcome during the 8-week intervention period between groups using Student's t-test, except for variables that did not follow a normal distribution (shoulder stiffness (VAS), shoulder muscle stiffness, and peripheral blood flow velocity of superficial vessels), which were analyzed using the Mann–Whitney U test. For categorical data analysis, Fisher's exact test was used to compare the groups based on safety assessment. Primary and secondary outcomes were also analyzed and stratified by sex and age (<51, ≥51 years). The age line was determined at 51 years because the average and median ages of the study participants were 51.6 and 52 years, respectively. In addition, we were interested in sex hormone effects. Data are expressed as mean ± SD or mean difference (95% confidence interval) in tables or mean ± SE in graphs. Statistical analyses were performed using IBM SPSS Statistics Version 22 (IBM, Armonk, NY, USA), with statistical significance set at $p < 0.05$.

3. Results

3.1. Population Characteristics

The flow of participants is shown in Figure 1. After screening the initial pool of applicants with an application form (first screening), 124 out of 258 participants attended the orientation session regarding the clinical trial. All 124 agreed to participate, 9 were excluded from the second screening, 2 withdrew their participation, and 113 underwent the third screening process, which included an ophthalmic examination. Finally, 100 subjects who met all the criteria were included in the study. One participant in the ginger group dropped out of the study during the last visit for personal reasons.

Table 1 summarizes the participants' backgrounds. Choline esterase only exhibited significant differences at baseline. Table 2 shows the baseline outcomes for each group and by sex. Despite randomized allocation, there was a significant difference in the VAS for eye fatigue, with higher baseline levels in the ginger group than in the placebo group.

Table 1. Characteristics of the study participants.

	Placebo (n = 49)	Ginger (n = 51)	p-Value
Age (years)	51.1 ± 12.0	52.0 ± 10.2	0.694
Male/Female	12/37	13/38	-
Height (cm)	159.7 ± 7.8	159.5 ± 6.8	0.902
Body weight (kg)	55.3 ± 11.9	56.6 ± 11.6	0.626
BMI (kg/m^2)	21.5 ± 3.3	22.1 ± 3.8	0.429
Body fat percentage (%)	24.8 ± 7.5	26.1 ± 8.1	0.482
Systolic blood pressure (mmHg)	109.9 ± 18.0	112.4 ± 15.2	0.673
Diastolic blood pressure (mmHg)	66.8 ± 12.9	68.3 ± 10.5	0.902
Heart rate (beats per min)	68.8 ± 12.5	69.7 ± 9.0	0.469
White blood cell count (×10^3/mL)	5.23 ± 1.55	5.45 ± 1.19	0.438
Red blood cell count (×10^6/mL)	4.57 ± 0.43	4.64 ± 0.45	0.480
Hemoglobin (g/dL)	13.6 ± 1.4	14.0 ± 1.3	0.102
Hematocrit (%)	42.3 ± 3.9	43.4 ± 3.7	0.151
Platelet count (×10^4/mL)	24.6 ± 6.3	25.4 ± 6.0	0.532
AST (IU/L)	21.3 ± 5.0	21.0 ± 6.0	0.797
ALT (IU/L)	18.9 ± 9.2	19.6 ± 12.9	0.746
γ-GTP (IU/L)	21.4 ± 8.7	28.2 ± 33.8	0.176
LDH(IU/L)	188 ± 26	188 ± 24	0.968
Choline esterase (IU/L)	316 ± 68	345 ± 70 *	0.041
Alkaline phosphatase (IU/L)	65.9 ± 19.1	67.5 ± 16.9	0.676
Amylase (IU/L)	80.1 ± 28.9	96.9 ± 92.1	0.227
Total protein (g/dL)	7.44 ± 0.45	7.41 ± 0.37	0.708
Total bilirubin (mg/dL)	0.79 ± 0.28	0.73 ± 0.22	0.233
Albumin (g/dL)	4.57 ± 0.28	4.53 ± 0.25	0.473
Uric acid (mg/dL)	4.69 ± 1.10	4.89 ± 1.39	0.436
Blood urea nitrogen (mg/dL)	13.5 ± 3.3	13.2 ± 4.4	0.720
Creatinine (mg/dL)	0.691 ± 0.131	0.690 ± 0.165	0.968
eGFR (mL/min/1.73 m^2)	98.9 ± 21.0	99.5 ± 21.9	0.886
Total cholesterol (mg/dL)	228 ± 42	232 ± 40	0.613
LDL cholesterol (mg/dL)	136 ± 35	141 ± 33	0.523
HDL cholesterol (mg/dL)	69.4 ± 20.4	70.8 ± 17.2	0.728
LDL/HDL ratio	2.13 ± 0.82	2.10 ± 0.65	0.846
Triglycerides (mg/dL)	110.9 ± 97.9	107.9 ± 63.6	0.856
Fasting blood glucose (mg/dL)	97.3 ± 8.7	95.5 ± 9.0	0.327

Data are expressed as mean ± SD. * Statistical difference versus placebo group by Student's t-test at $p < 0.05$.

The subjects' diary showed high compliance rates of 98.6 ± 2.2% in the ginger group and 98.8 ± 2.2% in the placebo group, with no notable difference between the two groups. After analyzing the subjects' dietary records, there were no significant differences in daily calorie intake changes between the groups (46.9 ± 432.0 kcal in the ginger group and 117.7 ± 323.7 kcal in the placebo group).

3.2. Ginger Enhances Peripheral Blood Flow Velocity

Ocular blood flow decreased during the ginger consumption period, with no significant difference between the groups (Figure 2A,B). The tendencies did not differ between the experimental groups when subgroups according to sex were analyzed. Figure 2C shows a statistically significant increase in the peripheral blood flow velocity of deep vessels after ginger consumption only in females ($p < 0.05$). This increase was contributed by those under 51 years of age (Table 3). By contrast, there was no significant change in superficial vessel blood flow velocity among all, males, and females (Figure 2D), but only among females ≥51 years (Table 3).

Table 2. The baseline values of each outcome.

	Placebo	Ginger	p-Value
Retinal blood flow			
All (n = 49, 51)	10.4 ± 3.9	9.4 ± 3.3	0.143
Male (n = 12, 13)	10.1 ± 3.0	9.5 ± 3.8	0.662
Female (n = 37, 38)	10.6 ± 4.2	9.4 ± 3.2	0.160
Blood flow in optic disc			
All (n = 49, 51)	34.7 ± 6.3	34.1 ± 6.3	0.588
Male (n = 12, 13)	30.6 ± 4.8	31.1 ± 5.8	0.819
Female (n = 37, 38)	36.1 ± 6.2	35.1 ± 6.2	0.480
Peripheral blood Flow Velocity in Deep Vessels			
All (n = 49, 51)	38.9 ± 15.1	36.6 ± 13.4	0.438
Male (n = 12, 13)	31.8 ± 13.5	38.0 ± 17.0	0.322
Female (n = 37, 38)	41.2 ± 15.1	36.2 ± 12.2	0.118
Peripheral blood Flow Velocity in Superficial Vessels			
All (n = 49, 51)	33.3 ± 7.7	31.5 ± 7.7	0.226
Male (n = 12, 13)	30.3 ± 7.8	30.6 ± 9.3	0.917
Female (n = 37, 38)	34.4 ± 7.5	31.8 ± 7.2	0.131
VAS of Eye Fatigue (mm)			
All (n = 49, 51)	57.8 ± 17.7	64.7 ± 14.4 *	0.035
Male (n = 12, 13)	58.9 ± 19.3	66.1 ± 16.5	0.328
Female (n = 37, 38)	57.4 ± 17.5	64.2 ± 13.8	0.065
VAS of Shoulder Stiffness (mm)			
All (n = 49, 51)	65.6 ± 20.2	68.6 ± 17.2	0.429
Male (n = 12, 13)	63.5 ± 24.2	67.0 ± 16.2	0.680
Female (n = 37, 38)	66.3 ± 19.1	69.2 ± 17.8	0.502
VAS of Body Warmth (mm)			
All (n = 49, 51)	52.4 ± 14.2	53 ± 16.5	0.834
Male (n = 12, 13)	54.5 ± 12.2	14.4 ± 4.2	0.999
Female (n = 37, 38)	51.7 ± 14.8	53 ± 17.4	0.740
Shoulder Muscle Stiffness			
All (n = 49, 51)	32.1 ± 4.8	32.4 ± 6.4	0.788
Male (n = 12, 13)	29.9 ± 2.6	29.1 ± 5.4	0.647
Female (n = 37, 38)	32.8 ± 5.1	33.5 ± 6.3	0.591

Data are expressed as mean ± SD. * Statistical difference versus placebo group by Student's t-test at $p < 0.05$.

Table 3. Age- and sex-dependent effects of ginger. Differences during the 8-week intervention period.

	Male		Female	
(n; Placebo, Ginger)	**≥51 Years Old (n = 9, 9)**	**<51 Years Old (n = 3, 4)**	**≥51 Years Old (n = 21, 20)**	**<51 Years Old (n = 16, 18)**
Retinal blood flow	−0.0 (−2.4, 2.4)	3.0 (1.5, 4.5) **	−0.2 (−1.1, 0.7)	−0.0 (−0.9, 0.8)
Blood flow in optic disc	0.7 (−3.2, 4.6)	2.4 (−1.9, 6.6)	−0.9 (−3.9, 2.1)	−1.7 (−4.5, 1.0)
Peripheral blood Flow Velocity in Deep Vessels	−12.4 (−27.9, 3.1)	2.0 (−9.9, 13.9)	2.8 (−5.2, 10.9)	10.9 (2.4, 19.5) *
Peripheral blood Flow Velocity in Superficial Vessels	−0.3 (−12.1, 11.5)	−3.1 (−12.1, 5.9)	4.3 (0.5, 8.1) *	−0.3 (−5.9, 5.4)
VAS of Eye Fatigue (mm)	−7.4 (−27.2, 12.4)	−4.6 (−31.4, 22.2)	−1.2 (−13.8, 11.3)	−16.8 (−30.9, −2.6) *
VAS of Shoulder Stiffness (mm)	−5.5 (−28.5, 17.5)	6.6 (−18.3, 31.6)	−5.8 (−19.2, 7.7)	−12.9 (−24.2, −1.7) *
VAS of Body Warmth (mm)	3.6 (−15.4, 22.5)	33.3 (9.6, 57.1) *	4.7 (−8.2, 17.7)	1.5 (−14.0, 17.0)
Shoulder Muscle Stiffness	−1.6 (−8.3, 5.1)	−3.3 (−6.7, 0.1)	0.8 (−3.4, 5.0)	−1.3 (−4.8, 2.1)

The data are the mean difference (95% confidence interval) of the ginger group versus the placebo group. * $p < 0.05$ and ** $p < 0.01$ compared to placebo group by Student's t-test.

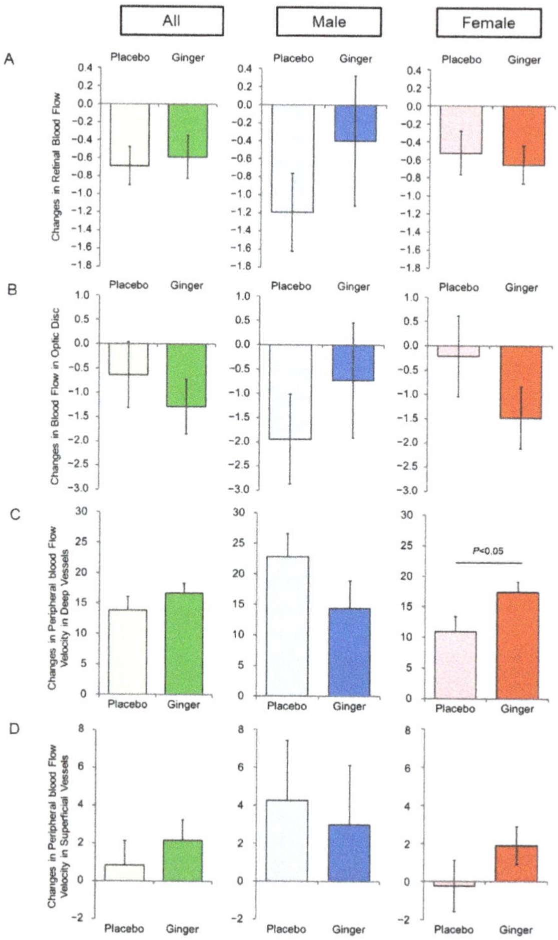

Figure 2. Changes in ocular and peripheral blood flow by ginger intake. (**A**) Changes in retinal blood flow; (**B**) changes in blood flow in the optic disc; (**C**) changes in the peripheral blood flow velocity of deep vessels; (**D**) changes in the peripheral blood flow velocity of superficial vessels during the 8-week intervention period. Data represent the mean ± SE.

3.3. *Ginger Alleviates Eye Fatigue and Shoulder Stiffness*

Figure 3 shows the results of three types of VAS and shoulder muscle stiffness measurements using a muscle hardness meter (TDM-NA1). Self-reported eye fatigue (VAS) was reduced in both groups; however, the degree was significantly greater in the ginger group than in the placebo group (Figure 3A, "All"). Shoulder stiffness in VAS also decreased in both groups, but the ginger group decreased more than the placebo group (p = 0.067, Figure 3B, "All").

Since this clinical trial was conducted from autumn to winter, self-reported body warmth was shifted toward the colder direction in the placebo group (Figure 3C). However, despite the same seasonal conditions as the parallel study, the VAS values for body warmth did not decrease from baseline in the ginger group, although there was no significant differences between the groups.

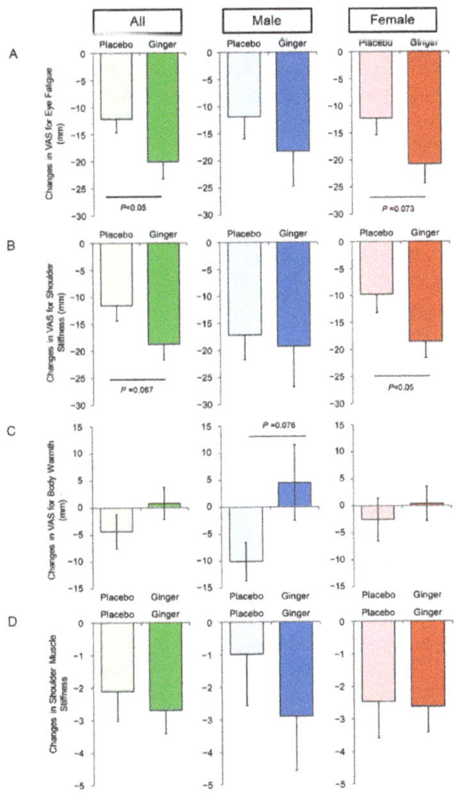

Figure 3. Changes in VAS and shoulder muscle stiffness by ginger intake. (**A**) Changes in VAS for eye fatigue; (**B**) changes in VAS for shoulder stiffness; (**C**) changes in VAS for body warmth; (**D**) changes in shoulder muscle stiffness during the 8-week intervention period. Data represent the mean ± SE.

As shown in Figure 3B, although an improvement in shoulder stiffness (VAS) was observed, there was no difference between intervention groups in the objective measurement of shoulder muscle stiffness using TDM-NA1 (Figure 3D).

Sex-dependent effects were also observed in VAS scores for eye fatigue and shoulder stiffness (Figure 3A,B). Similarly, the subgroup of younger females (<51 years) contributed to these improvements (Table 3).

3.4. Safety of Ginger

The amount of ginger used in this study did not exceed the range of average daily ginger consumption in Japan. Safety was assessed by the study subject's self-reported symptoms in daily records, physical examinations, and clinical questionnaires. No safety issues related to ginger consumption were addressed (Tables S1 and S2).

4. Discussion

In recent years, the rapid development and diffusion of computers, smartphones, and video games have increased the prevalence of VDT syndrome, a modern malady. More office work, inadequate exercise, and VDT increase complaints of dry eyes, eye fatigue, and shoulder and neck discomfort, reducing quality of life.

We evaluated whether ginger consumption improved blood flow and/or self-reported complaints, such as eye fatigue and shoulder stiffness. Ginger accelerated peripheral blood flow; however, this effect was limited to relatively young females (under 51 years old) in stratified subgroup analyses, indicating age- and sex-dependent responses. Ginger consumption can prevent hypertension [17,18]. In a cross-sectional study examining the association between ginger intake and the incidence of various chronic diseases, subgroup analyses separated by age groups showed a negative association between increased ginger intake and the incidence of hypertension in patients aged $\geq$ 18 years and $\geq$40 years, whereas the association was lost in those aged 60 years and older [17]. A systematic review indicated that ginger's blood pressure-lowering effects were observed only in studies with a mean age of 50 years or younger [18]. These results support the age-dependent effects of ginger on blood pressure. The mechanism of lowering blood pressure is not completely understood. However, it appears that the dilation of blood vessels may play a role based on the finding that ginger extract causes endothelium-dependent relaxation of porcine coronary arteries through the NO signaling pathway [31]. Although no change in blood pressure (systolic and diastolic) was observed during the intervention for all subgroups (stratified by sex or age) in this study, the participants were not a population with high blood pressure.

The effect of ginger on blood flow in young females implies the involvement of female hormones. Oral administration of ginger honey has been reported to induce estrogen and glutathione elevation in mice under stress conditions [32]. It has also been demonstrated that estrogen decreases cerebral vascular tone and increases cerebral blood flow by enhancing endothelial-derived NO and prostacyclin pathways, whereas testosterone has the opposite effect [33]. Furthermore, estrogen enhances NO production, drives blood vessel dilation, and increases blood flow [34,35]. Based on the evidence mentioned above, the increase in blood flow in young females in this study could be driven by blood vessel dilation from enhanced estrogen levels due to ginger consumption.

In this study, the enhancement of blood flow velocity by ginger consumption was detected mainly in the deep vessels but not superficial vessels. It is likely that superficial vessels are easily affected by the circumstances, and deep vessels more accurately reflect ginger's effects. In addition, blood flow increased overall, regardless of the intervention group. This trend might be the result of the participants becoming more relaxed as the clinical visit progressed. However, the effect of ginger on blood flow was detected beyond the overall increase.

Similar trends were observed for self-reported eye fatigue and shoulder stiffness. In other words, females aged <51 years showed significant improvements in eye fatigue and shoulder stiffness, as observed in peripheral blood flow. It appears that these improvements result from blood flow enhancement in young females.

The feeling of body warmth increased in the ginger group as the average in "All", "Male", and "Female" but was not significant. On the other hand, the feeling of body warmth shifted colder in the placebo group during the intervention. Ginger's effect on body warmth may be counteracted by changes in seasonal cold temperatures from autumn to winter. Although men under 51 years of age showed a significant increase over the placebo group in VAS for body warmth, these results must be clarified in future studies because the sample size of the subgroup was quite small.

The results were inconsistent between self-reported shoulder stiffness (VAS) and shoulder muscle hardness measured in terms of ginger effects, in which the former improved and the latter showed no significant difference. This finding may be due to the difficulty in measuring the exact same position on the shoulder during the 4-week interval measurements.

In this study, the ocular blood flow determined by LSFG-NAVI was not enhanced, but decreased in both groups, without significant differences between groups. In subgroup analyses, men under 51 years of age showed a statistical difference between the groups only in the retinal area but not in the optic area. However, similar to the results for body warmth, more studies are needed due to the small sample size. Considering that eye fatigue was significantly improved in the ginger group, it is possible that the optic nerve and surrounding tissue are delivered more oxygen and nutrients owing to improvements in ocular blood flow, thereby improving eye fatigue. This study was conducted from the beginning of autumn to winter; therefore, ocular blood flow may have been diminished by low temperatures, whereas peripheral blood flow increased under the same seasonal conditions. Reproducibility in ocular blood flow measurements in terms of variation between the measurer and different examination dates is a major concern that should be addressed in future studies.

The prevalence of myopia in middle-aged populations is relatively high in East Asia. It is more severe in preschool and school children, reflecting the rapid spread of VDT in recent years [36]. Myopia is a known risk factor for glaucoma [37]. Interestingly, the axial length in the ginger group decreased by 0.006 mm after 8 weeks of the intervention period in this study. From a clinical perspective, it seems insignificant, but if it continuously shortens, it would be −0.038 mm per year. Conversely, the placebo group showed an increase in axial length of 0.006 mm at 8 weeks, and a statistically significant difference was observed between the groups (p = 0.019). Moreover, the number of subjects whose axial length was reduced was significantly higher in the ginger group (17 of 51) than in the placebo group (6 of 49, p = 0.017 by Fisher's exact test). According to the single-center cohort study, which investigated myopia prevalence and progression at ages 20 and 28 in Western Australia, the axial length elongated to 0.02 mm/year as an average in eight years [38]. Therefore, future clinical studies with a longer intervention period are expected to confirm the meaningful reduction in axial length by ginger consumption since it would be beneficial for myopia from a longitudinal perspective. If this is the case, ginger may potentially contribute to maintaining eye health.

The current study has three limitations. First, the number of male participants was relatively small, which could have affected the accuracy of the subgroup analysis by sex and age. Second, the degree of inter- and intra-measurer variability of ocular blood flow assessed using the LSFG-NAVI was not negligible for comparison over the intervention period. Therefore, it is possible that ocular blood flow was also increased by ginger consumption but could not be detected under the study conditions. Finally, the baseline VAS score for eye fatigue was significantly higher in the ginger group than in the placebo group. Baseline shoulder stiffness was also slightly higher in the ginger group, but the difference was not statistically significant. These were the results of randomization stratified by sex and not at baseline levels. However, the average at week 8 in both VAS scores for eye fatigue and shoulder stiffness is lower in the ginger group than in the placebo group in the "All", "Female", and "Female under 51 years old" subgroups. In addition, analysis of covariance (ANCOVA) for eye fatigue using the baseline value as a covariate showed significant differences between groups.

Our research was conducted using a representative Japanese population. However, future research with larger and more diverse populations, considering factors such as age, sex, ethnicity, cultural differences, socioeconomic status, and geographical location, would improve the generalizability of our findings.

5. Conclusions

Ginger is safe and beneficial for improving eye fatigue and shoulder stiffness by increasing blood flow velocity, especially for females under 51 years of age. These benefits are crucial to enhance quality of life since these symptoms are often understated despite being significant for the individual.

6. Patents

After obtaining the results of this clinical study, Hiroshima University and Ikeda Food Research Co., Ltd. jointly submitted patents for using ginger for eye fatigue and shoulder stiffness. F.H. and Y.K. are co-inventors of these patents.

Supplementary Materials: The following supporting information can be downloaded at: https://www.mdpi.com/article/10.3390/nu16162715/s1, Table S1: Number of subjects showing adverse events during the intervention., Table S2: Frequency of self-reported symptoms during the intervention.

Author Contributions: Conceptualization, F.H. and Y.K.; data curation, F.H., Y.N., H.L., L.L., K.K., K.O.-O. and Y.K.; investigation, F.H., Y.N., H.L., L.L., K.K., K.O.-O. and Y.K.; methodology, F.H. and Y.K.; writing—original draft, F.H.; writing—review and editing, K.K. and Y.K. All authors have read and agreed to the published version of the manuscript.

Funding: This study was funded by Ikeda Food Research Co., Ltd., Hiroshima, Japan. The experimental capsules were provided by the company.

Institutional Review Board Statement: The study was conducted in accordance with the guidelines of the Declaration of Helsinki and approved by the Institutional Review Board of Hiroshima University (C-329-1, 5 August 2021).

Informed Consent Statement: Written informed consent was obtained from all subjects involved in the study.

Data Availability Statement: The raw data supporting the conclusions of this article will be made available by the authors upon request with the right intent.

Conflicts of Interest: F.H. and Y.K. are co-inventors of the ginger patent applications. The other authors have no conflicts of interest to declare other than study funding. The funding source had no role in the design, execution, interpretation, or writing of this study.

References

1. Ahmad, B.; Rehman, M.U.; Amin, I.; Arif, A.; Rasool, S.; Bhat, S.A.; Afzal, I.; Hussain, I.; Bilal, S.; Mir, M.U.R. A Review on Pharmacological Properties of Zingerone (4-(4-Hydroxy-3-methoxyphenyl)-2-butanone). *Sci. World J.* **2015**, *2015*, 816364. [CrossRef]
2. Li, F.; Nitteranon, V.; Tang, X.; Liang, J.; Zhang, G.; Parkin, K.L.; Hu, Q. In vitro antioxidant and anti-inflammatory activities of 1-dehydro-[6]-gingerdione, 6-shogaol, 6-dehydroshogaol and hexahydrocurcumin. *Food Chem.* **2012**, *135*, 332–337. [CrossRef]
3. Danwilai, K.; Konmun, J.; Sripanidkulchai, B.-O.; Subongkot, S. Antioxidant activity of ginger extract as a daily supplement in cancer patients receiving adjuvant chemotherapy: A pilot study. *Cancer Manag. Res.* **2017**, *9*, 11–18. [CrossRef] [PubMed]
4. Li, H.; Liu, Y.; Luo, D.; Ma, Y.; Zhang, J.; Li, M.; Yao, L.; Shi, X.; Liu, X.; Yang, K. Ginger for health care: An overview of systematic reviews. *Complement. Ther. Med.* **2019**, *45*, 114–123. [CrossRef]
5. Borrelli, F.; Capasso, R.; Aviello, G.; Pittler, M.H.; Izzo, A.A. Effectiveness and Safety of Ginger in the Treatment of Pregnancy-Induced Nausea and Vomiting. *Obstet. Gynecol.* **2005**, *105*, 849–856. [CrossRef]
6. Ding, M.; Leach, M.; Bradley, H. The effectiveness and safety of ginger for pregnancy-induced nausea and vomiting: A systematic review. *Women Birth* **2013**, *26*, e26–e30. [CrossRef] [PubMed]
7. Stanisiere, J.; Mousset, P.-Y.; Lafay, S. How Safe Is Ginger Rhizome for Decreasing Nausea and Vomiting in Women during Early Pregnancy? *Foods* **2018**, *7*, 50. [CrossRef]
8. Thomson, M.; Corbin, R.; Leung, L. Effects of Ginger for Nausea and Vomiting in Early Pregnancy: A Meta-Analysis. *J. Am. Board Fam. Med.* **2014**, *27*, 115–122. [CrossRef]
9. Viljoen, E.; Visser, J.; Koen, N.; Musekiwa, A. A systematic review and meta-analysis of the effect and safety of ginger in the treatment of pregnancy-associated nausea and vomiting. *Nutr. J.* **2014**, *13*, 20. [CrossRef]
10. Anh, N.H.; Kim, S.J.; Long, N.P.; Min, J.E.; Yoon, Y.C.; Lee, E.G.; Kim, M.; Kim, T.J.; Yang, Y.Y.; Son, E.Y.; et al. Ginger on Human Health: A Comprehensive Systematic Review of 109 Randomized Controlled Trials. *Nutrients* **2020**, *12*, 157. [CrossRef] [PubMed]
11. Attari, V.E.; Mahdavi, A.M.; Javadivala, Z.; Mahluji, S.; Vahed, S.Z.; Ostadrahimi, A. A systematic review of the anti-obesity and weight lowering effect of ginger (*Zingiber officinale Roscoe*) and its mechanisms of action. *Phytother. Res.* **2018**, *32*, 577–585. [CrossRef]
12. Maharlouei, N.; Tabrizi, R.; Lankarani, K.B.; Rezaianzadeh, A.; Akbari, M.; Kolahdooz, F.; Rahimi, M.; Keneshlou, F.; Asemi, Z. The effects of ginger intake on weight loss and metabolic profiles among overweight and obese subjects: A systematic review and meta-analysis of randomized controlled trials. *Crit. Rev. Food Sci. Nutr.* **2019**, *59*, 1753–1766. [CrossRef] [PubMed]
13. Mazidi, M.; Gao, H.-K.; Rezaie, P.; Ferns, G.A. The effect of ginger supplementation on serum C-reactive protein, lipid profile and glycaemia: A systematic review and meta-analysis. *Food Nutr. Res.* **2016**, *60*, 32613. [CrossRef]
14. Pourmasoumi, M.; Hadi, A.; Rafie, N.; Najafgholizadeh, A.; Mohammadi, H.; Rouhani, M.H. The effect of ginger supplementation on lipid profile: A systematic review and meta-analysis of clinical trials. *Phytomedicine* **2018**, *43*, 28–36. [CrossRef] [PubMed]
15. Zhu, J.; Chen, H.; Song, Z.; Wang, X.; Sun, Z. Effects of Ginger *(Zingiber officinale Roscoe)* on Type 2 Diabetes Mellitus and Components of the Metabolic Syndrome: A Systematic Review and Meta-Analysis of Randomized Controlled Trials. *Evid.-Based Complement. Altern. Med.* **2018**, *2018*, 5692962. [CrossRef] [PubMed]
16. Wang, Y.; Yu, H.; Zhang, X.; Feng, Q.; Guo, X.; Li, S.; Li, R.; Chu, D.; Ma, Y. Evaluation of daily ginger consumption for the prevention of chronic diseases in adults: A cross-sectional study. *Nutrition* **2017**, *36*, 79–84. [CrossRef]
17. Hasani, H.; Arab, A.; Hadi, A.; Pourmasoumi, M.; Ghavami, A.; Miraghajani, M. Does ginger supplementation lower blood pressure? A systematic review and meta-analysis of clinical trials. *Phytother. Res.* **2019**, *33*, 1639–1647. [CrossRef]

18. Chen, C.X.; Barrett, B.; Kwekkeboom, K. Efficacy of oral ginger (*Zingiber officinale*) for dysmenorrhea: A systematic review and meta-analysis. *Evid. Based Compl. Altern. Med.* **2016**, *2016*, 6295737. [CrossRef]
19. Daily, J.W.; Zhang, X.; Kim, D.S.; Park, S. Efficacy of Ginger for Alleviating the Symptoms of Primary Dysmenorrhea: A Systematic Review and Meta-analysis of Randomized Clinical Trials. *Pain Med.* **2015**, *16*, 2243–2255. [CrossRef]
20. Lakhan, S.E.; Ford, C.T.; Tepper, D. *Zingiberaceae* extracts for pain: A systematic review and meta-analysis. *Nutr. J.* **2015**, *14*, 50. [CrossRef]
21. Terry, R.; Posadzki, P.; Watson, L.K.; Ernst, E. The Use of Ginger (*Zingiber officinale*) for the Treatment of Pain: A Systematic Review of Clinical Trials. *Pain Med.* **2011**, *12*, 1808–1818. [CrossRef] [PubMed]
22. Wilson, P.B. Ginger (*Zingiber officinale*) as an Analgesic and Ergogenic Aid in Sport: A Systemic Review. *J. Strength Cond. Res.* **2015**, *29*, 2980–2995. [CrossRef]
23. Fjærvoll, H.; Fjærvoll, K.; Magno, M.; Moschowits, E.; Vehof, J.; Dartt, D.A.; Utheim, T.P. The association between visual display terminal use and dry eye: A review. *Acta Ophthalmol.* **2022**, *100*, 357–375. [CrossRef]
24. Kawashima, M.; Yamatsuji, M.; Yokoi, N.; Fukui, M.; Ichihashi, Y.; Kato, H.; Nishida, M.; Uchino, M.; Kinoshita, S.; Tsubota, K. Screening of dry eye disease in visual display terminal workers during occupational health examinations: The Moriguchi study. *J. Occup. Health* **2015**, *57*, 253–258. [CrossRef] [PubMed]
25. Miljanović, B.; Dana, R.; Sullivan, D.A.; Schaumberg, D.A. Impact of Dry Eye Syndrome on Vision-Related Quality of Life. *Am. J. Ophthalmol.* **2007**, *143*, 409–415. [CrossRef]
26. Zeitz, O.; Galambos, P.; Wagenfeld, L.; Wiermann, A.; Wlodarsch, P.; Praga, R.; Matthiessen, E.T.; Richard, G.; Klemm, M. Glaucoma progression is associated with decreased blood flow velocities in the short posterior ciliary artery. *Br. J. Ophthalmol.* **2006**, *90*, 1245–1248. [CrossRef] [PubMed]
27. Shiga, Y.; Aizawa, N.; Tsuda, S.; Yokoyama, Y.; Omodaka, K.; Kunikata, H.; Yasui, T.; Kato, K.; Kurashima, H.; Miyamoto, E.; et al. Preperimetric Glaucoma Prospective Study (PPGPS): Predicting Visual Field Progression with Basal Optic Nerve Head Blood Flow in Normotensive PPG Eyes. *Transl. Vis. Sci. Technol.* **2018**, *7*, 11. [CrossRef]
28. Shimada, N.; Ohno-Matsui, K.; Harino, S.; Yoshida, T.; Yasuzumi, K.; Kojima, A.; Kobayashi, K.; Futagami, S.; Tokoro, T.; Mochizuki, M. Reduction of retinal blood flow in high myopia. *Graefe's Arch. Clin. Exp. Ophthalmol.* **2004**, *242*, 284–288. [CrossRef] [PubMed]
29. Knobloch, K.; Kraemer, R.; Lichtenberg, A.; Jagodzinski, M.; Gosling, T.; Richter, M.; Krettek, C. Microcirculation of the Ankle after Cryo/Cuff Application in Healthy Volunteers. *Int. J. Sports Med.* **2006**, *27*, 250–255. [CrossRef]
30. Li, H.; Yoshizaki, T.; Liang, L.; Iwahashi, M.; Kawahara, A.; Shirai, A.; Arimitsu, J.; Ito, M.; Tsumura, N.; Ogawa-Ochiai, K. Assessing the effects of Kampo medicine on human skin texture and microcirculation. *Artif. Life Robot.* **2022**, *27*, 64–69. [CrossRef]
31. Wu, H.; Horng, C.; Tsai, S.; Lee, Y.; Hsu, S.; Tsai, Y.; Tsai, F.; Chiang, J.; Kuo, D.; Yang, J. Relaxant and vasoprotective effects of ginger extracts on porcine coronary arteries. *Int. J. Mol. Med.* **2018**, *41*, 2420–2428. [CrossRef] [PubMed]
32. Usman, A.N.; Raya, I.; Yasmin, R.; Dirpan, A.; Arsyad, A.; Permatasari, A.E.; Sumidarti, A.; Umami, N. Ginger honey affects cortisol, estrogen and glutathione levels; preliminary study to target preconceptional women. *Gac. Sanit.* **2021**, *35*, S251–S253. [CrossRef] [PubMed]
33. Krause, D.N.; Duckles, S.P.; Pelligrino, D.A. Influence of sex steroid hormones on cerebrovascular function. *J. Appl. Physiol.* **2006**, *101*, 1252–1261. [CrossRef] [PubMed]
34. Van Buren, G.A.; Yang, D.-S.; Clark, K.E. Estrogen-induced uterine vasodilatation is antagonized by L-nitroarginine methyl ester, an inhibitor of nitric oxide synthesis. *Am. J. Obstet. Gynecol.* **1992**, *167*, 828–833. [CrossRef] [PubMed]
35. Weiner, C.P.; Lizasoain, I.; A Baylis, S.; Knowles, R.G.; Charles, I.G.; Moncada, S. Induction of calcium-dependent nitric oxide synthases by sex hormones. *Proc. Natl. Acad. Sci. USA* **1994**, *91*, 5212–5216. [CrossRef] [PubMed]
36. Meng, W.; Butterworth, J.; Malecaze, F.; Calvas, P. Axial Length of Myopia: A Review of Current Research. *Ophthalmologica* **2011**, *225*, 127–134. [CrossRef] [PubMed]
37. Marcus, M.W.; de Vries, M.M.; Montolio, F.G.J.; Jansonius, N.M. Myopia as a Risk Factor for Open-Angle Glaucoma: A Systematic Review and Meta-Analysis. *Ophthalmology* **2011**, *118*, 1989–1994.e2. [CrossRef]
38. Lee, S.S.-Y.; Lingham, G.; Sanfilippo, P.G.; Hammond, C.J.; Saw, S.-M.; Guggenheim, J.A.; Yazar, S.; Mackey, D.A. Incidence and Progression of Myopia in Early Adulthood. *JAMA Ophthalmol.* **2022**, *140*, 162–169. [CrossRef] [PubMed]

nutrients

MDPI

Article

Quinoa Polyphenol Extract Alleviates Non-Alcoholic Fatty Liver Disease via Inhibiting Lipid Accumulation, Inflammation and Oxidative Stress

Wenjun Yao, Mingcong Fan, Haifeng Qian, Yan Li and Li Wang *

State Key Laboratory of Food Science and Technology, School of Food Science and Technology, Wuxi 214026, China; 15675122924@163.com (W.Y.); fanmingcong@jiangnan.edu.cn (M.F.); qianhaifeng@jiangnan.edu.cn (H.Q.); liyan0520@jiangnan.edu.cn (Y.L.)
* Correspondence: wl0519@163.com

Abstract: Recently, the incidence of NAFLD has exploded globally, but there are currently no officially approved medications for treating the condition. The regulation of NAFLD through plant-derived active substances has become a new area of interest. Quinoa (*Chenopodium quinoa* Willd.) has been discovered to contain a large quantity of bioactive compounds. In this study, we established a free fatty acid (FFA)-induced steatosis model and explored the effects of quinoa polyphenol extract (QPE) on the major hallmarks of NAFLD. The results indicated that QPE significantly reduced intracellular triglyceride (TG) and total cholesterol (TC) levels. Additionally, QPE remarkably elevated the levels of superoxide dismutase (SOD), catalase (CAT) and glutathione (GSH) and lowered levels of malondialdehyde (MDA). Further examination revealed that QPE attenuated intracellular inflammation, which was verified by the reduced levels of pro-inflammatory cytokines. Mechanistically, QPE inhibited fatty acid biosynthesis mainly by targeting de novo lipogenesis (DNL) via the AMPK/SREBP-1c signaling pathway. Moreover, network pharmacology was used to analyze key targets for NAFLD mitigation by ferulic acid (FA), a major component of QPE. Taken together, this study suggests that QPE could ameliorate NAFLD by modulating hepatic lipid metabolism and alleviating oxidative stress and inflammation.

Keywords: non-alcoholic fatty liver disease; oxidative stress; AMP-activated protein kinase

1. Introduction

Non-alcoholic fatty liver disease (NAFLD) is a metabolic disease identified by excessive fatty buildup in the liver induced by factors excluding alcohol consumption and other known liver-damaging factors [1]. The main features include steatosis, liver inflammation, hepatocyte vacuolation and, in severe cases, pathomorphological changes such as hepatocyte necrosis or apoptosis and liver fibrosis. NAFLD has captured widespread interest due to its increasing incidence annually. Currently, the prevalence of NAFLD hovers at approximately 25% worldwide, with rates exceeding 30% in South America and the Middle East [2]. However, there is still a lack of a specific medication to treat NAFLD in clinics. Existing drugs are mainly used to improve the metabolic syndrome caused by obesity, but the disadvantages of poor specificity and side effects make it difficult for them to be widely used. Therefore, finding effective and food-derived bioactive compounds to improve NAFLD is of great importance.

Previous studies have confirmed that hepatic lipogenesis and fatty acid β-oxidation play pivotal roles in regulating lipid deposition in the liver [3], which is linked to oxidative stress and the severity of NAFLD. Therefore, the acceleration of lipid consumption and the inhibition of lipid synthesis are considered a beneficial tactic for diminishing fat buildup in the liver. De novo lipogenesis (DNL) is a biological pathway where acetyl-CoA is transformed into fatty acids through the actions of acetyl-CoA carboxylase (ACC) and fatty acid synthase (FAS) [4]. DNL serves as a critical process in lipid metabolism, and the abnormal activation of this process may trigger hepatic steatosis. It has been reported that key lipogenic enzymes involved in DNL can be modulated at the transcriptional level by sterol regulatory element-binding protein (SREBP). Notably, SREBP-1c mainly controls triglyceride (TG)synthesis and can undergo post-transcriptional modifications by adenosine monophosphate-activated protein kinase (AMPK). AMPK is considered an important energy sensor, serving as a central enzyme protein that modulates cellular metabolism and impacts lipid metabolism balance [5,6]. Recent studies have found that many herbs or food extracts can reduce hepatic steatosis by phosphorylating and activating AMPK and inhibiting the expression of SREBP-1 [7], indicating that enhancing AMPK activity could be a useful therapeutic approach to alleviating NAFLD.

Quinoa (*Chenopodium quinoa* Willd.) is a pseudo-cereal renowned for its nutritional benefita and has been identified as a source of numerous bioactive compounds, including flavonoids, phenolic acids, saponins and polysaccharides. Although there is growing evidence that the intake of quinoa is positively associated with a reduced risk of NAFLD [8], the underlying mechanism and main biological components remain unclear [9], making breeding high-quality quinoa varieties and developing high-quality products challenging. Polyphenols extracted from quinoa have been proved to have remarkable antioxidant capacity and anti-inflammatory activity. It was previously reported that quinoa ethanol extract showed potent antioxidant activity, which was related to the high flavonoid content of the extract [10]. In a study, quinoa seeds were found to have high phenolic contents and excellent antioxidant properties based on 1,1-diphenyl-2-picrylhydrazyl (DPPH), ferric reducing antioxidant power (FRAP) and β-carotene bleaching assays [11]. An in vitro experiment also reported that quinoa polyphenols can downregulate interleukin-1β (IL-1β), IL-8 and tumor necrosis factor-α (TNF-α) cytokines in Caco-2 cells [12]. Given that oxidative stress and inflammation are the main factors in the generation and development of NAFLD, it was hypothesized that quinoa polyphenols may have an ameliorative effect on NAFLD. Although the role of quinoa polyphenols in the alleviation of NAFLD is gaining attention, studies on their specific effects are insufficient, and the molecular mechanisms involved require further investigation.

Based on this context, the current study aimed to find out the therapeutic effects of quinoa polyphenol extract (QPE) and its major phenolic acids on NAFLD. To this end, QPE was obtained by ultrasound-assisted extraction, and its phenolic composition was identified by ultraperformance liquid chromatography-coupled quadrupole time-of-flight mass spectrometry (UPLC-Q-TOF-MS). The effects of QPE on lipid accumulation, oxidative stress indicators and inflammatory cytokines were evaluated in $HepG_2$ cells. Considering that AMPK regulated DNL through multiple mechanisms, we conducted an investigation into the changes in AMPK and its downstream substrates before and after QPE treatment in the cells. Moreover, a network pharmacology analysis was performed to determine the potential targets and molecular mechanisms of the main phenolic acids in QPE to alleviate NAFLD. Our results may expand the active functions of quinoa and meet the demand for effective dietary supplements to ameliorate NAFLD.

2. Materials and Methods

2.1. Materials

Black quinoa seeds were kindly provided by the zonlife company (Shuozhou, China). Quinoa seeds were ground and sieved through 60 mesh, and quinoa powders were stored in polyethylene bags sealed at −20 °C until use. Phenolic acid standards were obtained from Macklin Inc. (Shanghai, China). HPLC-grade acetonitrile and formic acid were purchased from Merck (Darmstadt, Germany). Kits for measuring total cholesterol (TC) and triglyceride (TG) were acquired from the Jiancheng Bioengineering Institute (Nanjing, China). The bicinchoninic acid (BCA) protein quantification kit, HiScript® III RT SuperMix for the qPCR reverse transcription kit and ChamQ Universal SYBR qPCR Master Mix kit were provided by Vazyme Biotech Co., Ltd. (Nanjing, China). Modified Dulbecco medium (DMEM) and fetal bovine serum (FBS) were purchased from Thermo Fisher Scientific Inc. (Waltham, MA, USA). Sodium oleate and sodium palmitate for cell experiments were purchased from Mreda (Beijing, China). FFA-free bovine serum albumin (BSA) was purchased from Solarbio (Beijing, China). Antibodies against FAS, AMPK, phosphorylated AMPK (*p*-AMPK) and GAPDH were purchased from Cell Signaling Technology (Danvers, MA, USA). Anti-SREBP-1c was purchased from Santa Cruz Biotechnology (Dallas, TX, USA). Omni-ECL Femto Light Chemiluminescence kit was purchased from Epizyme Biotech (Shanghai, China). Human hepatoma $HepG_2$ cells were collected from the cell bank of the Chinese Academy of Sciences (Shanghai, China).

2.2. Extraction of QPE

The quinoa powders were degreased by stirring with hexane and evaporated to dryness. A total of 100 g of quinoa powders was extracted with 1 L of 80% acetone in an ultrasonic bath (KQ-500ES, Kunshan, China) operating at a frequency of 40 kHz for 30 min. The extract was centrifuged (Hitachi CR-GIII, Hitachi Ltd., Tokyo, Japan) for 15 min at 4 °C and 8000× *g*. The extraction was repeated twice, and the resulting supernatants were combined. After adjusting the pH to 1.5–2.0, the extract was concentrated at 45 °C using a rotary evaporator (BUCHI R-300, BUCHI Ltd., Flawil, Switzerland). The extract was then extracted 2–3 times with ethyl acetate and was concentrated at 37 °C. Finally, the extract was re-dissolved with ultrapure water and was lyophilized in a lyophilizer (LGJ-10E, Sihuan Ltd., Beijing, China). The lyophilized samples were subsequently stored in a −20 °C freezer until use.

2.3. UPLC Q-TOF-MS Analysis of Phenolic Compounds in QPE

The separation by chromatography was carried out on a Waters ACQUITY UPLC system (Waters, Milford, MA, USA) equipped with a BEH C18 analytical column (2.1 mm × 100 mm, 1.7 μm). The mobile phase consisted of (A) acetonitrile and (B) 125 mM formic acid with the following gradient: 0–0.5 min, 2% A; 0.5–10 min, 2–20% A; 10–18 min, 20–100% A; 18–21 min, 100% A; 21–21.5 min, 100–0% A. The injection flow rate was 0.3 mL/min, and the column temperature was 40 °C. The mass spectrometry data acquired by the Q-TOF-MS detector (Waters, MA, USA) were used to detect phenolic substances in the QPE. The electrospray was set to negative ion mode with a mass scan range of m/z 50–1200. The capillary voltage was 3 kV, while the cone voltage was 40 V. Nitrogen (N_2) and helium (He) were selected as the desolvation gas and cone gas, with flow rates of 800 L/h and 50 L/h, respectively. A data analysis was conducted with the help of MassLynx v4.2 software. The identified compounds were quantified using standard substances.

2.4. Cell Culture and Treatment

$HepG_2$ cells were cultured in complete medium (90% DMEM, 10% FBS, 1% Penicillin-Streptomycin solution). Cells were placed in an incubator set at 37 °C with 5% CO_2. At the stage of 80–90% cell fusion, the cells were digested and passaged for subsequent experiments. The steatosis $HepG_2$ cell model was induced with FFA (sodium oleate/sodium palmitate = 2/1) to stimulate excessive lipid synthesis according to the previously reported method [13]. $HepG_2$ cells were exposed to varying concentrations of FFA and QPE in a medium supplemented with 1% FFA-free BSA for 24 h. The control group was complete medium containing a final concentration of 1% FFA-free BSA.

2.5. Cell Viability

The cell viability was determined by MTT assay. Briefly, $HepG_2$ cells were seeded into 96-well plates at 1×10^5 cells/well and then exposed to different concentrations of FFA (0, 150, 300, 450, 600, 750, 900 μmol/L) and QPE (0, 10, 20, 40, 80, 160, 320, 640, 1280, 2560 μg/mL) for 24 h. Next, 10 μL of MTT solution (Merck KGaA, Darmstadt, Germany) was added to each well and allowed to incubate for 4 h. After that, the cells were incubated with 150 μL of DMSO solution, and the absorbance was measured at 490 nm using a microplate reader (BioTek Ltd., Winooski, VT, USA). Each treatment was replicated three times.

2.6. Oil Red O Staining

The cell-staining process was performed as previously described [14]. In brief, $HepG_2$ cells were immobilized by 4% formalin for 30 min and stained with Oil Red O reagent for 30 min at 4 °C. The cells were rinsed with sterile water 3–4 times to clear excess staining solution. The washed plates were then observed under a fluorescent inverted microscope (Axio Vert A1, Carl Zeiss AG, Oberkochen, Germany) and photographed. After observation, isopropanol was added to the plates, and the eluates were used for the quantification of Oil Red O content at a wavelength of 490 nm.

2.7. Measurement of Intracellular TC and TG

After treatments, cell lysis solution (2% Triton X-100 lysis for 30 min) was added to the cell sediment to completely lyse the cells. The concentration of proteins was determined by BCA assay, and the intracellular TC and TG contents were quantified according to the methods described in the TC and TG kit instructions.

2.8. Measurement of Oxidative Stress

Oxidative stress can be detected by measuring intracellular superoxide dismutase (SOD), malondialdehyde (MDA), glutathione (GSH) and catalase (CAT) levels. Measurements were obtained using commercial kits purchased from Solarbio Co. (Beijing, China).

2.9. Real-Time Quantitative Polymerase Chain Reaction (RT-qPCR) Analysis

Total cellular RNA was obtained with Trizol reagent (Takara Bio, Beijing, China) and converted to cDNA following the kit instructions. An amount of 4.6 μL of cDNA was used in each qPCR reaction, and the number of qPCR cycles was 40. The implementation of the PCR analysis was conducted on the Applied Biosystems QuantStudio™3 (Thermo Fisher Scientific Inc., Waltham, MA, USA) with the employment of QuantStudio™ design and analysis software. The PCR primers were synthesized by Shangya Biotechnology Co., Ltd. (Shanghai, China), and their sequences can be found in Table S1 of the Supplementary File. The calculation of relative gene expressions was determined by the method of $2^{-\triangle\triangle Ct}$ with the use of GAPDH as the internal reference gene.

2.10. Western Blot Analysis

A total of 1×10^6 $HepG_2$ cells were seeded in 6-well plates. After treatment, the cultured cells were collected and lysed. Next, the extracted protein samples were separated by 10% SDS-PAGE electrophoresis and subsequently transferred onto PVDF membranes. The membranes were blocked with 5% skim milk for 1 h and washed with Tris-buffered saline (TBS)–Tween. After completion of the blotting and blocking steps, membranes were incubated with one of the following primary antibodies at 4 °C overnight: anti-FAS (1:1000, 3180), anti-SREBP-1c (1:1000, sc365513), anti-*p*-AMPK (1:1000, 2535), anti-AMPK (1:1000, 2532) and anti-GAPDH (1:4000, 97166), followed by another 1 h incubation with an appropriate secondary antibody. Finally, the optical density values of the protein bands were measured with ImageJ 1.54 software and normalized to GAPDH.

2.11. Network Pharmacology Study

2.11.1. Identification of Potential Targets of Ferulic Acid (FA) and Protocatechuic Acid (PCA)

The target prediction of FA and PCA was performed using SwissTargetPrediction (www.SwissTargetPrediction.ch, accessed on 18 October 2023), PubChem (https://pubchem.ncbi.nlm.nih.gov/, accessed on 18 October 2023) and Pharm Mapper (http://www.lilab-ecust.cn/pharmmapper/, accessed on 19 October 2023). The results were standardized with the help of the UniProt database (https://www.uniprot.org/, accessed on 19 October 2023).

2.11.2. Collection of Core Targets of NAFLD

The targets associated with NAFLD were collected from the GeneCards database (www.genecards.org, accessed on 20 October 2023) and the OMIM database (https://omim.org/, accessed on 20 October 2023).

2.11.3. Construction of the Protein–Protein Interaction (PPI) Network

With the aim of exploring the possible mechanism between the two phenolic compounds and targets related to NAFLD, we integrated the relevant target information into the STRING database (https://string-db.org, accessed on 26 October 2023). Subsequently, the interaction networks between these targets were mapped and visualized with the help of Cytoscape 3.9.1 software. The Centiscape plug-in was then employed to compute the degree and betweenness of each gene in the network. Targets were labeled as key if their degree and betweenness values were equal to or higher than the average.

2.11.4. Gene Ontology (GO) and Kyoto Encyclopedia of Genes and Genomes (KEGG) Pathway Enrichment Analysis

The collected intersection targets of the phenolic compounds and NAFLD were entered into the DAVID database (https://david.ncifcrf.gov/, accessed on 26 October 2023). GO analysis is a powerful tool to systematically describe the function of genes and their protein products. It involves three main levels: molecular function (MF), biological process (BP) and cellular component (CC) analyses. The enriched terms of BP, MF and CC were sorted according to *p*-value, and the top 20 terms were filtered and plotted as bubble charts. In addition, the KEGG pathway enrichment analysis is a key technique for exploring potential signaling pathways related to the candidate targets in the improvement of NAFLD.

2.12. Molecular Docking

The top eight proteins were identified as receptors and FA molecules as ligands. The 3D structures of the proteins were firstly obtained from the Protein Data Bank (PDB) (https://www.rcsb.org/, accessed on 1 June 2024). The MOL2 format of FA was obtained from the TCMSP database (https://old.tcmsp-e.com/tcmsp.php, accessed on 1 June 2024) and was converted to the PDB format by Autodock. Water removal and hydrogenation were performed using AutodockTools 1.5.7 software, and the results were saved in PDBQT format. The docking box coordinates were then determined and molecular docking operations were performed using Autodock vina software. Finally, pymol 2.1.0 was used for visualization to obtain 3D analytical charts.

2.13. Statistical Analysis

SPSS 26.0 software and GraphPad Prism 9.0 were employed to conduct a statistical analysis. Experimental data were reported as mean $\pm$ standard deviation (SEM) from a minimum of three independent experiments. The statistical analysis was examined with a one-way analysis of variance (ANOVA), followed by Fisher's least significant difference (LSD) test. $p < 0.05$ was deemed to be statistically significant.

3. Results

3.1. Polyphenolic Composition of QPE

The phenolic composition of the QPE was analyzed by UPLC Q-TOF-MS. As revealed in Table 1, seven phenolic acids were successfully identified based on the mass spectrometry data of these substances, specifically, vanillic acid, PCA, caffeic acid, *p*-hydroxybenzoic acid, *p*-coumaric acid, FA and sinapic acid. In addition, two flavan-3-ol monomers, catechin and epicatechin, were detected in the QPE. The identified compounds were quantitatively analyzed by comparison with standard substances (see Table S2 for details). The results of the study showed that the main phenolic substances with a high content in QPE were PCA and FA. As reported, PCA was the dominant phenolic acid both in red and black quinoa, and black quinoa had the highest phenolic acids concentration among white, red and black quinoa [15]. A recent study also reported that black and red grains had markedly higher contents of p-coumaric acid and FA [16]. These results were consistent with our study.

Table 1. UPLC Q-TOF-MS analysis of polyphenolic components in QPE.

No.	Compound	RT (min)	$[M-H]^-$ (m/z)	Fragment Ions (m/z)
1	Vanillic acid	4.50	167.0391	152.0116, 108.0229
2	Protocatechuic acid	4.53	153.0188	109.0297, 108.0218
3	Caffeic acid	5.48	179.0422	135.0458
4	p-Hydroxybenzoic acid	6.07	137.0302	93.0341
5	p-Coumaric acid	6.78	163.0401	119.0509
6	Ferulic acid	7.60	193.0555	178.0267, 149.0601, 134.0368
7	(-)-Catechin	8.06	289.0862	175.0351, 137.0212, 134.0440, 123.0479
8	(-)-Epicatechin	8.07	289.0862	137.0243, 123.0448, 109.0295
9	Sinapic acid	8.15	223.0689	194.0116, 165.0168, 147.0482

3.2. QPE Attenuated FFA-Induced Lipid Accumulation in $HepG_2$ Cells

Prior to performing the experiments, we screened the FFA concentrations. Up to 600 μM, the MTT results confirmed that FFA did not have any cytotoxic effects (Figure 1a). Therefore, 600 μM of FFA was selected as the modeling concentration in the following experiments. Subsequently, $HepG_2$ cells were subjected to QPE at different concentrations (0, 10, 20, 40, 80, 160, 320, 640, 1280, 2560 μg/mL) to detect cell viability. As shown in Figure 1b, the proliferation of $HepG_2$ cells was significantly decreased after treatment with 640 μg/mL of QPE, suggesting that the concentrations of QPE used in this experiment (100 μg/mL and 200 μg/mL) were safe. In addition, Oil Red O staining was used to visualize the impact of QPE on FFA-induced lipid deposition, and the relative lipid accumulation was calculated by quantifying the OD value at 490 nm. The results revealed a significant rise in lipid droplets in the model cells as opposed to the control group, with QPE notably decreasing FFA-induced lipid deposition (Figure 1c,d). Consistently, the TG and TC levels in the model group were markedly elevated compared with the control group, indicating the successful establishment of a steatosis cell model by stimulating cells with 600 μM FFA. A significant reduction in TG and TC contents was observed after QPE treatment, as opposed to the FFA group (Figure 1e,f). The findings showed that QPE was successful in lowering intracellular TG and TC levels and reducing lipid accumulation in $HepG_2$ cells.

3.3. QPE Attenuated Oxidative Stress Caused by Lipid Accumulation in $HepG_2$ Cells

Oxidative stress occurs when there is an imbalance between the oxidative and antioxidant systems of cells and tissues, leading to an overproduction of oxygen radicals and reactive oxygen species (ROS). To evaluate the extent of oxidative stress in cells after liver injury, an evaluation of MDA, SOD, CAT and GSH levels in $HepG_2$ cells was conducted. In comparison to the untreated cells, the antioxidant enzymes were downregulated, and the MDA content was significantly elevated in the model group, indicating that FFA-induced excessive oxidative stress occurred in the $HepG_2$ cells. Treatment with QPE remarkably increased the activities of SOD and CAT and the GSH content (Figure 2a–c). Meanwhile, the QPE groups displayed a significant decline in MDA content compared with the model group (Figure 2d). This suggested that lipid buildup exacerbated oxidative stress in $HepG_2$ cells, while QPE was found to notably alleviate oxidative stress.

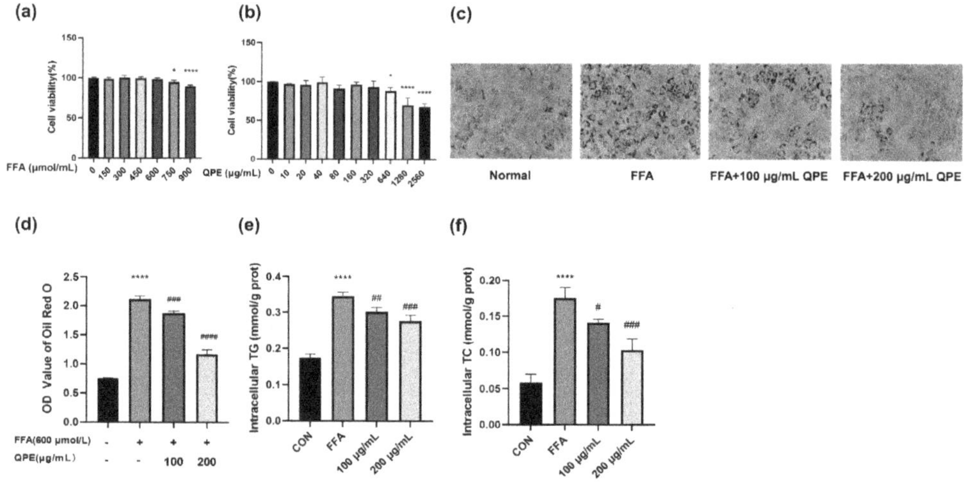

Figure 1. (**a**) Effect of FFA on cell viability. (**b**) Effect of QPE on cell viability. (**c**) Oil red O staining microscope photographs taken for normal control, FFA- and QPE-treated groups at 200× magnification. (**d**) Lipid accumulation was quantified by colorimetric method. (**e**,**f**) Effect of QPE on intracellular TG and TC levels. Data are presented as means ± SD (n = 3), * $p < 0.05$, **** $p < 0.0001$ compared to control group and # $p < 0.05$, ## $p < 0.01$, ### $p < 0.001$, #### $p < 0.0001$ compared to model group.

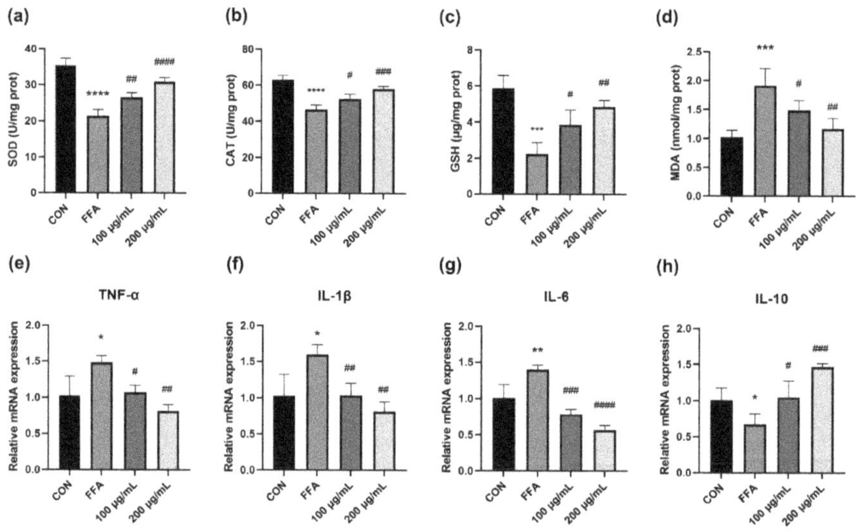

Figure 2. The evaluation of oxidative stress and inflammation in $HepG_2$ cells treated with QPE. (**a**,**b**) The activity of SOD and CAT. (**c**) The GSH content. (**d**) The MDA content. (**e**–**h**) The relative mRNA expressions of TNF-α, IL-1β, IL-6 and IL-10. Data are presented as means ± SD (n = 3), * $p < 0.05$, ** $p < 0.01$, *** $p < 0.001$, **** $p < 0.0001$ compared to control group and # $p < 0.05$, ## $p < 0.01$, ### $p < 0.001$, #### $p < 0.0001$ compared to model group.

3.4. QPE Alleviated FFA-Induced Inflammatory Response

Several studies have confirmed a relationship between NAFLD and the release of pro-inflammatory cytokines [17,18]. To delve deeper into the impact of QPE on the inflammatory response, we evaluated the levels of several major inflammatory cytokines.

Interleukin-1β (IL-1β), IL-6 and tumor necrosis factor-α (TNF-α) are pro-inflammatory factors secreted by macrophages and are positively correlated with the level of inflammation. Compared to the untreated cells, the FFA-induced group exhibited a considerable increase in relative mRNA levels of IL-1β, IL-6, and TNF-α, while the levels of these elevated pro-inflammatory cytokines were significantly lowered after QPE intervention (Figure 2e–g). Notably, QPE remarkably upregulated the expression of mRNA for IL-10 compared to the model group (Figure 2h). By inhibiting pro-inflammatory cytokine synthesis and blocking NF-κB activity, IL-10 serves as an important anti-inflammatory mediator [19]. The combined findings demonstrated that QPE has the potential to effectively alleviate NAFLD through the regulation of oxidative stress and inflammation.

3.5. Effect of QPE on mRNA Expression of Lipid Metabolism-Related Enzymes in NAFLD Cell Models

In order to explore how QPE alleviates NAFLD, we studied the gene levels responsible for lipid metabolism in $HepG_2$ cells. The relative mRNA expressions of SREBP-1c, FAS, ACC, SREBP-2 and 3-hydroxy-3-methylglutaryl-CoA reductase (HMGCR) in the FFA group were significantly increased, whereas the relative mRNA expressions of carnitine palmitoyltransterase-1 (CPT-1) and peroxisome proliferators-activated preceptor α (PPARα) were significantly lower in the FFA group than in the control group (Figure 3a–g). As shown in (Figure 3a–c), QPE significantly downgraded the mRNA levels of the SREBP-1c, FAS and ACC genes responsible for DNL compared to the model group. QPE also significantly increased the mRNA levels of the CPT-1 and PPARα genes involved in fatty acid β-oxidation (Figure 3f,g). Altogether, these results suggest that QPE decreased the excessive lipid buildup by upregulating the mRNA expressions of lipolysis-related genes and downregulating the mRNA expressions of lipogenesis-related genes. Moreover, the influence of QPE on AMPK activity was assessed. Immunoblotting studies demonstrated that QPE reversed the reduction in phosphorylated AMPK, which in turn decreased the protein expression levels of SREBP-1c and FAS, leading to the inhibition of TG synthesis in $HepG_2$ cells (Figure 3h,k).

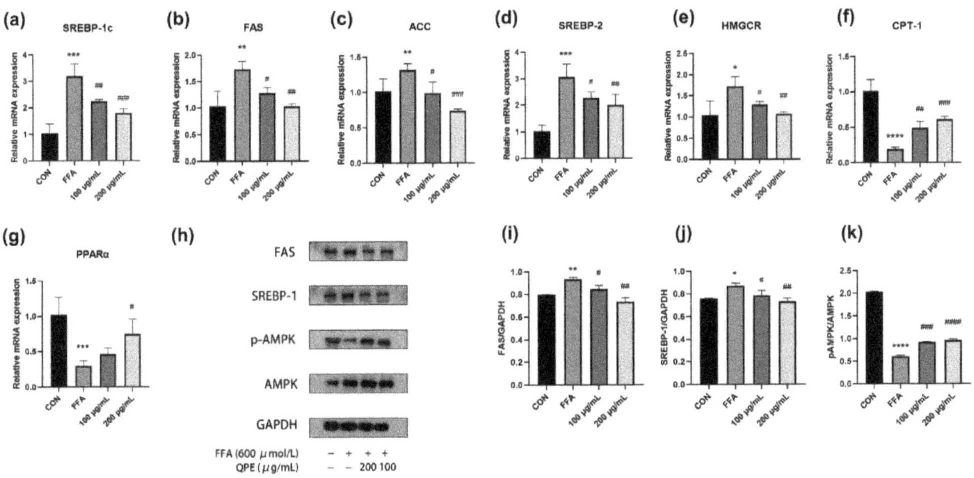

Figure 3. (**a**–**g**) RT-PCR was conducted to detect relative mRNA expressions of genes responsible for lipid metabolism in $HepG_2$ cells. (**h**) The protein expressions of FAS, SREBP-1c, *p*-AMPK and AMPK in $HepG_2$ cells were detected by Western blot. (**i**–**k**) The gray analysis was analyzed by ImageJ 1.54 software. Data are presented as means ± SD ($n = 3$), * $p < 0.05$, ** $p < 0.01$, *** $p < 0.001$, **** $p < 0.0001$ compared to control group and # $p < 0.05$, ## $p < 0.01$, ### $p < 0.001$, #### $p < 0.0001$ compared to model group.

3.6. Target Network Analysis

Considering that FA and PCA were the two main phenolic acids in QPE, the present study preliminarily studied the molecular mechanism of FA and PCA alleviating NAFLD by network pharmacology. By analyzing the structures of FA and PCA (Figure 4a), their target genes were predicted using SwissTargetPrediction and the Pharm Mapper database, and a total of 234 FA and 229 PCA target genes were obtained. A Venn diagram was constructed to obtain 40 common targets of FA and NAFLD, and 10 common targets of PCA and NAFLD (Figure 4c). The Cytoscape plug-in PPI network, based on the STRING database and topological data analysis, was used to construct a PPI network that had 37 connected nodes and 172 relationship pairs (Figure 4e). The network analysis showed that the degree average value and the betweenness average value were 9.30 and 36.05, respectively. Targets with an above-average degree and betweenness were regarded as key targets that may have important roles in regulating NAFLD-related biological processes [20]. The eight key targets meeting this selection criterion, listed in descending order of betweenness (Table S3), were tumor protein p53 (TP53), epidermal growth factor receptor (EGFR), matrix metalloproteinase-9 (MMP9), amyloid beta precursor protein (APP), MMP2, signal transducer and activator of transcription 3 (STAT3), interferon gamma (IFNG) and NF-κB subunit p65 (RELA).

3.7. Pathway Enrichment Analysis of FA Target Genes

Common targets were analyzed by employing the GO and pathway enrichment analysis functions within the DAVID database. The top 20 enriched terms of BP, MF and CC were selected based on p-value and screened to draw dot bubble charts. The BP analysis revealed that FA acts mainly through the positive regulation of interleukin-6 production, positive regulation of gene expression and positive regulation of NF-κB transcription factor activity (Figure 5a). The CC analysis revealed that the targets are mainly associated with the cytoplasm, mitochondrion and plasma membrane (Figure 5b). Moreover, the MF analysis indicated that FA exerted its function by interacting primarily with enzyme binding, protein homodimerization activity, identical protein binding, protein kinase binding transcription factor activity and sequence-specific DNA binding (Figure 5c). Based on the KEGG enrichment analysis, it could be seen that the alleviating effect of FA on NAFLD mainly involved ROS, the HIF-1 signaling pathway, lipids and atherosclerosis, insulin resistance, and the PI3K-Akt signaling pathway, which mediated the potential mechanism of FA intervention in NAFLD (Figure 5d).

3.8. Molecular Docking of FA with Core Targets

To further verify the accuracy of the core targets (APP, EGFR, IFNG, MMP2, MMP9, RELA, STAT3 and TP53) obtained in the network, a molecular docking analysis between core targets and the FA molecule was performed in Autodock vina (Table 2). According to the binding energy, the top three target proteins (MMP9, MMP2 and EGFR) were selected for visual analysis (Figure 6). Figure 6 showed the non-bonding interactions, including hydrogen bonding (indicated by the green dashed line), the π-π stacking effect (indicated by the red dashed line) of the FA molecule with the surrounding amino acid residues, hydrophobic interactions (indicated by the gray dashed lines) and the space between the FA molecule and the protein pocket position.

Table 2. Docking information of core targets with FA.

Targets	PDBID	Binding Energy (kcal·mol^{-1})
APP	1AAP	−5.2
EGFR	3POZ	−6.2
IFNG	3BES	−5.5
MMP2	1CK7	−6.4
MMP9	5UE3	−7.3
RELA	1NFI	−5.8
STAT3	6NJS	−5.8
TP53	2BIM	−5.0

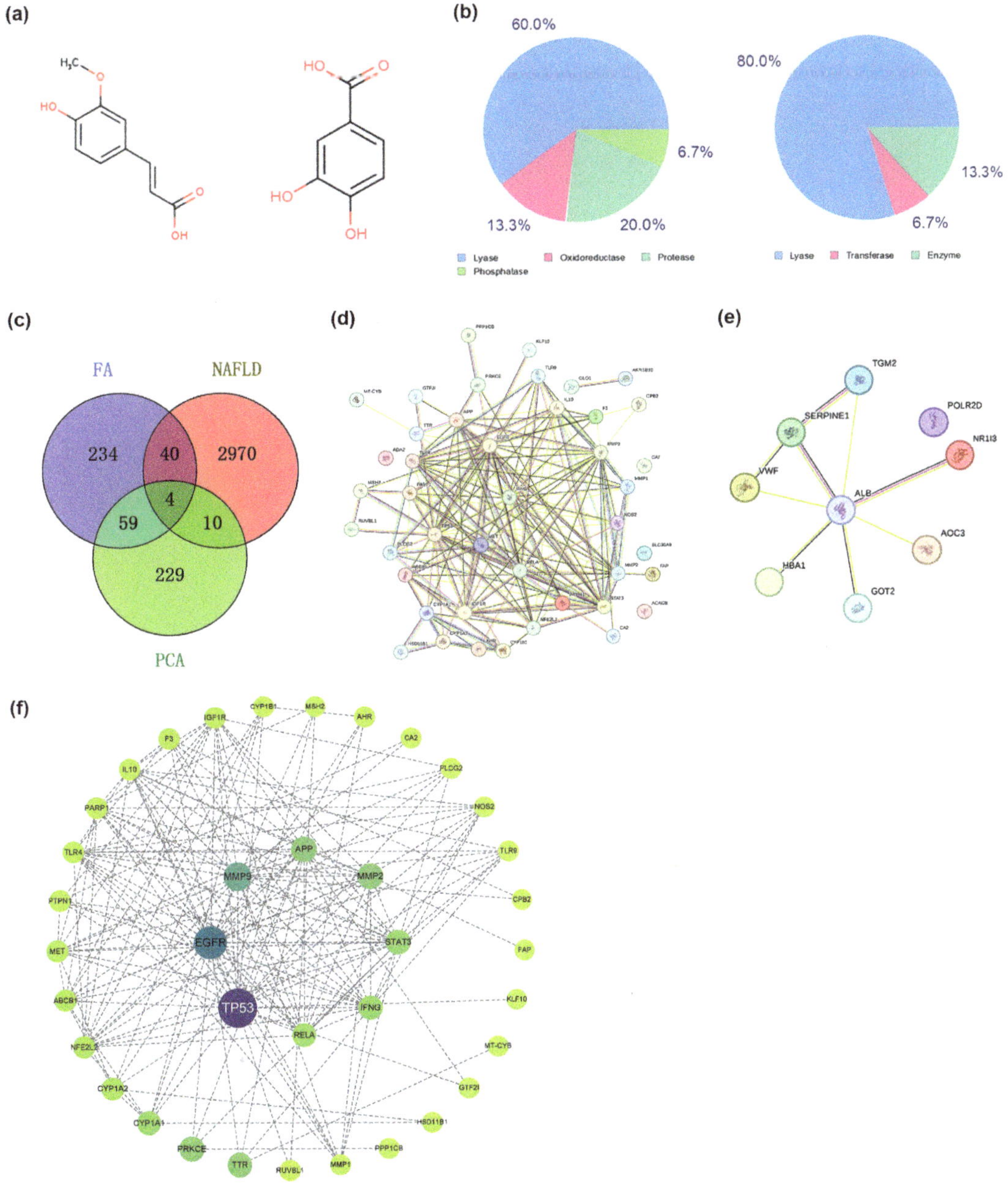

Figure 4. Predicted effects of phenolic acids against NAFLD. (**a**) Chemical structures of FA and PCA. (**b**) Target classes of FA and PCA. (**c**) Venn diagram of FA and PCA target genes crossed with genes related to NAFLD. (**d**) The PPI network of FA target genes. (**e**) The PPI network of PCA target genes. (**f**) The PPI network for FA acting on NAFLD. The target network consisted of 37 nodes and 172 edges, with the nodes symbolizing the targets of FA acting on NAFLD and the edges denoting relationships between the targets.

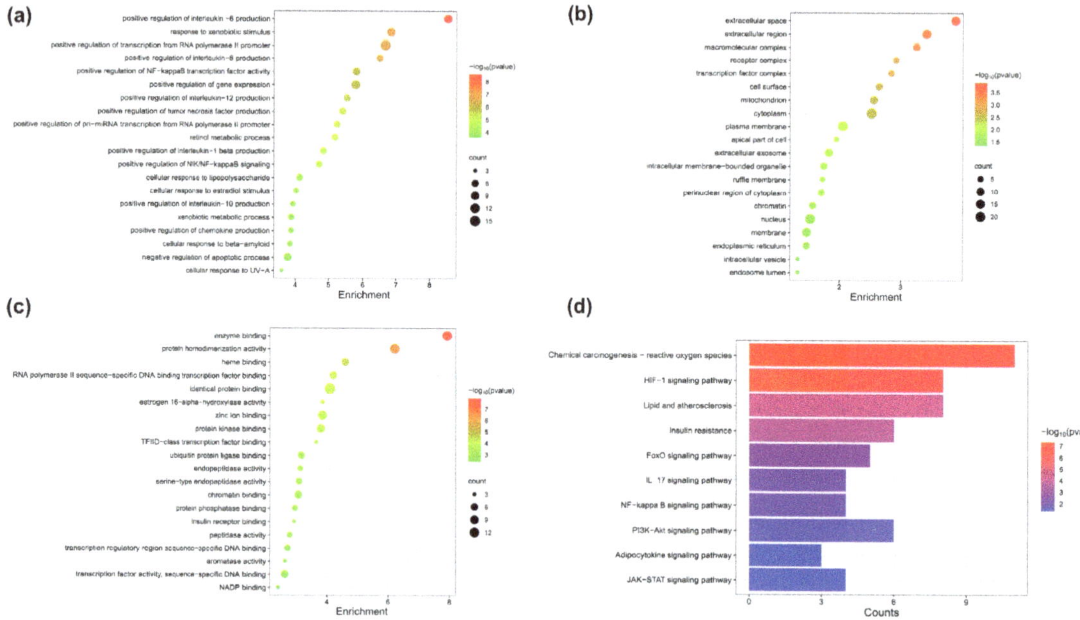

Figure 5. Functional enrichment analysis. (**a**) The BP analysis. (**b**) The CC analysis. (**c**) The MF analysis. (**d**) The KEGG enrichment analysis.

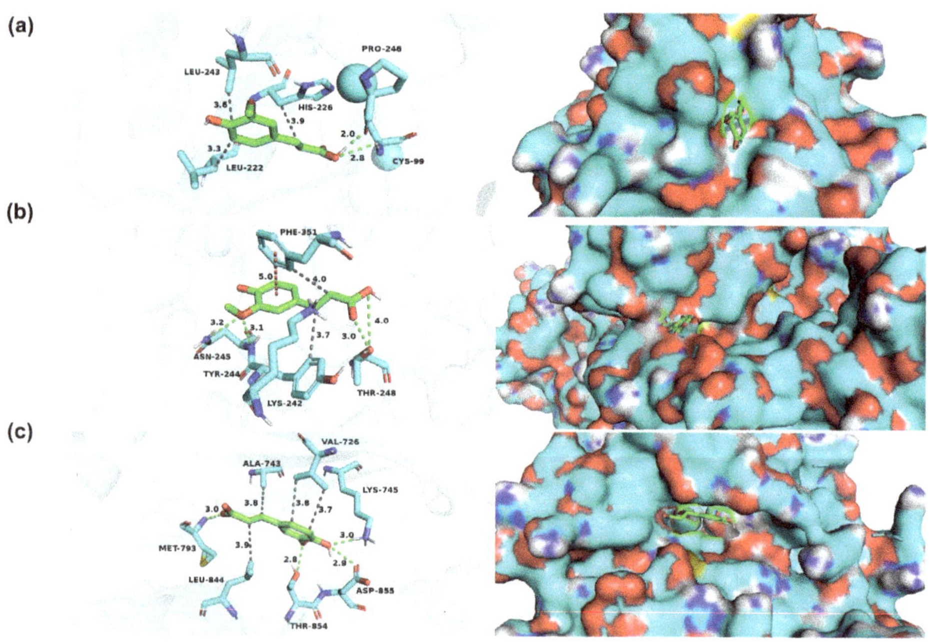

Figure 6. Visualization of molecular docking. (**a**) MMP9. (**b**) MMP2. (**c**) EGFR.

4. Discussion

NAFLD is now recognized as a prevalent and rising liver disease globally, although its pathogenesis is currently unclear. Hepatic steatosis is an indispensable initiator of NAFLD and has a profound impact on the pathology of NAFLD. The Oil Red O staining results clearly indicated a notable rise in intracellular lipid levels in the model group and a significant decrease in intracellular lipid content following QPE treatment, which implied that QPE might lessen the lipid accumulation induced by FFA (Figure 1a–c). The results also showed that QPE intervention greatly reduced the intracellular TG and TC contents increased by FFA (Figure 1d,e). Therefore, it can be said that QPE shows significant physiological lipid-lowering activity.

Oxidative stress plays a crucial role in the occurrence and progression of NAFLD by impairing mitochondrial function, causing an imbalance between intracellular lipid synthesis and catabolism and ultimately leading to cellular steatosis. The degree of oxidative stress correlates significantly with the severity of NAFLD, and an abnormal expression of oxidative stress-related markers is frequently present in the liver of NAFLD patients. Previous studies reported that quinoa seeds slowed down fat peroxidation, effectively reduced plasma MDA concentrations and maintained SOD, CAT and GPx activities in the normal range [21]. Researchers found that red and yellow quinoa sprout extract was effective in reducing MDA and enhancing GSH and SOD activities in rats. This result suggested that the phenolic and flavonoid components contained in red sprouts may have potent bioactivities in attenuating oxidative stress, as well as hepatic inflammatory responses [22]. Our research showed that QPE significantly improved the activity of SOD, CAT and GSH in $HepG_2$ cells (Figure 2a–c). When the body undergoes oxidative stress, a large number of free radicals are generated, leading to the oxidation of fatty acids and their breakdown into a series of lipid peroxides such as MDA. MDA generated through lipid peroxidation can damage cell membranes and lead to impaired cell function, making it a key indicator of the severity of cellular damage. SOD is the main antioxidant enzyme responsible for the scavenging of superoxide anion, which is essential for protection against oxidative-induced injuries and inflammatory reactions. As mentioned above, the increase in SOD, CAT and GSH activity coupled, with the decrease in MDA, after QPE indicated an alleviation of oxidative stress, thereby improving NAFLD.

Elevated levels of IL-1β, IL-6 and TNF-α were found to be strongly correlated with an increased risk of NAFLD in a meta-analysis [15]. TNF-α not only promotes inflammation itself, but also exacerbates the inflammatory reaction by inducing the synthesis of other inflammatory cytokines. Previous studies have found that IL-10, a key anti-inflammatory cytokine, can efficiently inhibit the release of various inflammatory cytokines by T cells [23]. Upon investigation, it was observed that QPE remarkably decreased the mRNA levels of IL-1β, IL-6 and TNF-α, while increasing the mRNA expression of IL-10 (Figure 2e–h). Collectively, the present study indicated that QPE might have a positive influence on alleviating NAFLD by decreasing lipid accumulation, relieving oxidative stress and regulating inflammatory cytokines. Therefore, we further investigated the molecular mechanisms involved.

Hepatic fat accumulation is viewed as a major contributor to the development of NAFLD and can be triggered by several causes, including elevated hepatic FFA absorption, impaired fatty acid β-oxidation and elevated DNL. Considering DNL is a complex regulatory process, the regulation of pivotal nuclear transcription factors and enzymes in DNL is critical for the control of lipid metabolism. As a key enzyme in fatty acids synthesis, ACC regulates the production of malonyl-CoA, which is an allosteric inhibitor of CPT1 [24]. Previous studies suggest that resveratrol ameliorated NAFLD induced by high-fat diets, and this effect was associated with a reduction in the hepatic mRNA expressions of SREBP1, FAS, ACC and PPARγ in rats [25]. In our study, it was observed that QPE caused a notable reduction in the mRNA levels of SREBP-1c, ACC and FAS (Figure 3a–c), alongside an elevation in the mRNA levels of CPT1 and PPARα, as opposed to the model group (Figure 3f,g). These results implied that QPE could effectively reduce intracellular lipid buildup by modulating the expression of genes that play a role in lipid metabolism. Notably, an elevated SREBP-2 mRNA expression level was measured in the steatosis state of $HepG_2$ cells, implying that SREBP-2 may be involved in the induction of NAFLD (Figure 3d). In contrast to SREBP1, SREBP-2 mainly controls TC synthesis and can regulate the expression of proteins associated with cholesterol biosynthesis, including the important rate-limiting enzyme HMGCR. This study identified a substantial increase in the mRNA levels of SREBP-2 and HMGCR in the model group as opposed to untreated cells, possibly leading to increased TC synthesis (Figure 3d,e). Earlier research revealed that berberine regulated cholesterol synthesis by targeting the SREBP-2-HMGCR signal pathway [26]. It was consistent with our findings that mRNA levels of SREBP-2 and HMGCR were greatly reduced after QPE, suggesting that the decreased intracellular TC synthesis was likely mediated by regulating the expression of SREBP-2 and HMGCR.

AMPK signaling is one of the key factors regulating lipid homeostasis and is considered as an effective therapeutic target for NAFLD. According to a recent study, a substantial increase in the activity of the SREBP-1c/FAS pathway was exhibited in NAFLD mice [27]. Additionally, experiments have provided strong evidence for the connection between the suppression of the SREBP-1c/FAS pathway and a decline in hepatic lipid synthesis [28]. As reported, AMPK-dependent phosphorylation controls the protein degradation and nuclear localization of SREBP-1c [25], which further inhibits the expression of downstream target genes. In our investigation, QPE remarkably upregulated AMPK phosphorylation, while decreasing the expression of SREBP-1c and FAS in comparison to the FFA-only group (Figure 3h–k). Consistent with previous studies, the activation of AMPK inhibited the activity of SREBP-1c and further suppressed the transcription of DNL-related genes, thereby reducing adipogenesis and ultimately slowing down lipid accumulation [29]. These results imply an ameliorative effect of QPE on FFA-induced hepatic steatosis by modulating the AMPK/SREBP-1c signaling pathway.

FA was found to be one of the major polyphenols of QPE and was reported to possess various hepatoprotective, anti-inflammatory, antioxidant and anti-tumor effects [30]. Network pharmacology has become a new approach for investigating the effects and mechanisms of biologically active nutrients [31]. Therefore, we finally analyzed the potential targets and molecular mechanisms of FA for alleviating NAFLD by network pharmacology. The PPI network analysis showed that there were 37 nodes and 172 edges in the network of FA acting on NAFLD. Eight key genes were screened based on degree and betweenness: TP53, EGFR, MMP9, APP, MMP2, STAT3, IFNG and RELA. The interaction of FA with core proteins was predicted by molecular docking experiments. Smaller values of molecular binding energy indicate a tighter binding. A binding energy <-5.0 kcal·mol^{-1} was considered to indicate a strong binding of the ligand to the target site, and a binding energy <-7.0 kcal·mol^{-1} suggests a stronger affinity between the two [32]. The results showed that the three protein targets that bound most strongly to FA were MMP9, MMP2 and EGFR. FA formed hydrogen bonds with the PRO-246 and CYS-99 sites of MMP9 and the THR-248 site of MMP2 (Figure 6a,b). It was also noted that FA formed hydrogen bonds with four different sites of EGFR (Figure 6c). MMP-9 played an important role in promoting the formation of NAFLD and the progression of liver fibrosis [33]. One study reported that MMP9 could distinguish patients at risk of progression from non-alcoholic steatohepatitis to hepatocellular carcinoma [34]. It was also reported that EGFR may inhibit lipid accumulation and liver fibrosis through mechanisms involving the regulation of oxidative stress [35]. In addition, the GO analysis showed that targets in the PPI network were primarily associated with the regulation of inflammatory cytokines and gene expression, including IL-1β, IL-6, IL-8, IL-10, IL-12 and chemokine. Moreover, the KEGG enrichment analysis showed that FA mainly functioned in ROS, the HIF-1 signaling pathway, lipids and atherosclerosis, insulin resistance, and the PI3K-Akt signaling pathway. As previously mentioned, oxidative stress induced by ROS and inflammation is an important trigger of NAFLD. Our data provide evidence to further explore the above key targets and signaling pathways.

Taken together, the present study demonstrated that QPE effectively decreased lipid accumulation, reduced oxidative stress and alleviated inflammatory response in a steatosis cell model. The alleviating effect of QPE on NAFLD required AMPK activation to hamper the maturation of SREBP-1c and consequently decrease the lipid accumulation derived from DNL. These findings may offer valuable insights into how quinoa can alleviate hepatic steatosis and establish a theoretical basis for the integration of quinoa in functional food research and development. Notwithstanding the findings of this study, it is crucial to address its limitations. This is mainly due to the fact that the single cell line model ($HepG_2$ cells) used in the study may pose a constraint on the generalizability of the results. In order to overcome this limitation, future studies could consider the inclusion of primary hepatocytes or multiple different hepatocyte cell lines. At the same time, an in vivo model could be introduced to validate the results of the in vitro study and further assess the bioavailability and metabolic pathways of QPE.

5. Conclusions

To conclude, this study sought to analyze the impact and molecular pathway through which QPE and its major phenolic acids alleviate NAFLD. Cellular experiments confirmed that QPE could effectively alleviate NAFLD from three angles: alleviating lipid accumulation, lowering oxidative stress markers and modulating inflammatory cytokine levels. Notably, the reduced intracellular TG synthesis was likely mediated by the activation of the AMPK/SREBP-1c signaling pathway. Furthermore, the application of network pharmacology helped anticipate the core targets and molecular pathways of FA in mitigating NAFLD. The enrichment analysis results indicated that the improvement mechanism of FA was closely related to the inhibition of oxidative stress, insulin resistance and the regulation of inflammatory cytokines. The overall results suggest that QPE is a potential dietary supplement in the treatment of NAFLD, as it can reduce oxidative stress, decrease hepatic inflammation and inhibit hepatic steatosis by activating the AMPK pathway. Nevertheless, additional studies are required to understand how QPE exerts beneficial effects in animal models of NAFLD and the regulatory mechanisms involved.

Supplementary Materials: The following supporting information can be downloaded at: https://www.mdpi.com/article/10.3390/nu16142276/s1, Table S1: Primer sequences used in RT-qPCR. Table S2: Content of compounds in QPE. Table S3: Targets with higher-than-average betweenness and degree in PPI network.

Author Contributions: W.Y.: Conceptualization, Methodology, Data curation, Software, Writing—original draft. M.F.: Writing—review and editing. H.Q.: Validation. Y.L.: Conceptualization, Writing—review and editing. L.W.: Conceptualization, Writing—review and editing, Funding acquisition. All authors have read and agreed to the published version of the manuscript.

Funding: This research was funded by the Earmarked Fund for China Agriculture Research System, grant number CARS-08-G19, the National Natural Science Foundation of China, grant number 32072254 and 32071166, the Young Elite Scientists Sponsorship Program by CAST, grant number 2020QNRC001, the Key Technology Research and Development Program in Xinjiang Uygur Autonomous Region, grant number 2022A02009-3, and the "Qing Lan Project in Jiangsu Province" program.

Institutional Review Board Statement: Not applicable.

Informed Consent Statement: Not applicable.

Data Availability Statement: The data can be accessed on request.

Conflicts of Interest: The authors have confirmed that they do not have any competing financial interests associated with this manuscript.

References

1. Rinella, M.E. Nonalcoholic fatty liver disease: A systematic review. *JAMA-J. Am. Med. Assoc.* **2015**, *314*, 1521. [CrossRef] [PubMed]
2. Younossi, Z.; Anstee, Q.M.; Marietti, M.; Hardy, T.; Henry, L.; Eslam, M.; George, J.; Bugianesi, E. Global burden of NAFLD and NASH: Trends, predictions, risk factors and prevention. *Nat. Rev. Gastroenterol. Hepatol.* **2018**, *15*, 11–20. [CrossRef] [PubMed]

3. Yang, J.S.; Tongson, J.; Kim, K.H.; Park, Y. Piceatannol attenuates fat accumulation and oxidative stress in steatosis-induced HepG2 cells. *Curr. Res. Food Sci.* **2020**, *3*, 92–99. [CrossRef]
4. Batchuluun, B.; Pinkosky, S.L.; Steinberg, G.R. Lipogenesis inhibitors: Therapeutic opportunities and challenges. *Nat. Rev. Drug Discov.* **2022**, *21*, 283–305. [CrossRef]
5. Ahmad, B.; Serpell, C.J.; Fong, I.L.; Wong, E.H. Molecular Mechanisms of Adipogenesis: The Anti-adipogenic Role of AMP-Activated Protein Kinase. *Front. Mol. Biosci.* **2020**, *7*, 76. [CrossRef]
6. Rajan, P.; Natraj, P.; Ranaweera, S.S.; Dayarathne, L.A.; Lee, Y.J.; Han, C.H. Anti-adipogenic effect of the flavonoids through the activation of AMPK in palmitate (PA)-treated HepG2 cells. *J. Vet. Sci.* **2022**, *23*, e42022. [CrossRef] [PubMed]
7. Lee, G.H.; Peng, C.; Park, S.A.; Hoang, T.H.; Lee, H.Y.; Kim, J.; Kang, S.I.; Lee, C.H.; Lee, J.S.; Chae, H.J. Citrus Peel Extract Ameliorates High-Fat Diet-Induced NAFLD via Activation of AMPK Signaling. *Nutrients* **2020**, *12*, 673. [CrossRef]
8. Noratto, G.D.; Murphy, K.; Chew, B.P. Quinoa intake reduces plasma and liver cholesterol, lessens obesity-associated inflammation, and helps to prevent hepatic steatosis in obese db/db mouse. *Food Chem.* **2019**, *287*, 107–114. [CrossRef]
9. Ren, G.X.; Teng, C.; Fan, X.; Guo, S.Y.; Zhao, G.; Zhang, L.Z.; Liang, Z.; Qin, P.Y. Nutrient composition, functional activity and industrial applications of quinoa (*Chenopodium quinoa* Willd.). *Food Chem.* **2023**, *410*, 135290. [CrossRef]
10. Park, J.H.; Lee, Y.J.; Kim, Y.H.; Yoon, K.S. Antioxidant and Antimicrobial Activities of Quinoa (*Chenopodium quinoa* Willd.) Seeds Cultivated in Korea. *Prev. Nutr. Food Sci.* **2017**, *22*, 195–202.
11. Marmouzi, I.; Madani, N.; Charrouf, Z.; Cherrah, Y.; Faouzi, M.Y.A. Analyse approximative et composition en acides gras et minéraux de Chenopodium quinoa Willd. Marocain, et propriétés antioxydantes selon la polarité. *Phytothérapie* **2015**, *13*, 110–117. [CrossRef]
12. Noratto, G.; Carrion-Rabanal, R.; Medina, G.; Mencia, A.; Mohanty, I.; Gonzalez, D.; Murphy, K. Quinoa protective effects against obesity-induced intestinal inflammation. *FASEB J.* **2015**, *29*, 602–609. [CrossRef]
13. Chen, S.N.; Che, S.Y.; Li, S.Q.; Ruan, Z. The combined impact of decabromodiphenyl ether and high fat exposure on non-alcoholic fatty liver disease in vivo and in vitro. *Toxicology* **2021**, *464*, 153015. [CrossRef] [PubMed]
14. Lee, M.R.; Park, K.I.; Ma, J.Y. Leonurus japonicus Houtt Attenuates Non-alcoholic Fatty Liver Disease in Free Fatty Acid-Induced $HepG_2$ Cells and Mice Fed a High-Fat Diet. *Nutrients* **2017**, *10*, 20. [CrossRef]
15. Liu, M.J.; Zhu, K.L.; Yao, Y.; Chen, Y.H.; Guo, H.M.; Ren, G.X.; Yang, X.S.; Li, J.C. Antioxidant, anti-inflammatory, and antitumor activities of phenolic compounds from white, red, and black *Chenopodium quinoa* seed. *Cereal Chem.* **2020**, *97*, 703–713. [CrossRef]
16. Qian, G.T.; Li, X.Y.; Zhang, H.; Zhang, H.L.; Zhou, J.W.; Ma, X.H.; Sun, W.; Yang, W.; He, R.K.; Wahab, A.T.; et al. Metabolomics analysis reveals the accumulation patterns of flavonoids and phenolic acids in quinoa (*Chenopodium quinoa* Willd.) grains of different colors. *Food Chem.-X* **2023**, *17*, 100594. [CrossRef]
17. Duan, Y.M.; Pan, X.F.; Luo, J.Y.; Xiao, X.; Li, J.Y.; Bestman, P.L.; Luo, M.Y. Association of Inflammatory Cytokines with Non-Alcoholic Fatty Liver Disease. *Front. Immunol.* **2022**, *13*, 880298. [CrossRef] [PubMed]
18. Arai, N.; Miura, K.; Aizawa, K.; Sekiya, M.; Nagayama, M.; Sakamoto, H.; Maeda, H.; Morimoto, N.; Iwamoto, S.; Yamamoto, H. Probiotics suppress non-alcoholic steatohepatitis and carcinogenesis progression in hepatocyte-specific PTEN knockout mice. *Sci. Rep.* **2022**, *12*, 16206. [CrossRef]
19. Li, H.; Hu, D.; Fan, H.M.; Zhang, Y.; LeSage, G.D.; Caudle, Y.; Stuart, C.; Liu, Z.M.; Yin, D.L. β-Arrestin 2 Negatively Regulates Toll-like Receptor 4 (TLR4)-triggered Inflammatory Signaling via Targeting p38 MAPK and Interleukin 10. *J. Biol. Chem.* **2014**, *289*, 23075–23085. [CrossRef]
20. Bonte, M.A.; El Idrissi, F.; Gressier, B.; Devos, D.; Belarbi, K. Protein network exploration prioritizes targets for modulating neuroinflammation in Parkinson's disease. *Int. Immunopharmacol.* **2021**, *95*, 107526. [CrossRef]
21. Pasko, P.; Barton, H.; Zagrodzki, P.; Izewska, A.; Krosniak, M.; Gawlik, M.; Gawlik, M.; Gorinstein, S. Effect of Diet Supplemented with Quinoa Seeds on Oxidative Status in Plasma and Selected Tissues of High Fructose-Fed Rats. *Plant Foods Hum. Nutr.* **2010**, *65*, 146–151. [CrossRef] [PubMed]
22. Al-Qabba, M.M.; El-Mowafy, M.A.; Althwab, S.A.; Alfheeaid, H.A.; Aljutaily, T.; Barakat, H. Phenolic Profile, Antioxidant Activity, and Ameliorating Efficacy of *Chenopodium quinoa* Sprouts against CCl_4-Induced Oxidative Stress in Rats. *Nutrients* **2020**, *12*, 2904. [CrossRef]
23. Holan, V.; Zajicova, A.; Javorkova, E.; Trosan, P.; Chudickova, M.; Pavlikova, M.; Krulova, M. Distinct cytokines balance the development of regulatory T cells and interleukin-10-producing regulatory B cells. *Immunology* **2014**, *141*, 577–586. [CrossRef] [PubMed]
24. Ke, R.; Xu, Q.C.; Li, C.; Luo, L.Y.; Huang, D.Q. Mechanisms of AMPK in the maintenance of ATP balance during energy metabolism. *Cell Biol. Int.* **2018**, *42*, 384–392. [CrossRef]
25. Tejada, S.; Capo, X.; Mascaro, C.M.; Monserrat-Mesquida, M.; Quetglas-Llabres, M.M.; Pons, A.; Tur, J.A.; Sureda, A. Hepatoprotective Effects of Resveratrol in Non-Alcoholic Fatty Live Disease. *Curr. Pharm. Des.* **2021**, *27*, 2558–2570. [CrossRef]
26. Shan, M.Y.; Dai, Y.; Ren, X.D.; Zheng, J.; Zhang, K.B.; Chen, B.; Yan, J.; Xu, Z.H. Berberine mitigates nonalcoholic hepatic steatosis by downregulating SIRT1-FoxO1-SREBP2 pathway for cholesterol synthesis. *J. Integr. Med.-JIM* **2021**, *19*, 545–554. [CrossRef] [PubMed]
27. An, J.P.; Choi, J.H.; Huh, J.; Lee, H.J.; Han, S.; Noh, J.R.; Kim, Y.H.; Lee, C.H.; Oh, W.K. Anti-hepatic steatosis activity of *Sicyos angulatus* extract in high-fat diet-fed mice and chemical profiling study using UHPLC-qTOF-MS/MS spectrometry. *Phytomedicine* **2019**, *63*, 152999. [CrossRef]

28. Fang, K.; Wu, F.; Chen, G.; Dong, H.; Li, J.B.; Zhao, Y.; Xu, L.J.; Zou, X.; Lu, F.E. Diosgenin ameliorates palmitic acid-induced lipid accumulation via AMPK/ACC/CPT-1A and SREBP-1c/FAS signaling pathways in LO2 cells. *BMC Complement. Altern. Med.* **2019**, *19*, 255. [CrossRef] [PubMed]
29. Guo, Y.; Sun, Q.; Wang, S.; Zhang, M.; Lei, Y.; Wu, J.; Wang, X.; Hu, W.; Meng, H.; Li, Z.; et al. Corydalis saxicola Bunting total alkaloids improve NAFLD by suppressing de novo lipogenesis through the AMPK-SREBP1 axis. *J. Ethnopharmacol.* **2023**, *319 Pt 1*, 117162. [CrossRef]
30. Zduńska, K.; Dana, A.; Kolodziejczak, A.; Rotsztejn, H. Antioxidant Properties of Ferulic Acid and Its Possible Application. *Ski. Pharmacol. Physiol.* **2018**, *31*, 332–336. [CrossRef]
31. Cui, K.L.; Zhang, L.C.; La, X.; Wu, H.L.; Yang, R.P.; Li, H.Q.; Li, Z.Y. Ferulic Acid and P-Coumaric Acid Synergistically Attenuate Non-Alcoholic Fatty Liver Disease through HDAC1/PPARG-Mediated Free Fatty Acid Uptake. *Int. J. Mol. Sci.* **2022**, *23*, 15297. [CrossRef] [PubMed]
32. Yeerjiang, A.; Maimaitiyiming, D.; Yang, T.; Fang, L.; Aihemaitituoheti, A.; Aimaiti, M.; Zhang, X.Y.; Nijiati, Y. Pomegranate Peel in the Amelioration of High-Altitude Disease: A Network Pharmacology and Molecular Docking Study of Underlying Mechanisms. *J. Food Biochem.* **2023**, *2023*, 7186747. [CrossRef]
33. Ljumovic, D.; Diamantis, I.; Alegakis, A.K.; Kouroumalis, E.A. Differential expression of matrix metalloproteinases in viral and non-viral chronic liver diseases. *Clin. Chim. Acta* **2004**, *349*, 203–211. [CrossRef] [PubMed]
34. Coilly, A.; Desterke, C.; Guettier, C.; Samuel, D.; Chiappini, F. FABP4 and MMP9 levels identified as predictive factors for poor prognosis in patients with nonalcoholic fatty liver using data mining approaches and gene expression analysis. *Sci. Rep.* **2019**, *9*, 19785. [CrossRef]
35. Liang, D.D.; Chen, H.J.; Zhao, L.P.; Zhang, W.X.; Hu, J.; Liu, Z.G.; Zhong, P.; Wang, W.; Wang, J.Y.; Liang, G. Inhibition of EGFR attenuates fibrosis and stellate cell activation in diet-induced model of nonalcoholic fatty liver disease. *Biochim. Biophys. Acta (BBA) Mol. Basis Dis.* **2018**, *1864*, 133–142. [CrossRef]

nutrients

MDPI

Article

Effect of the Administration of *Cordyceps militaris* Mycelium Extract on Blood Markers for Anemia in Long-Distance Runners

Akira Nakamura [1], Eri Shinozaki [2,3], Yoshio Suzuki [3], Kazuki Santa [4,5], Yoshio Kumazawa [6,7], Fumio Kobayashi [8], Isao Nagaoka [5,9,*] and Natsue Koikawa [3]

1 Faculty of Health and Sports Science, Juntendo University, Chiba 270-1695, Japan; aknaka@juntendo.ac.jp
2 Koyama Memorial Hospital, Ibaraki 314-0030, Japan
3 Graduate School of Health and Sports Science, Juntendo University, Chiba 270-1695, Japan; yssuzuki@juntendo.ac.jp (Y.S.); nkoikawa@juntendo.ac.jp (N.K.)
4 Department of Biotechnology, Tokyo College of Biotechnology, Tokyo 114-0032, Japan; k-santa@juntendo.ac.jp
5 Faculty of Medical Science, Juntendo University, Chiba 279-0013, Japan
6 Department of Biochemistry, School of Medicine, Juntendo University, Tokyo 113-8421, Japan; kumazawa@vsj.co.jp
7 Vino Science Japan Inc., Kanagawa 210-0855, Japan
8 La Vie En Sante Ltd., Ibaraki 315-0014, Japan; f_kobayashi@nifty.com
9 Department of Biochemistry and Systems Biomedicine, Graduate School of Medicine, Juntendo University, Tokyo 113-8421, Japan
* Correspondence: nagaokai@juntendo.ac.jp; Tel.: +81-47-354-3311

Abstract: In the present study, we conducted a placebo-controlled, double-blind, parallel-group comparison trial in which an extract of *Cordyceps militaris* (CM) mycelium was administered to long-distance runners for 16 weeks during the pre-season training period and blood test markers for anemia were investigated. The results indicated that the change rates of serum ferritin levels were moderately increased in the CM group (n = 11) but decreased in the placebo group (n = 11) during the study period, and the levels were significantly increased in the CM group compared with those in the placebo group at 4 weeks and 8 weeks after the test food intake ($p < 0.05$). Moreover, the change rates of hemoglobin and hematocrit were significantly increased in the CM group compared with those in the placebo group at 8 weeks after the test food intake ($p < 0.05$). These observations suggest that the intake of test food containing *Cordyceps militaris* mycelium extract is expected to effectively maintain the hemoglobin and hematocrit levels in long-distance runners, possibly via the suppression of the decrease in iron storage, which is reflected by serum ferritin, during pre-season training. Furthermore, the levels of creatine kinase were increased above the normal range in both the placebo and CM groups at registration. Interestingly, the creatine kinase levels were significantly decreased in the CM group compared with those in the placebo group at 16 weeks after the test food intake ($p < 0.05$). These results suggest that *Cordyceps militaris* mycelium extract exhibits a protective action on the muscle damage observed in long-distance runners and may suppress muscle injury. Together, these observations suggest that *Cordyceps militaris* mycelium extract exhibits an improving effect on the markers for not only anemia, but also muscle injury in long-distance runners during pre-season training.

Keywords: Dongchong-hongxiacao; long-distance runner; anemic marker; ferritin; hemoglobin; hematocrit; creatine kinase

1. Introduction

Ophiocordyceps sinensis, also known as *Cordyceps sinensis* or Dong Chong Xia Cao (winter worm summer grass), is an entomopathogenic fungus with a club-shaped fruiting body originally found in the alpine region of China at an altitude of 3000–5000 m [1–4]. The host of the fungus is the larvae of the Chinese moth (*Hepialus armoricanns* Oben).

Ophiocordyceps sinensis infects the larva in winter, slowly grows inside the larva, utilizes the nutrients of the larva and emerges from the ground in summer with the distinctive shape of "Dongchong-hongxiacao", retaining the larva in the ground.

Since the Chinese moth (Oben) that is susceptible to *Ophiocordyceps sinensis* does not naturally live in Japan, a variety of fungi including *Ophiocordyceps sobolifera*, which grows in the larva of *Platypleura kaempferi*, and *Cordyceps militaris*, which grows in the larvae of the moths, have been used for Dongchong-hongxiacao [4,5].

Some research has already been conducted on the effect of a supplement containing *Cordyceps sinensis* on exercise performance. In one study, 10 healthy untrained males were administered with an extract of *Cordyceps sinensis* mycelium for one week and subjected to a treadmill exercise load test. The results indicated that, with the administration of the *Cordyceps sinensis* mycelium extract, the blood glucose level was maintained during exercise, whereas the blood lactic acid level was decreased, and the increase in blood sugar was suppressed after the exercise [6]. Furthermore, 18 male long-distance runners were administered with *Cordyceps sinensis*–containing supplement for two weeks during high-altitude training. Interestingly, with the administration, the treadmill exercise times were significantly prolonged and aerobic capacity was increased in the runners [7]. Moreover, 14 male middle- and long-distance runners were administered with *Cordyceps sinensis* extract for two months, and the results indicated that reticulocytes were increased after the administration [8]. These observations suggest that the administration of *Cordyceps sinensis* extract may enhance aerobic capacity in athletes, possibly by increasing reticulocytes and improving oxygen transport. However, the values of red blood cell count, hematocrit and hemoglobin were not significantly changed with the administration of *Cordyceps sinensis* extract in the study by Chen et al. [7].

During the pre-season training that is performed before the official season, endurance runners are likely to develop sports anemia because of iron loss, which is associated with sweating and foot-strike hemolysis [9,10]. Based on the above findings, we hypothesized that the administration of Dongchong-hongxiacao may ameliorate anemia observed in endurance runners during pre-season training. Thus, in the present study, we conducted a placebo-controlled, double-blind, parallel-group comparison trial in which the extract of *Cordyceps militaris* mycelium was administered to long-distance runners for 16 weeks during the pre-season training period, and the blood test markers for anemia were investigated. We utilized extracts of *Cordyceps militaris* mycelium instead of *Cordyceps sinensis* extracts, although the effects of *Dongchong-hongxiacao* on exercise performance have been previously evaluated using supplements containing *Cordyceps sinensis* [6–8]. This is because the Chinese moth (Oben) that is susceptible to *Cordyceps sinensis* does not naturally live in Japan, so extracts of other fungi that infect and grow in the larvae of insects, including *Cordyceps militaris*, are used for Dongchong-hongxiacao in Japan [4,5].

2. Materials and Methods

2.1. Subjects

A total of 22 healthy male long-distance runners participated in this study. The inclusion criteria included male long-distance runners aged from 18 to 24 years old belonging to the Faculty of Health and Sports Science, Juntendo University (Chiba, Japan). The exclusion criteria included individuals with significant anxiety about the intake of test foods, which could disturb their normal daily life; individuals suffering from diseases to be treated, including anemia (judged by a preliminary blood test); individuals taking medicines (including iron supplements) prescribed by a physician during the test period; individuals who donated a blood component or 200 mL of whole blood within one month prior to the start of this study; individuals who donated 400 mL of blood in the four months prior to the start of this study; individuals whose blood collection volume exceeded 800 mL in the previous 12 months, including the blood collection volume in this study; individuals who were participating in other trials or had completed a similar trial in the previous four weeks; individuals taking medication or supplements aimed at improving anemia;

individuals with anemia-related diseases or conditions; and individuals who were judged to be inappropriate for participating in this study by the principal investigator.

Participants who responded to the recruitment for the study were provided with a research consent document and a thorough explanation of the research content. They were required to submit written voluntary consent to participate in the study. In addition, if the participants were minors, written consents were obtained from their guardians.

All 22 subjects completed the test food intake and measurements; however, two subjects (one each from the placebo group and the *Cordyceps militaris* (CM) group) did not participate in the 5000 m run conducted after the study period, so they were excluded from the 5000 m record. Since there were no defects in other measured values, all 22 subjects were included in the analysis (Figure 1). The age of the subjects at the time of registration was 19.7 ± 0.9 years in the placebo group and 20.2 ± 1.1 years in the CM group, and the height of subjects was 170.6 ± 6.6 cm in the placebo group and 172.0 ± 5.4 cm in the CM group. Table 1 shows the weight, body mass index (BMI), body fat percentage, skeletal muscle percentage and basal metabolic rate of the subjects during the study period (0 week at registration, 4 weeks, 8 weeks and 16 weeks after the intake of test foods).

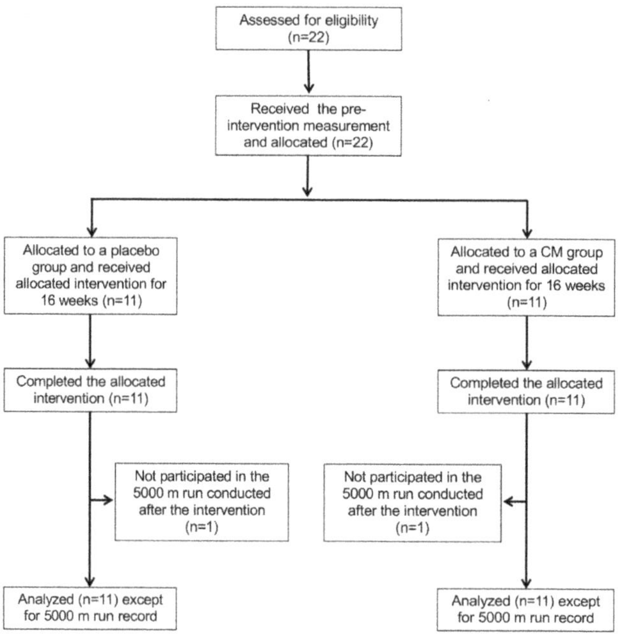

Figure 1. Flow diagram of the subjects who participated in the study.

Table 1. Body weight, body mass index, body fat percentage, skeletal muscle percentage and basal metabolic rate of the subjects in the placebo and CM groups during the study period.

	Groups	0 Week	4 Weeks	8 Weeks	16 Weeks
Body weight (kg)	Placebo	56.6 ± 4.4	56.4 ± 4.8	56.8 ± 4.8	57.3 ± 5.0
	CM	57.2 ± 4.3	57.0 ± 4.0	57.1 ± 3.8	57.7 ± 3.8
Body mass index (kg/m^2)	Placebo	19.5 ± 0.9	19.4 ± 1.0	19.5 ± 1.1	19.7 ± 1.0
	CM	19.4 ± 1.3	19.3 ± 1.2	19.4 ± 1.2	19.6 ± 1.4
Body fat percentage (%)	Placebo	14.5 ± 2.1	14.0 ± 2.3	14.4 ± 2.5	14.4 ± 2.3
	CM	14.0 ± 2.5	13.7 ± 2.5	14.7 ± 2.7	14.0 ± 2.9
Skeletal muscle percentage (%)	Placebo	41.8 ± 1.4	42.3 ± 1.5	42.0 ± 1.6	42.1 ± 1.4
	CM	41.8 ± 1.3	42.1 ± 1.6	41.6 ± 1.6	42.0 ± 1.9
Basal metabolic rate (kcal)	Placebo	1452.6 ± 74.7	1451.6 ± 80.5	1455.7 ± 81.1	1466.1 ± 85.6
	CM	1463.7 ± 70.3	1461.2 ± 65.2	1459.9 ± 63.1	1473 4 ± 62.4

Values of the placebo (n = 11) and CM (n = 11) groups are shown as the mean ± SD.

This study was reviewed and approved by the Research Ethics Committee of the Faculty of Sports and Health Sciences, Juntendo University (Juntendo University Ethics Committee No. 31-5; Date of approval, 18 July 2019), and was conducted in accordance with the Declaration of Helsinki.

2.2. Research Protocol

This study was a placebo-controlled, double-blind, parallel-group comparison trial. Based on the results of the measurements performed at registration (18 July 2019), the subjects were assigned to the placebo group or the CM group to ensure that there were no significant differences in ages, levels of hemoglobin and erythropoietin, or seasonal best scores in 5000 m run. Thereafter, they started ingesting the placebo or the CM food for 16 weeks from 2 August 2019 to 22 November 2019. All subjects were instructed to take the placebo or the CM food (6 capsules per day; 3 capsules in the morning and 3 capsules in the evening) with water. In addition, if the subjects forgot to take the placebo or the CM food on one day, they were instructed not to take 2 days of doses on the following day. During the study period, they were allowed to eat and exercise as usual, and were prohibited from taking any medications or supplements intended to improve anemia. The placebo and the CM foods were distributed every month, and at the same time, the empty food bags were collected to check the intake status.

During the study period, the subjects recorded their intake of the placebo or the CM food in a diary. The diaries were distributed every month, and the diaries for the previous month were collected at the same time. Adherence to the intervention was evaluated on the basis of the consumption record in the study diary, and <80% adherence was considered a protocol violation. In this study, the adherence was >99% in both the placebo and CM groups.

In addition to the measurement performed at registration (0 week), blood tests and physical measurements were taken at 4 weeks, 8 weeks and 16 weeks after the test food intake (2 August 2019). However, height was measured only at registration. Body weight, body mass index (BMI), body fat percentage, skeletal muscle percentage and basal metabolic rate were measured during the study period using the Omron HBF-208IT body weight and body composition meter (Omron Healthcare Co., Ltd., Kyoto, Japan) based on the impedance method.

A dietary survey using a brief-type self-administered diet history questionnaire (BDHQ) was conducted at registration, and at 4 weeks, 8 weeks, 12 weeks and 16 weeks after the test food intake. BDHQ data was analyzed by the DHQ Support Center (Gender Medical Research Co., Ltd., Tokyo, Japan). In addition, official records for the 5000 m run were measured at registration (July 2019) and after finishing the test food intake (November 2019).

2.3. Test Foods

The test food containing *Cordyceps militaris* was produced by La Vie En Sante Ltd. (Ibaraki, Japan) as a *Cordyceps militaris* mycelium extraction powder (patent registered strain of KT165514). This extraction powder is a food product that has passed the anti-doping certification program (INFORMED-CHOICE) administered by LGC Ltd. (Laboratory of the Government Chemist, Teddington, UK), an international anti-doping certification organization.

Cordyceps militaris mycelium extraction powder (300 mg) was contained in each capsule so that the intake amount was 1800 mg per day in 6 capsules. In a previous study, the erythropoietin level was increased at a dose of 25 mg/kg of *Cordyceps sinensis* in mice [11]. Thus, the intake amount was calculated to be 1500 mg in humans, based on the body weight of the subjects, which was approximately 60 kg. In this study, the sufficient intake amount was set at 1800 mg per day. The placebo food was also produced by La Vie En Sante Ltd. The test food capsule (containing 300 mg of *Cordyceps militaris* mycelium extraction powder, 6.8 mg of silicon dioxide, 17 mg of calcium stearate, and 16.2 mg of potato starch) and the placebo food capsule (containing approximately 300 mg of potato starch) had the same appearance so were indistinguishable from each other.

2.4. Blood Tests

Blood tests were performed at 6:40 AM. After waking up, the subjects were allowed to drink only water, asked to skip breakfast and instructed to walk, not run, to the laboratory. The measured blood test markers are as follows: red blood cell (normal range, 427–500 × 10^4/μL), hemoglobin (13.5–17.6 mg/dL), hematocrit (39.8–51.8%), serum iron (54–200 μg/dL), transferrin saturation index (TSAT; Fe ÷ TIBC × 100) (>20%), unsaturated iron-binding capacity (UIBC; 104–259 μg/dL), total iron-binding capacity (TIBC; 253–365 μg/dL), ferritin (39.4–340 ng/mL), erythropoietin (4.2–23.7 mIU/mL), white blood cell (3900–9800/μL), total protein (6.7–8.3 g/dL), triglyceride (50–149 mg/dL), total cholesterol (150–219 mg/dL), HDL cholesterol (40–86 mg/dL), creatine kinase (62–287 U/L), γ-glutamyl transpeptidase (GT; <70 IU/L), aspartate aminotransferase (AST; 10–40 U/L), alanine aminotransferase (ALT; 5–40 U/L), C-reacting protein (<0.14 mg/dL), urea nitrogen (8–22 mg/dL), uric acid (3.7–7.0 mg/dL), creatinine (0.61–1.04 mg/dL), testosterone (1.31–8.71 ng/mL), sodium (136–147 mEq/L), potassium 3.5–5.0 mEq/L), calcium (8.5–10.2 mg/dL), magnesium (1.8–2.6 mg/dL) and chloride (98–109 mEq/L). The blood tests were performed by SRL, Inc. (Tokyo, Japan).

2.5. Statistical Analysis

The data were shown as mean ± SD. In the case of hemoglobin, hematocrit, ferritin and erythropoietin, the change rates were calculated by comparing the values at 4 weeks, 8 weeks and 16 weeks after the test food intake with those at registration (0 week) and expressed as percentage; the change in the values at 4 weeks, 8 weeks and 16 weeks were divided by those at 0 week and multiplied by 100. Since some datasets did not meet the assumptions of normality, non-parametric methods were used for the statistical analysis. The Shapiro-Wilk test was used to determine normality in this study. The Wilcoxon signed–rank test or the Friedman test (p values adjusted by Bonferroni) was used for the intra-group comparison, and the Mann–Whitney U test was used for comparisons between the two independent (placebo and CM) groups. Statistical analysis was performed using SPSS software version 29 (IBM Corporation, Chicago, IL, USA). The significance level was set at $p < 0.05$. Since this study was designed to evaluate the effect of the CM intake, the authors did not set a primary endpoint, and did not perform the power analysis beforehand.

3. Results

3.1. Background Characteristics of the Subjects during Study Period

Monthly running distances of the subjects from August to November were 320~490 km in the placebo and CM groups, and the total running distances of the subjects were 1732.0 ± 23.9 km in the placebo group and 1623.5 ± 369.1 km in the CM group (Table 2). There were no significant differences between the two groups in the monthly running distances and total running distances. Regarding the 5000 m running time, the record time was significantly shortened after the test food intake (November 2019) compared with that at the registration (July 2019) in both the placebo and CM groups ($p < 0.001$); however, there was no significant difference between the two groups (Table 3). Moreover, the amounts of dietary intake of iron and vitamin C, which affects the absorption of iron in the gastrointestinal tract, were compared between the placebo and CM groups during study period based on the dietary survey using BDHQ. The results indicated that there was no significant difference in the dietary intake of iron and vitamin C between the two groups at all time points during the study period (0 week, at the registration; 4 weeks, 8 weeks, 12 weeks and 16 weeks after the test food intake) (Table 4). Furthermore, no adverse health effects attributable to the test food intake were observed during 16 weeks of the study period.

Table 2. Monthly running distance of the subjects in the placebo and CM groups during the study period.

Groups	August	September	October	November	Total
Placebo (km)	485.1 ± 127.5	432.0 ± 54.3	488.7 ± 44.3	326.2 ± 66.2	1732.0 ± 231.9
CM (km)	474.3 ± 107.5	369.8 ± 133.9	456.3 ± 115.2	323.0 ± 83.8	1623.5 ± 389.1

Values of the placebo (n = 11) and CM (n = 11) groups are shown as the mean ± SD.

Table 3. Measurements of the 5000 m running time of the subjects in the placebo and CM groups before and after the intervention.

Groups	Pre-Intervention	Post-Intervention	p
Placebo (km)	15:18.82 ± 00:31.60	14:54.44 ± 00:32.00	<0.001
CM (km)	15:22.75 ± 00:35.31	14:55.98 ± 00:33.93	<0.001

Table 4. Intake of dietary iron and vitamin C in the placebo and CM groups during the study period.

Dietary Components	Weeks	Placebo Group	CM Group
Iron (mg/1000 kcal)	0 week	4.35 ± 0.94	4.29 ± 0.87
	4 weeks	3.98 ± 0.85	3.78 ± 0.67
	8 weeks	4.10 ± 0.65	4.26 ± 1.01
	12 weeks	4.14 ± 0.68	3.80 ± 0.65
	16 weeks	4.24 ± 0.76	4.19 ± 0.67
Vitamin C (mg/1000 cal)	0 week	60.55 ± 19.43	55.45 ± 16.08
	4 weeks	50.39 ± 23.94	48.55 ± 15.67
	8 weeks	50.35 ± 19.17	50.94 ± 21.06
	12 weeks	55.53 ± 23.78	54.58 ± 16.22
	16 weeks	55.45 ± 21.76	59.79 ± 20.51

Values of the placebo (n = 11) and CM (n = 11) groups are shown as the mean ± SD.

The official record for the 5000 m run were measured at registration (pre-intervention), and after finishing the test food intake (post-intervention). However, two subjects (one each in the placebo group and the CM group) did not participate in the 5000 m run conducted after the intervention. Therefore, those two subjects were excluded from the 5000 m record. Thus, the values of the placebo (n = 10) and CM (n = 10) groups are shown as the mean ± SD, and compared between pre- and post-intervention.

3.2. Blood Test Markers Related to Oxygen Transport Capacity

The levels of red blood cell, hemoglobin, hematocrit and TIBC did not essentially change during the study period in both the placebo and CM groups (Table 5). In contrast, the levels of serum iron and transferrin saturation index (TSAT; Fe ÷ TIBC × 100) were decreased during the study period in both the placebo and CM groups; however, these changes were not significant during the study period or between the two groups. The level of UIBC was more increased in the CM group compared with that in the placebo group during the study period, and the level was significantly increased in the CM group at 16 weeks after the test food intake compared with that at registration ($p < 0.05$). Interestingly, the serum ferritin level was decreased in the placebo group but was increased in the CM group during the study period, and the level was significantly decreased in the placebo group at 8 weeks after the food intake compared with that at registration ($p < 0.001$) (Figure 2A; Table 5). Moreover, the erythropoietin levels were significantly increased in both the placebo and CM groups at 16 weeks after the food intake compared with those at registration ($p < 0.05$) (Figure 2B; Table 5). However, there were no significant differences between the two groups during the study period in relation to the levels of UIBC, serum ferritin and erythropoietin.

Table 5. Changes in blood test markers in the subjects of the placebo and CM groups during the study period.

	Groups	0 Week	4 Weeks	8 Weeks	16 Weeks
Red blood cells (10^4/mL)	Placebo	487.36 ± 40.26	487.36 ± 41.26	485.00 ± 38.61	492.82 ± 34.90
	CM	489.09 ± 35.00	491.73 ± 39.37	502.55 ± 37.50	495.64 ± 34.56
	Mann–Whitney U	NS	NS	NS	NS
Hemoglobin (g/dL)	Placebo	14.85 ± 1.14	14.83 ± 1.04	14.84 ± 1.14	14.96 ± 1.00
	CM	14.85 ± 0.79	14.92 ± 0.78	15.33 ± 0.98	15.00 ± 0.94
	Mann–Whitney U	NS	NS	NS	NS
Hematocrit (%)	Placebo	44.01 ± 3.08	43.81 ± 2.83	43.55 ± 3.01	44.87 ± 2.68
	CM	44.22 ± 1.90	44.36 ± 2.40	45.05 ± 2.30	45.46 ± 2.37
	Mann–Whitney U	NS	NS	NS	NS
Iron (mg/mL)	Placebo	112.45 ± 37.45	110.00 ± 24.42	110.00 ± 37.62	89.82 ± 25.96
	CM	128.64 ± 27.93	120.45 ± 23.66	127.82 ± 26.62	94.82 ± 33.94
	Mann–Whitney U	NS	NS	NS	NS
TSAT (%)	Placebo	34.28 ± 11.6	33.28 ± 7.6	32.22 ± 9.52	28.07 ± 7.97
	CM	40.29 ± 8.94	37.73 ± 8.77	38.62 ± 9.39	29.62 ± 9.49
	Mann–Whitney U	NS	NS	NS	NS
UIBC (mg/dL)	Placebo	217.45 ± 44.62	222.27 ± 35.40	226.82 ± 27.51	230.73 ± 32.35
	CM	192.82 ± 40.45	204.09 ± 48.76	206.36 ± 41.90	222.82 ± 34.03 *
	Mann–Whitney U	NS	NS	NS	NS
TIBC (mg/dL)	Placebo	329.91 ± 22.54	332.27 ± 28.02	336.82 ± 31.91	320.55 ± 22.78
	CM	321.45 ± 34.49	324.55 ± 39.83	334.18 ± 25.43	317.64 ± 37.10
	Mann–Whitney U	NS	NS	NS	NS
Ferritin (ng/mL)	Placebo	56.42 ± 33.06	51.46 ± 25.54	39.02 ± 21.79 ***	51.06 ± 35.43
	CM	60.28 ± 32.13	68.86 ± 32.80	64.89 ± 39.94	67.43 ± 36.15
	Mann–Whitney U	NS	NS	NS	NS
Erythropoietin (mIU/mL)	Placebo	6.75 ± 1.74	6.82 ± 1.99	7.58 ± 1.87	9.16 ± 1.98 *
	CM	6.98 ± 2.14	6.44 ± 1.71	8.05 ± 2.17	10.55 ± 2.96 *
	Mann–Whitney U	NS	NS	NS	NS
White blood cells (/mL)	Placebo	7127 ± 1861	6081 ± 1031	5100 ± 1037 **	5918 ± 643
	CM	5627 ± 716	5518 ± 753	5327 ± 752	5236 ± 452
	Mann–Whitney U	<0.05	NS	NS	<0.05
Total protein (g/dL)	Placebo	7.32 ± 0.35	7.34 ± 0.37	7.17 ± 0.33	7.14 ± 0.34
	CM	7.24 ± 0.30	7.30 ± 0.17	7.35 ± 0.38	7.19 ± 0.25
	Mann–Whitney U	NS	NS	NS	NS
Triglyceride (mg/dL)	Placebo	47.82 ± 29.23	41.36 ± 16.16	53.55 ± 19.59	82.09 ± 35.77 *
	CM	50.27 ± 21.74	47.55 ± 14.43	61.91 ± 29.87	77.91 ± 32.63 *
	Mann–Whitney U	NS	NS	NS	NS
Total cholesterol (mg/dL)	Placebo	182.27 ± 32.05	184.00 ± 33.37	185.64 ± 31.33	188.73 ± 29.07
	CM	172.27 ± 18.55	175.64 ± 19.61	177.64 ± 22.38	177.82 ± 22.95
	Mann–Whitney U	NS	NS	NS	NS
HDL cholesterol (mg/dL)	Placebo	77.36 ± 15.23	79.18 ± 14.30	80.64 ± 15.64	75.45 ± 13.49
	CM	68.73 ± 14.54	71.91 ± 12.96	71.18 ± 14.28	69.18 ± 14.93
	Mann–Whitney U	NS	NS	NS	NS
Creatine kinase (U/L)	Placebo	427.91 ± 399.60	645.73 ± 636.14	280.45 ± 164.85	384.64 ± 188.84
	CM	336.73 ± 249.79	402.00 ± 239.84	203.18 ± 113.12 *	225.82 ± 109.49
	Mann–Whitney U	NS	NS	NS	<0.05

Values of the placebo (n = 11) and CM (n = 11) groups are shown as the mean ± SD. The Mann–Whitney U test was used for comparisons between the placebo and CM groups. The Friedman test was used for the intra-group comparison during the study period (comparison between 0 week and 4 weeks, 8 weeks, 12 weeks or 16 weeks). * $p < 0.05$, ** $p < 0.01$, *** $p < 0.001$. NS, not significant.

Furthermore, the change rates (%) in hemoglobin, hematocrit, ferritin and erythropoietin were calculated by comparing the values at 4 weeks, 8 weeks and 16 weeks with those at registration (0 week) (Figure 3). Importantly, the change rates of hemoglobin and hematocrit were significantly increased in the CM group compared with those in the placebo group at 8 weeks after the test food intake ($p < 0.05$) (Figure 3A,B). Moreover, the change rates of ferritin were increased in the CM group but decreased in the placebo group, and the levels were significantly decreased in the placebo group compared with those of the CM group at 4 weeks and 8 weeks after the test food intake ($p < 0.05$) (Figure 3C). In contrast, the change rates of erythropoietin were increased during the study period in both the placebo and CM groups, and there was no significant difference between the two groups at 4 weeks, 8 weeks and 16 weeks after the test food intake (Figure 3D).

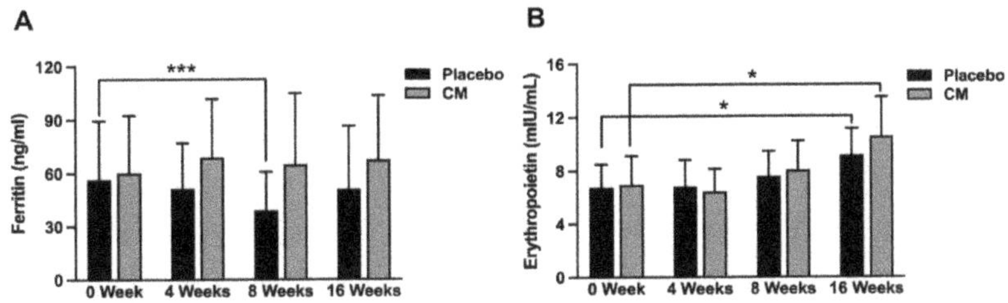

Figure 2. Serum levels of ferritin and erythropoietin in the placebo and CM groups during the study period. Serum levels of ferritin (**A**) and erythropoietin (**B**) were measured in the placebo (n = 11) and CM (n = 11) groups during the study period (0 week, at registration; 4 weeks, 8 weeks, 12 weeks and 16 weeks after the test food intake). Values are shown as the mean ± SD, comparing 0 week with 8 weeks, 12 weeks or 16 weeks. * $p < 0.05$, *** $p < 0.001$.

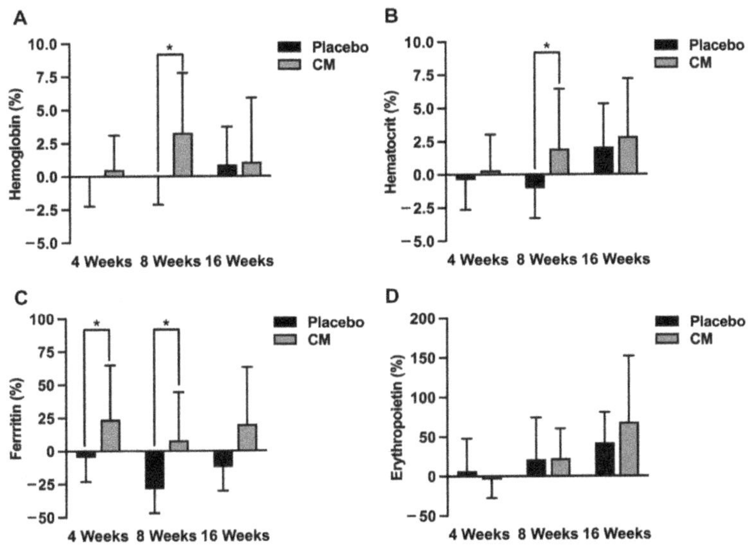

Figure 3. Change rates in the levels of hemoglobin, hematocrit, ferritin and erythropoietin in the placebo and CM groups during the study period. The change rates were calculated by comparing the values at 4 weeks, 8 weeks and 16 weeks after the test food intake with those at registration (0 week) in hemoglobin (**A**), hematocrit (**B**), ferritin (**C**) and erythropoietin (**D**), and expressed as a percentage. Data are shown as the mean ± SD, and compared between the placebo (n = 11) and CM (n = 11) groups. * $p < 0.05$.

3.3. *Other Blood Test Markers*

The level of white blood cells was significantly lower in the CM group than in the placebo group at registration and at 16 weeks after the test food intake ($p < 0.05$) (Table 5). Moreover, the white blood cell level was significantly decreased in the placebo group at 8 weeks during study period ($p < 0.01$). The level of C-reacting protein was significantly decreased at 8 weeks after the test food intake in the placebo group ($p < 0.01$)

(Table 6). The urea nitrogen level was significantly decreased at 8 weeks and 16 weeks after the test food intake in both the placebo and CM groups ($p < 0.05$). The uric acid level was significantly decreased at 16 weeks after the test food intake in the placebo group ($p < 0.05$). In contrast, the triglyceride level was significantly increased at 16 weeks after the study food intake in both the placebo and CM groups ($p < 0.05$). However, there were no significant differences between the two groups during the study period in relation to the levels of C-reacting protein, urea nitrogen, uric acid and triglyceride. Regarding total protein, total cholesterol, HDL cholesterol, GT, AST, ALT, creatinine, testosterone, sodium, potassium, calcium, magnesium and chloride, there were no significant differences found during the study period (0 week, 4 weeks, 8 weeks and 16 weeks) in the placebo and CM groups, or between the two groups during the study period (Tables 5 and 6).

Table 6. Changes in blood test markers in the subjects of the placebo and CM groups during the study period.

	Groups	0 Week	4 Weeks	8 Weeks	16 Weeks
GT (IU/L)	Placebo	22.73 ± 5.35	24.55 ± 8.04	23.45 ± 7.93	22.00 ± 5.50
	CM	21.45 ± 5.65	24.73 ± 10.90	24.09 ± 8.13	21.09 ± 5.99
	Mann–Whitney U	NS	NS	NS	NS
AST (U/L)	Placebo	39.45 ± 22.15	46.00 ± 27.04	32.00 ± 10.14	38.55 ± 13.84
	CM	29.27 ± 8.91	33.27 ± 12.77	26.00 ± 6.26	28.55 ± 6.68
	Mann–Whitney U	NS	NS	NS	NS
ALT (U/L)	Placebo	7.32 ± 0.35	7.34 ± 0.37	7.17 ± 0.33	7.14 ± 0.34
	CM	7.24 ± 0.30	7.30 ± 0.17	7.35 ± 0.38	7.19 ± 0.25
	Mann–Whitney U	NS	NS	NS	NS
C-reacting protein (mg/dL)	Placebo	0.36 ± 0.89	0.05 ± 0.06	0.02 ± 0.01 **	0.05 ± 0.02
	CM	0.05 ± 0.03	0.04 ± 0.01	0.04 ± 0.01	0.06 ± 0.03
	Mann–Whitney U	NS	NS	NS	NS
Urea nitrogen (mg/dL)	Placebo	19.85 ± 5.93	18.51 ± 4.56	15.09 ± 2.99 ***	15.62 ± 3.41 **
	CM	18.92 ± 6.37	17.75 ± 5.12	14.32 ± 3.28 ***	15.21 ± 4.78 *
	Mann–Whitney U	NS	NS	NS	NS
Uric acid (mg/dL)	Placebo	5.78 ± 0.80	5.92 ± 0.95	5.51 ± 0.83	4.95 ± 0.66 *
	CM	5.85 ± 0.89	5.86 ± 0.65	5.34 ± 0.65	4.94 ± 0.78
	Mann–Whitney U	NS	NS	NS	NS
Creatinine (mg/dL)	Placebo	0.78 ± 0.08	0.78 ± 0.09	0.75 ± 0.07	0.78 ± 0.08
	CM	0.82 ± 0.06	0.83 ± 0.08	0.79 ± 0.06	0.80 ± 0.05
	Mann–Whitney U	NS	NS	NS	NS
Testosterone (ng/mL/L)	Placebo	6.25 ± 1.85	6.09 ± 2.14	6.05 ± 1.83	6.09 ± 1.95
	CM	7.24 ± 2.39	7.05 ± 2.33	7.12 ± 2.16	7.01 ± 1.76
	Mann–Whitney U	NS	NS	NS	NS
Sodium (mEq/L)	Placebo	140.36 ± 1.29	140.18 ± 0.87	140.00 ± 1.00	140.91 ± 0.94
	CM	141.18 ± 1.17	140.73 ± 1.27	140.45 ± 1.04	141.27 ± 1.35
	Mann–Whitney U	NS	NS	NS	NS
Potassium (mEq/L)	Placebo	4.35 ± 0.41	4.17 ± 0.28	4.14 ± 0.29	4.32 ± 0.24
	CM	4.12 ± 0.15	4.15 ± 0.29	4.15 ± 0.20	4.39 ± 0.34
	Mann–Whitney U	NS	NS	NS	NS
Calcium (mg/dL)	Placebo	9.41 ± 0.23	9.35 ± 0.25	9.45 ± 0.23	9.41 ± 0.21
	CM	9.41 ± 0.20	9.44 ± 0.31	9.52 ± 0.20	9.51 ± 0.29
	Mann–Whitney U	NS	NS	NS	NS
Magnesium (mg/dL)	Placebo	2.31 ± 0.11	2.30 ± 0.13	2.23 ± 0.13	2.32 ± 0.10
	CM	2.25 ± 0.09	2.26 ± 0.12	2.23 ± 0.12	2.29 ± 0.11
	Mann–Whitney U	NS	NS	NS	NS
Chloride (mEq/L)	Placebo	103.27 ± 1.10	103.64 ± 0.92	103.09 ± 1.30	103.45 ± 1.13
	CM	103.55 ± 1.21	103.00 ± 1.34	103.00 ± 1.57	103.82 ± 1.25
	Mann–Whitney U	NS	NS	NS	NS

Values of the placebo (n = 11) and CM (n = 11) groups are shown as the mean ± SD. The Mann–Whitney U test was used for comparisons between the placebo and CM groups. The Friedman test was used for the intra-group comparison during the study period (comparison between 0 week and 4 weeks, 8 weeks, 12 weeks or 16 weeks). * $p < 0.05$, ** $p < 0.01$, *** $p < 0.001$. NS, not significant.

Notably, the levels of creatine kinase were increased to above the normal range (62–287 U/L) in both the placebo and CM groups at registration (Table 5). Interestingly, the creatine kinase level did not significantly change in the placebo group during the test period; however, the level was significantly decreased in the CM group at 8 weeks after the test food intake ($p < 0.05$) (Table 5). Moreover, the creatine kinase level was significantly decreased in the CM group compared with that in the placebo group at 16 weeks after the test food intake ($p < 0.05$) (Figure 4, Table 5).

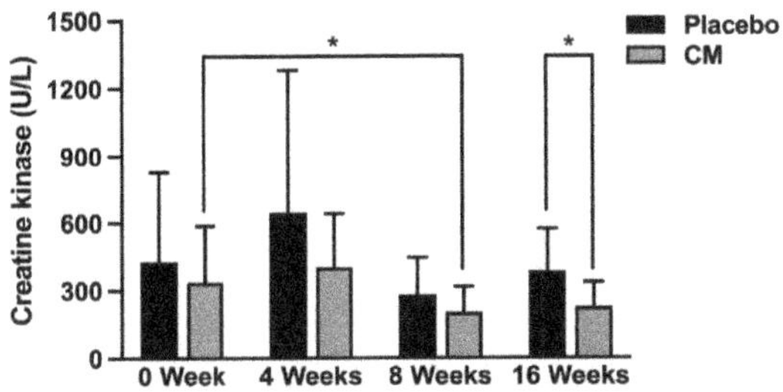

Figure 4. Serum level of serum creatin kinase in the placebo and CM groups during the study period. The serum levels of serum creatin kinase were measured in the placebo (n = 11) and CM (n = 11) groups during the study period (0 week, at registration; 4 weeks, 8 weeks, 12 weeks and 16 weeks after the test food intake). Values are shown as the mean ± SD, comparing 0 week with 8 weeks, 12 weeks or 16 weeks, and comparing the placebo and CM groups. * $p < 0.05$.

Except for creatine kinase, the abovementioned changes during the study period were within the normal range.

4. Discussion

In this study, to investigate the effect of *Cordyceps militaris* (CM) mycelium extract on blood markers for anemia, a placebo-controlled, double-blind, parallel-group comparison trial was conducted, involving test foods (a placebo food and a CM extract–containing food) being administered to long-distance runners for 16 weeks during the pre-season training period. The values of the following parameters measured in the subjects were not significantly different between the placebo and CM groups during the study period: body weight, BMI and body fat percentage (Table 1); monthly running distances and total running distances (Table 2); and the amounts of dietary intake of iron and vitamin C (Table 4). In contrast, the 5000 m running time was significantly shortened after the test food intake compared with that at registration in both the placebo and CM groups; however, there was no significant difference between the two groups (Table 3). Furthermore, there were no adverse health effects observed that were attributable to the test foods during the study period.

It is possible that ambient temperatures and seasonal changes may have affected the performance of the athletes, the hematological markers and other physiological indicators recorded in the log test period (16 weeks). However, we confirmed that the changes in the blood tests and hematological markers were within the normal range during the test period (Tables 5 and 6). Moreover, the body measurement markers (body weight, body mass index, body fat percentage, skeletal muscle percentage and basal metabolic rate) were not essentially changed during the test periods (Table 1). In contrast, the performance of the athletes, as evaluated by their 5000 m running time, was significantly faster in both the placebo and CM groups owing to the pre-season training (Table 3). Therefore, we believe that the effects of ambient temperatures and seasonal changes were minimal on the hematological markers and physiological indicators during the log test period (16 weeks) in this study.

Regarding the effect of the *Cordyceps sinensis* supplement on exercise performance, consistent results were not obtained. Specifically, some studies have indicated that the

Cordyceps sinensis supplement improves exercise performance in healthy older subjects [12] and aerobic performance in long-distance track and field athletes [7]. In contrast, other studies have shown that the *Cordyceps sinensis* supplement has no effect on aerobic exercise performance in physically inactive (sedentary) young adults [13] and endurance-trained cyclists [14–16]. In the present study, the 5000 m running time was significantly shortened in not only the CM group, but also the placebo group after the test food intake, and the administration of the *Cordyceps militaris* mycelium extract did not exhibit a distinctive effect on endurance performance (5000 m running) (Table 3), although the administration exhibited an improving effect on the markers for anemia and muscle injury in long-distance runners, as described below. However, it may be difficult to simply compare the effects of different *Cordyceps sinensis* supplement and *Cordyceps militaris* mycelium extract on the exercise performance.

The total amount of iron in the body is approximately 4–5 g; 65% functions as the heme of hemoglobin in red blood cells, 4% functions as the heme of myoglobin in muscle, and 15–30% is complexed with ferritin and stored in the liver and other organs [17,18]. Iron metabolism in the human body is a semi-closed circuit with no active excretion mechanism. Thus, only 1 to 2 mg of iron is lost per day in healthy individuals, through the mechanisms of sweat and the detachment of mucous membranes and epithelial cells [17,18]. Factors contributing to enhanced iron excretion include increased iron loss in sweat; increased excretion of red blood cells, hemoglobin and myoglobin in urine; and gastrointestinal bleeding [17,18]. Notably, the half-life of iron is shorter in long-distance runners than in non-athlete controls, suggesting that iron turnover is enhanced in runners [9,10]. In addition, iron demand is thought to increase in athletes, owing to increased blood volume and increased iron-containing enzymes and myoglobin in muscle [9,10]. Moreover, it is possible that gastrointestinal function is decreased because of intense training, which may reduce iron absorption from the intestines [9,10]. This study was conducted during pre-season training, in which long-distance runners perform intensive running training before the official season to improve their endurance capacity. The total distance covered by the long-distance runners participating in this study was more than 1600 km (from July to November) (Table 3), and their 5000 m running records were shortened in both the placebo and CM groups (Table 2). Thus, it is assumed that the endurance performance of the subjects was increased, and the iron loss and demand were possibly enhanced in the long-distance runners during the study period.

Iron deficiency anemia is the most common type of anemia [17,18]. Prolonged iron deficiency leads to a depletion in stored iron, followed by decreased serum iron levels, and finally resulting in iron deficiency anemia accompanied by reduced hemoglobin. The state in which stored iron is reduced is called latent iron deficiency, the state in which serum iron is reduced is labeled overt iron deficiency, and the state in which hemoglobin is reduced is identified as iron deficiency anemia [17,18]. Interestingly, endurance athletes experience a decreased exercise performance when their serum iron levels are low, even if they do not develop iron deficiency anemia [9,10]. The amount of iron stored in the body is reflected in the serum ferritin levels [19,20]. In this study, the serum ferritin level was slightly decreased in the placebo group during the study period and was significantly decreased at 8 weeks after the food intake compared with that at registration ($p < 0.001$) (Figure 2A; Table 5). In contrast, the serum ferritin level was moderately increased in the CM group during the study period, although there was no significant difference during the study period (0 week, 4 weeks, 8 weeks, 12 weeks and 16 weeks after the test food intake) (Figure 2A; Table 5). Moreover, the serum ferritin levels were not significantly different between the placebo and CM groups during the study period. Interestingly, however, when the change rates were evaluated during the study period, the serum ferritin levels were moderately increased in the CM group but decreased in the placebo group, and the levels were significantly increased in the CM group compared with those in the placebo group at 4 weeks and 8 weeks after the test food intake ($p < 0.05$) (Figure 3C). These results suggest that the test food containing *Cordyceps militaris* mycelium extract has the potential to suppress the decrease in iron storage (as evidence by the reduction in serum ferritin) in endurance athletes (long-distance runners).

In a healthy individual, the lifespan of red blood cells is approximately 120 days. Interestingly, the serum level of erythropoietin (a hematopoietic hormone) was significantly increased at 16 weeks after the test food intake compared with that at registration in both the placebo and CM groups ($p < 0.05$) (Figure 2B; Table 5). Moreover, when the change rates were evaluated during the study period, the erythropoietin levels were gradually increased at 8 weeks and 16 weeks after the test food intake in both the placebo and CM group, and there was no significant difference between the two groups during the study period (Figure 3D). These observations suggest that erythropoietin levels are likely increased in both the placebo and CM groups during the study period, possibly accompanied by the loss of iron in the long-distance runners (as demonstrated by the decrease in serum iron and TSAT). However, the intake of test food containing *Cordyceps militaris* mycelium extract did not exhibit a distinctive effect on erythropoietin levels in the long-distance runners.

Erythropoietin stimulates the production of red blood cells and increases hemoglobin and hematocrit levels [21]. In the present study, the levels of red blood cells, hemoglobin and hematocrit did not essentially change during the study period in both the placebo and test food groups (Table 5). However, when the change rates were evaluated during the study period, the levels of hemoglobin and hematocrit were significantly increased in the CM group compared with those in the placebo group at 8 weeks after the test food intake ($p < 0.05$) (Figure 3A,B). Moreover, ferritin levels were significantly increased in the CM group compared with those in the placebo group at 4 weeks and 8 weeks after the test food intake ($p < 0.05$) (Figure 3C). Based on these observations, it could be speculated that, although the erythropoietin levels were increased in both the placebo and CM groups, possibly accompanied by iron loss, the hemoglobin and hematocrit levels were increased or maintained in the CM group owing to the suppression of iron storage loss, whereas the hemoglobin and hematocrit levels were decreased in the placebo group owing to the decrease in iron storage (as demonstrated by the reduction in serum ferritin). Thus, the intake of the test food containing *Cordyceps militaris* mycelium extract is expected to effectively maintain the hemoglobin and hematocrit levels in long-distance runners by suppressing the decrease in iron storage during pre-season training.

The results of the present study indicate that the change rates in the levels of hemoglobin, hematocrit and ferritin significantly increased in the CM group compared with those in the placebo group, although the absolute values of these parameters were within the normal range and were not significantly different between the two groups during the test period. This is possibly based on the findings that the effect of *Cordyceps militaris* mycelium extract is minimal, just increasing the change rates of hemoglobin, hematocrit and ferritin, but not exceeding the normal range of these markers.

Intense physical exercise such as endurance running induces an inflammatory response in muscle, and results in muscle damage accompanied with an increase in serum creatine kinase (a biomarker for inflammatory response in muscle) [22–24]. In this context, it has been reported that the serum creatine kinase level is increased during or immediately after exercise in long-distance runners such as marathon runners [22–24]. Notably, in the present study, the serum creatine kinase levels were increased above the normal range (62–287 U/L) in both the placebo and CM groups at registration (Table 4), suggesting that inflammation and damage were induced in the muscle of the subjects participating in this study. Interestingly, the level of creatine kinase was significantly decreased in the CM group at 8 weeks after the test food intake ($p < 0.05$) (Figure 4, Table 5), and the level was significantly decreased in the CM group compared with that in the placebo group at 16 weeks after the test food intake ($p < 0.05$) (Figure 4, Table 5). Since *Cordyceps sinensis* contains substances with anti-inflammatory and antioxidant potential [1–4,25,26], it could be speculated that the *Cordyceps militaris* mycelium extract administered in this study exhibits anti-inflammatory and antioxidant actions on muscle, thereby protecting muscle injury in long-distance runners during pre-season training.

The results of the present study indicate that the level of C-reacting protein was significantly decreased at 8 weeks in the placebo group; however, the level was not essentially changed in the CM group. Since the administration of the *Cordyceps militaris* mycelium extract significantly decreased the level of CK (a biomarker for inflammatory response in muscle), it could be speculated that *Cordyceps militaris* mycelium extract exhibits anti-inflammatory action on injured muscle as evaluated by CK but not C-reacting protein.

This study has some limitations. First, when the change rates of hemoglobin and hematocrit were evaluated during the study period, these anemic markers were significantly increased in the CM group compared with those in the placebo group at 8 weeks after the test food intake ($p < 0.05$) (Figure 3A,B). However, the values of hemoglobin and hematocrit themselves were not significantly changed during the study period in both the placebo and test food groups (Table 5). This could be explained by the fact that the subjects participating in this study were long-distance runners belonging to the track and field team of a university, and they were well nourished without any evidence of anemia, making it difficult to determine the clear effect of the test food on the anemic markers (hemoglobin and hematocrit). To clarify the effect of the test food, studies should be conducted using subjects with a risk of anemia (such as uncontrolled amateur athletes). Second, the present study revealed the potential of *Cordyceps militaris* mycelium to suppress a decrease in iron storage (as demonstrated by a decrease in serum ferritin levels) in long-distance runners during the pre-season training period. However, the mechanism for the action of the test food is not clear. Moreover, it is unclear which components are responsible for the action of the *Cordyceps militaris* mycelium extract. Although the effects of Dongchong-hongxiacao (*Cordyceps)* on exercise performance have been mostly evaluated using supplements containing *Cordyceps sinensis* [6–8], in this study, we utilized extracts of *Cordyceps militaris* mycelium. *Cordyceps* contains various kinds of chemical constituents including nucleotides/nucleotide derivatives, polysaccharides, sterols and fatty acids, and other compounds [1]. Although the pharmacologically active components of *Cordyceps* are still unresolved, at least two chemical constituents, cordycepin and cordycepic acid have been identified and proposed as important active constituents [1]. Interestingly, cordycepin and cordycepic acid are contained in both *Cordyceps militaris* and *Cordyceps sinensis* as common components [1]. In the future, it will be necessary to elucidate the mechanism for the action of *Cordyceps militaris* mycelium extract and to identify the components of *Cordyceps militaris* mycelium that contribute to the suppression of muscle injury and the decrease in iron storage. Third, in the present study, the study population was limited to long-distance runners belonging to a university. In future, it would be interesting to evaluate the effect of *Cordyceps militaris* mycelium extract using athletes from other sports or even non-athletes.

5. Conclusions

The present study has shown that *Cordyceps militaris* mycelium extract is expected to effectively maintain the hemoglobin and hematocrit levels in long-distance runners by suppressing the decrease in iron storage during pre-season training. Moreover, the extract was found to alleviate muscle injury (as demonstrated by the decrease in serum creatine kinase levels) in long-distance runners, possibly owing to its anti-inflammatory and antioxidant potential.

Author Contributions: Conceptualization: I.N., Y.K. and F.K.; investigation and methodology: A.N., E.S. and N.K.; supervision: I.N. and N.K.; data curation: Y.S., I.N. and N.K.; writing—original draft: Y.S., K.S. and I.N.; writing—review and editing: Y.S. and I.N. All authors have read and agreed to the published version of the manuscript.

Funding: This research was funded by La Vie En Sante Ltd. (Ibaraki, Japan), grant numbers L20180426 and L20190325.

Institutional Review Board Statement: The study was conducted in accordance with the Declaration of Helsinki and approved by the Institutional Review Board of Juntendo University Ethics Committee (No. 31-5; Date of approval, 18 July 2019) for studies involving humans.

Informed Consent Statement: Informed consent was obtained from all subjects involved in the study. Written informed consent has been obtained from the patient(s) to publish this paper.

Data Availability Statement: Data are contained within the article.

Acknowledgments: The authors sincerely appreciate the participation of all subjects in this study.

Conflicts of Interest: The present study was supported by La Vie En Sante Ltd., which produced the test supplements used in this study. However, the company had no role in the design of the study; in the collection, analyses, or interpretation of data; in the writing of the manuscript; or in the decision to publish the results. Author Yoshio Kumazawa was employed by the company Vino Science Japan Inc. The remaining authors declare that the research was conducted in the absence of any commercial or financial relationships that could be construed as a potential conflict of interest.

Abbreviations

CM, *Cordyceps militaris;* BMI, body mass index; BDHQ, brief-type self-administered diet history questionnaire; TSAT, transferrin saturation index; UIBC, unsaturated iron-binding capacity; TIBC, total iron-binding capacity; GT, γ-glutamyl transpeptidase; AST, aspartate aminotransferase; ALT, alanine aminotransferase.

References

1. Yue, K.; Ye, M.; Zhou, Z.; Sun, W.; Lin, X. The genus *Cordyceps*: A chemical and pharmacological review. *J. Pharm. Pharmacol.* **2013**, *65*, 474–493. [CrossRef] [PubMed]
2. Chen, P.X.; Wang, S.; Nie, S.; Marcone, M. Properties of *Cordyceps sinensis*: A review. *J. Funct. Foods* **2013**, *5*, 550–569. [CrossRef] [PubMed]
3. Xu, J.; Hang, Y.; Chen, X.X.; Zheng, S.C.; Chen, P.; Mo, M.H. The Mechanisms of pharmacological activities of *Ophiocordyceps sinensis* fungi. *Phytother. Res.* **2016**, *30*, 1572–1583. [CrossRef] [PubMed]
4. Olatunji, O.J.; Tang, J.; Tola, A.; Auberon, F.; Oluwaniyi, O.; Ouyang, Z. The genus *Cordyceps*: An extensive review of its traditional uses, phytochemistry and pharmacology. *Fitoterapia* **2018**, *129*, 293–316. [CrossRef] [PubMed]
5. Yahagi, N. Illustrated catalogue of Japanese *Cordyceps* (*Entomonogenous* fungi): The Yahagi collection of Japanese Cordyceps stored in the Tohoku University museum. *Bull. Tohoku Univ. Mus.* **2008**, *8*, 29–89.
6. Nagata, A.; Tajima, T.; Moriyasu, S. Effectiveness on ingestion with *Cordyceps sinensis* drinks during running exercise of human. *J. Ex. Sports Physiol.* **2002**, *9*, 85–92.
7. Chen, C.Y.; Hou, C.W.; Bernard, J.R.; Chen, C.C.; Hung, T.C.; Cheng, L.L.; Liao, Y.H.; Kuo, C.H. *Rhodiola crenulata*- and Cordyceps sinensis-based supplement boosts aerobic exercise performance after short-term high altitude training. *High Alt. Med. Biol.* **2014**, *15*, 371–379. [CrossRef] [PubMed]
8. Muramatsu, I.; Omagari, S. Effectiveness on ingestion with edible sweet potato tops and *Codyceps sinensis* on male mid- and long-distance runners. *Ann. Fitness Sports Sci.* **2016**, *52*, 1–11.
9. Clénin, G.; Cordes, M.; Huber, A.; Schumacher, Y.O.; Noack, P.; Scales, J.; Kriemler, S. Iron deficiency in sports—Definition, influence on performance and therapy. *Swiss Med. Wkly.* **2015**, *145*, w14196. [CrossRef]
10. Damian, M.T.; Vulturar, R.; Login, C.C.; Damian, L.; Chis, A.; Bojan, A. Anemia in sports: A narrative review. *Life* **2021**, *11*, 987. [CrossRef]
11. Manabe, N.; Azuma, Y.; Sugimoto, M.; Uchio, K.; Miyamoto, M.; Taketomo, N.; Tsuchita, H.; Miyamoto, H. Effects of the mycelial extract of cultured *Cordyceps sinensis* on in vivo hepatic energy metabolism and blood flow in dietary hypoferric anaemic mice. *Br. J. Nutr.* **2000**, *83*, 197–204. [CrossRef] [PubMed]
12. Chen, S.; Li, Z.; Krochmal, R.; Abrazado, M.; Kim, W.; Cooper, C.B. Effect of Cs-4 (*Cordyceps sinensis*) on exercise performance in healthy older subjects: A double-blind, placebo-controlled trial. *J. Altern. Complement. Med.* **2010**, *16*, 585–590. [CrossRef] [PubMed]
13. Liao, Y.H.; Chao, Y.C.; Sim, B.Y.; Lin, H.M.; Chen, M.T.; Chen, C.Y. *Rhodiola/Cordyceps*-based herbal supplement promotes endurance training-improved body composition but not oxidative stress and metabolic biomarkers: A preliminary randomized controlled study. *Nutrients* **2019**, *11*, 2357. [CrossRef] [PubMed]
14. Earnest, C.P.; Morss, G.M.; Wyatt, F.; Jordan, A.N.; Colson, S.; Church, T.S.; Fitzgerald, Y.; Autrey, L.; Jurca, R.; Lucia, A. Effects of a commercial herbal-based formula on exercise performance in cyclists. *Med. Sci. Sports Exerc.* **2004**, *36*, 504–509. [CrossRef] [PubMed]

15. Parcell, A.C.; Smith, J.M.; Schulthies, S.S.; Myrer, J.W.; Fellingham, G. *Cordyceps sinensis* (CordyMax Cs-4) supplementation does not improve endurance exercise performance. *Int. J. Sport Nutr. Exerc. Metab.* **2004**, *14*, 236–242. [CrossRef]
16. Colson, S.N.; Wyatt, F.B.; Johnston, D.L.; Autrey, L.D.; FitzGerald, Y.L.; Earnest, C.P. *Cordyceps sinensis*- and *Rhodiola rosea*-based supplementation in male cyclists and its effect on muscle tissue oxygen saturation. *J. Strength Cond. Res.* **2005**, *19*, 358–363. [PubMed]
17. Andrews, N.C. Disorders of iron metabolism. *N. Engl. J. Med.* **1999**, *341*, 1986–1995. [CrossRef] [PubMed]
18. Hentze, M.W.; Muckenthaler, M.U.; Andrews, N.C. Balancing acts: Molecular control of mammalian iron metabolism. *Cell* **2004**, *117*, 285–297. [CrossRef] [PubMed]
19. Knovich, M.A.; Storey, J.A.; Coffman, L.G.; Torti, S.V.; Torti, F.M. Ferritin for the clinician. *Blood Rev.* **2009**, *23*, 95–104. [CrossRef] [PubMed]
20. Wang, W.; Knovich, M.A.; Coffman, L.G.; Torti, F.M.; Torti, S.V. Serum ferritin: Past, present and future. *Biochim. Biophys. Acta* **2010**, *1800*, 760–769. [CrossRef]
21. Jelkmann, W. Erythropoietin after a century of research: Younger than ever. *Eur. J. Haematol.* **2007**, *78*, 183–205. [CrossRef] [PubMed]
22. Bird, S.R.; Linden, M.; Hawley, J.A. Acute changes to biomarkers as a consequence of prolonged strenuous running. *Ann. Clin. Biochem.* **2014**, *51*, 137–150. [CrossRef] [PubMed]
23. Bernat-Adell, M.D.; Collado-Boira, E.J.; Moles-Julio, P.; Panizo-González, N.; Martínez-Navarro, I.; Hernando-Fuster, B.; Hernando-Domingo, C. Recovery of inflammation, cardiac, and muscle damage biomarkers after running a marathon. *J. Strength Cond. Res.* **2021**, *35*, 626–632. [CrossRef] [PubMed]
24. Da Ponte, A.; Giovanelli, N.; Antonutto, G.; Nigris, D.; Curcio, F.; Cortese, P.; Lazzer, S. Changes in cardiac and muscle biomarkers following an uphill-only marathon. *Res. Sports Med.* **2018**, *26*, 100–111. [CrossRef]
25. Qian, G.M.; Pan, G.F.; Guo, J.Y. Anti-inflammatory and antinociceptive effects of cordymin, a peptide purified from the medicinal mushroom *Cordyceps sinensis*. *Nat. Prod. Res.* **2012**, *26*, 2358–2362. [CrossRef]
26. Liu, Y.; Wang, J.; Wang, W.; Zhang, H.; Zhang, X.; Han, C. The chemical constituents and pharmacological actions of *Cordyceps sinensis*. *Evid. Based Complement. Alternat. Med.* **2015**, *2015*, 575063.

nutrients

MDPI

Review

Moringa oleifera and Blood Pressure: Evidence and Potential Mechanisms

Francesca Menichetti [1], Chiara Berteotti [2], Vittoria Schirinzi [3], Carolina Poli [4], Roberta Arrighi [1] and Alessandro Leone [1,5,*]

[1] International Center for the Assessment of Nutritional Status and the Development of Dietary Intervention Strategies (ICANS-DIS), Department of Food, Environmental and Nutritional Sciences (DeFENS), University of Milan, 20133 Milan, Italy
[2] PRISM Lab, Department of Biomedical and Neuromotor Sciences, Alma Mater Studiorum University of Bologna, 40126 Bologna, Italy
[3] Endocrinology and Care of Diabetes Unit-Azienda Ospedaliero-Universitaria S. Orsola Malpighi, Alma Mater Studiorum University of Bologna, 40126 Bologna, Italy
[4] Professional Development and Implementation of Research in Health Professions Unit, IRCCS Azienda Ospedaliero, Universitaria di Bologna, 40126 Bologna, Italy
[5] IRCCS Istituto Auxologico Italiano, Clinical Nutrition Unit, Department of Endocrine and Metabolic Medicine, 20100 Milan, Italy
* Correspondence: alessandro.leone1@unimi.it

Abstract: The prevalence of hypertension is increasing worldwide, in particular in developing countries. Anti-hypertensive drugs are commonly used to treat hypertension. However, in developing countries, where access to health care is scarce and the supply system is poor, anti-hypertensive drugs may not always be available. *Moringa oleifera* is a plant widely found in developing countries, with its leaves, seeds, flowers, roots, and pods used both for nutritional purposes and in traditional medicine to treat various diseases, including hypertension. This review summarizes the evidence, both in animal and human models, about the antihypertensive effects of different parts of *M. oleifera*, discusses possible mechanisms of action, explores its bioactive compounds with potential antihypertensive properties, and highlights the limitations of its use as a hypotensive agent. Many preclinical studies attribute antihypertensive properties to *M. oleifera*, particularly the leaves. However, it is premature to draw firm conclusions, as there is a great lack of randomized controlled trials demonstrating its real efficacy. The mechanisms of action and the compounds responsible for the hypotensive effect have not yet been fully elucidated. Therefore, further clinical trials showing its efficacy are strongly required before promoting Moringa for therapeutic purposes. At present, Moringa remains a plant with nutritional and pharmacological potential.

Keywords: *Moringa oleifera*; hypertension; blood pressure; traditional medicine; developing countries

1. Introduction

Hypertension, defined as a systolic blood pressure of 140 mm Hg or higher or a diastolic blood pressure of 90 mm Hg or higher [1], is a leading preventable risk factor for cardiovascular disease (CVD) and all-cause mortality worldwide [2]. Between 1990 and 2019, the global prevalence of hypertension nearly doubled, reaching 1.13 billion individuals, with the highest burden observed in low- and middle-income countries [3].

Lifestyle modifications, including salt restriction, the moderation of alcohol consumption, the consumption of vegetables, fruits, and low-fat dairy products, weight reduction, regular physical exercise, and smoking cessation, have proven effective in reducing blood pressure. However, implementing these changes can be challenging and not implemented [4], or not sufficient to bring blood pressure values back to normal limits. Consequently, the use of oral medications is recommended [1]. These drugs are effective but can have side effects and may not always be available, especially in developing countries with fragile healthcare systems and inadequate supply chains [5].

The food environment offers another promising avenue for the prevention and treatment of hypertension. Medicinal plants, used in traditional medicine for centuries, contain bioactive compounds that can help regulate blood pressure. These plants are affordable, accessible, and have minimal side effects, making them an attractive option, especially in developing countries. Among them, *Moringa oleifera*, a plant widely cultivated in tropical and subtropical regions, has gained attention for its nutritional [6] and medicinal properties [7,8]. In particular, its leaves are abundant in proteins, minerals (potassium, calcium, magnesium, iron), vitamins (β-carotene, α-tocopherol), dietary fiber [9–11], and bioactive compounds [6,12,13]. Due to this rich composition, they are widely utilized in traditional medicine across developing countries to treat various ailments, including diabetes, cardiovascular diseases, and hypertension [14–16].

While several reviews have examined the health benefits of *M. oleifera*, including its effects on cardiac function [17] and cardiometabolic disorders [18], to our knowledge, no recent review has specifically focused on its hypotensive effects by analyzing both preclinical and clinical studies. This review provides a comprehensive overview of the evidence regarding *Moringa*'s impact on blood pressure, explores the potential physiological mechanisms and bioactive compounds responsible for its hypotensive effects, and discusses the limitations of the current research. We also address challenges in using *M. oleifera* as an antihypertensive therapy and propose directions for future studies.

2. Physiological Regulation of Blood Pressure

Arterial blood pressure is regularly measured in patients to assess cardiovascular health. It is expressed in millimeters of mercury and consists of systolic and diastolic measurements. Systolic pressure represents the maximum pressure in the arteries when the heart contracts to pump blood, while diastolic pressure is the minimum pressure when the heart relaxes between beats [19]. Arterial pressure is closely related to cardiac output, arterial elasticity, and peripheral vascular resistance. It can be easily influenced by various activities, and ideally, blood pressure should range from 90/60 mmHg to 120/80 mmHg. Maintaining this range is crucial for health. Stage 1 hypertension is classified between 140/80 mmHg and 159/99 mmHg [20], while stage 2 hypertension falls within the range of 160/100 mmHg to 179/109 mmHg [21]. Hypertensive urgency occurs with readings over 180/120 mmHg, and hypertensive emergency involves life-threatening symptoms and organ damage [22]. Hypotension is defined as a blood pressure lower than 90/60 mmHg [23]. The body uses several mechanisms to regulate blood pressure, including the baroreceptor reflex, antidiuretic hormone, and the renin–angiotensin–aldosterone system (RAAS).

2.1. Baroreceptor Reflex

Baroreceptors, located in blood vessels, play a key role in regulating blood pressure by responding to vessel wall stretch. These mechanoreceptors send sensory information to the central nervous system, influencing vascular resistance and cardiac output. There are high-pressure and low-pressure baroreceptors. High-pressure baroreceptors are found in the carotid sinus and aortic arch. They respond to blood pressure changes, sending signals via the glossopharyngeal and vagus nerves, respectively.

Activation of these receptors leads to a response that influences sympathetic activity: increased blood pressure suppresses sympathetic activity, while decreased blood pressure (e.g., in hypovolemic shock) reduces baroreceptor firing, raising sympathetic activity to increase blood pressure [24]. Low-pressure baroreceptors are located in large veins, pulmonary vessels, and the right atrium and ventricle, responding mainly to volume changes. Decreased firing from these receptors triggers the release of antidiuretic hormone, renin, and aldosterone to regulate blood pressure [25]. Although baroreceptors control short-term blood pressure fluctuations, their role in long-term regulation is limited, as they reset to a new pressure level over time. However, experimental studies suggest they can still influence long-term blood pressure, especially by modulating kidney sympathetic nerve activity [26]. In hypertension, baroreceptor sensitivity decreases due to carotid sinus stiffness, raising the threshold and reducing their responsiveness to pressure changes. Sinoaortic denervation can cause temporary or prolonged hypertension [27,28].

2.2. Antidiuretic Hormone

Antidiuretic hormone (ADH), also known as vasopressin, is synthesized in the hypothalamus, primarily by neurons in the supraoptic nuclei and, to a lesser extent, by neurons in the paraventricular nuclei, which mainly produce oxytocin. ADH is transported along the hypothalamic–hypophysial tract to the posterior pituitary, where it is released into the bloodstream via fenestrated capillaries. ADH production and release are triggered by several factors: high plasma osmolarity (detected by osmoreceptors in the hypothalamus), low blood volume (causing reduced tension in low-pressure baroreceptors), decreased blood pressure (leading to reduced stretch in high-pressure baroreceptors), and angiotensin II.

The primary function of ADH is to increase water reabsorption in the collecting ducts of the kidneys, raising plasma volume and arterial pressure. High concentrations of ADH can also induce moderate vasoconstriction, which increases peripheral resistance and further raises arterial pressure [29,30]. A detailed description of ADH action is reported in Figure 1.

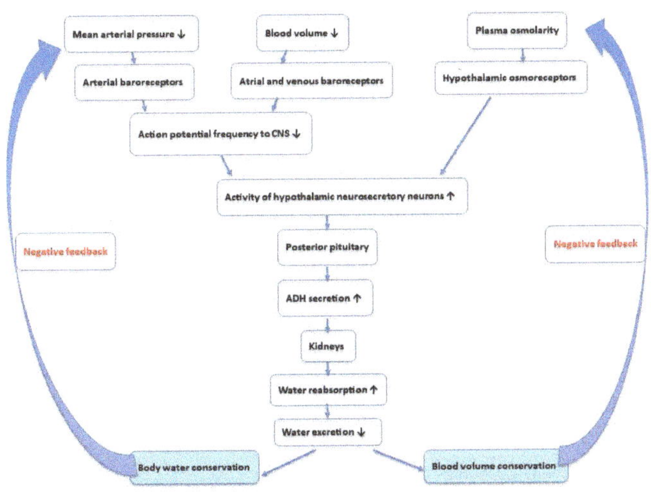

Figure 1. Mechanisms controlling the secretion of antidiuretic hormone (ADH, or vasopressin) and its effects on the body's water volume, and consequently, on the circulating volume, blood pressure, and body fluid osmolarity. The black arrows indicate the direction of change in physiological parameters.

2.3. *Renin–Angiotensin–Aldosterone System (RAAS)*

The renin–angiotensin–aldosterone system (RAAS) plays a critical role in regulating arterial blood pressure by increasing blood volume and peripheral resistance through hormonal actions. It begins when juxtaglomerular cells in the kidneys release renin in response to low blood pressure, increased sympathetic activity, or reduced sodium levels in the distal convoluted tubules. Renin converts angiotensinogen, produced by the liver, into angiotensin I, which is then converted into angiotensin II in the pulmonary vessels by the angiotensin-converting enzyme (ACE).

Angiotensin II raises arterial pressure by acting as a potent vasoconstrictor, constricting efferent arterioles in the kidney glomerulus to maintain the glomerular filtration rate, increasing sodium reabsorption in the kidneys (leading to water retention), and stimulating the release of ADH from the posterior pituitary and aldosterone from the adrenal cortex. Aldosterone increases sodium reabsorption and potassium secretion in the kidneys, enhancing water retention and further raising blood pressure. A detailed description of angiotensin II action is reported in Figure 2.

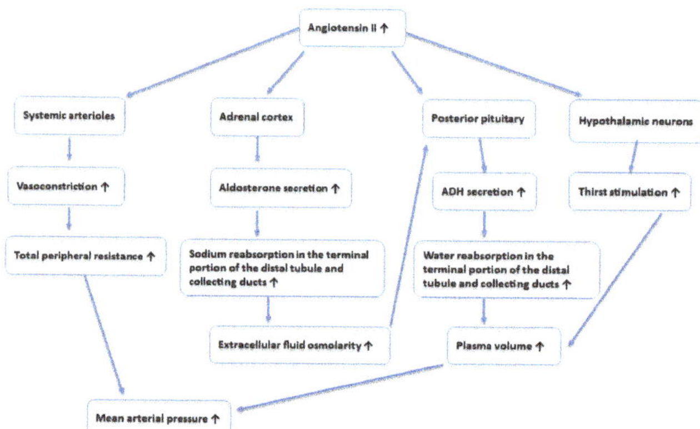

Figure 2. Angiotensin II mechanisms of blood pressure control. The black arrows indicate the direction of change in physiological parameters.

While the baroreceptor reflex provides short-term pressure regulation, the RAAS handles both acute and chronic regulation.

The goal of arterial pressure regulation is to maintain adequate tissue perfusion without causing damage. In cases of acute hypotension, the baroreflex works to stabilize blood pressure. Chronic hypertension, often without a clear cause, is known as essential hypertension and accounts for around 95% of hypertension cases. This condition can lead to severe complications in the brain, heart, and kidneys [31–33].

3. Search Strategy and Study Selection

The search for studies was conducted using the PubMed database, employing the following search string: "moringa oleifera" [tiab] AND ("blood pressure" [tiab] OR "hypertension" [tiab]). Additional studies were retrieved from the references of the selected studies. The search included studies published up to December 2024. To be included, studies had to be original articles published in English, investigating the effects of *Moringa oleifera* (in its whole form, extract, or specific component) on blood pressure in either animal or human models, or examining the mechanisms through which *Moringa oleifera* might modulate blood pressure.

4. Effect of *Moringa oleifera* on Blood Pressure

4.1. Animal Studies

Various studies have investigated both acute and chronic effects of *M. oleifera* on blood pressure in both healthy and hypertensive animal models. These experiments, detailed in Table 1, primarily involved the administration of *M. oleifera* leaves, seeds, or their extracts.

Table 1. Effects of *Moringa oleifera* on blood pressure in animal studies.

Studies	Part of Moringa	Experimental Model	Results
Abrogoua et al. [34]	Aqueous extract of *Bidens pilosa* and fresh leaves of *M. oleifera*	Healthy rabbits were treated with increasing doses of the traditional dietary supplement (5×10^{-8} to 5×10^{-2} mg/kg bw) or acetylcholine.	The extract produced a dose-dependent hypotensive effect, reducing blood pressure by 7.14 ± 4% to 100 ± 7.5% compared to normal levels in rabbits.
Aekthammarat et al. [35]	Aqueous leaf extract	Six male Wistar rats received acetylcholine (control), followed by leaf extract (1, 3, 10, 30 mg/kg). Six male Wistar rats were pretreated with L-NAME, followed by the same leaf extract doses.	Acute intravenous injection of *M. oleifera* extract caused a dose-dependent reduction in the mean arterial pressure in the normotensive rats, with reductions of 12.87 ± 1.45%, 21.52 ± 1.27%, 27.83 ± 0.64%, and 29.87 ± 2.34%, respectively. Significant differences were observed at all doses compared to 1 mg/kg. L-NAME pretreatment significantly reduced the BP-lowering effect of the extract, with reductions of 2.31 ± 0.61%, 6.09 ± 0.78%, 8.43 ± 1.23%, and 8.57 ± 1.43% at the respective doses.
Faizi et al. [36]	Ethanolic and hot water extracts and relative fractions and isolates of pods, seeds, pulp, and leaves	Normotensive Wistar rats were treated with fractions (10 and 30 mg/kd) and isolates (3 and 10 mg/kg) of *M. oleifera* pod, seed, pulp and leaf extract.	Ethanolic extracts of *M. oleifera* pods and seeds reduced blood pressure by 41% and 43% at 30 mg/kg. The aqueous fraction was inactive. The neutral and acidic sub-fractions of the ethyl acetate phase reduced pressure by 37.6% and 25.5%. Isolated compounds also lowered blood pressure. Hot water extracts of pods and leaves showed similar effects at 30 mg/kg.
Attakpa et al. [37]	Aqueous leaf extract	A total of 20 Wistar–Kyoto normotensive rats (WKYs) and 20 spontaneously hypertensive rats (SHRs) followed a control diet for 16 weeks, then were divided into four groups and treated for 8 weeks. Group 1 was treated only with diet. Groups 2 to 4 received a control diet + *M. oleifera* leaf extract (200, 400, and 600 mg/kg).	The extract reduced BP in the SHR rats in a dose-dependent manner. Significant differences were found between group 2 and group 3, but not between group 3 and group 4. No effects were seen in the normotensive rats.
Aekthammarat et al. [38]	Aqueous leaf extract	A total of 48 male Wistar rats were split into 6 groups. Groups 1 and 2 were normal rats, while groups 3 to 6 were L-NAME-induced hypertensive rats. They were treated daily for 3 weeks with the following: • Group 1: distilled water (1 mL/kg/day); • Group 2: *M. oleifera* extract (60 mg/kg); • Group 3: distilled water (1 mL/kg/day); • Group 4: Captopril (5 mg/kg); • Group 5: *M. oleifera* extract (30 mg/kg); • Group 6: *M. oleifera* extract (60 mg/kg).	Daily intragastrically administration of *M. oleifera* leaf extract decreased the SBP in a dose-dependent manner in the L-NAME hypertensiverats. The highest dose resulted in a lowering of pressure as early as one week into treatment. *M. oleifera* extract (60 mg/kg/day) did not affect blood pressure or heart rate in the normal rats.

Table 1. *Cont.*

Studies	Part of Moringa	Experimental Model	Results
Acuram et al. [39]	Methanolic and ethyl acetate leaf extracts	A total of 35 female ICR mice were divided into 7 groups and treated for 25 days: • Group 1: Control—distilled water; • Group 2: Solvent/vehicle; • Group 3: Captopril (20 mg/kg/day); • Group 4: Methanol extract (0.3 g/kg/day); • Group 5: Methanol extract (0.01 g/kg/day); • Group 6: Ethyl acetate extract (0.3 g/kg/day); • Group 7: Ethyl acetate extract (0.01 g/kg/day). Hypertension was induced in groups 2–7 by L-NAME treatment (30 mg/kg/day).	Methanolic extract reduced SBP from 102.35 ± 1.55 mm Hg to 90.97 ± 0.80 mm Hg. The ethanolic extract significantly reduced SBP to values comparable to those in the control group. No significant difference in BP was observed at either dosage (0.01 g/kg/day and 0.3 g/kg/day)
Chen et al. [40]	Leaf extract	**Acute study**: A total of 48 male Wistar rats (26 control and 22 with monocrotaline-induced pulmonary hypertension) were treated for 3 weeks with 1.5, 4.5, or 15 mg/kg of *M. oleifera* extract. **Chronic study**: A total of 22 male Wistar rats (7 control and 15 with monocrotaline-induced pulmonary hypertension) were treated for 3 weeks. On days 14–20, the control group received saline injection, and half of the monocrotaline-induced hypertensive rats received 4.5 mg/kg of *M. oleifera* extract.	**Acute study**: In the control rats, no significant difference was found in pulmonary arterial pressure at any dose. In the monocrotaline-induced hypertensive group, pulmonary arterial pressure decreased after Moringa extract administration. The 4.5 mg/kg dose resulted in an 80% reduction in pulmonary arterial pressure. **Chronic study**: Compared to the control group, MCT administration increased pulmonary arterial pressure. Repeated administrations of Moringa extract during the last week significantly reversed the monocrotaline-induced hypertension to a level similar to that of the control group.
Randriamboavonjy et al. [41]	Seed powder	A total of 12 spontaneous hypertensive rats were treated for 8 weeks. The experimental group received *M. oleifera* seed powder mixed into food (750 mg/d/rat), while the control group received normal food.	The treatment had no effect on diurnal and nocturnal SBP and DBP in the hypertensive rats. The treatment reduced the nocturnal heart rate during wakefulness.

Abrogoua et al. [34] tested the hypotensive effect of an aqueous extract, including salt, *Bidens pilosa* whole plant, and fresh *M. oleifera* leaves (20% of weight), on healthy rabbits. The extract, administered via injection, induced a dose-dependent reduction in blood pressure. Similarly, Aekthammarat et al. [35] observed that intravenous administration of the aqueous extract of *M. oleifera* leaves at doses of 1, 3, 10, and 30 mg/kg caused a rapid and dose-dependent reduction in the mean arterial pressure in normotensive rats and in rats pretreated with *N*ω-nitro-L-arginine methyl ester (L-NAME) to induce hypertension. In the normotensive rats, the highest dose of *M. oleifera* extract produced the greatest reduction in blood pressure (−30%), maintained for 37 min. Treatment with the leaf extract also reduced the mean arterial pressure in the hypertensive rats, though to a lesser extent than in the normotensive rats (−8.5% at the 30 mg/kg dose). In addition, Faizi et al. [36] assessed the acute hypotensive activity of ethanolic and aqueous extracts of *M. oleifera* pods, seeds, and leaves, along with their relative fractions and isolates, in normotensive WKY rats. They discovered that the ethanolic extracts of whole pods and seeds, administered at a dose of 30 mg/kg, led to reductions of 41% and 43%, respectively, in the mean arterial blood pressure. Specifically, the neutral and acidic subfractions of the ethyl acetate phase of the ethanolic extract of *M. oleifera* pods exhibited antihypertensive effects, while the aqueous fraction was inactive. β-sitosterol, methyl ester of p-hydroxybenzoic acid, and p-hydroxybenzaldehyde were identified among the isolates from these extracts as having a hypotensive effect. Additionally, extracts in the hot water of pods and leaves also demonstrated hypotensive activity. Regarding the chronic effect, Attakpa et al. [37] investigated the impact of the aqueous extract of *M. oleifera* leaves on male normotensive and spontaneous hypertensive rats (SHRs). The animals underwent a pretreatment with a standard diet for 16 weeks, and then were divided into groups receiving increasing amounts of *M. oleifera* leaves extract (200, 400, and 600 mg/kg) for 8 weeks. They noted a dose-dependent reduction in blood pressure in the SHRs, with significant hypotensive effects observed at doses of 400 and 600 mg/kg compared to the control diet, without a significant difference between the two doses. No effect of *M. oleifera* was observed in the WKY rats. Aekthammarat et al. [38] administered the aqueous extract of *M. oleifera* leaves to normotensive and hypertensive-induced WKY rats at doses of 30 or 60 mg/kg/day for three weeks. Hypertension was induced by adding 50 mg/kg/day of L-NAME to the drinking water for the same duration. They observed a dose-dependent decrease in systolic and diastolic blood pressure, as well as heart rate, in the hypertensive rats treated with *M. oleifera* compared to the untreated rats. However, treatment with *M. oleifera* did not affect blood pressure or heart rate in the normotensive rats. Acuram et al. [39] conducted a study on the antihypertensive activity of methanolic and ethyl acetate extracts of *M. oleifera* leaves in female mice. The animals were divided into several groups and treated for 45 days. Group 1 received distilled water orally (control group); group 2 received solvent or vehicle; group 3 was administered captopril (20 mg/kg/day); groups 4 and 5 received low and high doses of methanol extract of *M. oleifera* (0.01 g/kg/day and 0.3 g/kg/day); groups 6 and 7 were given low and high doses of ethyl acetate extract of *M. oleifera* (0.01 g/kg/day and 0.3 g/kg/day). Hypertension was induced in groups 2–7 by L-NAME treatment (30 mg/kg/day). The L-NAME treatment significantly increased blood pressure. The methanolic extract of *M. oleifera* led to a progressive and significant reduction in blood pressure, comparable to that of the control group by the end of the treatment period. Similar results were observed with the ethyl acetate extracts of *M. oleifera*, although a significant effect was only observed at the end of the treatment period. There was no significant difference in blood pressure between the high (0.3 g/kg/day) and low (0.01 g/kg/day) doses of *M. oleifera* extracts. Chen et al. [40] investigated the acute and chronic effects of *M. oleifera* leaf extract in the

WKY rats with induced pulmonary hypertension via subcutaneous injection of monocrotaline (MCT, 60 mg/kg). Acute administration of 4.5 mg/kg of the *M. oleifera* extract reduced pulmonary arterial pressure to around 80% of the MCT control. Chronic supplementation with the *M. oleifera* extract for one week at the same dose reversed the MCT-induced increase in pulmonary arterial pressure. Finally, Randriamboavonjy et al. [41] studied the impact of *M. oleifera* seed powder on cardiac function in SHRs. The animals were divided into two groups: one receiving a standard diet and the other a standard diet supplemented with 750 mg/d/rat of *M. oleifera* seed powder for 8 weeks. The treatment did not alter the diurnal or nocturnal systolic and diastolic arterial pressures. However, it led to a reduction in the nocturnal heart rate, without affecting the diurnal rate, when the animals were awake and active.

Numerous studies have validated the antihypertensive properties of *M. oleifera*, especially its leaves. However, evidence supporting the effects of other parts, like the seeds and pods, is limited. Moreover, the antihypertensive effects appear more pronounced in hypertensive animal models, while results in healthy animals are more varied.

4.2. Human Studies

We only found four studies examining the effects of *M. oleifera* on blood pressure in humans. The first research was conducted on healthy individuals, while the other three studies focused on participants with diabetes. Notably, none of the studies included subjects with hypertension. A detailed summary of human study is reported in Table 2.

Chan Sun et al. [42] reported that the consumption of cooked *M. oleifera* leaves led to a reduction in postprandial blood pressure among healthy subjects. This study was a prospective, placebo-controlled clinical trial involving a random sample of 41 healthy participants. Those in the treated group consumed 120 g of the plant's cooked leaves, while the control group received a placebo. Blood pressure measurements were taken at baseline (prior to the meal) and at regular intervals over the next 24 h (2, 4, 6, 10, 20, and 24 h after the meal). Additionally, all participants maintained a food diary during the week preceding the study, allowing researchers to estimate their total daily salt intake. The results show a significant decrease in diastolic blood pressure from baseline to the 2 h postprandial evaluation in the experimental group, but not in the control group. There were no significant differences observed in systolic blood pressure between baseline and postprandial measurements in either group. Moreover, among the participants in the experimental group with a high salt intake (7 g/day) during the week prior to the study, there was a notable decrease in both their systolic and diastolic blood pressure following the consumption of *Moringa oleifera* leaves. Conversely, higher blood pressure values were recorded in the participants with increased salt consumption in the control group. Afiaenyi et al. [43] employed a double-blind, parallel-group randomized controlled design for their study. The research involved 40 diabetic subjects, comprising 12 men and 28 women, who were randomized into four groups. The control group received an isocaloric diet based on the caloric distribution recommended by the American Diabetes Association (50–60% of daily caloric intake from carbohydrates, 25–30% from fat, and 15–20% from protein) [44]. The experimental groups received daily doses of 20 g, 40 g, and 60 g of Moringa leaves, respectively, in addition to the prescribed diet, for a duration of 14 days. The study findings revealed a notable reduction in systolic blood pressure (by -13 mm Hg, from 136.40 ± 7.66 to 123.90 ± 13.82 mm Hg) in the group treated with 40 g of *M. oleifera* leaves. However, this reduction was not observed in the other groups. Taweerutchana et al. [45] conducted a prospective randomized placebo-controlled study involving individuals with diabetes. The participants were randomly allocated to receive either 8 g per day of *M. oleifera* leaf capsules or a placebo for a duration of 4 weeks. At the conclusion of the treatment period, the researchers did not observe significant changes in systolic or diastolic blood pressure in either the treatment group or the placebo group. Finally, Diaz-Prieto et al. [46] conducted a double-blind, randomized, placebo-controlled, parallel-group study involving 73 patients with prediabetes. The 12-week intervention consisted of a daily administration of six capsules, each containing 400 mg of *M. oleifera* dry leaf powder or a placebo. At the end of the study, no significant effects were observed on systolic or diastolic blood pressure.

Table 2. Effects of *Moringa oleifera* on blood pressure in human studies.

Human Studies			
Studies	**Part of Moringa**	**Experimental Model**	**Results**
Chan Sun et al. [42]	Cooked leaves	A total of 41 participants aged 18–65 years (14 males, 27 females) were randomized into two groups: • The experimental group (n = 23) consumed 120 g of sautéed *M. oleifera*; • The control group (n = 18) consumed an equivalent amount of placebo. SBP and DBP were measured at baseline and postprandially at intervals up to 24 h (2, 4, 6, 10, 20, and 24 h after the meal).	Both the case and control groups showed decreased systolic blood pressure postprandially, but no significant difference was observed compared to baseline. Diastolic blood pressure decreased overall postprandially for both groups, with a significant difference noted between 2 h and baseline only in the experimental group.
Afiaenyi et al. [43]	Steamed leaves	A total of 40 adults (12 males, 28 females) with type 2 diabetes were split into groups and treated for 14 days: Group 1: Standard diet; Group 2: Standard diet + 20 g/day *M. oleifera* leaves; Group 3: Standard diet + 40 g/day *M. oleifera* leaves; Group 4: Standard diet + 60 g/day *M. oleifera* leaves.	Group 3 showed a significant decrease in SBP from 136.40 ± 7.66 mm Hg to 123.90 ± 13.82 mm Hg, with a mean decrease of 12.5 mm Hg. Group 4 did not show a significant reduction in SBP (−7.8 mm Hg). No significant reduction in DBP was observed in group 3 or 4 (−4.7 mm Hg and 3.3 mm Hg, respectively).
Taweerutchana et al. [45]	Leaf powder	RCT with placebo involving 32 people with type 2 diabetes. They were treated for 4 weeks with 8 g/day of *M. oleifera* leaf powder (experimental group) or placebo (control group).	No effect on SBP and DBP was observed.
Diaz-Prieto et al. [46]	Leaf powder	A double-blind RCT with placebo involving 73 patients with prediabetes. Patients were treated for 12 weeks with six capsules, each containing 400 mg of *M. oleifera* dry leaf powder (experimental group) or placebo (control group).	No effect on SBP and DBP was observed.

5. Possible Mechanisms of Action

Several studies have proposed different physiological mechanisms to explain the hypotensive effects of *M. oleifera* leaves and seeds.

It has been suggested that *M. oleifera* can induce vasorelaxation through both endothelium-dependent and endothelium-independent mechanisms. These mechanisms are summarized and shown in Table 3 and Figure 3, respectively.

Endothelium-dependent relaxation is a fundamental process in the regulation of vasodilation, mediated by the release of three major factors: nitric oxide (NO), prostacyclin (PGI_2), and endothelium-derived hyperpolarizing factors (EDHFs) [47]. These mediators act on vascular smooth muscle cells (VSMCs), promoting relaxation and facilitating blood flow. Several experimental studies have indicated that *M. oleifera* leaf extract induces vasodilation in isolated mesenteric arterial beds from both healthy and hypertensive rats [35,38]. The vasodilatory effect of the *M. oleifera* extract is largely endothelium-dependent, as demonstrated by a significant but not complete reduction in efficacy following endothelial removal [35,38]. This suggests a predominant, though not exclusive, role of endothelial mediators in its hypotensive action. The vasodilatory effect of *M. oleifera* leaf extract appears to be linked to its ability to stimulate NO production [35] and reduce oxidative stress [38]. In particular, a study on human pulmonary artery endothelial cells treated with increasing concentrations of *M. oleifera* leaf extract have shown an enhancement in NO production, an effect abolished by L-NAME, a non-selective inhibitor of endothelial nitric oxide synthase (eNOS) [35]. This finding suggests that *M. oleifera* leaf extract activates eNOS, increasing NO availability. A further study on aortic sections from middle-aged rats indicated that the eNOS activation induced by *M. oleifera* seed extract might be mediated by the upregulation of protein kinase B (Akt), which phosphorylates and activates eNOS, and the downregulation of arginase-1. Reduced arginase-1 expression increases the availability of L-arginine, the substrate required for NO biosynthesis, thereby contributing to the vasodilatory effect of the *M. oleifera* extracts [48].

Table 3. Summary of the mechanisms of action by which *Moringa oleifera* influences blood pressure.

Category	Mechanism		Effect	Final Result
Endothelium-Dependent	(+) eNOS (+) Protein kinase B (AKT) (-) Arginase-1		(+) NO biosynthesis	(+) Vasorelaxation
	(-) Reactive oxygen species (ROS) (+) Superoxide dismutase (SOD) (+) Catalase (CAT) (-) NADPH oxidase	(-) oxidative stress	(+) NO availability	
	(+) Endothelium-derived hyperpolarizing factors (EDHF) bioavailability		Hyperpolarization of VSMC	
Non-Endothelium-Dependent	(-) Receptor-operated calcium channels (ROCCs) (-) Voltage-operated calcium channels (VOCCs) (-) Inositol trisphosphate (IP3) receptor		(-) Intracellular Ca^{2+} in VSMC	
Systemic Regulatory Mechanisms	Inhibition of the renin–angiotensin–aldosterone system (RAAS)		(-) Systemic vascular resistance	

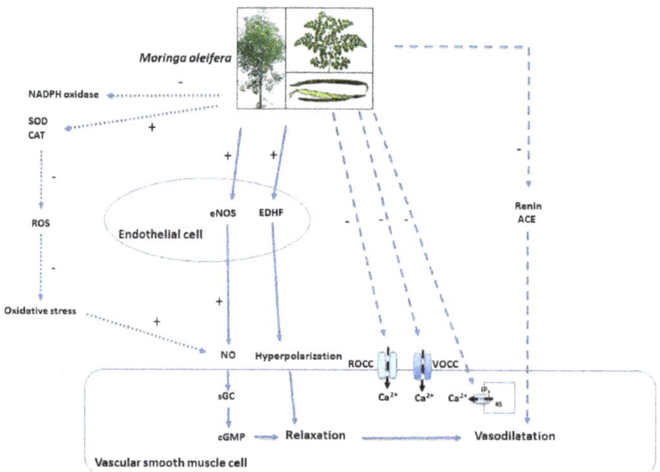

Figure 3. Overview of the mechanisms by which *Moringa oleifera* influences blood pressure. Abbreviation: eNOS, endothelial nitric oxide synthase; NO, nitric oxide; EDHF, endothelium-derived hyperpolarizing factors; sGC, soluble guanylate cyclase; cGMP, cyclic guanosine monophosphate; VOCCs, voltage-operated calcium channels; ROCCs, receptor-operated calcium channels; IP3, inositol trisphosphate, ACE, angiotensin-converting enzyme; SOD, superoxide dismutase; CAT, catalase; ROS, reactive oxygen species.

Oxidative stress impairs endothelial function by reducing NO bioavailability due to its reaction with superoxide anion (O_2^-), leading to the formation of peroxynitrite ($ONOO^-$), a potent oxidant that uncouples eNOS and inhibits its Akt-mediated activation [49,50]. A study demonstrated that treatment with *M. oleifera* leaf extract reduced O_2^- production and enhanced the activity of antioxidant enzymes, such as superoxide dismutase (SOD) and catalase (CAT), which neutralize free radicals [38]. Increased SOD activity was also confirmed in hypertensive rats treated with *M. oleifera* seed extract, which additionally reduced the expression of regulatory subunits of NADPH oxidase, an enzyme involved in ROS production [51]. These findings suggest that *M. oleifera* extract may reduce oxidative stress, thereby increasing NO availability. This, in turn, promotes the relaxation of VSMCs by activating soluble guanylate cyclase (sGC), leading to the production of cyclic guanosine monophosphate (cGMP), a key mediator of vasodilation [35].

Beyond NO-induced vasorelaxation, *M. oleifera* leaf extract also appears to induce vasodilation via EDHFs [52]. EDHFs act by opening potassium (K^+) channels in VSMCs, causing K^+ efflux and inducing membrane hyperpolarization. This hyperpolarization leads to the closure of voltage-operated calcium channels (VOCCs), reducing Ca^{2+} entry and consequently inhibiting VSMC contraction. Experimental evidence has shown that *M. oleifera* leaf extract induces dose-dependent relaxation even in arterial preparations pretreated with L-NAME and indomethacin, inhibitors of eNOS and cyclooxygenases (enzymes responsible for PGI2 synthesis), respectively. However, endothelium-dependent vasodilation was significantly reduced when contraction was induced using a high K^+ solution, a condition that inhibits EDHF-mediated responses [52]. This suggests that *M. oleifera* leaf extract induces vasodilation through a mechanism involving VSMC membrane hyperpolarization. The exact identity of EDHFs remains unclear, but a study suggested that hydrogen sulfide (H_2S) may be involved [53].

Nonendothelium-dependent mechanisms are physiological processes that regulate vascular function without directly involving the endothelium, but act directly on VSMCs. They primarily involve calcium homeostasis, ion channel activity, and neurogenic control of vascular function. The contractile state of VSMCs is governed by intracellular calcium (Ca^{2+}) levels, which are regulated by VOCCs, receptor-operated calcium channels (ROCCs), and intracellular calcium stores controlled by inositol trisphosphate (IP3) receptors. An increase in intracellular Ca^{2+} triggers vasoconstriction, whereas its reduction leads to relaxation. Another critical component of non-endothelium-dependent regulation is neurogenic control, particularly the adrenergic system, where sympathetic activation enhances vasoconstriction via α_1-adrenoceptor activation, whereas NO-containing nerves counteract this effect through axo-axonal inhibition of adrenergic signaling. *M. oleifera* leaf extract has been shown to exert direct effects on VSMCs via non-endothelium-dependent mechanisms [52]. Recent studies on hypertensive rat models have demonstrated that *M. oleifera* leaf extract reduces vascular tone by inhibiting extracellular Ca^{2+} influx and intracellular Ca^{2+} mobilization, leading to decreased contractility. Specifically, *M. oleifera* leaf extract blocks VOCCs and ROCCs, thereby limiting the Ca^{2+} entry required for contraction. Additionally, *M. oleifera* leaf extract modulates IP3-mediated calcium release from the sarcoplasmic reticulum, further attenuating intracellular Ca^{2+} accumulation. Notably, while some vasodilatory agents act by opening K^+ channels, the most recent findings indicate that MOE-mediated relaxation does not involve potassium channel activation, as evidenced by the fact that K^+ channel blockers did not alter its vasodilatory effect. Instead, *M. oleifera* leaf extract primarily functions as a calcium channel blocker, displaying a mechanism comparable to that of nifedipine, a well-characterized VOCC inhibitor [52]. Furthermore, in L-NAME-induced hypertension, *M. oleifera* leaf extract has been found to mitigate neurogenic vasoconstriction, likely through oxidative stress reduction, which may preserve NO availability from perivascular nerves and counteract sympathetic overactivation.

Another proposed mechanism to explain the blood pressure-lowering effects of *M. oleifera* is the inhibition of the renin–angiotensin–aldosterone system. Several studies have tested the ACE-inhibitory effect of different protein fractions and phenolic compounds [39,54]. One study [54] found that protein hydrolysates from *M. oleifera* leaves, obtained through enzymatic digestion with Alcalase, exhibit significant inhibitory activity against both angiotensin-converting enzyme (ACE) and renin, with maximum inhibition rates of 84.71% and 43.72%, respectively, for peptides with a molecular weight of <1 kDa. Two bioactive peptides, Leu-Gly-Phe-Phe (LGF) and Gly-Leu-Phe-Phe (GLFF), were isolated and characterized, showing IC_{50} values of 0.29 mM and 0.31 mM for ACE, along with concurrent renin inhibition. Their oral administration to spontaneously hypertensive rats led to a reduction in both systolic and diastolic blood pressure, with the most pronounced effect observed 6 h post-administration, suggesting their potential as natural antihypertensive agents. Another study [39] focused on the methanolic and ethyl acetate extracts of *M. oleifera* leaves, assessing their ability to inhibit ACE in vitro. The ethyl acetate extract demonstrated the highest inhibitory activity and was, therefore, subjected to biofractionation to identify the compound(s) responsible for its bioactivity. This process led to the isolation of two flavonoids, quercetin-3-O-glucoside and kaempferol-3-O-glucoside, which were identified using HPLC and NMR spectroscopy. Notably, quercetin-3-O-glucoside exhibited dose-dependent ACE inhibition, reaching 75.74% at 28 μg/mL. However, the bioactivity of kaempferol-3-O-glucoside could not be assessed due to its low yield.

These findings highlight that the hypotensive effects of *M. oleifera* appear to result from a combination of endothelium-dependent and independent mechanisms, primarily involving NO- and EDHF- mediated vasorelaxation, oxidative stress reduction, calcium channel blockade, and renin–angiotensin system inhibition. Experimental studies highlight its ability to enhance endothelial function, reduce vascular resistance, and modulate neurogenic and hormonal pathways involved in blood pressure regulation.

6. Compounds with Hypotensive Potential

The hypotensive properties of *Moringa oleifera* have been studied since the 1990s, with the isolation of various bioactive compounds from leaves and pods using ethanolic and aqueous extracts. The first study [55] isolated, through ethanolic extraction of fresh leaves, thiocarbamate glycosides, including niazinin A, niazinin B, niazimicin, and the mixture of niaziminin A and B. These compounds, purified via TLC and HPLC, exhibited dose-dependent hypotensive activity when injected into normotensive Wistar rats. At a dose of 1 mg/kg, all compounds reduced blood pressure by 14–22%, whereas at 3 mg/kg, the reduction ranged from 40% to 65%. A second study [56] expanded research on ethanolic leaf extracts, isolating an isothiocyanate, such as 4-[(4′-O-acetyl-α-L-rhamnosyloxy)benzyl]isothiocyanate, thiocarbamate glycosides, including niaziminin A, and niaziminin B, as well as two nitrile glycosides, niazirin and niazirinin. In vivo tests in normotensive Wistar rats confirmed that only (4-[(4′-O-acetyl-α-L-rhamnosyloxy)benzyl]isothiocyanate, niaziminin A, and niaziminin B) were active, reducing blood pressure by 15–20% at 1 mg/kg and by 35–40% at 3 mg/kg, whereas the nitriles (niazirin and niazirinin) showed no hypotensive effects up to 5 mg/kg. A third study [57] isolated, from ethanolic leaf extracts, two carbamate glycosides, including niazimin A, and niazimin B, and two thiocarbamate glycosides, including niazicin A and niazicin B. Following intravenous injection into normotensive Wistar rats, niazimin A, niazimin B, niazicin A, and niazicin B reduced blood pressure by 15–20% at a dose of 1 mg/kg, while at

3 mg/kg, the reduction was 35–40%. A fourth study [58] confirmed the role of thiocarbamate glycosides. O-methyl, 4-[(2′,3′,4′-tri-O-acetyl-α-L-rhamnosyloxy)benzyl]thiocarbamate, O-ethyl, 4-[(2′,3′,4′-tri-O-acetyl-α-L-rhamnosyloxy)benzyl]thiocarbamate, and niazimicin B were isolated from the ethanolic extract of *Moringa oleifera* leaves. After administration via the jugular vein in normotensive Wistar rats, all thiocarbamates reduced blood pressure by 10–20% at a dose of 1 mg/kg, while at 3 mg/kg, the reduction ranged from 30% to 40%. In parallel, research extended to the plant's pods and seeds. A further study [36] examined the hypotensive activity of ethanolic and aqueous pod extracts. The aqueous extract exhibited hypotensive effects at 30 mg/kg. Fractionation of the ethanolic extract led to the isolation of several hypotensive compounds. p-Hydroxybenzaldehyde showed the highest efficacy, reducing blood pressure by 40% at 3 mg/kg and by 75% at 10 mg/kg. Methyl p-hydroxybenzoate, at a dose of 10 mg/kg, caused a 47% reduction, while β-sitosterol, at 3 mg/kg, led to a 43% decrease. Tests further revealed that hypotensive activity was greater in seeds (43% at 30 mg/kg) than in the pericarp, which exhibited a biphasic response, whereas the pulp was inactive. A further study [59] confirmed significant hypotensive effects of niazinin A, niazinin B, niazimicin, and niaziminin A and B obtained from ethanolic extract of *M. oleifera* leaf. Intravenous administration of these compounds (1–10 mg/kg) in anesthetized rats induced a dose-dependent reduction in both systolic and diastolic blood pressure. To investigate the underlying mechanism, guinea pig atria were pretreated with atropine (1 mg/kg), which abolished the hypotensive response to acetylcholine but did not affect the response to the Moringa compounds, ruling out muscarinic receptor involvement. Additionally, a further in vitro experiment on rabbit aorta showed reductions in the contraction force and rate, while in isolated rabbit aorta preparations, the compounds inhibited K^+-induced contractions. These findings suggest that the hypotensive effect of these compounds is primarily due to a direct depressant action on cardiac and smooth muscle tissues.

More recent studies have investigated the hypotensive properties of the protein fraction [54] and certain phenolic compounds [39]. As previously described, specific peptides (LGF and GLFF) and a flavonoid glycoside (quercetin-3-O-glucoside) have shown ACE-inhibitory effects.

Finally, it is widely known that *M. oleifera* is a plant rich in bioactive compounds, including β-carotene, phenolic acids, flavonoids, and isothiocyanates, which confer significant antioxidant properties [6]. Several studies have demonstrated that *Moringa oleifera* leaf extract effectively reduces oxidative stress by neutralizing excessive ROS, which are responsible for cellular damage and chronic inflammation. This antioxidant capacity is particularly relevant for cardiovascular health, as oxidative stress plays a key role in the development of hypertension and other cardiovascular diseases.

These studies demonstrate that *M. oleifera* contains numerous hypotensive compounds, with thiocarbamates and isothiocyanates as the primary contributors to the effect. Additionally, certain phenols and sterols contribute to the hypotensive activity, although efficacy varies depending on the plant part and the type of extract used.

7. Limitations of Using *Moringa oleifera* as an Antihypertensive Therapy

M. oleifera possesses a potential antihypertensive effect. However, the use of *M. oleifera* as an alternative therapeutic for hypertension must consider several limitations. Several preclinical studies have suggested the hypotensive potential of *M. oleifera*. However, translating results from animal studies to humans is challenging. Differences in metabolism, cardiovascular regulation, and drug absorption among species can significantly impact how *M. oleifera* affects blood pressure in humans compared to animal models. Additionally, the doses used in animal studies may not be feasible or safe for human consumption. Most animal models of hypertension rely on induced conditions that may not fully represent the complexity of human hypertension, making it difficult to predict real-world clinical effects. Therefore, there is a need to demonstrate the hypotensive effects of *M. oleifera* in humans with appropriate clinical studies. Clinical evidence is currently quite limited, and the results of existing studies are conflicting and inconclusive. The studies conducted so far have primarily involved healthy individuals or patients with diabetes, rather than those with diagnosed hypertension. Some trials have indicated a mild reduction in blood pressure, particularly in subjects with high salt intake, while others have reported no significant effects. Given these inconsistencies, the current data do not allow for definitive conclusions about *M. oleifera* as an antihypertensive agent. Further well-designed, randomized controlled trials involving hypertensive individuals are necessary to clarify its efficacy and determine appropriate dosages. Furthermore, to ensure the safe and effective use of *Moringa oleifera*, it is essential to elucidate the mechanism(s) underlying its antihypertensive effects. Only a limited number of studies, primarily conducted by the same research groups, have addressed this topic. Therefore, the current knowledge requires further validation, preferably through independent studies, to confirm and expand upon the existing findings. Moreover, as described above, the pharmacological effect seems to be related to the numerous secondary metabolites present in the leaves, as well as in other parts of the plant. It is important to note that the concentrations of these molecules depend on numerous factors, such as the variety of the plant and the environmental growth conditions [60], making standardization of the product difficult. Therefore, unlike a drug with a standardized concentration, *M. oleifera* may exhibit variable concentrations of these bioactive components, potentially impacting its efficacy. Moreover, there is currently no consensus on the optimal dosage of Moringa required to achieve antihypertensive effects. As a food product, it is likely that a high intake of Moringa is necessary to achieve effects comparable to those of a pharmaceutical drug. However, high consumption may be impractical because Moringa can alter the sensory characteristics of foods [13], particularly their taste, which could limit individuals' willingness to consume it in sufficient quantities for a therapeutic effect. Additionally, high intake may cause gastrointestinal side effects [11], limiting its feasibility as a long-term therapy. This can be obviated by identifying the specific molecule(s) responsible for the hypotensive effect. While some studies—mostly outdated—have investigated this aspect, several important considerations must be taken into account. The effects of these molecules have primarily been evaluated using in vitro assays (e.g., enzyme or cell-based assays) or through intravenous administration, bypassing the issue of bioavailability. However, it is well established that secondary metabolites, such as polyphenols and isothiocyanates, exhibit low bioavailability when administered orally. Therefore, in addition to validating previous findings, future research should focus on evaluating the hypotensive potential of these compounds following oral administration to better reflect physiological conditions.

All these aspects currently limit the use of *M. oleifera* as a potential therapy for hypertension. Despite these challenges, smaller amounts of *M. oleifera* could be useful for hypertension prevention or as an adjunct to antihypertensive therapy. However, for this latter point, it is crucial to ensure that there are no interactions with medications, particularly antihypertensive drugs, and to confirm the absence of adverse effects on liver or kidney function. Studies in this area are almost entirely lacking, and therefore, caution is advised when considering *M. oleifera* as an antihypertensive therapy.

8. Conclusions and Future Directions

Preclinical studies support the hypotensive properties of *M. oleifera*. Animal studies suggest that various parts of *M. oleifera*, particularly its leaves, may contribute to blood pressure reduction through multiple mechanisms, including NO and EDHF modulation, calcium channel inhibition, and regulation of the renin–angiotensin–aldosterone system. These effects appear to be associated with the presence of thiocarbamates, isothiocyanates, flavonoids, peptides, and other secondary metabolites. However, findings from human studies are limited and inconsistent. Notably, there is a lack of randomized controlled trials specifically targeting hypertensive patients or assessing blood pressure as a primary outcome, which would be necessary to confirm preclinical results.

Further investigations are needed to elucidate the exact mechanisms of action and to identify the specific bioactive compounds responsible for the antihypertensive effects of *M. oleifera*. Given that human administration occurs orally, it is crucial to consider the bioavailability of these compounds, as this could significantly influence their efficacy. Moreover, determining the optimal dosage at which *M. oleifera* exerts its antihypertensive effects is essential to ensure both efficacy and safety. Additionally, for safe clinical use, potential interactions between *M. oleifera* and antihypertensive medications must be thoroughly examined. Addressing these critical aspects will be fundamental to defining the therapeutic potential of *M. oleifera* in hypertension management.

In conclusion, *Moringa oleifera* shows potential as a natural antihypertensive agent, but current evidence is insufficient to support its widespread use for this purpose. Further rigorous research is essential to validate its efficacy, ensure its safety, and establish standardized guidelines for its application in clinical settings.

Author Contributions: Conceptualization, A.L.; methodology, C.B., F.M. and A.L.; writing—original draft preparation, C.B., F.M., V.S., C.P., R.A. and A.L.; writing—review and editing, C.B. and A.L.; supervision, C.B. and A.L. All authors have read and agreed to the published version of the manuscript.

Funding: This research received no external funding.

Conflicts of Interest: The authors declare no conflicts of interest.

References

1. McEvoy, J.W.; McCarthy, C.P.; Bruno, R.M.; Brouwers, S.; Canavan, M.D.; Ceconi, C.; Christodorescu, R.M.; Daskalopoulou, S.S.; Ferro, C.J.; Gerdts, E.; et al. 2024 ESC Guidelines for the management of elevated blood pressure and hypertension: Developed by the task force on the management of elevated blood pressure and hypertension of the European Society of Cardiology (ESC) and endorsed by the European Society of Endocrinology (ESE) and the European Stroke Organisation (ESO). *Eur. Heart J.* **2024**, *45*, 3912–4018. [CrossRef] [PubMed]
2. Mills, K.T.; Stefanescu, A.; He, J. The global epidemiology of hypertension. *Nat. Rev. Nephrol.* **2020**, *16*, 223–237. [CrossRef]
3. NCD Risk Factor Collaboration (NCD-RisC). Worldwide trends in hypertension prevalence and progress in treatment and control from 1990 to 2019: A pooled analysis of 1201 population-representative studies with 104 million participants. *Lancet* **2021**, *398*, 957–980. [CrossRef]
4. Cuspidi, C.; Tadic, M.; Grassi, G.; Mancia, G. Treatment of hypertension: The ESH/ESC guidelines recommendations. *Pharmacol. Res.* **2018**, *128*, 315–321. [CrossRef]
5. Chow, C.K.; Teo, K.K.; Rangarajan, S.; Islam, S.; Gupta, R.; Avezum, A.; Bahonar, A.; Chifamba, J.; Dagenais, G.; Diaz, R.; et al. Prevalence, awareness, treatment, and control of hypertension in rural and urban communities in high-, middle-, and low-income countries. *JAMA* **2013**, *310*, 959–968. [CrossRef] [PubMed]
6. Leone, A.; Fiorillo, G.; Criscuoli, F.; Ravasenghi, S.; Santagostini, L.; Fico, G.; Spadafranca, A.; Battezzati, A.; Schiraldi, A.; Pozzi, F.; et al. Nutritional Characterization and Phenolic Profiling of *Moringa oleifera* Leaves Grown in Chad, Sahrawi Refugee Camps, and Haiti. *Int. J. Mol. Sci.* **2015**, *16*, 18923–18937. [CrossRef]
7. Leone, A.; Spada, A.; Battezzati, A.; Schiraldi, A.; Aristil, J.; Bertoli, S. *Moringa oleifera* Seeds and Oil: Characteristics and Uses for Human Health. *Int. J. Mol. Sci.* **2016**, *17*, 2141. [CrossRef]

8. Leone, A.; Spada, A.; Battezzati, A.; Schiraldi, A.; Aristil, J.; Bertoli, S. Cultivation, Genetic, Ethnopharmacology, Phytochemistry and Pharmacology of *Moringa oleifera* Leaves: An Overview. *Int. J. Mol. Sci.* **2015**, *16*, 12791–12835. [CrossRef]
9. Nova, E.; Redondo-Useros, N.; Martínez-García, R.M.; Gómez-Martínez, S.; Díaz-Prieto, L.E.; Marcos, A. Potential of *Moringa oleifera* to Improve Glucose Control for the Prevention of Diabetes and Related Metabolic Alterations: A Systematic Review of Animal and Human Studies. *Nutrients* **2020**, *12*, 2050. [CrossRef]
10. Brilhante, R.S.N.; Sales, J.A.; Pereira, V.S.; Castelo-Branco, D.S.C.M.; Cordeiro, R.A.; de Souza Sampaio, C.M.; de Araújo Neto Paiva, M.; Santos, J.B.F.D.; Sidrim, J.J.C.; Rocha, M.F.G. Research advances on the multiple uses of *Moringa oleifera*: A sustainable alternative for socially neglected population. *Asian Pac. J. Trop. Med.* **2017**, *10*, 621–630. [CrossRef]
11. Barichella, M.; Pezzoli, G.; Faierman, S.A.; Raspini, B.; Rimoldi, M.; Cassani, E.; Bertoli, S.; Battezzati, A.; Leone, A.; Iorio, L.; et al. Nutritional characterisation of Zambian *Moringa oleifera*: Acceptability and safety of short-term daily supplementation in a group of malnourished girls. *Int. J. Food Sci. Nutr.* **2019**, *70*, 107–115. [CrossRef] [PubMed]
12. Leone, A.; Di Lello, S.; Bertoli, S.; Ravasenghi, S.; De Amicis, R.; Menichetti, F.; Fico, G.; Santagostini, L.; Mohamed-Iahdih, B.; Mohamed Lamin Saleh, S.; et al. *Moringa oleifera* leaf powder enhances glycemic control in sahrawi women with type 2 diabetes: Findings from a 3-month unblinded randomized controlled trial. *PharmaNutrition* **2025**, *31*, 100434. [CrossRef]
13. Leone, A.; Bertoli, S.; Di Lello, S.; Bassoli, A.; Ravasenghi, S.; Borgonovo, G.; Forlani, F.; Battezzati, A. Effect of *Moringa oleifera* Leaf Powder on Postprandial Blood Glucose Response: In Vivo Study on Saharawi People Living in Refugee Camps. *Nutrients* **2018**, *10*, 1494. [CrossRef]
14. Arora, S. Nutritional significance and therapeutic potential of *Moringa oleifera*: The wonder plant. *J. Food Biochem.* **2021**, *45*, e13933. [CrossRef]
15. Matic, I.; Guidi, A.; Kenzo, M.; Mattei, M.; Galgani, A. Investigation of medicinal plants traditionally used as dietary supplements: A review on. *J. Public. Health Afr.* **2018**, *9*, 841. [CrossRef]
16. Anwar, F.; Latif, S.; Ashraf, M.; Gilani, A.H. *Moringa oleifera*: A food plant with multiple medicinal uses. *Phytother. Res.* **2007**, *21*, 17–25. [CrossRef]
17. Alia, F.; Putri, M.; Anggraeni, N.; Syamsunarno, M. The Potency of *Moringa oleifera* Lam. as Protective Agent in Cardiac Damage and Vascular Dysfunction. *Front. Pharmacol.* **2021**, *12*, 724439. [CrossRef]
18. Louisa, M.; Patintingan, C.G.H.; Wardhani, B.W.K. *Moringa oleifera* Lam. in Cardiometabolic Disorders: A Systematic Review of Recent Studies and Possible Mechanism of Actions. *Front. Pharmacol.* **2022**, *13*, 792794. [CrossRef]
19. Shahoud, J.S.; Sanvictores, T.; Aeddula, N.R. Physiology, Arterial Pressure Regulation. In *StatPearls*; StatPearls Publishing LLC.: Tampa, FL, USA, 2023.
20. Whelton, P.K.; Carey, R.M.; Aronow, W.S.; Casey, D.E., Jr.; Collins, K.J.; Dennison Himmelfarb, C.; DePalma, S.M.; Gidding, S.; Jamerson, K.A.; Jones, D.W.; et al. 2017 ACC/AHA/AAPA/ABC/ACPM/AGS/APhA/ASH/ASPC/NMA/PCNA Guideline for the Prevention, Detection, Evaluation, and Management of High Blood Pressure in Adults: A Report of the American College of Cardiology/American Heart Association Task Force on Clinical Practice Guidelines. *J. Am. Coll. Cardiol.* **2018**, *71*, e127–e248. [CrossRef]
21. Reboussin, D.M.; Allen, N.B.; Griswold, M.E.; Guallar, E.; Hong, Y.; Lackland, D.T.; Miller, E.P.R., 3rd; Polonsky, T.; Thompson-Paul, A.M.; Vupputuri, S. Systematic Review for the 2017 ACC/AHA/AAPA/ABC/ACPM/AGS/APhA/ASH/ASPC/NMA/PCNA Guideline for the Prevention, Detection, Evaluation, and Management of High Blood Pressure in Adults: A Report of the American College of Cardiology/American Heart Association Task Force on Clinical Practice Guidelines. *Circulation* **2018**, *138*, e595–e616. [CrossRef]
22. Aronow, W.S. Treatment of hypertensive emergencies. *Ann. Transl. Med.* **2017**, *5*, S5. [CrossRef] [PubMed]
23. Brzezinski, W.A. Blood Pressure. In *Clinical Methods: The History, Physical, and Laboratory Examinations*; Walker, H.K., Hall, W.D., Hurst, J.W., Eds.; Butterworth Publishers, a Division of Reed Publishing: Boston, MA, USA, 1990.
24. Sanders, J.S.; Mark, A.L.; Ferguson, D.W. Importance of aortic baroreflex in regulation of sympathetic responses during hypotension. Evidence from direct sympathetic nerve recordings in humans. *Circulation* **1989**, *79*, 83–92. [CrossRef] [PubMed]
25. Gelman, S. Venous function and central venous pressure: A physiologic story. *Anesthesiology* **2008**, *108*, 735–748. [CrossRef] [PubMed]
26. Malpas, S.C. What sets the long-term level of sympathetic nerve activity: Is there a role for arterial baroreceptors? *Am. J. Physiol. Regul. Integr. Comp. Physiol.* **2004**, *286*, R1–R12. [CrossRef]
27. Hall, J.E.; Hall, M.E. *Guyton and Hall Textobook of Medical Physiology*; Elsevier: Amsterdam, The Netherlands, 2020; Volume 14.
28. Bruce, M.; Koeppen, B.A.S. *Berne&Levy Fisiologia*; Casa Editrice Ambrosiana: Rozzano, Italy, 2018; Volume VII, p. 943.
29. McClure, J.M.; Rossi, N.F.; Chen, H.; O'Leary, D.S.; Scislo, T.J. Vasopressin is a major vasoconstrictor involved in hindlimb vascular responses to stimulation of adenosine A(1) receptors in the nucleus of the solitary tract. *Am. J. Physiol. Heart Circ. Physiol.* **2009**, *297*, H1661–H1672. [CrossRef]

30. Henderson, K.K.; Byron, K.L. Vasopressin-induced vasoconstriction: Two concentration-dependent signaling pathways. *J. Appl. Physiol.* **2007**, *102*, 1402–1409. [CrossRef]
31. Zhang, R.; Behbehani, K.; Crandall, C.G.; Zuckerman, J.H.; Levine, B.D. Dynamic regulation of heart rate during acute hypotension: New insight into baroreflex function. *Am. J. Physiol. Heart Circ. Physiol.* **2001**, *280*, H407–H419. [CrossRef]
32. Carretero, O.A.; Oparil, S. Essential hypertension. Part I: Definition and etiology. *Circulation* **2000**, *101*, 329–335. [CrossRef]
33. Oparil, S.; Zaman, M.A.; Calhoun, D.A. Pathogenesis of hypertension. *Ann. Intern. Med.* **2003**, *139*, 761–776. [CrossRef]
34. Abrogoua, D.P.; Dano, D.S.; Manda, P.; Adepo, A.J.; Kablan, B.J.; Goze, N.B.; Ehoulé, K. Effect on blood pressure of a dietary supplement containing traditional medicinal plants of Côte d'Ivoire. *J. Ethnopharmacol.* **2012**, *141*, 840–847. [CrossRef]
35. Aekthammarat, D.; Tangsucharit, P.; Pannangpetch, P.; Sriwantana, T.; Sibmooh, N. *Moringa oleifera* leaf extract enhances endothelial nitric oxide production leading to relaxation of resistance artery and lowering of arterial blood pressure. *Biomed. Pharmacother.* **2020**, *130*, 110605. [CrossRef]
36. Faizi, S.; Siddiqui, B.S.; Saleem, R.; Aftab, K.; Shaheen, F.; Gilani, A.H. Hypotensive constituents from the pods of *Moringa oleifera*. *Planta Med.* **1998**, *64*, 225–228. [CrossRef] [PubMed]
37. Attakpa, E.S.; Bertin, G.A.; Chabi, N.W.; Ategbo, J.M.; Seri, B.; Khan, N.A. *Moringa oleifera*-rich diet and T cell calcium signaling in spontaneously hypertensive rats. *Physiol. Res.* **2017**, *66*, 753–767. [CrossRef]
38. Aekthammarat, D.; Pannangpetch, P.; Tangsucharit, P. *Moringa oleifera* leaf extract lowers high blood pressure by alleviating vascular dysfunction and decreasing oxidative stress in L-NAME hypertensive rats. *Phytomedicine* **2019**, *54*, 9–16. [CrossRef]
39. Acuram, L.K.; Chichioco Hernandez, C.L. Anti-hypertensive effect of *Moringa oleifera* Lam. *Cogent Biol.* **2019**, *5*, 1596526. [CrossRef]
40. Chen, K.H.; Chen, Y.J.; Yang, C.H.; Liu, K.W.; Chang, J.L.; Pan, S.F.; Lin, T.B.; Chen, M.J. Attenuation of the extract from *Moringa oleifera* on monocrotaline-induced pulmonary hypertension in rats. *Chin. J. Physiol.* **2012**, *55*, 22–30. [CrossRef]
41. Randriamboavonjy, J.I.; Loirand, G.; Vaillant, N.; Lauzier, B.; Derbré, S.; Michalet, S.; Pacaud, P.; Tesse, A. Cardiac Protective Effects of *Moringa oleifera* Seeds in Spontaneous Hypertensive Rats. *Am. J. Hypertens.* **2016**, *29*, 873–881. [CrossRef]
42. Chan Sun, M.; Ruhomally, Z.B.; Boojhawon, R.; Neergheen-Bhujun, V.S. Consumption of *Moringa oleifera* Lam Leaves Lowers Postprandial Blood Pressure. *J. Am. Coll. Nutr.* **2020**, *39*, 54–62. [CrossRef]
43. Afiaenyi, C.I.; Ngwu, K.E.; Okafor, M.A.; Ayogu, R.N. Effects of *Moringa oleifera* leaves on the blood glucose, blood pressure, and lipid profile of type 2 diabetic subjects: A parallel group randomized clinical trial of efficacy. *Nutr. Health* **2025**, *31*, 281–291. [CrossRef]
44. Bantle, J.P.; Wylie-Rosett, J.; Albright, A.L.; Apovian, C.M.; Clark, N.G.; Franz, M.J.; Hoogwerf, B.J.; Lichtenstein, A.H.; Mayer-Davis, E.; Mooradian, A.D.; et al. Nutrition recommendations and interventions for diabetes: A position statement of the American Diabetes Association. *Diabetes Care* **2008**, *31* (Suppl. S1), S61–S78. [CrossRef]
45. Taweerutchana, R.; Lumlerdkij, N.; Vannasaeng, S.; Akarasereenont, P.; Sriwijitkamol, A. Effect of *Moringa oleifera* Leaf Capsules on Glycemic Control in Therapy-Naïve Type 2 Diabetes Patients: A Randomized Placebo Controlled Study. *Evid. Based Complement. Altern. Med.* **2017**, *2017*, 6581390. [CrossRef]
46. Díaz-Prieto, L.E.; Gómez-Martínez, S.; Vicente-Castro, I.; Heredia, C.; González-Romero, E.A.; Martín-Ridaura, M.D.C.; Ceinos, M.; Picón, M.J.; Marcos, A.; Nova, E. Effects of *Moringa oleifera* Lam. Supplementation on Inflammatory and Cardiometabolic Markers in Subjects with Prediabetes. *Nutrients* **2022**, *14*, 1937. [CrossRef] [PubMed]
47. Loh, Y.C.; Tan, C.S.; Ch'ng, Y.S.; Yeap, Z.Q.; Ng, C.H.; Yam, M.F. Overview of the Microenvironment of Vasculature in Vascular Tone Regulation. *Int. J. Mol. Sci.* **2018**, *19*, 120. [CrossRef]
48. Randriamboavonjy, J.I.; Heurtebise, S.; Pacaud, P.; Loirand, G.; Tesse, A. *Moringa oleifera* seeds Improve Aging-Related Endothelial Dysfunction in Wistar Rats. *Oxid. Med. Cell. Longev.* **2019**, *2019*, 2567198. [CrossRef] [PubMed]
49. Kukongviriyapan, U.; Kukongviriyapan, V.; Pannangpetch, P.; Donpunha, W.; Sripui, J.; Sae-Eaw, A.; Boonla, O. Mamao Pomace Extract Alleviates Hypertension and Oxidative Stress in Nitric Oxide Deficient Rats. *Nutrients* **2015**, *7*, 6179–6194. [CrossRef] [PubMed]
50. Xu, J.; Zou, M.H. Molecular insights and therapeutic targets for diabetic endothelial dysfunction. *Circulation* **2009**, *120*, 1266–1286. [CrossRef]
51. Randriamboavonjy, J.I.; Rio, M.; Pacaud, P.; Loirand, G.; Tesse, A. *Moringa oleifera* seeds Attenuate Vascular Oxidative and Nitrosative Stresses in Spontaneously Hypertensive Rats. *Oxid. Med. Cell. Longev.* **2017**, *2017*, 4129459. [CrossRef]
52. Aekthammarat, D.; Pannangpetch, P.; Tangsucharit, P. *Moringa oleifera* leaf extract induces vasorelaxation via endothelium-dependent hyperpolarization and calcium channel blockade in mesenteric arterial beds isolated from L-NAME hypertensive rats. *Clin. Exp. Hypertens.* **2020**, *42*, 490–501. [CrossRef]

53. Aekthammarat, D.; Tangsucharit, P.; Pannangpetch, P. Hydrogen sulfide as a mediator of endothelium-dependent relaxation evoked by *Moringa oleifera* leaf extract in mesenteric arterial beds isolated from L-NAME hypertensive rats. *J. Complement. Integr. Med.* **2020**, *18*, 287–293. [CrossRef]
54. Ma, K.; Wang, Y.; Wang, M.; Wang, Z.; Wang, X.; Ju, X.; He, R. Antihypertensive activity of the ACE–renin inhibitory peptide derived from *Moringa oleifera* protein. *Food Funct.* **2021**, *12*, 8994–9006. [CrossRef]
55. Faizi, S.; Siddiqui, B.S.; Saleem, R.; Siddiqui, S.; Aftab, K.; Gilani, A.-u.-H. Isolation and structure elucidation of novel hypotensive agents, niazinin A, niazinin B, niazimicin and niaziminin A + B from *Moringa oleifera*: The first naturally occurring thiocarbamates. *J. Chem. Soc. Perkin Trans.* **1992**, *1*, 3237–3241. [CrossRef]
56. Faizi, S.; Siddiqui, B.S.; Saleem, R.; Siddiqui, S.; Aftab, K.; Gilani, A.H. Isolation and structure elucidation of new nitrile and mustard oil glycosides from *Moringa oleifera* and their effect on blood pressure. *J. Nat. Prod.* **1994**, *57*, 1256–1261. [CrossRef] [PubMed]
57. Faizi, S.; Siddiqui, B.S.; Saleem, R.; Siddiqui, S.; Aftab, K.; Gilani, A.-u.-H. Novel hypotensive agents, niazimin A, niazimin B, Niazicin A and Niazicin B from *Moringa oleifera*: Isolation of first naturally occurring carbamates. *J. Chem. Soc. Perkin Trans.* **1994**, *1*, 3035–3040. [CrossRef]
58. Faizi, S.; Siddiqui, B.S.; Saleem, R.; Siddiqui, S.; Aftab, K.; Gilani, A.H. Fully acetylated carbamate and hypotensive thiocarbamate glycosides from *Moringa oleifera*. *Phytochemistry* **1995**, *38*, 957–963. [CrossRef]
59. Gilani, A.H.; Aftab, K.; Suria, A.; Siddiqui, S.; Salem, R.; Siddiqui, B.S.; Faizi, S. Pharmacological studies on hypotensive and spasmolytic activities of pure compounds from *Moringa oleifera*. *Phytother. Res.* **1994**, *8*, 87–91. [CrossRef]
60. Foster, M.C.; Hwang, S.J.; Massaro, J.M.; Hoffmann, U.; DeBoer, I.H.; Robins, S.J.; Vasan, R.S.; Fox, C.S. Association of subcutaneous and visceral adiposity with albuminuria: The Framingham Heart Study. *Obesity* **2011**, *19*, 1284–1289. [CrossRef]

nutrients MDPI

Review

A Narrative Review of Quercetin's Role as a Bioactive Compound in Female Reproductive Disorders

Yasaman Khamineh [1], Mahsa Ghiasvand [1,2], Sanaz Panahi-Alanagh [3], Parisa Rastegarmand [4], Samaneh Zolghadri [5,*] and Agata Stanek [6,*]

1 Department of Animal Sciences and Marine Biology, Faculty of Life Sciences and Biotechnology, Shahid Beheshti University, Tehran 1983969411, Iran; yasaman.khamine@gmail.com (Y.K.); mahsaghiasvandd1998m@gmail.com (M.G.)
2 Department of Stem Cells and Developmental Biology, Cell Science Research Centre, Royan Institute for Stem Cell Biology and Technology, Academic Center for Education, Culture and Research (ACECR), Tehran 3365166571, Iran
3 Department of Plant and Animal Biology, Faculty of Biological Science and Technology, University of Isfahan, Isfahan 817467344, Iran; sanazpanahialanagh@gmail.com
4 Department of Microbiology, College of Science, Shiraz Branch, Islamic Azad University, Shiraz 1477893780, Iran; p.rastegar1991@gmail.com
5 Department of Biology, Jahrom Branch, Islamic Azad University, Jahrom 7414785318, Iran
6 Department of Internal Medicine, Metabolic Diseases and Angiology, Faculty of Health Sciences in Katowice, Medical University of Silesia, Ziolowa 45/47 St., 40-635 Katowice, Poland
* Correspondence: z.jahromi@ut.ac.ir (S.Z.); astanek@tlen.pl (A.S.); Tel.: +98-715437200 (S.Z.); +48-604119099 (A.S.)

Abstract: Lifestyle, nutrition, and metabolic status are central to maintaining women's reproductive health. With the rising prevalence of infertility, the need for effective strategies to preserve and enhance women's reproductive well-being has become increasingly urgent. Quercetin, a plant-derived polyphenol, has attracted growing interest for its potential to support reproductive health, regulate the hormonal balance, and improve fertility. This narrative review examines Quercetin's role in women's reproductive health and delineates its possible mechanisms of action in female reproductive system disorders, including polycystic ovary syndrome, recurrent miscarriage, and cervical, ovarian, and endometrial cancer (EC). By highlighting the biological pathways through which quercetin may exert its effects, this article underscores the need for further research and clinical trials to validate its therapeutic potential and its applications as a bioactive compound in foods aimed at enhancing women's reproductive health.

Keywords: female reproductive disorders; quercetin; polycystic ovary syndrome; gynecological cancers; pregnancy loss

1. Introduction

Concerns regarding female fertility and long-term reproductive health have escalated in response to the increasing prevalence of conditions such as polycystic ovary syndrome (PCOS) [1], various gynecological cancers [2], and pregnancy challenges such as recurrent miscarriages [3]. A substantial body of epidemiological and clinical evidence suggests that plant-based diets can reduce the risk of chronic diseases, including cancer [4,5]. Bioactive compounds derived from natural sources have garnered attention for their potential to address these multifactorial challenges. Among these bioactive compounds, Quercetin

[2-(3,4-dihydroxyphenyl)-3,5,7-trihydroxy-4-Hchromen-4-one] is a widely consumed dietary flavonoid present in a variety of foods, including fruits, green leafy vegetables, seeds, buckwheat, nuts, flowers, barks, broccoli, olive oil, apples, onions, green tea, red grapes, red wine, dark cherries, and berries like blueberries and cranberries [6]. In addition, numerous studies have shown that Quercetin, when taken in acceptable amounts, may provide beneficial biological effects, including antioxidant, anticancer, and anti-inflammatory properties [7]. By scavenging reactive oxygen species (ROS) and reducing inflammation, Quercetin could enhance the health of reproductive tissues and lower the risk of related conditions [8]. Moreover, Quercetin has shown promise in balancing hormones and reducing excess androgens [9]. Additionally, by mitigating inflammation and potentially improving how the body uses insulin, Quercetin could help regularize women's periods [10].

Quercetin also has the potential to affect various pathological processes associated through multiple targets and pathways [11], making it a promising candidate for addressing these health issues. Quercetin decreases apoptosis by blocking Akt/PKB phosphorylation, minimizing mitochondrial cyst release, and downregulating Cu–Zn peroxidase dismutase to suppress the ROS reaction [12]. Similarly, it was observed that Quercetin protects primordial follicles in mice by inhibiting the activation of the PI3K/Akt/FOXO3a pathway [13]. Recently, researchers are boosting Quercetin's efficacy through encapsulation, combining it with antioxidants, or selectively breeding specific fruits and vegetables offers the potential to naturally increase the Quercetin content, allowing for the development of tailored, Quercetin-rich foods for specific health benefits [9,10,14].

Despite the existing studies on the benefits of quercetin, there remains a significant gap in the literature regarding a comprehensive review specifically focused on its effects on the female reproductive system. In this narrative review, we will explore a diverse array of research on Quercetin, a bioactive compound derived from plants, and its effects on female reproductive health issues, including PCOS, pregnancy loss, and gynecological cancers. Additionally, we will examine the potential of Quercetin-based functional foods as an innovative and accessible strategy to enhance women's reproductive health. Our review will include an analysis of in vitro/vivo studies, and clinical trial research, along with insights into the origin, metabolism, and pharmacokinetics properties of Quercetin.

2. Methods

This narrative review conducted a literature search across four principal scientific databases: PubMed, ScienceDirect, Google Scholar, and Web of Science, focusing on relevant studies up to 2025. The search strategy utilized to identify applicable articles was as follows: (((("plant-based diet") OR ("polyphenol")) OR ("quercetin-based foods")) OR ("quercetin")) AND ((((((((((("polycystic ovary syndrome") OR ("PCOS")) OR ("pregnancy")) OR ("pregnancy loss")) OR ("miscarriage")) OR ("gynecological cancer")) OR ("cervical cancer")) OR ("ovarian cancer")) OR ("endometrial cancer")) OR ("anticancer")) OR ("antioxidant")) OR ("anti-inflammatory")). All abstracts generated from this search were screened to pinpoint relevant studies. Moreover, a manual search was performed to answer secondary research questions. The inclusion criteria encompassed original research articles, in vitro and in vivo studies, clinical trials, and narrative or systematic reviews that investigated quercetin's mechanisms of action and its therapeutic potential in female reproductive health. Studies were excluded if they did not correlate with reproductive function, failed to examine mechanistic pathways, or centered on compounds unrelated to quercetin.

3. Effect of Quercetin on Pregnancy and Miscarriage

Recent multinational research has indicated a growing prevalence of herbal medicine use during pregnancy [15]. However, this trend raises concerns, as many women lack sufficient awareness of the phytochemical properties of these products, leading to improper usage, and, consequently, they may inadvertently jeopardize their health and that of their unborn children [16]. Spontaneous pregnancy loss prior to viability, commonly referred to as miscarriage, represents a significant challenge in reproductive health. The absence of a universally standardized definition for this condition complicates the precise assessment of its prevalence, with reported rates varying between 1% and 5% [17]. Recurrent pregnancy loss (RPL), defined as the occurrence of multiple consecutive miscarriages, is estimated to affect 2% to 5% of couples, often resulting in profound emotional distress and disrupting family planning endeavors. Etiological factors associated with RPL include chromosomal anomalies, defective placentation, thrombotic disorders, and unfavorable uterine conditions [18–20]. Among these, oxidative stress has been identified as a critical factor in early pregnancy failure. Evidence suggests that premature and disorganized maternal blood flow to the placenta is associated with elevated oxidative damage in placental tissues, further contributing to pregnancy loss [21], and disruptions in the equilibrium between oxidative stress and inflammatory processes have been implicated in the pathogenesis of these pregnancy-related immune disorders [22]. Oxidative stress (OS) has been shown to impair placental function and disrupt fetal development through multiple mechanisms. These include the dysregulation of critical nutrient transporters, such as Slc2a1 and Slc38a1, as well as the induction of cellular apoptosis [23–25]. Such disruptions can lead to severe pregnancy complications, including embryonic resorption, recurrent pregnancy loss, intrauterine growth restriction (IUGR), and fetal demise [26]. In women with recurrent abortions, the increased generation of radical species by leukocytes was demonstrated via increased granulocyte spontaneous chemiluminescence [27]. Studies have shown that Quercetin plays a vital role in reducing oxidative stress during trophoblast syncytialization, a critical process in placental development [28]. Disruptions in syncytialization, often caused by oxidative stress and mitochondrial dysfunction, are implicated in pregnancy-related complications, including hypertensive disorders of pregnancy (HDP). In HDP-affected placentas, mitochondrial dysfunction results in reactive oxygen species (ROS) overproduction, which further impairs syncytialization [29,30]. Recent studies have demonstrated that Quercetin treatment (5 μM) for 48 h facilitates trophoblast fusion by upregulating syncytialization markers and enhancing mitochondrial fusion and mitophagy, as evidenced by immunofluorescence analysis. Although cell fusion inherently generates ROS, Quercetin effectively counteracts oxidative stress by regulating key antioxidant pathways, thereby supporting placental health and function [28]. In vitro studies conducted by Wang et al. revealed that 1 μM, 5 μM, and 10 μM of Quercetin have the potential to reduce the incidence of spontaneous abortion (SA) by modulating inflammatory responses and apoptotic pathways in HTR-8/SVneo cells exposed to lipopolysaccharide (LPS). Inflammatory responses, especially those triggered by LPS-induced immune activation, are widely acknowledged as a significant cause of preterm birth. Emerging evidence indicates that Quercetin, a naturally occurring polyphenol, may offer protective benefits against preterm labor by inhibiting inflammatory pathways and improving fetal survival rates [30]. Several studies have also investigated the effects of Quercetin on pregnancy and miscarriage in vivo. Wu et al. conducted a study using an LPS-induced SA mouse model, revealing that gavaging with low-dose Quercetin (0.25 mg/mL) has the potential to decrease embryo loss rates and moderately increase the average embryo weight. The researchers highlighted that Quercetin may promote the expulsion or resorption of non-viable embryos post-miscarriage and support the uterus in returning to its pre-pregnancy condition [31]. In a murine model of LPS-induced preterm labor, the administration of Quercetin at a dose of 90 mg/kg via oral gavage significantly reduced the incidence of preterm labor by 63.5% and improved the neonatal survival rates to 83.76% [32]. Mechanistically, Quercetin achieved these protective effects by inhibiting the activation of Nuclear Factor Kappa B (NF-κB) and Activator protein 1 (AP-1), two critical transcription factors involved in mediating inflammatory responses. The study revealed that Quercetin downregulated the expression of NF-κB/P65, AP-1/C-JUN, Cyclooxygenase-2/Prostaglandin-Endoperoxide Synthase 2 (COX-2/PTGS2), and Interleukin 6 (IL-6) at both the mRNA and protein levels in the myometrium. This suppression of inflammatory pathways contributed to reduced uterine inflammation and played a key role in preventing the onset of preterm labor [33]. Liu et al. investigated the mechanisms underlying Quercetin's protective effects using a pregnant mouse model exposed to PM2.5. Their research demonstrated that gavaged Quercetin (100 mg/kg) effectively prevents miscarriage by suppressing the expression of pro-inflammatory cytokines, such as IL-6 and Interleukin 8 (IL-8), while upregulating the levels of Heme Oxygenase-1 (HO-1) in peripheral blood [34]. Network pharmacology and UPLC-Q/TOF-MS analyses identified Quercetin as a key active component in BYLY, highlighting its potential role in enhancing pregnancy viability. In in vitro trophoblast models, Quercetin (2 μM) was shown to counteract hypoxia-induced apoptosis, mitochondrial dysfunction, and impaired cell proliferation, all of which are critical factors in recurrent spontaneous abortion [35] pathology [36]. Further mechanistic studies have revealed that Quercetin regulates the balance between mitochondrial fission and fusion by downregulating Drp1 expression through miR-34a-5p modulation, thereby supporting placental cell survival and function [37]. Notably, Quercetin's potential benefits have been explored in clinical trials. A recent clinical trial involving 480 patients with recurrent SA demonstrated that a quadri-combination therapy (BYLY: Bushen, Yiqi, Lixue, Yangtai) significantly lowered early miscarriage rates when it used alongside duphaston, outperforming either treatment administered alone [36]. Despite the limited number of human clinical studies, these findings highlight Quercetin's diverse roles in modulating immune responses, hormonal balance, and cellular processes. However, some studies have reported inconsistent results, indicating that Quercetin may also lead to side effects. For instance, doses of 50 μM of Quercetin were found to impair embryonic development in mice, causing a 20–30% reduction in morula and blastocyst formation rates [38]. Moreover, offspring of mice that were exposed to Quercetin (302 mg/kg feed) during pregnancy displayed a 40% increase in hepatic iron storage in adulthood, which was associated with alterations in cytokine expression levels, specifically IL-1β, IL-6, and IL-10 [38]. This prenatal exposure also induced hypermethylation of repetitive DNA elements, which may have implications for long-term gene expression modifications [39].

Thus, while the effects of Quercetin may vary depending on dosage and physiological context, these findings underscore the importance of conducting large-scale clinical trials in humans to further investigate its potential role in addressing recurrent spontaneous abortion and improving pregnancy outcomes.

4. Effect of Quercetin on Polycystic Ovary Syndrome

The ovarian microenvironment is essential for maintaining normal ovarian function and promoting female fertility [40]. Disruptions within this environment, as seen in PCOS, can have significant consequences. PCOS is a prevalent and complex endocrine disorder affecting approximately 5–20% of women of reproductive age, with the precise prevalence varying based on diagnostic criteria and the population studied [40,41]. It is a leading cause of anovulatory infertility, accounting for approximately 80% of cases [41] and is frequently associated with metabolic conditions such as insulin resistance (IR), obesity, and an increased risk of type 2 diabetes and cardiovascular disease [42–44]. PCOS is marked by a complex interplay of reproductive hormone imbalances. A hallmark of the condition is an elevated luteinizing hormone (LH)-to-follicle-stimulating hormone ratio [45]. In women with PCOS, the follicle-stimulating hormone [45] levels tend to be low to normal compared to those in normally cycling women during the early follicular phase of the menstrual cycle and lack the typical cyclic fluctuations necessary for ovulation. This hormonal dysregulation contributes to the development of enlarged, polycystic ovaries and clinical manifestations, including menstrual irregularities, infertility, and hirsutism [46]. Emerging evidence highlights the significant roles of inflammation and oxidative stress in PCOS pathophysiology. Oxidative stress and inflammation in PCOS operate within a self-perpetuating cycle. Specifically, oxidative stress can induce inflammation through the activation of NF-κB, a key transcription factor that promotes the expression of inflammatory cytokines such as Tumor Necrosis Factor-alpha (TNF-α) and IL-6 [47,48]. Inflammation, in turn, can amplify oxidative stress by enhancing ROS production [48]. This reciprocal interplay exacerbates IR and hyperandrogenemia, both of which are central to PCOS pathophysiology [48,49]. Furthermore, PCOS development is often linked to disruptions in key signaling pathways like Phosphoinositide 3 Kinase/Akt (PI3K/Akt), Transforming Growth Factor β/Suppressor of Mothers against Decapentaplegic (TGF-β/Smads), Wnt/β-catenin, and Hippo/YAP, which play a significant role in the disease's progression [50]. Since, there is no standardized treatment for PCOS [41]. Clinical management focuses on personalized medication tailored to individual symptoms, particularly hormonal treatments. However, these therapies frequently have common side effects. For example, anti-estrogen medications, such as clomiphene citrate, are frequently used as the first-line treatment for anovulatory infertility in women with PCOS. It is important to note that obese women with PCOS may experience reduced effectiveness and lower pregnancy rates when using these medications to induce ovulation [51]. Therefore, it is evident that current treatment options primarily address specific aspects of PCOS, and they come with notable limitations. Given Quercetin's anti-inflammatory and antioxidant effects, it has been widely studied as a possible PCOS treatment [6].

In vitro studies suggest that Quercetin protects granulosa cells from oxidative stress and apoptosis induced by various stressors. Quercetin treatment also reduced ROS levels and increased antioxidant and anti-apoptotic protein expression in ovary cells [52]. For instance, in hydrogen peroxide-induced oxidative stress in bovine granulosa cells, 10 uM of granulosa decreased the ROS levels, while it increased NF-E2-related factor 2 (Nrf2), thereby repairing cell damage [53]. Adding 2 ug/mL Quercetin to the maturation media enhanced the bovine oocytes' quality and protected them from early apoptosis. The Quercetin-enriched media also strengthened cumulus cells, reducing their apoptosis and significantly increasing oocyte survival, with the upregulation of Octamer binding Transcription Factor 4 (OCT-4) and the receptors for the Insulin-like Growth Factor (IGF2R) and B-cell Lymphoma-2 (Bcl-2) proteins [54]. Several studies have also investigated Quercetin's effects on PCOS in vivo. Wang et al. found that 2 mL of Quercetin (100 mg/kg) lowered the levels of inflammatory cytokines such as Interleukin-1 beta (IL-1β), IL-6, and TNFα, decreased NF-κB activation (including the nuclear translocation of NF-κBp65), and significantly reduced the phosphorylation of Insulin Receptor Substrate-1 (IRS-1) tyrosine in Dehydroepiandrosterone (DHEA)-induced PCOS in female Wistar rats. These results suggest Quercetin's mechanism of action involves inhibiting the TLR/NF-κB signaling pathway, thereby improving the ovarian inflammatory microenvironment in PCOS [55]. Another study showed that the levels of the antioxidant enzymes Superoxide Dismutase

(SOD), catalase, Glutathione S Transferase (GST), and reduced glutathione were significantly lower in PCOS rats. However, 100 mg/kg BW Quercetin significantly increased the levels of these enzymes in DHEA-induced PCOS in Wistar rats [56]. Quercetin treatment (30 mg/kg) in letrozole-induced PCOS in female Sprague Dawley (SD) rats led to a notable reduction in both the ovarian and cystic follicle diameters. Additionally, Quercetin demonstrated strong antioxidant properties, contributing to the recovery of ovarian cysts and promoting the health of follicles. Quercetin markedly regulated steroidogenesis, decreasing the testosterone and estradiol levels and increasing the progesterone levels [57]. In DHEA-induced PCOS rat models, oral administration with Quercetin (25 mg/kg) improved ovarian follicle development (increased preantral, antral, and preovulatory follicles and corpora lutea) and reduced follicular atresia and cyst formation, and modulated apoptosis markers (Bax and Bcl-2) in the ovaries. Additionally, Quercetin lowered the serum free testosterone and the LH/FSH ratio, mirroring the effects of metformin [58]. Shah et al. demonstrated that 125 mg/kg Quercetin in letrozole-induced PCOS Parkes strain mice models effectively normalized the elevated LH/FSH ratios and boosted estrogen levels. Notably, the study revealed that Quercetin played a vital role in preserving ovarian follicles by promoting the corpus luteum regeneration and eliminating cystic follicles, which ultimately helped reset the estrous cycle [59]. In a study using a DHEA-induced PCOS rat model, gavage daily administration of 2 mL of a quercetin solution (100 mg/kg) reduced serum testosterone, estradiol, LH, and the LH/FSH ratio, while it increased serum FSH. These effects were similar to those observed in a separate study using metformin in a similar DHEA-induced PCOS rat model [60]. Another study found that a Quercetin-rich extract from bitter melon could act as an insulin sensitizer and enhance ovulation, potentially aiding in the management of letrozole-induced PCOS in Swiss albino female rats. The hormonal analysis showed significant reductions in the LH, insulin, and testosterone levels in the treatment groups, along with improved FSH levels [61]. Hyperglycemia a common comorbidity of PCOS, primarily driven by insulin resistance. Research also indicates that bitter melon may possess hypoglycemic properties [62]. In a letrozole-induced PCOS rat model, *Fagonia indica* extract, rich in quercetin, improved PCOS symptoms. This plant extract reduced body weight, ovarian cysts, and improved follicular growth. Furthermore, it restored hormonal balance, lipid profiles, liver function markers, and increased antioxidant enzyme levels [63].

Most research on Quercetin's effects utilizes animal models; however, there are few studies involving human patients with PCOS. This is significant considering that adiponectin levels are often reduced in individuals with PCOS. In this regard, Rezvan et al. Showed the effects of oral Quercetin supplementation in women with PCOS. Quercetin was effective on insulin sensitivity and hormone levels in women with PCOS. Compared to a placebo group, 1 g daily Quercetin supplementation slightly increased the total and high-molecular-weight adiponectin levels, significantly reduced the testosterone and LH levels, and also lowered insulin resistance (HOMA-IR) levels [64]. A randomized, double-blind, placebo-controlled trial investigated the effects of 1000 mg/day quercetin supplementation were investigated in overweight and obese women with PCOS. The study found that quercetin significantly reduced plasma resistin concentrations, mRNA levels, testosterone, and LH levels compared to the placebo group. Although fasting blood glucose, insulin, and HOMA-IR levels were decreased in the quercetin group, these changes were not statistically significant compared to the placebo [65]. Vaez et al. also found that Quercetin (500 mg) reduced inflammatory markers and LH levels in women with PCOS, while also improving the oocyte and embryo quality and increasing pregnancy rates [66]. In a study, researchers used network pharmacology and molecular docking to examine the mechanisms of BUSHEN HUATAN (BHHD), a Chinese medicine which consists of eight different herbs for treating PCOS patients. They found that it may improve insulin resistance and hormonal imbalances through various components and pathways, with Quercetin identified as a key component in its effectiveness [67]. Moreover, Yi-Jing Decoction (YJD), a traditional Chinese medicine, has been utilized for patients with PCOS. Research has identified quercetin as one of its potentially beneficial constituents. The findings suggest that YJD may treat PCOS by regulating levels of androgens and insulin, as well as by reducing inflammation. These effects are thought to result from interactions with key genes that are implicated in the pathogenesis of PCOS [68]. Notably, studies found no serious adverse events, reporting only mild gastrointestinal discomfort [69]. While these trials provided valuable insights into the therapeutic role of quercetin, they did not comprehensively assess broader clinical outcomes [6].

Collectively, Quercetin shows promise as a PCOS treatment due to its antioxidant and anti-inflammatory properties, supported by positive in vitro and animal studies. However, larger clinical trials are needed to confirm its efficacy and optimal dosage (Figure 1).

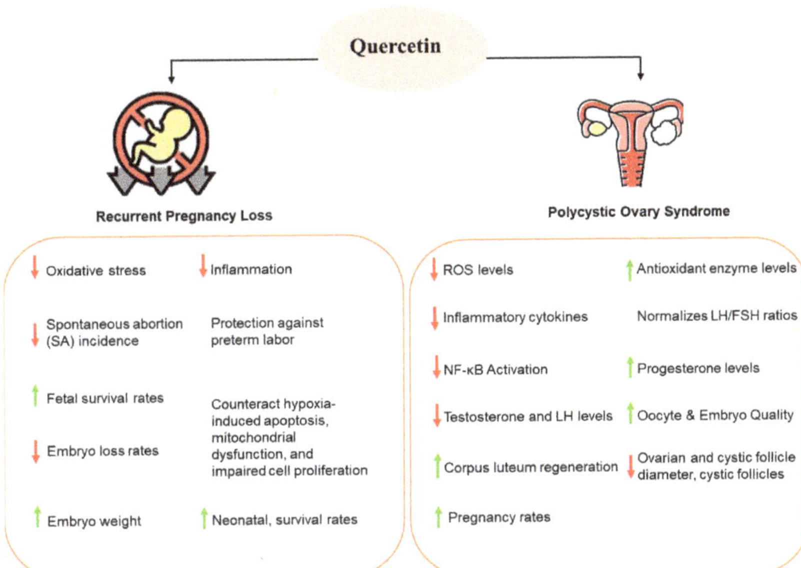

Figure 1. Effect of Quercetin on PCOS and pregnancy loss: potential mechanisms by which Quercetin alleviates PCOS symptoms and improves pregnancy outcomes.

5. Effect of Quercetin on Gynecological Cancers

Gynecological cancers including ovarian, endometrial, and cervical cancers pose a major global health challenge for women [70,71]. Despite advances in conventional treatments such as surgery, radiotherapy, and chemotherapy, these approaches often suffer from significant side effects and variable efficacy among patients [72,73]. This has driven growing interest in the potential of dietary interventions, particularly functional foods rich in plant bioactive compounds, to complement standard cancer therapies. Epidemiological studies have linked dietary patterns high in plant-based compounds to a reduced risk of various cancers [74,75]. As Quercetin has garnered significant interest for its potent anticancer properties, the following sections explore its effects on ovarian, cervical, and endometrial cancer. A summary of these effects is presented in Table 1.

Table 1. Quercetin's effect on gynecological cancers.

Cancer Type	Sample/Model	Effect of Quercetin	Study Type	References
Cervical	HeLa, SiHa cells	↓ cell viability (dose-dependent), G2/M arrest, p53-dependent mitochondrial apoptosis, ↓ NF-κB (p50, p65), ↓ CXCL8, MYC, IL-2, IL-1A	In vitro	[76–78]
Cervical	Nude mouse model (xenograft)	↓ tumor growth, alters tumor endothelial ultrastructure, potential anti-angiogenic effects	In vivo	[79]
Cervical	U14 tumor-bearing mice + PEG-Que-NLs	Improved cytotoxicity vs. free quercetin; higher tumor inhibition rate with PEGylated liposomes	In vivo	[80]
Ovarian	SKOV-3 cells	Dose/time-dependent ↓ in cell proliferation, G0/G1 arrest, ↓ survivin, ↑ apoptosis	In vitro	[81]
Ovarian	PA-1 cell line (human metastatic)	↓ Bcl-2, Bcl-xL; ↑ Bax, caspase-3/9, cytochrome c → promotes mitochondrial apoptosis	In vitro	[82]
Ovarian	OVCAR-3 TOV-112D A2780	Overcomes cisplatin resistance and radiosensitization; pro-apoptotic, anti-proliferative, anti-inflammatory	In vitro	[83–85]
Ovarian	SKOV-3 /mouse xenograft	Low-dose Quercetin reduces chemo cytotoxicity; high dose is pro-apoptotic (↑ antioxidant enzymes, ↓ oxidative damage)	In vitro In vivo	[83]
Ovarian	Cisplatin-resistant SKOV-3/CDDP	Re-sensitizes resistant cells to cisplatin, blocks PI3K/Akt/mTOR, ↓ Nrf2 and SOD2, promotes mitochondrial apoptosis, pro-oxidant effect	In vitro	[86,87]
Ovarian	Phase I trial (advanced cancers)	IV quercetin safe, anecdotal ↓ CA-125 in an ovarian cancer patient; no follow-up Phase II specific to OC	Clinical (Phase I)	[88]
Endometrial	Tumors	Quercetin (0.01–10 μM) → dose-dependent suppression of colony formation	In vitro	[89]
Endometrial	Ishikawa, HEC-1 A cells	↓ proliferation, invasion, migration; ↑ apoptosis; modulates ATF5/JUN/PI3K/AKT/mTOR, induces autophagy	In vitro	[90]
Endometrial	Human endometriotic epithelial and stromal cells) + Animal model (mouse)	↓ proliferation, suppressed multiple pathways (EGFR/c-Myc/survivin, mTOR), ↓ lesion size in mouse model	In vitro In vivo	[91]
Endometrial	HEC-1-A cells	↓ proliferation, migration; ↑ apoptosis, cell cycle arrest; triggers ferroptosis	In vitro	[92]

NF-Kb—Nuclear Factor Kappa B; CXCL8—C-X-C motif chemokine ligand 8; IL-2—interleukin 1; IL-1A—interleukin 1A; PI3K/Akt/mTOR—phosphoinositide 3 kinase; Nrf2—nuclear factor erythroid 2-related factor 2; SOD2—superoxide dismutase 2; CA-125—cancer antigen 125; OC—ovarian cancer; ATF5/JUN/PI3K/AKT/mTOR—activating Transcription Factor 5; EGFR—epidermal growth factor receptor; ↓—decrease; ↑— increase. → leads to or results in.

5.1. Cervical Cancer

Cervical cancer is the fourth most frequently diagnosed malignancy in women and the fourth leading cause of cancer-related deaths worldwide [74]. In 2022, more than 662,000 new cases were reported globally, with approximately 349,000 deaths, highlighting its significant impact on female mortality [93]. Chronic inflammation and oxidative stress are recognized as key drivers in cervical carcinogenesis, contributing to processes such as cell proliferation, dysregulation of the cell cycle, migration, and apoptosis, and even epigenetic alterations [94–96]. Inflammation, while critical for tissue repair and immune defense, becomes detrimental when sustained over a prolonged period. In the context of cervical cancer, persistent inflammation, often initiated by human papillomavirus (HPV) infection, leads to the continuous secretion of pro-inflammatory cytokines such as TNF-α, Interferon gamma (IFN-γ), IL-1, and IL-8. In addition, molecules including Hypoxia-Inducible Factor (HIF), Inducible Nitric Oxide Synthase (iNOS), COX, Matrix Metalloproteinases (MMPs), and TGF-β, along with the activation of signaling pathways like NF-κB and Janus Kinase/signal Transducers and Activators of Transcription (JAK/STAT) [97], collectively promote tumor initiation, transformation, progression, and metastasis [98–100].

Quercetin has emerged as a promising natural agent in cervical cancer prevention and treatment due to its potent anti-inflammatory [101] and antioxidant [102] properties. Several in vitro studies using cervical cancer cell lines, such as SiHa Cells [76] and Hela cells [77], have demonstrated that Quercetin can suppress cell viability in a dose-dependent manner. It is observed that Quercetin treatment induces G2/M phase cell cycle arrest and triggers mitochondrial apoptosis through a p53-dependent mechanism [78,103]. This apoptotic effect is further reinforced by Quercetin's capacity to downregulate key NF-κB family members (p50 and p65) and inhibit the NF-κB-mediated transcription of anti-apoptotic genes, thereby disrupting survival pathways and sensitizing cancer cells to programmed cell death [104].

Moreover, Quercetin has been shown to modulate the expression of inflammatory mediators involved in cervical carcinogenesis. In HeLa cells, Quercetin treatment (25–50 μM) leads to the decreased expression of Chemokine (C-X-C motif) Ligand 8 (CXCL8), MYC Proto-Oncogene, BHLH Transcription Factor (MYC), IL-2, and IL-1A, molecules that play crucial roles in sustaining the inflammatory microenvironment and promoting cancer progression [101]. These in vitro results indicate that Quercetin may disrupt inflammatory and survival pathways crucial for cervical cancer progression. Given its demonstrated positive effects in several in vitro studies, Quercetin shows promise as a functional food ingredient to support female reproductive health. Moreover, Quercetin has been reported to influence the epidermal growth factor receptor (EGFR) pathway. While several studies have indicated that Quercetin downregulates EGFR expression, thereby impeding cancer cell proliferation, some evidence suggests that Quercetin may also activate specific phosphorylation sites (such as Tyr1068) on EGFR, potentially diminishing its anticancer efficacy [76,105]. This contradictory evidence highlights the complexity of Quercetin's molecular interactions and emphasizes the need for further research to clarify its precise role in EGFR signaling within cervical cancer cells.

In vivo studies, though limited in cervical cancer-specific models, support Quercetin's anti-inflammatory and antioxidant effects observed in vitro. For example, Wei et al. investigated Quercetin's effects on cervical cancer growth in a nude mouse model. The study found that Quercetin, at doses of 50 and 100 mg/kg administered orally, significantly inhibited tumor growth and altered the ultrastructure of tumor endothelial cells [79]. In addition, another study aiming to overcome Quercetin's poor water solubility encapsulated Quercetin in PEGylated Liposomes (PEG-Que-NLs). The optimized formulation demonstrated a slow-release profile and significantly enhanced cytotoxicity against HeLa cells in vitro compared to those of free Quercetin and conventional liposomes. Furthermore, in vivo experiments in this study using U14 cervical carcinoma-bearing mice showed that intravenous injection of PEG-Que-NLs resulted in a significantly higher tumor inhibition rate than that achieved with free Quercetin or non-PEGylated liposomes, highlighting the potential of this delivery system for cervical cancer treatment [80].

Despite its potential benefits in cervical cancer, no clinical trials specifically examining Quercetin's efficacy in this disease were identified in the search results. However, considering Quercetin's safety profile and observed effects in other cancers, future clinical investigations are warranted. Well-designed clinical studies are essential for determining whether Quercetin, administered as a dietary supplement or through Quercetin-rich functional foods, can improve treatment outcomes for cervical cancer patients.

5.2. Ovarian Cancer

Ovarian cancer (OC) ranks as the third most prevalent and the deadliest cancer affecting the female reproductive system. Approximately 70% of patients are diagnosed at advanced stages, characterized by the presence of distant metastases [106]. Researchers have focused on diet quality as a promising option for therapy because of the fewer side effects associated with it [107].

Although the connections between diet, metabolism, and ovarian cancer are not fully clear, many bioactive compounds in functional foods possess antioxidant and anti-inflammatory properties. Therefore, functional foods may help prevent DNA damage and suppress the uncontrolled growth of cancer cells [108,109]. Regarding Quercetin's antioxidant and anti-inflammatory properties, extensive experimental evidence has suggested that Quercetin can inhibit ovarian cancer cell proliferation and induce apoptosis, while also enhancing chemosensitivity and radiosensitivity and overcoming Cisplatin resistance [81,83,110–114].

For instance, Ren et al. examined Quercetin's effects on the human ovarian cancer cell line SKOV-3. Their study found that treating these cells with Quercetin (0–30 mg/mL) led to a dose- and time-dependent reduction in cell proliferation. In addition, they discovered that Quercetin not only triggered apoptosis but also caused the cells to arrest in the G0/G1 phase of the cell cycle, with fewer cells progressing to the G2/M phase. Higher doses of Quercetin were associated with reduced levels of survivin, a protein that normally helps cells evade apoptosis [81]. In addition, a recent in vitro study by Teekaraman et al. explored the Quercetin's anticancer on the PA-1 human metastatic ovarian cancer cell line. In their study, treating PA-1 cells with Quercetin at concentrations between 0 and 200 μM for 24 h led to a dose-dependent decrease in cell viability, with the most pronounced effects observed at 50 and 75 μM. On a molecular level, this treatment shifted the balance between apoptotic regulators by reducing anti-apoptotic proteins (Bcl-2 and Bcl-xL) while increasing pro-apoptotic markers (caspase-3, caspase-9, Bax, and cytochrome c). These findings suggest that Quercetin promotes cell death via the mitochondrial apoptotic pathway, underscoring its potential to inhibit metastatic ovarian cancer cell growth [82]. These pro-apoptotic and anti-proliferative effects have been observed in other lines as well, including OVCAR-3 [84], TOV-112D [85], and A2780 [83], indicating Quercetin's ability to induce ovarian cancer cell death in vitro [115].

Beyond its direct cytotoxicity, Quercetin modulates key inflammatory and oxidative stress pathways in OC cells. Hasan et al. examined the impact of Quercetin on the ovarian adenocarcinoma SKOV-3 cell line and its cisplatin-resistant variant (SKOV-3/CDDP). They reported that treating the resistant cells with 100 μM Quercetin, which notably reduced cell viability, led to a marked suppression of genes encoding key antioxidant enzymes (SOD2, CAT, GPX1, and HO-1), the transcription factor Nrf2, and critical kinases in the Phosphoinositide 3 Kinase/Akt/mammalian target of Rapamycin (PI3K/Akt/mTOR) signaling pathway [86]. In their next study, Hasan et al. demonstrated that pre-treatment with Quercetin re-sensitizes cisplatin-resistant ovarian cancer SKOV-3/CDDP cells by suppressing the overexpression of antioxidant enzymes and the PI3K/Akt/mTOR signaling pathway, both of which are linked to cisplatin resistance. They showed that optimal Quercetin dosing (15–100 μM) not only arrests the cell cycle but also induces apoptosis through a pro-oxidant effect by inhibiting the Thioredoxin (Trx/TrxR) system, thereby increasing ROS production and activates the mitochondrial apoptotic cascade, as evidenced by the cleavage of caspases and Poly ADP-ribose polymerase (PARP) [87].

In vivo studies using animal models largely corroborate these in vitro findings. For instance, Li et al. demonstrated that, in ovarian cancer cell lines, low concentrations of Quercetin (5–30 μM) can significantly reduce the cytotoxic effects of chemotherapy drugs such as cisplatin, taxol, pirarubicin, and 5-fluorouracil, whereas higher doses (40–100 μM) are pro-apoptotic. This antagonistic effect is mediated by Quercetin's capacity to mitigate ROS-induced injury and enhance endogenous antioxidant enzyme expression, ultimately diminishing drug-induced cell death. These in vitro results were corroborated in a xenograft mouse model, where a low-dose Quercetin pre-treatment (20 mg/kg, oral administration) reduced cisplatin's efficacy by alleviating oxidative damage in tumor tissues, suggesting that Quercetin supplementation during ovarian cancer therapy may compromise treatment outcomes [114].

Clinical trial evidence for Quercetin's efficacy in OC remains limited. An early Phase I trial evaluating intravenous Quercetin in advanced cancers, which included an ovarian cancer patient, reported acceptable safety profiles and an anecdotal reduction in the CA-125 tumor marker. Despite promising experimental findings, no subsequent Phase II trials have specifically evaluated the efficacy of quercetin in ovarian cancer, revealing a notable gap in the translation of research to clinical practice [88]. Numerous in vitro and in vivo studies have demonstrated that quercetin exerts multifaceted anticancer effects in ovarian cancer, including pro-apoptotic, anti-proliferative, anti-inflammatory, and anti-metastatic mechanisms. However, in contrast to earlier research suggesting the beneficial effects of quercetin, an experimental study found that quercetin may diminish the efficacy of certain antineoplastic agents, such as cisplatin, 5-fluorouracil, taxol, and pirarubicin. At low concentrations, quercetin displayed anti-apoptotic properties, reducing ROS-mediated damage from these drugs and increasing the activity of antioxidant enzymes in tumor cells [114]. To validate these findings in human populations, well-designed clinical trials are essential, as are strategies to optimize dosing and delivery systems to enhance quercetin's low bioavailability.

5.3. Endometrial Cancer

Endometrial cancer (EC) represents the most prevalent form of gynecological cancer in developed countries, predominantly affecting postmenopausal women. Several risk factors have been identified, including obesity, nulliparity, late menopause, and specific genetic predispositions [116,117]. Treatment strategies for EC typically involve a combination of surgery, radiation, chemotherapy, and hormone therapy, determined by the cancer's stage and subtype [118]. However, the increasing incidence of resistance to conventional therapies has intensified the focus on developing effective preventive measures and complementary treatments. This context has positioned functional foods as promising candidates for cancer prevention and management [119].

Quercetin has garnered attention for its potential chemopreventive and therapeutic effects in EC. In an in vitro study, Scambia et al. investigated Quercetin's ability to inhibit colony formation in nine primary gynecological tumors (four ovarian and five endometrial). Quercetin (dissolved in solvent) alone exhibited a dose-dependent suppression of tumor cell proliferation (0.01–10 μM) [89]. In another study, Yang and Ma explored how Quercetin inhibited the EC cell development by targeting the Expression of Activating Transcription

Factor 5 (ATF5)/JUN/PI3K/AKT/mTOR pathway and enhancing autophagy. Using network pharmacology and cellular experiments with the Ishikawa and HEC-1 A cell lines, they demonstrated that Quercetin suppresses cell proliferation, invasion, and migration while promoting apoptosis. These antitumor effects were closely linked to autophagy modulation through PI3K/AKT/mTOR pathway downregulation, highlighting Quercetin's potential as a therapeutic agent for EC [90]. Zhang et al. conducted both in vitro and in vivo studies to examine how the flavonoids kaempferol and Quercetin, which directly bind to Nuclear Receptor 4A1 (NR4A1), can hinder the advancement of endometriosis. By inhibiting NR4A1, these compounds reduced the proliferation of human endometriotic epithelial and stromal cells, as well as of Ishikawa EC cells, through suppressing multiple growth and survival pathways (EGFR/c-Myc/survivin, mTOR) and fibrotic signaling, while also modifying oxidative stress pathways. In in vivo experiments using a mouse model of endometriosis, kaempferol and Quercetin (100 mg/kg/day, oral administration) effectively decreased the endometriotic lesion size without affecting the body weight, highlighting their potential as a nutritional therapy for endometriosis [91]. Li et al. conducted an in vitro study on HEC-1-A EC cells to evaluate Quercetin's impact on cell viability, proliferation, and apoptosis, and the possible role of ferroptosis in these processes. Their results showed that 100 μM Quercetin inhibited proliferation and migration, induced cell cycle arrest, and promoted apoptosis of HEC-1-A cells. Furthermore, Quercetin's antitumor effects appeared to be strongly linked to triggering ferroptosis, suggesting a potential therapeutic avenue for EC [92]. Nevertheless, the use of Quercetin in EC raises concerns due to its estrogenic properties. It has shown that Quercetin can produce significant estrogenic effects, increasing serum estradiol levels by up to 22.48%. Since EC is typically estrogen-sensitive, this estrogenic activity may diminish its potential anticancer benefits for certain patients [120]. Given EC's multifaceted nature, a personalized approach that considers genetic and hormonal factors could further refine Quercetin's clinical application. However, the absence of clinical trials investigating quercetin's effects on endometrial cancer is notable.

6. Limitations and Challenges of Quercetin Usage

Promising findings from clinical trial studies have been observed, suggesting that quercetin may have beneficial effects on various conditions such as hyperuricemia [121], PCOS [64], obesity [122], and blood pressure [123]. However, there is a notable lack of clinical research focusing specifically on gynecological cancers and pregnancy-related issues, which is significant as it limits our understanding of quercetin's efficacy in these critical domains. Preclinical studies have identified several limitations that impede the therapeutic application of quercetin in the female reproductive system. One of the most important challenges is its low bioavailability, which restricts optimal therapeutic outcomes [124]. Joseph et al. demonstrated that quercetin's clinical application is hindered by poor water solubility and limited oral absorption, prompting the development of advanced hybrid hydrogel delivery systems designed to enhance its bioavailability [125]. Furthermore, studies have shown that quercetin undergoes rapid phase II metabolism, primarily through glucuronidation and sulfation shortly after absorption, significantly affecting its systemic availability and therapeutic window [126–128]. In response to these challenges, researchers are exploring innovative drug delivery systems, including quercetin-loaded gels, polymeric micelles [129], nanoparticles [129], and glucan-quercetin conjugates [130]. However, a notable methodological weakness has been identified in these studies due to the lack of standardization concerning the source of quercetin utilized [131]. Additionally, mostly studies which are reviewed in this article, have been conducted over short durations, ranging from weeks to a few months, which limits the evaluation of long-term efficacy and safety regarding reproductive disorders. This limitation is particularly concerning given the substantial discrepancy between pharmacological doses used in research, up to 945 mg/m^2 intravenously [88]. In contrast, a study conducted in Japan found that the median intake in a typical Western diet is closer to 10 mg/day, with primary sources being onions, apples, and green tea [132]. This disparity underscores the critical distinction between quercetin's role as a dietary component and its potential as a pharmaceutical agent. Addressing these gaps highlights an urgent need for further large-scale, randomized controlled trials to establish quercetin's clinical efficacy and safety while clarifying optimal dosages and administration routes in women's reproductive health.

7. Conclusions

Quercetin demonstrates compelling potential in managing various female reproductive health conditions, including pregnancy-related challenges, PCOS, and gynecological cancers. Its antioxidant, anti-inflammatory, and hormone-modulating properties have been highlighted across numerous in vitro and in vivo studies, with limited clinical trials indicating early but promising benefits. Moreover, incorporating quercetin into diets could offer a practical, patient-friendly strategy to enhance the substance's bioavailability and therapeutic efficacy. Future investigations should focus on well-structured clinical trials to confirm these findings, optimize dosing, and address potential interactions with conventional therapies, ultimately advancing Quercetin's role as a valuable component in women's reproductive healthcare.

Author Contributions: Conceptualization, S.Z. and A.S.; writing—original draft preparation, Y.K., M.G., S.P.-A. and P.R.; writing—review and editing, Y.K., M.G., S.P.-A., P.R., A.S. and S.Z.; supervision, A.S. and S.Z. All authors have read and agreed to the published version of the manuscript.

Funding: This research received no external funding.

Institutional Review Board Statement: Not applicable.

Informed Consent Statement: Not applicable.

Data Availability Statement: No new data were created or analyzed in this study. Data sharing does not apply to this article.

Conflicts of Interest: The authors declare no conflicts of interest.

References

1. Szilágyi, A.; Szabó, I. *Endocrine Characteristics of Polycystic Ovary Syndrome (PCOS)*; NISCAIR-CSIR: New Delhi, India, 2003.
2. Keyvani, V.; Kheradmand, N.; Navaei, Z.N.; Mollazadeh, S.; Esmaeili, S.-A. Epidemiological trends and risk factors of gynecological cancers: An update. *Med. Oncol.* **2023**, *40*, 93.
3. Laijawala, R.A. Recurrent Pregnancy Loss: Immunological aetiologies and associations with mental health. *Brain Behav. Immun. -Health* **2024**, *41*, 100868.
4. Madigan, M.; Karhu, E. The role of plant-based nutrition in cancer prevention. *J. Unexplored Med. Data* **2018**, *3*, 9.
5. DeClercq, V.; Nearing, J.T.; Sweeney, E. Plant-Based Diets and Cancer Risk: What is the Evidence? *Curr. Nutr. Rep.* **2022**, *11*, 354–369. [CrossRef]
6. Pourteymour Fard Tabrizi, F.; Hajizadeh-Sharafabad, F.; Vaezi, M.; Jafari-Vayghan, H.; Alizadeh, M.; Maleki, V. Quercetin and polycystic ovary syndrome, current evidence and future directions: A systematic review. *J. Ovarian Res.* **2020**, *13*, 11.
7. Li, Y.; Yao, J.; Han, C.; Yang, J.; Chaudhry, M.T.; Wang, S.; Liu, H.; Yin, Y. Quercetin, inflammation and immunity. *Nutrients* **2016**, *8*, 167. [CrossRef]
8. Vašková, J.; Klepcová, Z.; Špaková, I.; Urdzík, P.; Štofilová, J.; Bertková, I.; Kľoc, M.; Rabajdová, M. The importance of natural antioxidants in female reproduction. *Antioxidants* **2023**, *12*, 907. [CrossRef]

9. Valentová, K.; Šíma, P.; Rybková, Z.; Křížan, J.; Malachová, K.; Křen, V. (Anti)mutagenic and immunomodulatory properties of quercetin glycosides. *J. Sci. Food Agric.* **2016**, *96*, 1492–1499. [CrossRef]
10. Deepika; Maurya, P.K. Health Benefits of Quercetin in Age-Related Diseases. *Molecules* **2022**, *27*, 2498. [CrossRef]
11. Ding, J.; Mei, S.; Cai, M.; Zhang, D.; Yu, J. Integrated network pharmacology and clinical study to reveal the effects and mechanisms of bushen huoxue huatan decoction on polycystic ovary syndrome. *Evid. -Based Complement. Altern. Med.* **2022**, *2022*, 2635375.
12. Sharma, H.; Sen, S.; Singh, N. Molecular pathways in the chemosensitization of cisplatin by quercetin in human head and neck cancer. *Cancer Biol. Ther.* **2005**, *4*, 949–955. [CrossRef]
13. Li, J.; Long, H.; Cong, Y.; Gao, H.; Lyu, Q.; Yu, S.; Kuang, Y. Quercetin prevents primordial follicle loss via suppression of PI3K/Akt/Foxo3a pathway activation in cyclophosphamide-treated mice. *Reprod. Biol. Endocrinol.* **2021**, *19*, 63.
14. Lai, W.-F.; Wong, W.-T. Design and optimization of quercetin-based functional foods. *Crit. Rev. Food Sci. Nutr.* **2022**, *62*, 7319–7335. [CrossRef]
15. Kennedy, D.A.; Lupattelli, A.; Koren, G.; Nordeng, H. Herbal medicine use in pregnancy: Results of a multinational study. *BMC Complement. Altern. Med.* **2013**, *13*, 355.
16. Ożarowski, M.; Mikołajczak, P.Ł.; Kujawski, R.; Wielgus, K.; Klejewski, A.; Wolski, H.; Seremak-Mrozikiewicz, A. Pharmacological effect of quercetin in hypertension and its potential application in pregnancy-induced hypertension: Review of in vitro, in vivo, and clinical studies. *Evid. -Based Complement. Altern. Med.* **2018**, *2018*, 7421489.
17. Tomkiewicz, J.; Darmochwał-Kolarz, D. The diagnostics and treatment of recurrent pregnancy loss. *J. Clin. Med.* **2023**, *12*, 4768. [CrossRef]
18. Melo, P.; Dhillon-Smith, R.; Islam, M.A.; Devall, A.; Coomarasamy, A. Genetic causes of sporadic and recurrent miscarriage. *Fertil. Steril.* **2023**, *120*, 940–944.
19. Carbonnel, M.; Pirtea, P.; de Ziegler, D.; Ayoubi, J.M. Uterine factors in recurrent pregnancy losses. *Fertil. Steril.* **2021**, *115*, 538–545.
20. Practice Committee of the American Society for Reproductive Medicine. Evaluation and treatment of recurrent pregnancy loss: A committee opinion. *Fertil. Steril.* **2012**, *98*, 1103–1111.
21. Hempstock, J.; Jauniaux, E.; Greenwold, N.; Burton, G.J. The contribution of placental oxidative stress to early pregnancy failure. *Hum. Pathol.* **2003**, *34*, 1265–1275.
22. Obeagu, E.; Obeagu, G. Enhancing maternal and fetal well-being: The role of antioxidants in pregnancy. *Elite J. Med. Sci.* **2024**, *2*, 76–87.
23. Araújo, J.R.; Correia-Branco, A.; Pereira, A.C.; Pinho, M.J.; Keating, E.; Martel, F. Oxidative stress decreases uptake of neutral amino acids in a human placental cell line (BeWo cells). *Reprod. Toxicol.* **2013**, *40*, 76–81. [CrossRef]
24. Bartho, L.A.; Holland, O.J.; Moritz, K.M.; Perkins, A.V.; Cuffe, J.S. Maternal corticosterone in the mouse alters oxidative stress markers, antioxidant function and mitochondrial content in placentas of female fetuses. *J. Physiol.* **2019**, *597*, 3053–3067. [CrossRef]
25. Umekawa, T.; Sugiyama, T.; Kihira, T.; Murabayashi, N.; Zhang, L.; Nagao, K.; Kamimoto, Y.; Ma, N.; Yodoi, J.; Sagawa, N. Overexpression of thioredoxin-1 reduces oxidative stress in the placenta of transgenic mice and promotes fetal growth via glucose metabolism. *Endocrinology* **2008**, *149*, 3980–3988. [CrossRef]
26. Webster, J.; Miller, M.; Vemulapalli, R. Encephalitozoon cuniculi-associated placentitis and perinatal death in an alpaca (Lama pacos). *Vet. Pathol.* **2008**, *45*, 255–258. [CrossRef]
27. Safronova, V.; Matveeva, N.; Avkhacheva, N.; Sidel'nikova, V.; Van'ko, L.; Sukhikh, G. Changes in regulation of oxidase activity of peripheral blood granulocytes in women with habitual abortions. *Bull. Exp. Biol. Med.* **2003**, *136*, 257–260. [CrossRef]
28. Yoshida, K.; Kusama, K.; Shinohara, G.; Sato, S.; Yoshie, M.; Tamura, K. Quercetin stimulates trophoblast fusion via the mitochondrial function. *Sci. Rep.* **2024**, *14*, 287. [CrossRef]
29. Takashima, M.; Tanaka, W.; Matsuyama, H.; Tajiri, H.; Sakakibara, H. Maternal quercetin consumption during pregnancy may help regulate total cholesterol/HDL-cholesterol ratio without effect on cholesterol levels in male progeny consuming high-fat diet. *Nutrients* **2021**, *13*, 1242. [CrossRef]
30. Wang, D.; Li, X.; Li, Y.; Wang, R.; Wang, C.; Li, Y. New molecular mechanisms of quercetin in improving recurrent spontaneous abortion based on in-depth network pharmacology and molecular docking. *Front. Chem.* **2024**, *12*, 1407667. [CrossRef]
31. Wu, S.; Tian, Y.; Zhang, Q.; Fu, Z.; Lan, H.; Zhou, X.; Ma, L.; Lou, Y. Protective effect of quercetin on lipopolysaccharide-induced miscarriage based on animal experiments and network pharmacology. *Mol. Med. Rep.* **2024**, *29*, 99. [CrossRef]
32. Lin, X.; Peng, Q.; Zhang, J.; Li, X.; Huang, J.; Duan, S.; Zhang, W. Quercetin prevents lipopolysaccharide-induced experimental preterm labor in mice and increases offspring survival rate. *Reprod. Sci.* **2020**, *27*, 1047–1057. [CrossRef]
33. Dong, J.; Young, P.J.; Se, T.; Yahweh; Hwi, L.M. Quercetin inhibits NF-κB and AP-1 activation through induction of heme oxygenase-1 and attenuation of Src mediated PI3K/Akt, p38 and c-jun N-terminal protein kinase phosphorylations in raw 264.7

cells. In Proceedings of the 2012 Winter Symposium of the Korean Society for Laboratory Animal Science, Jeju, Republic of Korea, 28–30 June 2012; p. 97.

34. Liu, W.; Zhang, M.; Feng, J.; Fan, A.; Zhou, Y.; Xu, Y. The influence of quercetin on maternal immunity, oxidative stress, and inflammation in mice with exposure of fine particulate matter during gestation. *Int. J. Environ. Res. Public Health* **2017**, *14*, 592. [CrossRef] [PubMed]
35. Ahmadi, R.; Ziaei, S.; Parsay, S. Association between nutritional status with spontaneous abortion. *Int. J. Fertil. Steril.* **2016**, *10*, 337.
36. Zhou, J.; Li, L.; Pan, X.; Wang, J.; Qi, Q.; Sun, H.; Li, C.; Wang, L. The effect of a traditional Chinese quadri-combination therapy and its component quercetin on recurrent spontaneous abortion: A clinical trial, network pharmacology and experiments-based study. *Front. Pharmacol.* **2022**, *13*, 965694. [CrossRef]
37. Wang, H.; Lin, H.; Kang, W.; Huang, L.; Gong, S.; Zhang, T.; Huang, X.; He, F.; Ye, Y.; Tang, Y. miR-34a/DRP-1-mediated mitophagy participated in cisplatin-induced ototoxicity via increasing oxidative stress. *BMC Pharmacol. Toxicol.* **2023**, *24*, 16. [CrossRef]
38. Yu, S.; Long, H.; Lyu, Q.F.; Zhang, Q.H.; Yan, Z.G.; Liang, H.X.; Chai, W.R.; Yan, Z.; Kuang, Y.P.; Qi, C. Protective effect of quercetin on the development of preimplantation mouse embryos against hydrogen peroxide-induced oxidative injury. *PLoS ONE* **2014**, *9*, e89520. [CrossRef]
39. Vanhees, K.; Godschalk, R.W.; Sanders, A.; van Waalwijk van Doorn-Khosrovani, S.B.; van Schooten, F.J. Maternal quercetin intake during pregnancy results in an adapted iron homeostasis at adulthood. *Toxicology* **2011**, *290*, 350–358. [CrossRef] [PubMed]
40. Greff, D.; Juhász, A.E.; Váncsa, S.; Váradi, A.; Sipos, Z.; Szinte, J.; Park, S.; Hegyi, P.; Nyirády, P.; Ács, N. Inositol is an effective and safe treatment in polycystic ovary syndrome: A systematic review and meta-analysis of randomized controlled trials. *Reprod. Biol. Endocrinol.* **2023**, *21*, 10. [CrossRef]
41. Teede, H.J.; Misso, M.L.; Costello, M.F.; Dokras, A.; Laven, J.; Moran, L.; Piltonen, T.; Norman, R.J. Recommendations from the international evidence-based guideline for the assessment and management of polycystic ovary syndrome. *Hum. Reprod.* **2018**, *33*, 1602–1618. [CrossRef] [PubMed]
42. Zhu, T.; Cui, J.; Goodarzi, M.O. Polycystic ovary syndrome and risk of type 2 diabetes, coronary heart disease, and stroke. *Diabetes* **2021**, *70*, 627–637. [CrossRef]
43. Shrivastava, S.; Conigliaro, R.L. Polycystic ovarian syndrome. *Med. Clin. N. Am.* **2023**, *107*, 227–234. [CrossRef] [PubMed]
44. Zehravi, M.; Maqbool, M.; Ara, I. Polycystic ovary syndrome and infertility: An update. *Int. J. Adolesc. Med. Health* **2022**, *34*, 1–9. [CrossRef]
45. Tousizadeh, S.; Mohammadi-Moghadam, F.; Mohammadian-Hafshejani, A.; Sadeghi, R. Comparison of zinc levels in mothers with and without abortion: A systematic review and meta-analysiss. *Heliyon* **2024**, *10*, e30605. [CrossRef]
46. Dapas, M.; Dunaif, A. Deconstructing a syndrome: Genomic insights into PCOS causal mechanisms and classification. *Endocr. Rev.* **2022**, *43*, 927–965. [CrossRef] [PubMed]
47. Li, W.; Liu, C.; Yang, Q.; Zhou, Y.; Liu, M.; Shan, H. Oxidative stress and antioxidant imbalance in ovulation disorder in patients with polycystic ovary syndrome. *Front. Nutr.* **2022**, *9*, 1018674. [CrossRef] [PubMed]
48. Mancini, A.; Bruno, C.; Vergani, E.; d'Abate, C.; Giacchi, E.; Silvestrini, A. Oxidative stress and low-grade inflammation in polycystic ovary syndrome: Controversies and new insights. *Int. J. Mol. Sci.* **2021**, *22*, 1667. [CrossRef]
49. Mazloomi, S.; Sheikh, N.; Sanoee Farimani, M.; Pilehvari, S. Association of Prx4, total oxidant status, and inflammatory factors with insulin resistance in polycystic ovary syndrome. *Int. J. Endocrinol.* **2021**, *2021*, 9949753. [CrossRef] [PubMed]
50. Wang, K.; Li, Y. Signaling pathways and targeted therapeutic strategies for polycystic ovary syndrome. *Front. Endocrinol.* **2023**, *14*, 1191759. [CrossRef]
51. Legro, R.S.; Arslanian, S.A.; Ehrmann, D.A.; Hoeger, K.M.; Murad, M.H.; Pasquali, R.; Welt, C.K. Diagnosis and treatment of polycystic ovary syndrome: An Endocrine Society clinical practice guideline. *J. Clin. Endocrinol. Metab.* **2013**, *98*, 4565–4592. [CrossRef]
52. Ma, C.; Xiang, Q.; Song, G.; Wang, X. Quercetin and polycystic ovary syndrome. *Front. Pharmacol.* **2022**, *13*, 1006678. [CrossRef]
53. Khadrawy, O.Z.S. *Modulation of Nrf2-Mediated Oxidative Stress Response in Bovine Granulosa Cells and Preimplantation Embryos*; Universitäts-und Landesbibliothek Bonn: Bonn, Germany, 2019.
54. Davoodian, N.; Kadivar, A.; Davoodian, N.; Ahmadi, E.; Nazari, H.; Mehrban, H. The effect of quercetin in the maturation media on cumulus-granulosa cells and the developmental competence of bovine oocytes. *Theriogenology* **2022**, *189*, 262–269. [CrossRef] [PubMed]
55. Wang, Z.; Zhai, D.; Zhang, D.; Bai, L.; Yao, R.; Yu, J.; Cheng, W.; Yu, C. Quercetin Decreases Insulin Resistance in a Polycystic Ovary Syndrome Rat Model by Improving Inflammatory Microenvironment. *Reprod. Sci.* **2017**, *24*, 682–690. [CrossRef] [PubMed]

56. Olaniyan, O.T.; Bamidele, O.; Adetunji, C.O.; Priscilla, B.; Femi, A.; Ayobami, D.; Okotie, G.; Oluwaseun, I.; Olugbenga, E.; Mali, P.C. Quercetin modulates granulosa cell mRNA androgen receptor gene expression in dehydroepiandrosterone-induced polycystic ovary in Wistar rats via metabolic and hormonal pathways. *J. Basic Clin. Physiol. Pharmacol.* **2020**, *31*, 4.
57. Jahan, S.; Abid, A.; Khalid, S.; Afsar, T.; Shaheen, G.; Almajwal, A.; Razak, S. Therapeutic potentials of Quercetin in management of polycystic ovarian syndrome using Letrozole induced rat model: A histological and a biochemical study. *J. Ovarian Res.* **2018**, *11*, 26. [CrossRef]
58. Mahmoud, A.A.; Elfiky, A.M.; Abo-Zeid, F.S. The anti-androgenic effect of quercetin on hyperandrogenism and ovarian dysfunction induced in a dehydroepiandrosterone rat model of polycystic ovary syndrome. *Steroids* **2022**, *177*, 108936. [CrossRef] [PubMed]
59. Shah, M.Z.u.h.; Shrivastva, V.k.; Mir, M.A.; Sheikh, W.M.; Ganie, M.A.; Rather, G.A.; Shafi, M.; Bashir, S.M.; Ansari, M.A.; Al-Jafary, M.A. Effect of quercetin on steroidogenesis and folliculogenesis in ovary of mice with experimentally-induced polycystic ovarian syndrome. *Front. Endocrinol.* **2023**, *14*, 1153289. [CrossRef]
60. Zheng, S.; Chen, Y.; Ma, M.; Li, M. Mechanism of quercetin on the improvement of ovulation disorder and regulation of ovarian CNP/NPR2 in PCOS model rats. *J. Formos. Med. Assoc.* **2022**, *121*, 1081–1092. [CrossRef]
61. Hussain, L.; Aamir, N.; Hussain, M.; Asif, M.; Chauhdary, Z.; Manzoor, F.; Siddique, R.; Riaz, M. Therapeutic investigation of standardized aqueous methanolic extract of bitter melon (*Momordica charantia* L.) for its potential against polycystic ovarian syndrome in experimental animals' model: In vitro and in vivo studies. *Evid. -Based Complement. Altern. Med.* **2022**, *2022*, 5143653. [CrossRef]
62. Joseph, B.; Jini, D. Antidiabetic effects of Momordica charantia (bitter melon) and its medicinal potency. *Asian Pac. J. Trop. Dis.* **2013**, *3*, 93–102.
63. Younas, A.; Hussain, L.; Shabbir, A.; Asif, M.; Hussain, M.; Manzoor, F. Effects of fagonia indica on letrozole-induced polycystic ovarian syndrome (PCOS) in young adult female rats. *Evid. -Based Complement. Altern. Med.* **2022**, *2022*, 1397060. [CrossRef]
64. Rezvan, N.; Moini, A.; Janani, L.; Mohammad, K.; Saedisomeolia, A.; Nourbakhsh, M.; Gorgani-Firuzjaee, S.; Mazaherioun, M.; Hosseinzadeh-Attar, M.J. Effects of Quercetin on Adiponectin-Mediated Insulin Sensitivity in Polycystic Ovary Syndrome: A Randomized Placebo-Controlled Double-Blind Clinical Trial. *Horm. Metab. Res.* **2017**, *49*, 115–121. [CrossRef] [PubMed]
65. Khorshidi, M.; Moini, A.; Alipoor, E.; Rezvan, N.; Gorgani-Firuzjaee, S.; Yaseri, M.; Hosseinzadeh-Attar, M.J. The effects of quercetin supplementation on metabolic and hormonal parameters as well as plasma concentration and gene expression of resistin in overweight or obese women with polycystic ovary syndrome. *Phytother. Res.* **2018**, *32*, 2282–2289. [CrossRef]
66. Vaez, S.; Parivr, K.; Amidi, F.; Rudbari, N.H.; Moini, A.; Amini, N. Quercetin and polycystic ovary syndrome; inflammation, hormonal parameters and pregnancy outcome: A randomized clinical trial. *Am. J. Reprod. Immunol.* **2023**, *89*, e13644. [CrossRef] [PubMed]
67. Hong, Y.-L.; Wu, F. Effect of Bushen Huatan Recipe on the Akt signal pathway in polycystic ovarian syndrome model rats with insulin resistance: An experimental research. *Zhongguo Zhong Xi Yi Jie He Za Zhi = Chin. J. Integr. Tradit. West. Med.* **2014**, *34*, 230–234.
68. Lin, Y.; Xiang, L.; Li, X.; Tang, Q.; Meng, F.; Chen, W. Exploring the mechanism of Yi-Jing decoction in treating polycystic ovary syndrome by using network pharmacology. *Curr. Med. Chem.* **2023**, *30*, 2463–2474. [CrossRef] [PubMed]
69. Egert, S.; Bosy-Westphal, A.; Seiberl, J.; Kürbitz, C.; Settler, U.; Plachta-Danielzik, S.; Wagner, A.E.; Frank, J.; Schrezenmeir, J.; Rimbach, G.; et al. Quercetin reduces systolic blood pressure and plasma oxidised low-density lipoprotein concentrations in overweight subjects with a high-cardiovascular disease risk phenotype: A double-blinded, placebo-controlled cross-over study. *Br. J. Nutr.* **2009**, *102*, 1065–1074. [CrossRef]
70. Zhu, G.; Li, Z.; Tang, L.; Shen, M.; Zhou, Z.; Wei, Y.; Zhao, Y.; Bai, S.; Song, L. Associations of Dietary Intakes with Gynecological Cancers: Findings from a Cross-Sectional Study. *Nutrients* **2022**, *14*, 5026. [CrossRef]
71. Ferlay, J.; Colombet, M.; Soerjomataram, I.; Parkin, D.M.; Piñeros, M.; Znaor, A.; Bray, F. Cancer statistics for the year 2020: An overview. *Int. J. Cancer* **2021**, *149*, 778–789. [CrossRef]
72. Tiwary, S.; Hussain, M. Functional foods for prevention and treatment of cancer. *Asian. J. Pharm. Clin. Res.* **2021**, *14*, 4–10. [CrossRef]
73. Serna-Thomé, G.; Castro-Eguiluz, D.; Fuchs-Tarlovsky, V.; Sánchez-López, M.; Delgado-Olivares, L.; Coronel-Martínez, J.; Molina-Trinidad, E.M.; de la Torre, M.; Cetina-Pérez, L. Use of functional foods and oral supplements as adjuvants in cancer treatment. *Rev. Investig. Clin.* **2018**, *70*, 136–146. [CrossRef]
74. Saslow, D.; Solomon, D.; Lawson, H.W.; Killackey, M.; Kulasingam, S.L.; Cain, J.; Garcia, F.A.; Moriarty, A.T.; Waxman, A.G.; Wilbur, D.C.; et al. American Cancer Society, American Society for Colposcopy and Cervical Pathology, and American Society for Clinical Pathology screening guidelines for the prevention and early detection of cervical cancer. *CA Cancer J. Clin.* **2012**, *62*, 147–172. [CrossRef] [PubMed]

75. Sak, K. Chemotherapy and dietary phytochemical agesnts. *Chemother. Res. Pract.* **2012**, *2012*, 282570. [CrossRef]
76. Chen, X.; Xu, P.; Zhang, H.; Su, X.; Guo, L.; Zhou, X.; Wang, J.; Huang, P.; Zhang, Q.; Sun, R. EGFR and ERK activation resists flavonoid quercetin-induced anticancer activities in human cervical cancer cells in vitro. *Oncol. Lett.* **2021**, *22*, 754. [CrossRef] [PubMed]
77. He, C.; Lu, X.; Li, J.; Shen, K.; Bai, Y.; Li, Y.; Luan, H.; Tuo, S. The effect of quercetin on cervical cancer cells as determined by inducing tumor endoplasmic reticulum stress and apoptosis and its mechanism of action. *Am. J. Transl. Res.* **2021**, *13*, 5240–5247.
78. Vidya Priyadarsini, R.; Senthil Murugan, R.; Maitreyi, S.; Ramalingam, K.; Karunagaran, D.; Nagini, S. The flavonoid quercetin induces cell cycle arrest and mitochondria-mediated apoptosis in human cervical cancer (HeLa) cells through p53 induction and NF-κB inhibition. *Eur. J. Pharmacol.* **2010**, *649*, 84–91. [CrossRef]
79. Wei, W.; Liu, T.; Ding, B.; Cao, S. Study on relationship of quercetin on cervical carcinoma in nude mice model of tumor growth and the expression of heparanase. *Chin. J. Biochem. Pharm.* **2015**, *26–29*, 32.
80. Li, J.; Li, Z.; Gao, Y.; Liu, S.; Li, K.; Wang, S.; Gao, L.; Shi, M.; Liu, Z.; Han, Z.; et al. Effect of a Drug Delivery System Made of Quercetin Formulated into PEGylation Liposomes on Cervical Carcinoma In Vitro and In Vivo. *J. Nanomater.* **2021**, *2021*, 9389934. [CrossRef]
81. Ren, M.X.; Deng, X.H.; Ai, F.; Yuan, G.Y.; Song, H.Y. Effect of quercetin on the proliferation of the human ovarian cancer cell line SKOV-3 in vitro. *Exp. Ther. Med.* **2015**, *10*, 579–583. [CrossRef]
82. Teekaraman, D.; Elayapillai, S.P.; Viswanathan, M.P.; Jagadeesan, A. Quercetin inhibits human metastatic ovarian cancer cell growth and modulates components of the intrinsic apoptotic pathway in PA-1 cell line. *Chem. -Biol. Interact.* **2019**, *300*, 91–100. [CrossRef]
83. Zhou, J.; Gong, J.; Ding, C.; Chen, G. Quercetin induces the apoptosis of human ovarian carcinoma cells by upregulating the expression of microRNA-145. *Mol. Med. Rep.* **2015**, *12*, 3127–3131. [CrossRef]
84. Luo, H.; Jiang, B.-H.; King, S.M.; Chen, Y.C. Inhibition of cell growth and VEGF expression in ovarian cancer cells by flavonoids. *Nutr. Cancer* **2008**, *60*, 800–809.
85. Xintaropoulou, C.; Ward, C.; Wise, A.; Marston, H.; Turnbull, A.; Langdon, S.P. A comparative analysis of inhibitors of the glycolysis pathway in breast and ovarian cancer cell line models. *Oncotarget* **2015**, *6*, 25677–25695. [CrossRef] [PubMed]
86. Hasan, A.A.S.; Kalinina, E.V.; Tatarskiy, V.V.; Volodina, Y.L.; Petrova, A.S.; Novichkova, M.D.; Zhdanov, D.D.; Shtil, A.A. Suppression of the Antioxidant System and PI3K/Akt/mTOR Signaling Pathway in Cisplatin-Resistant Cancer Cells by Quercetin. *Bull. Exp. Biol. Med.* **2022**, *173*, 760–764. [CrossRef] [PubMed]
87. Hasan, A.A.; Kalinina, E.; Nuzhina, J.; Volodina, Y.; Shtil, A.; Tatarskiy, V. Potentiation of Cisplatin Cytotoxicity in Resistant Ovarian Cancer SKOV3/Cisplatin Cells by Quercetin Pre-Treatment. *Int. J. Mol. Sci.* **2023**, *24*, 10960. [CrossRef] [PubMed]
88. Ferry, D.R.; Smith, A.; Malkhandi, J.; Fyfe, D.W.; deTakats, P.G.; Anderson, D.; Baker, J.; Kerr, D.J. Phase I clinical trial of the flavonoid quercetin: Pharmacokinetics and evidence for in vivo tyrosine kinase inhibition. *Clin. Cancer Res.* **1996**, *2*, 659–668.
89. Scambia, G.; Ranelletti, F.O.; Panici, P.B.; Piantelli, M.; Bonanno, G.; De Vincenzo, R.; Ferrandina, G.; Maggiano, N.; Capelli, A.; Mancuso, S. Inhibitory effect of quercetin on primary ovarian and endometrial cancers and synergistic activity with cis-diamminedichloroplatinum(II). *Gynecol. Oncol.* **1992**, *45*, 13–19. [CrossRef]
90. Yang, L.; Ma, H. Quercetin inhibits the biological activity of endometrial cancer by regulating autophagy: A network pharmacology analysis and cellular experimental validation. *J. Funct. Foods* **2025**, *125*, 106657. [CrossRef]
91. Zhang, L.; Mohankumar, K.; Martin, G.; Mariyam, F.; Park, Y.; Han, S.J.; Safe, S. Flavonoids Quercetin and Kaempferol Are NR4A1 Antagonists and Suppress Endometriosis in Female Mice. *Endocrinology* **2023**, *164*, bqad133. [CrossRef]
92. Li, X.; Zhu, Q.; Ma, M.; Guo, H. Quercetin inhibits the progression of endometrial HEC-1-A cells by regulating ferroptosis—A preliminary study. *Eur. J. Med. Res.* **2022**, *27*, 292. [CrossRef]
93. Bray, F.; Laversanne, M.; Sung, H.; Ferlay, J.; Siegel, R.L.; Soerjomataram, I.; Jemal, A. Global cancer statistics 2022: GLOBOCAN estimates of incidence and mortality worldwide for 36 cancers in 185 countries. *CA Cancer J. Clin.* **2024**, *74*, 229–263.
94. Preci, D.P.; Almeida, A.; Weiler, A.L.; Franciosi, M.L.M.; Cardoso, A.M. Oxidative damage and antioxidants in cervical cancer. *Int. J. Gynecol. Cancer* **2021**, *31*, 265–271. [CrossRef] [PubMed]
95. Hemmat, N.; Bannazadeh Baghi, H. Association of human papillomavirus infection and inflammation in cervical cancer. *Pathog. Dis.* **2019**, *77*, ftz048. [CrossRef]
96. Holub, K.; Biete, A. Impact of systemic inflammation biomarkers on the survival outcomes of cervical cancer patients. *Clin. Transl. Oncol.* **2019**, *21*, 836–844. [CrossRef]
97. Gutiérrez-Hoya, A.; Soto-Cruz, I. Role of the JAK/STAT pathway in cervical cancer: Its relationship with HPV E6/E7 oncoproteins. *Cells* **2020**, *9*, 2297. [CrossRef]
98. Suarez-Carmona, M.; Lesage, J.; Cataldo, D.; Gilles, C. EMT and Inflammation: Inseparable Actors of Cancer Progression. *Mol. Oncol.* **2017**, *11*, 805–823. [CrossRef]

99. Yeung, Y.T.; Aziz, F.; Guerrero-Castilla, A.; Arguelles, S. Signaling pathways in inflammation and anti-inflammatory therapies. *Curr. Pharm. Des.* **2018**, *24*, 1449–1484. [CrossRef] [PubMed]
100. Georgescu, S.R.; Mitran, C.I.; Mitran, M.I.; Caruntu, C.; Sarbu, M.I.; Matei, C.; Nicolae, I.; Tocut, S.M.; Popa, M.I.; Tampa, M. New insights in the pathogenesis of HPV infection and the associated carcinogenic processes: The role of chronic inflammation and oxidative stress. *J. Immunol. Res.* **2018**, *2018*, 5315816. [CrossRef] [PubMed]
101. Kedhari Sundaram, M.; Raina, R.; Afroze, N.; Bajbouj, K.; Hamad, M.; Haque, S.; Hussain, A. Quercetin modulates signaling pathways and induces apoptosis in cervical cancer cells. *Biosci. Rep.* **2019**, *39*, BSR20190720. [CrossRef]
102. Alrawaiq, N.S.; Abdullah, A. A review of flavonoid quercetin: Metabolism, bioactivity and antioxidant properties. *Int. J. Pharm.Tech. Res.* **2014**, *6*, 933–941.
103. Clemente-Soto, A.F.; Salas-Vidal, E.; Milan-Pacheco, C.; Sánchez-Carranza, J.N.; Peralta-Zaragoza, O.; González-Maya, L. Quercetin induces G2 phase arrest and apoptosis with the activation of p53 in an E6 expression-independent manner in HPV-positive human cervical cancer-derived cells. *Mol. Med. Rep.* **2019**, *19*, 2097–2106. [CrossRef]
104. Deng, S.; Yuan, P.; Sun, J. The role of NF-κB in carcinogenesis of cervical cancer: Opportunities and challenges. *Mol. Biol. Rep.* **2024**, *51*, 538. [CrossRef] [PubMed]
105. Pani, S.; Mohapatra, S.; Sahoo, A.; Baral, B.; Debata, P.R. Shifting of cell cycle arrest from the S-phase to G2/M phase and downregulation of EGFR expression by phytochemical combinations in HeLa cervical cancer cells. *J. Biochem. Mol. Toxicol.* **2022**, *36*, e22947. [PubMed]
106. Cortez, A.J.; Tudrej, P.; Kujawa, K.A.; Lisowska, K.M. Advances in ovarian cancer therapy. *Cancer Chemother. Pharmacol.* **2018**, *81*, 17–38.
107. Essa, M.M.; Bishir, M.; Bhat, A.; Chidambaram, S.B.; Al-Balushi, B.; Hamdan, H.; Govindarajan, N.; Freidland, R.P.; Qoronfleh, M.W. Functional foods and their impact on health. *J. Food Sci. Technol.* **2023**, *60*, 820–834. [CrossRef]
108. Nandi, S.; Sikder, R.; Rapior, S.; Arnould, S.; Simal-Gandara, J.; Acharya, K. A review for cancer treatment with mushroom metabolites through targeting mitochondrial signaling pathway: In vitro and in vivo evaluations, clinical studies and future prospects for mycomedicine. *Fitoterapia* **2024**, *172*, 105681. [PubMed]
109. Islam, S.M.R.; Siddiqua, T.J. 20—Functional foods in cancer prevention and therapy: Recent epidemiological findings. In *Functional Foods in Cancer Prevention and Therapy*; Kabir, Y., Ed.; Academic Press: Cambridge, MA, USA, 2020; pp. 405–433. [CrossRef]
110. Yi, L.; Zongyuan, Y.; Cheng, G.; Lingyun, Z.; Guilian, Y.; Wei, G. Quercetin enhances apoptotic effect of tumor necrosis factor-related apoptosis-inducing ligand (TRAIL) in ovarian cancer cells through reactive oxygen species (ROS) mediated CCAAT enhancer-binding protein homologous protein (CHOP)-death receptor 5 pathway. *Cancer Sci.* **2014**, *105*, 520–527. [CrossRef]
111. Ji, H.; Zhang, Z.; Chen, C.; Xu, W.; Liu, T.; Dong, Y.; Wang, J.; Wang, H.; Zhu, X. The impact of quercetin and paclitaxel combination on ovarian cancer cells. *iScience* **2024**, *27*, 110434. [CrossRef]
112. Hashemzaei, M.; Delarami Far, A.; Yari, A.; Heravi, R.E.; Tabrizian, K.; Taghdisi, S.M.; Sadegh, S.E.; Tsarouhas, K.; Kouretas, D.; Tzanakakis, G.; et al. Anticancer and apoptosis-inducing effects of quercetin in vitro and in vivo. *Oncol. Rep.* **2017**, *38*, 819–828. [CrossRef]
113. Dhanaraj, T.; Mohan, M.; Arunakaran, J. Quercetin attenuates metastatic ability of human metastatic ovarian cancer cells via modulating multiple signaling molecules involved in cell survival, proliferation, migration and adhesion. *Arch. Biochem. Biophys.* **2021**, *701*, 108795. [PubMed]
114. Li, N.; Sun, C.; Zhou, B.; Xing, H.; Ma, D.; Chen, G.; Weng, D. Low concentration of quercetin antagonizes the cytotoxic effects of anti-neoplastic drugs in ovarian cancer. *PLoS ONE* **2014**, *9*, e100314.
115. Reyes-Farias, M.; Carrasco-Pozo, C. The Anti-Cancer Effect of Quercetin: Molecular Implications in Cancer Metabolism. *Int. J. Mol. Sci.* **2019**, *20*, 3177. [CrossRef] [PubMed]
116. Peeri, N.C.; Bertrand, K.A.; Na, R.; De Vivo, I.; Setiawan, V.W.; Seshan, V.E.; Alemany, L.; Chen, Y.; Clarke, M.A.; Clendenen, T. Understanding risk factors for endometrial cancer in young women. *JNCI J. Natl. Cancer Inst.* **2025**, *117*, 76–88.
117. Park, S.L.; Goodman, M.T.; Zhang, Z.F.; Kolonel, L.N.; Henderson, B.E.; Setiawan, V.W. Body size, adult BMI gain and endometrial cancer risk: The multiethnic cohort. *Int. J. Cancer* **2010**, *126*, 490–499.
118. Kedzia, M.; Basta, P.; Czajkowski, K.; Gogacz, M.; Spaczynski, R.; Mroczkowska, B.; Stojko, R.; Szaflik, T.; Szubert, M.; Szyllo, K. Guidelines of the Polish Society of Gynecologists and Obstetricians on the management of women with endometriosis. *Ginekol. Pol.* **2024**, *95*, 729–758. [CrossRef] [PubMed]
119. de Neufville Lucas, A.R. Lifestyle Interventions for Endometrial Cancer Survivors: Feasibility and Efficacy of a Novel Mindfulness and Dietary Counseling Program. Ph.D. Thesis, The Ohio State University, Columbus, OH, USA, 2014.
120. Slighoua, M.; Amrati, F.E.; Chebaibi, M.; Mahdi, I.; Al Kamaly, O.; El Ouahdani, K.; Drioiche, A.; Saleh, A.; Bousta, D. Quercetin and Ferulic Acid Elicit Estrogenic Activities In Vivo and In Silico. *Molecules* **2023**, *28*, 5112. [CrossRef] [PubMed]

121. Shi, Y.; Williamson, G. Quercetin lowers plasma uric acid in pre-hyperuricaemic males: A randomised, double-blinded, placebo-controlled, cross-over trial. *Br. J. Nutr.* **2016**, *115*, 800–806. [CrossRef]
122. Lee, J.-S.; Cha, Y. J.; Lee, K.-H.; Yim, J.-E. Onion peel extract reduces the percentage of body fat in overweight and obese subjects: A 12-week, randomized, double-blind, placebo-controlled study. *Nutr. Res. Pract.* **2016**, *10*, 175–181.
123. Brüll, V.; Burak, C.; Stoffel-Wagner, B.; Wolffram, S.; Nickenig, G.; Müller, C.; Langguth, P.; Alteheld, B.; Fimmers, R.; Naaf, S.; et al. Effects of a quercetin-rich onion skin extract on 24 h ambulatory blood pressure and endothelial function in overweight-to-obese patients with (pre-)hypertension: A randomised double-blinded placebo-controlled cross-over trial. *Br. J. Nutr.* **2015**, *114*, 1263–1277. [CrossRef]
124. Li, H.; Li, M.; Fu, J.; Ao, H.; Wang, W.; Wang, X. Enhancement of oral bioavailability of quercetin by metabolic inhibitory nanosuspensions compared to conventional nanosuspensions. *Drug Deliv.* **2021**, *28*, 1226–1236. [CrossRef]
125. Joseph, A.; Shanmughan, P.; Balakrishnan, A.; Maliakel, B. Enhanced Bioavailability and Pharmacokinetics of a Natural Self-Emulsifying Reversible Hybrid-Hydrogel System of Quercetin: A Randomized Double-Blinded Comparative Crossover Study. *ACS Omega* **2022**, *7*, 46825–46832. [CrossRef]
126. Van Zanden, J.J.; van der Woude, H.; Vaessen, J.; Usta, M.; Wortelboer, H.M.; Cnubben, N.H.; Rietjens, I.M. The effect of quercetin phase II metabolism on its MRP1 and MRP2 inhibiting potential. *Biochem. Pharmacol.* **2007**, *74*, 345–351. [CrossRef] [PubMed]
127. Justino, G.C.; Santos, M.R.; Canário, S.; Borges, C.; Florêncio, M.H.; Mira, L. Plasma quercetin metabolites: Structure-antioxidant activity relationships. *Arch Biochem. Biophys* **2004**, *432*, 109–121. [CrossRef] [PubMed]
128. Day, A.J.; Mellon, F.; Barron, D.; Sarrazin, G.; Morgan, M.R.; Williamson, G. Human metabolism of dietary flavonoids: Identification of plasma metabolites of quercetin. *Free. Radic. Res.* **2001**, *35*, 941–952. [PubMed]
129. Dian, L.; Yu, E.; Chen, X.; Wen, X.; Zhang, Z.; Qin, L.; Wang, Q.; Li, G.; Wu, C. Enhancing oral bioavailability of quercetin using novel soluplus polymeric micelles. *Nanoscale Res. Lett.* **2014**, *9*, 684. [PubMed]
130. Singh, A.; Kureel, A.K.; Dutta, P.; Kumar, S.; Rai, A.K. Curcumin loaded chitin-glucan quercetin conjugate: Synthesis, characterization, antioxidant, in vitro release study, and anticancer activity. *Int. J. Biol. Macromol.* **2018**, *110*, 234–244.
131. Manzoor, M.F.; Hussain, A.; Sameen, A.; Sahar, A.; Khan, S.; Siddique, R.; Aadil, R.M.; Xu, B. Novel extraction, rapid assessment and bioavailability improvement of quercetin: A review. *Ultrason. Sonochem.* **2021**, *78*, 105686. [CrossRef]
132. Nishimuro, H.; Ohnishi, H.; Sato, M.; Ohnishi-Kameyama, M.; Matsunaga, I.; Naito, S.; Ippoushi, K.; Oike, H.; Nagata, T.; Akasaka, H.; et al. Estimated daily intake and seasonal food sources of quercetin in Japan. *Nutrients* **2015**, *7*, 2345–2358. [CrossRef]

nutrients MDPI

Review

Functional Foods in Preventing Human Blood Platelet Hyperactivity-Mediated Diseases—An Updated Review

Asim K. Duttaroy

Department of Nutrition, Institute of Basic Medical Sciences, Faculty of Medicine, University of Oslo, 0313 Oslo, Norway; a.k.duttaroy@medisin.uio.no

Abstract: Backgrounds/Objectives: Abnormal platelet functions are associated with human morbidity and mortality. Platelets have emerged as critical regulators of numerous physiological and pathological processes beyond their established roles in hemostasis and thrombosis. Maintaining physiological platelet function is essential to hemostasis and preventing platelet-associated diseases such as cardiovascular disease, cancer metastasis, immune disorders, hypertension, diabetes, sickle cell disease, inflammatory bowel disease, sepsis, rheumatoid arthritis, myeloproliferative disease, and Alzheimer's disease. Platelets become hyperactive in obesity, diabetes, a sedentary lifestyle, hypertension, pollution, and smokers. Platelets, upon activation, can trawl leukocytes and progenitor cells to the vascular sites. Platelets release various proinflammatory, anti-inflammatory, and angiogenic factors and shed microparticles in the circulation, thus promoting pathological reactions. These platelet-released factors also maintain sustained activation, further impacting these disease processes. Although the mechanisms are unknown, multiple stimuli induce platelet hyperreactivity but involve the early pathways of platelet activation. The exact mechanisms of how hyperactive platelets contribute to these diseases are still unclear, and antiplatelet strategies are inevitable for preventing these diseases. Reducing platelet function during the early stages could significantly impact these diseases. However, while this is potentially a worthwhile intervention, using antiplatelet drugs to limit platelet function in apparently healthy individuals without cardiovascular disease is not recommended due to the increased risk of internal bleeding, resistance, and other side effects. The challenge for therapeutic intervention in these diseases is identifying factors that preferentially block specific targets involved in platelets' complex contribution to these diseases while leaving their hemostatic function at least partially intact. Since antiplatelet drugs such as aspirin are not recommended as primary preventives, it is essential to use alternative safe platelet inhibitors without side effects. Methods: A systematic search of the PUBMED database from 2000 to 2023 was conducted using the selected keywords: "functional foods", "polyphenols", "fatty acids", "herbs", fruits and vegetables", "cardioprotective agents", "plant", "platelet aggregation", "platelet activation", "clinical and non-clinical trial", "randomized", and "controlled". Results: Potent natural antiplatelet factors have been described, including omega-3 fatty acids, polyphenols, and other phytochemicals. Antiplatelet bioactive compounds in food that can prevent platelet hyperactivity and thus may prevent several platelet-mediated diseases, including cardiovascular disease. Conclusions: This narrative review describes the work during 2000–2023 in developing functional foods from natural sources with antiplatelet effects.

Keywords: blood platelet; functional food; phytochemicals; bioactive; cardiovascular diseases; cancer; water-soluble tomato extract; Fruitflow®; polyphenols; omega-3 fatty acids; hypertension; kiwifruit extract; platelet aggregation; diabetes

1. Introduction

Maintaining the physiological function of blood platelets is crucial for overall hemostasis and several physiological processes [1,2]. Reduced activation response of blood platelets can lead to excessive bleeding, whereas hyperactivation of platelets contributes to thrombotic complications. Platelet hyperactivity is associated with several processes, such as inflammatory and immune responses, angiogenesis, atherosclerosis, regeneration of liver tissue, and cancer metastasis [3–6]. Platelet hyperactivity is related to cardiovascular disease (CVD) and many other human diseases, such as cancer, renal diseases, Alzheimer's disease, and microorganism infections. However, the mechanisms are not well known [4,6–8]. The Framingham Heart Study revealed that persistent platelet hyperactivity is also associated with future arterial and venous thrombosis [9]. Individuals with diabetes, a sedentary lifestyle, obesity, and insulin resistance have platelet hyperactivity, which contributes to atherosclerotic plaque development and other platelet-mediated diseases [10–12]. Figure 1 depicts the association of platelet hyperactivity with CVD. Platelet hyperactivity is not only associated with CVD and stroke because platelet inhibitors also slow down cancer progression and related morbidities [13]. Platelets play critical roles in inflammation and immune responses [14,15] by supporting the release of IL-6 and NFkB [16], circulating platelet microparticles [17,18], and managing CRP levels [15,19]. A hyperinflammatory status can compromise the body's response to external stresses and predispose it to diabetes or atherosclerosis.

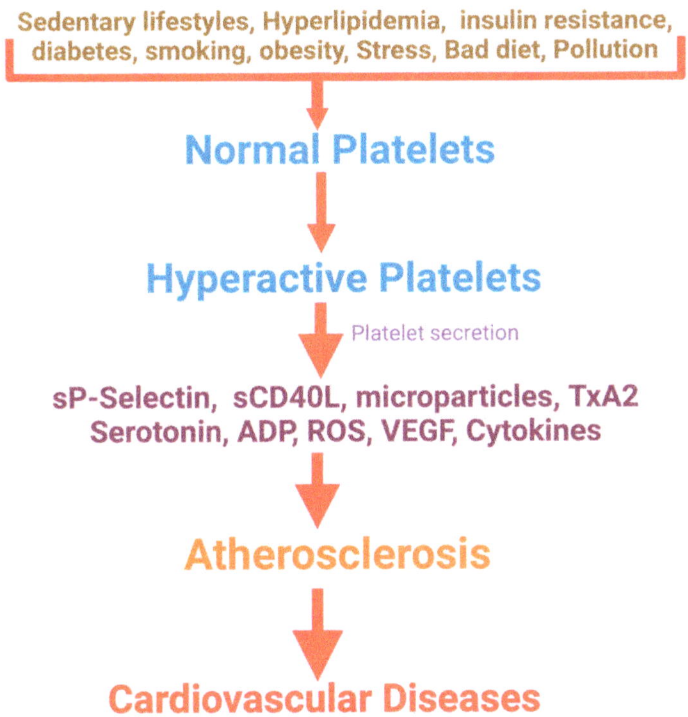

Figure 1. Hyperactivity of platelets and its impact on cardiovascular health.

Platelets play an essential role in CVD, both in the pathogenesis of atherosclerosis and in the development of acute thrombotic events. Although the mechanisms are unknown, platelets become hyperactive in insulin resistance, diabetes mellitus, obesity, smoking, dysbiosis, high-fat diet, pollution, and hyperlipidemia. Hyperactive platelets are involved in developing atherosclerosis through different mechanisms, such as membrane shedding, growth factor secretion, and the expression of several adhesive factors. In addition, hyperactive platelets are involved in the well-known penultimate thrombotic events.

Beyond the hemostatic process, platelets are involved in many processes through complicated interactions with many cells. Aspirin is the most used antiplatelet therapy for the secondary prevention of CVD [20], even though it causes several serious side effects. There are several reasons, including the fact that 25–30% of people are aspirin-resistant and the side effects, making aspirin unsuitable for the primary prevention of CVD [21]. Aspirin prophylaxis is not recommended in individuals without CVD, as per the European Guidelines on CVD prevention [22].

Maintaining regular platelet activity is critical in preventing platelet-associated diseases such as CVD, cancer metastasis, immune disorders, hypertension, diabetes mellitus, sickle cell disease, inflammatory diseases, bowel disease, rheumatoid arthritis, myeloproliferative disease, and Alzheimer's disease [23–28]. Understanding the causes and mechanisms of action of the modifying factors of platelet hyperactivity is also critical in preventing these diseases.

Consequently, there is growing interest in naturally occurring antiplatelet inhibitors that people can regularly consume. Many dietary antiplatelet components have been identified that can reduce platelet hyperactivity without side effects [29–33]. Dietary phytochemicals with antiplatelet activity become operative when continued platelet hyperactivity is experienced in response to inappropriate nutritional and lifestyle factors or exposure to smoke/air pollution [34–36], hyperglycemia and hyperlipidemia [37], and specific exercise patterns [38]. Earlier, we reviewed the mechanisms of diverse inhibitory action of various phytochemicals on platelet aggregation [4]. The bioactive compounds affect blood platelet function in multiple ways. Dietary omega-3 LCPUFAs modulate platelet function via TxB3 synthesis, modulation of platelet membranes, and increasing NO synthesis, whereas polyphenols suppress platelet activity via antioxidant activity and/or the GPIV-mediated pathway [4,29,32]. The mechanisms for individual phytochemicals are discussed in a later section. Figure 2 shows that platelet hyperactivity is related to hemostatic and non-hemostatic diseases. The relevance of platelet hyperactivity in the context of many diseases, including the growing epidemic nature of CVD, has strongly suggested the use of more natural approaches in the primary prevention of degenerative diseases. This narrative review provides an integrated summary of recent developments in platelet function in pathophysiology that connect hemostasis and other diseases. This narrative review describes the development of functional foods with antiplatelet factors during 2000–2023. A systematic search of the PUBMED database from 2000 to 2023 was conducted using the selected keywords: "functional foods", "polyphenols", "fatty acids", "herbs", "fruits and vegetables", "cardioprotective agents", "plant", "platelet aggregation", "platelet activation", "clinical and non-clinical trial", "randomized", and "controlled". This review highlights the development of bioactive compounds and their roles in preventing the hyperactivity of blood platelets and associated diseases. It suggests that targeting platelet hyperactivity early with antiplatelet regimes may prevent CVD and other diseases.

Platelets are versatile cells engaged in numerous pathophysiological processes, including inflammation and immunity, angiogenesis, regeneration, and carcinogenesis. Platelets become hyperactive under different conditions, and hyperactive platelets contribute to different diseases, as described in this diagram. Platelets are also crucial in thrombosis and hemostasis via various molecular and cellular events. This figure introduces the emerging role of platelets in the immune system, vascular biology, tumorigenesis, and beyond.

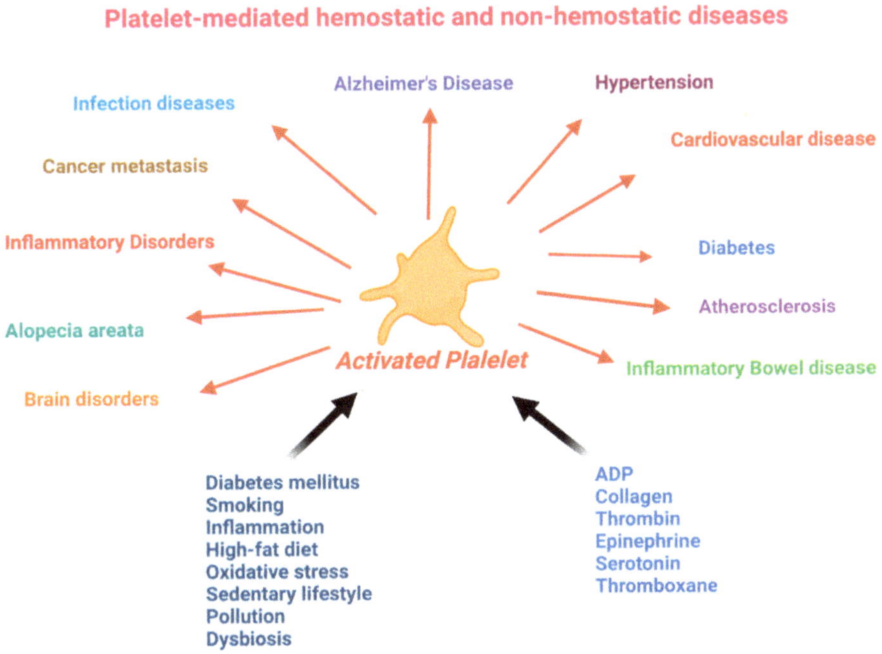

Figure 2. Roles of platelets in several hemostatic and non-hemostatic pathways.

2. Platelet Hyperactivity in Many Pathological Conditions

Human blood platelets are involved in hemostasis and thrombosis, including inflammation, infection, immunobiology, cancer metastasis, wound repair, and angiogenesis [39]. Platelets' vast capacity to regulate various physiological and pathological processes is primarily due to their granular storage and secretion of a wide range of biologically active agents and microparticles [40]. In addition, various platelet subpopulations exhibit biochemical and functional variability impacting these processes [41]. Therefore, multiple functions of platelets are possibly due to the apparent modulation of functions. Thus, platelets are no longer considered only for their roles in the hemostatic system. Platelet functional tests, such as platelet aggregation response and closure time, etc., are used to investigate the possible role of platelet hyperreactivity in the pathogenesis of vascular disorders and their complications.

Since platelet hyperreactivity increases in hyperlipidemia, hyperglycemia, oxidative stress, and cancers [42,43], understanding how platelets become hyperresponsive and contribute to CVD under these conditions is needed to prevent CVD [44]. Platelets maintain endothelial integrity; however, when activated, they disturb endothelium by interacting with their secretions [45,46]. Activated platelets secrete mRNA, nucleotides, enzymes, metal ions, microparticles, mitochondria, ATP, ADP, growth factors, chemokines, cytokines, protease inhibitors, adhesive glycoproteins serotonin, histamine, γ-aminobutyric acid, glutamate, epinephrine, dopamine, histamine, factor V, calcium, and many others [47–49]. Platelet microvesicles contain multiple RNAs and proteins involved in these processes [50,51]. In addition, platelets secrete microparticles and microvesicles that are empowered with angiogenic, immunosuppressive, and survival abilities [52–54]. The release of these factors by the activated platelets changes the cell membrane architecture and cell shape, including blood vessel walls, affecting the immediate milieu [30]. Platelet activation, aggregation, and the subsequent generation of an occlusive intra-arterial thrombus are essential in developing CVD and platelet-mediated diseases [55,56]. The most harmful consequence of sustained platelet hyperactivity is the widespread deposition of the micro aggregates on the vessel walls. Therefore, lowering baseline platelet activity may be necessary to impair platelet hyperactivity-mediated diseases.

Pathological Conditions Such as Metabolic Syndrome, Insulin Resistance, Obesity, Hypertension, and Tumors Enhance Platelet Hyperactivity

Platelets are activated by many agonists released in the circulation during pathologic conditions [57]. Platelet hyperactivity is also an underlying risk for diabetes, smoking, obesity, a sedentary lifestyle, pollution, dysbiosis, and other conditions. Inflammation may be exacerbated in patients with hypertension, CVD, and obesity, all associated with baseline platelet hyperreactivity [30,58]. Although the exact mechanism of platelet hyperactivity is not well known in these conditions, it could result from the sensitization of blood platelets to activation/aggregation by agonists [59] and/or due to the redistribution of young, more reactive platelets in the spleen [59] released into the circulation.

Metabolic syndrome (MetS) is a cluster of conditions related to abdominal obesity, insulin resistance, hyperlipidemia, hypertension, and inflammation [60]. MetS is associated with increased platelet reactivity, probably caused by associated hyperglycemia, dyslipidemia, and low-grade systemic inflammation. Platelet hyperactivity in MetS is induced by inflammation, obesity, dyslipidemia, hypertension, oxidative stress, and other metabolic disease [61]. Higher plasma levels of fibrinogen, PAI-1, thrombin, von Willebrand factor, factor VII, and other coagulation factors, as well as significant platelet aggregation, are also observed in MetS [62].

The MetS components increase platelet activation by increasing the calcium concentration and activating arachidonic acid, 20:4n-6 (ARA) signaling pathways. Platelet hyperactivity in dyslipidemia contributes to the thrombotic risk [63]. Platelet activation in dyslipidemia is induced via classic agonist receptor signaling pathways and pattern recognition receptors [63]. Platelets are stimulated by oxidized phospholipids present in low-density lipoproteins (LDLs) via specific pattern recognition receptors [64]. CD36/fatty acid translocase is platelets' scavenger receptor for oxidized lipids [64].

Oxidative stress may promote platelet hyperactivity by reducing physiologically accessible NO in MetS. Cigarette smoking and sedentary lifestyles also increase oxidative stress and platelet hyperactivity [35]. Platelets oxidize LDL by stimulating the production of reactive oxygen species (ROS) and degrading the LDL receptors by releasing proprotein convertase subtilisin/kexin type 9. Thus, platelet dysfunction and hyperlipidemia stimulate atherogenesis [65]. Moreover, reduced antiplatelet response to aspirin and higher platelet sensitivity toward agonists are observed in MetS. Therefore, hypolipidemic drugs modulate platelet function, whereas antiplatelet drugs normalize lipid metabolism. High levels of plasma leptin in obesity cause increased platelet aggregability [66]. The overall effect of MetS and obesity contributes to platelet activation [67]. Certain adipokines directly influence platelet function and, therefore, have the potential to serve as essential mediators of the cardiovascular consequences of obesity. Consistent with this, obesity is associated with elevations in platelet activation markers such as P-selectin expression and increased platelet microparticle shedding, resulting in increased platelet aggregation. The decreased adipose mass normalizes the markers of enhanced platelet activation. However, a causal role for platelet hyperactivity in obesity-related cardiovascular disorders is yet to be established.

Platelet function is influenced by ROS and nitric oxide (NO) metabolism [68,69]. Platelet aggregation is associated with increased glutathione disulfide levels and oxygen utilization. Changes may influence platelet-dependent thrombus formation in platelet or vascular redox status, antioxidants, ROS, and nitrogen species [70] creation. Hyperglycemia, dyslipidemia, and insulin resistance in diabetic conditions induce platelet hyperactivity, activation of the vascular wall, inflammation, and endothelial dysfunction. Hyperglycemia also causes the overproduction of superoxide and activates protein kinase C and nuclear factor kB (NFkB) [71]. NFkB stimulates the production of several inflammatory cytokines and increases cell adhesion molecules, such as CD40 ligand (CD40L). CD40L induces the production and release of proinflammatory cytokines [72]. Activated platelets express CD40L, indicating a link between hemostasis and inflammation [73].

Diabetic platelets have an increased intrinsic activation profile, whereas these platelets have the reduced influence of endogenous inhibitors and drugs. Thus, platelet hyperactivity in diabetes mellitus results from hypersensitivity to agonists and loss of the antiaggregatory mechanism. Diabetics' platelet hyperactivity is associated with increased circulating platelet microparticles and hypercoagulability [37]. Even though the usefulness of antiplatelet drugs in type 2 diabetes is not supported, diabetic patients still use low-dose aspirin or other antiplatelet drugs as a potential therapeutic therapy [74,75]. In diabetes mellitus, there is an imbalance between platelet inhibitors such as NO and prostacyclin (PGI_2) and increased production of platelet-activating and vasoconstricting substances. Decreased endothelium synthesis of PGI_2 [76] and reduced synthesis of NO was observed in type 2 diabetes mellitus [77]. Platelets express receptors for adhesion and increased synthesis of TxA_2, thrombin, and deranged calcium metabolism in diabetes. Platelets shed more platelet microparticles in type 2 diabetics and thus may play a role in inflammation and thrombosis. P-selectin-positive platelet microparticles may aid in the recruitment and adhesion of leucocytes, and platelets initiate the atherosclerosis process.

Spontaneous platelet activation is involved in hypertension [78–80]. High blood pressure also stimulates platelet activation via increasing the shear force on circulating platelets. Increased blood viscosity in patients with high blood pressure might also contribute to platelet hyperactivity. Under high-pressure flow, enhanced degranulation of platelets occurs [81]. Atherosclerotic lesions induce platelet activation, possibly due to the dysfunctional endothelium and local flow disturbances [82]. Numerous metabolic and physiologic changes occur in platelet reactivity in hypertension. Indeed, many studies have shown that various parameters of platelet activation are normalized with the treatment of hypertension [83]. Platelets from hypertensive patients tend to form aggregates [84], increased secretion of plasma β-thromboglobulin [85], high soluble and membrane expression of P-selectin [86], and increased intracellular levels of calcium [87]. However, the association between these markers and the degree of hypertension or responses to therapy are not well known [88]. Platelet activation and aggregation are also involved in the development of hypertension in different ways. Activated platelets release mediators, such as 5-hydroxytryptamine (5-HT or serotonin), ADP, ATP and lysophosphatidic acid [89]. Several of these agents enhance the intracellular Ca^{2+} concentration in vascular smooth muscle cells, promoting vasoconstriction and increasing the response of catecholamines.

Furthermore, the number of platelet α-adrenergic receptors increases in hypertension [90], which increases catecholamine responses. Catecholamines and angiotensin II increase intracellular Ca^{2+} concentration and promote contraction of vascular smooth muscle cells, platelet activation, and aggregation [90], which may participate in the genesis and maintenance of hypertension. Angiotensin II (Ang II) increases intracellular Ca^{2+} concentration and pH in platelets, which increases platelet sensitivity to aggregating agents [91–93]. Hypertensive platelets produce more reactive oxygen species (ROS) [85] that enhance platelet activity by reducing the bioavailability of NO and enhancing intracellular Ca^{2+} concentration. Inflammation is also exacerbated in hypertension, CVD, and obesity, all associated with baseline platelet hyperreactivity [30,58].

Endothelial dysfunction is associated with the reduced production of platelet inhibitors and vasodilators, and NO [94]. Therefore, the reduced synthesis of NO increases hypertension and platelet hyperactivity [95]. Similarly, dysfunctional endothelium produces less PGI_2 and increases platelet activity. Dysfunction of the endothelium in hypertension has a cross-talk with hyperactive platelets [83]. Similarly, increased platelet activation/aggregation in response to endothelin could contribute to thrombosis [96]. Hyperactive platelets are a critical earlier trigger for cancer-associated thrombotic events [97,98]. Interactions between platelets and tumor cells result in hyperactivity or activation of circulating blood platelets.

3. Modulation of Platelet Activity by Bioactive Compounds of Dietary Origin

Since the blockade of crucial platelet-activation pathways may prevent platelet hyperreactivity [99], a dietary antiplatelet agent is considered suitable for suppressing platelet hyperactivity in non-CVD people. Antiplatelet drugs would be inappropriate in such a public health setting. Reducing platelet function during the early stages could significantly impact the number of diseases. Natural antiplatelet functional foods have been developed to target platelet hyperactivity early and they have been investigated and may be able reduce several diseases. Nutritional modification of cellular functions by dietary lipids and other nutritive and non-nutritive factors offers an attractive avenue to correct, modify, or prevent many pathophysiological processes, including platelet hyperactivity [100]. Indeed, extensive in vitro and preclinical research demonstrates the efficacy of various food components in reducing platelet hyperactivity. The antiaggregatory effects of different aqueous fruit extracts on human platelets in vitro have been published previously [29]. However, there are only a small number of well-designed studies consistently demonstrating an antiplatelet benefit of only a few select dietary ingredients in healthy human subjects with measurable clinical outcomes. These include fish and fish oil, flavonoids in cocoa, and garlic. Various studies demonstrated that polyphenol supplementation affects platelet aggregation and function in vitro and in vivo, mainly neutralizing free radicals, inhibiting platelet activation via related signal transduction pathways, blocking TxA_2 receptors, and enhancing NO production. The effect of dietary polyphenols on platelet aggregation in vivo is often conflicting. Only flavanols mirrored in vivo showed efficacy in modulating platelet function in vitro [101]. In addition to fish oils, some plant oils may inhibit blood platelet activation. Since some plant oils contain linolenic acid, 18:3n-3, and phytosterols can prevent platelet hyperactivity [102] but require more human intervention trials for further confirmation.

Therefore, this review's objectives are two-fold: summarize the available clinical science to substantiate the antiplatelet efficacy of these ingredients and highlight recent and emerging clinical evidence for a new dietary antiplatelet component derived from fruits, vegetables, and fish oils. The antiplatelet benefits of these ingredients on humans, along with clearly defined outcomes related to the primary prevention of vascular events, namely platelet function, are discussed. Therefore, there is an increased interest in identifying bioactive compounds from edible sources with beneficial health effects, efficiency, and fewer adverse effects [4,30,103].

4. Omega-3 Fatty Acids

Since the first cross-cultural epidemiological studies in the 1970s, the CVD-preventive role of omega-3 long-chain polyunsaturated fatty acids (LCPUFAs), in particular docosahexaenoic acid, 22:6n-3 (DHA), and eicosapentaenoic acid, 20:5n-3 (EPA), has emerged [104]. Fish oil supplementation reduced platelet aggregation [105]. Essential fatty acids, linoleic acid, 18:2n-6 (LA), and alpha-linolenic acid, 18:3n-3 (ALA), in turn, compete for desaturase and elongase enzymes for their metabolism to LCPUFAs. A higher dietary intake of ALA compared to LA leads to an enhanced synthesis of EPA and DHA metabolites, resulting in a higher production of TxA_3 than the proaggregatory ARA-derived TxA_2. Prostaglandin H_2 is a precursor of other prostaglandins and thromboxane [106]. Antiplatelet mechanisms of action by DHA and EPA are thought to be mediated via inhibition of phospholipase A_2 activity, which would diminish the liberation of ARA from platelet plasma membrane phospholipids; inhibition of platelet cyclooxygenase 1 (COX-1), which would decrease the conversion of ARA to TxA_2; competition with ARA for platelet COX-1 and formation of less active TxA_3, or by alteration of platelet membrane fluidity state; and inhibition of TxA_2 induced platelet aggregation and decreased receptor affinity for TxA_2 [107].

Omega-3 LCPUFAs have gained considerable attention for their ability to improve cardiovascular health and prognosis. In contrast, the n-6 fatty acids such as linoleic acid, 18:2n-6, and ARA may increase platelet aggregation. Both EPA and DHA are incorporated into platelet membrane phospholipids, replacing ARA, thus decreasing platelet aggregation via reduced production of ARA-derived platelet-aggregating eicosanoids [29,108]. EPA also competes with ARA for COX, reducing ARA-derived metabolites. Therefore, EPA minimizes the synthesis of the proaggregatory ARA-derived TXA_2 [109,110]. EPA and DHA also alter membrane fluidity, regulating receptor expression and thrombin generation [111–113]. Resolvins produced from both EPA (resolvins E) and DHA (resolvins D) reduce and inhibit thromboxane-induced platelet aggregation [114]. Oxylipins (11-HDHA and 14-HDHA) derived from DHA also inhibited protein kinase A-mediated platelet activation and regulated agonist-induced platelet aggregation [115]. DHA and its 12-LOX-derived oxylipins also modulated collagen-induced platelet aggregation.

Several studies, such as in vitro, clinical trials, observational, epidemiological, and animal studies, investigated the impact of seafood consumption and omega-3 fatty acids on CVD. Human clinical studies showed that omega-3 LCPUFAs impart antiplatelet effects. Fischer et al. (1983) [116] showed that EPA supplementation at 4 gm per day through cod liver oil in eight healthy adult males for 25 days reduced platelet aggregation. In contrast, Gibney and Bolton-Smith (1988) [117] demonstrated that consumption of a low dose of EPA (2.25 gm) plus DHA (1.35 gm) per day did not affect platelet aggregation in response to collagen or low levels of ADP in eight healthy adult males for six weeks. However, there was a significant increase in platelet aggregation when higher levels of ADP were used.

Additionally, platelet TxB2 production was affected [117]. In contrast to other studies, the lack of DHA and EPA effect on platelet function may be due to the low dose of the omega-3 fatty acids used in this study. In a randomized, double-blind study by Li and Steiner (1991), 3, 6, or 9 gm EPA per day supplementation to fifteen healthy adults for three weeks reduced platelet adhesion to fibrinogen within the first week. Under low shear rates conditions, the 3 and 6 gm per day inhibited platelet adhesion by 81.7% and 85.5%, respectively, and the 9 gm dose inhibited rates of platelet adhesion at a similar level to the 3 gm dose. In contrast, platelet adhesion was maximally inhibited at high shear rates by the 3 gm of EPA per day [118].

Pirich and colleagues (1991) also demonstrated that supplementing twenty healthy adult subjects with EPA (216 mg) plus DHA (140 mg) per day for six weeks reduced TxB2 synthesis and significantly increased platelet survival time [119]. Indeed, the levels of DHA and EPA used were remarkably low, considering the positive benefits observed. However, this study's fish oil supplementation regimen also provided 390 mg of gamma-linolenic acid, 18:3n-6. So, whether the effects observed above were due to the combination of DHA and EPA or the three fatty acids is unclear.

In 2002, Svaneborg and colleagues showed that 10 gm of fish oil per day to eighteen healthy adults significantly decreased TxA_2 production and showed no change in the bleeding time [120]. In a more extensive randomized, double-blind study, Eschen et al. (2004) reported that EPA (3 gm) and DHA (2.9 gm) per day to sixty healthy adults for 12 weeks significantly decreased plasma P-selectin levels, used as an index of platelet activation [121]. Consuming omega-3 fatty acids for four weeks reduced platelet integrin (GPIIa/IIIb) activation, levels of fibrinogen, and factor V, but no effect on coagulation in healthy subjects [122]. In 2008, Din and colleagues showed that 500 gm per day of mackerel consumption for four weeks reduced platelet-monocyte aggregation by ~35%, which returned to baseline after cessation of fish consumption [123]. However, Eschen et al. (2004) found no change in soluble P-selectin levels [121]. More recently, an open-label 4-week sequential study showed that EPA (1.86 gm) and DHA (1.5 gm) per day supplementation to thirty healthy adults decreased GPIIa/IIIb activation and significantly reduced the expression of P-selectin [124]. Vericel and colleagues (1999) demonstrated that a low dose of EPA (30 mg) plus DHA (150 mg) per day for 42 days resulted in a reduction in platelet aggregation but not significantly [125]. These data contrast with those published by Croset et al. (1990) [126] and Driss et al. (1984) [127]. Therein, both investigators showed that low supplementation of EPA in elderly subjects significantly decreased platelet aggregation. In the study by Croset et al. (1990) [126], healthy elderly subjects were provided with the EPA from (1984), which provided 150 mg EPA per day for one month [127]. The discrepancy in the findings between the Vericel et al. study (1999) and that of Driss and colleagues (1984) and Croset and colleagues (1990) is most likely due to the level of EPA supplementation. In 2009, Guillot and coworkers [128] demonstrated that 400 and 800 mg DHA per day for two weeks to twelve healthy elderly subjects significantly reduced platelet reactivity and TxA_2 production. Still, this effect was reversed when 1600 mg DHA per day was consumed. DHA intake at 200 mg/day did not affect platelet reactivity or TxA_2 production. The lack of an effect of very high intakes of DHA and EPA in healthy elderly subjects on platelet activity is consistent with findings from Larson et al. (2008), who showed no inhibition of platelet aggregation with 4 gm of omega-3 LCPUFAs per day for 4 weeks [124]. Most studies support the antiplatelet effect of marine fish or oils in healthy human subjects; although the dose used appears to be key in dictating a benefit, low and high doses do not always show a benefit.

Indeed, a meta-analysis of 15 randomized controlled trials in humans has confirmed that omega-3 LCPUFAs inhibit platelet aggregation [110]. EPA has also reduced P-selectin, oxidized LDL (ox-LDL) antibodies, and glycoprotein IIb/IIIa expression on the platelet membranes [129]. Consuming 6.6 g of omega-3 LCPUFAs reduced serum P-selectin expression, which may help to decrease platelet activity [121]. However, the increase in the n-6/n-3 ratio has shifted the balance into a proaggregatory state.

The data on the primary and secondary prevention of CVD using omega-3 LCPUFAs are controversial. The latest meta-analysis suggests that regular intake of fish oil may be a risk factor for atrial fibrillation and stroke among the general population. However, it may be beneficial in certain CVD cases [130]. The published data support the use of omega-3 LCPUFAs in reducing the risk of CVD or CVD-related death. The expert guidelines consistently recommend consuming at least 250 mg/day of omega-3 LCPUFAs or at least two servings/week of oily fish for the general population [131]. However, the beneficial role of omega-3 LCPUFAs in CVD is still not sure [132–134]. The clinical trials showed limited or no effect on cardiovascular health, which may result from heterogeneous populations, background omega-3 LCPUFA status, and consumption discrepancies [135].

However, it is considered appropriate for all individuals to consume omega-3 LCPUFA daily as there are some benefits associated with CVD risk reduction and no adverse effects at the recommended levels. Epidemiological and intervention studies showed that dietary intakes between 0.4 g and 1.8 g/day of omega-3 LCPUFAs are optimum for cardiovascular health. Several systematic reviews, meta-analyses, and experts examined the role of omega-3 LCPUFAs on the cardiovascular system [131,136–142]. Expert recommendations generally support the cardiovascular health benefit of omega-3 LCPUFAs with a recommendation for a daily intake of 500 mg as DHA and EPA or 1–2 servings of seafood per week. The US Dietary Advisory Committee recommends at least two servings of seafood per week. American Heart Association recommends one to two seafood meals per week to prevent the risk of congestive heart failure, coronary heart disease, ischemic stroke, and sudden cardiac death [138].

Meta-analyses of several randomized trials indicated that omega-3 LCPUFAs positively affect CVD outcomes for primary and secondary prevention. Marine omega-3 LCPUFAs also improve CVD risk factors, including blood pressure, plasma lipids, and inflammation; however, many physicians do not recommend omega-3 fatty acids, mainly due to controversial results in randomized trials.

5. Plant Polyphenols

Plant polyphenols protect the cardiovascular system by reducing platelet hyperactivity and oxidative stress [143]. Since oxidative stress triggers inflammatory disorders, the basis for developing diseases such as immune disorders, atherosclerotic lesions, and plaque rupture, antioxidants are believed to slow the progression of many diseases, including CVD. Polyphenols can impart several health benefits, including protection from atherosclerosis, thrombosis, inflammation, and platelet hyperactivity [143–146]. The amount of polyphenols varies in plant-based foods, including fruits, chocolate, beverages, vegetables, and grains [101]. All polyphenols have the basic structure of an aromatic ring with a hydroxyl group. Polyphenols are mainly two groups, flavonoids, and nonflavonoids, despite numerous classes based on their carbon skeleton, phenol rings, and structural elements [101]. Flavonoids are further classified into flavonols, isoflavones, flavanones, anthocyanins, and flav-3-ols, whereas non-flavonoids consist of phenolic acids, hydrolyzable tannins, and stilbenes.

There is accumulating epidemiological and clinical evidence demonstrating that flavanol-rich foods can positively influence hemostasis through mechanisms that directly or indirectly affect platelet function and, in this way, ultimately decrease the risk for hypertension and stroke [147,148]. Plant-derived foods and beverages like red wine, tea, grapes, grape juice, cocoa, and chocolate are typically flavonol-rich and affect platelet aggregation.

Hamed et al. (2008) proposed that flavonoids can competitively inhibit binding to platelet-derived growth factor and TxA_2 receptors, negating the effects of ARA—and collagen-induced platelet aggregation [149]. In addition to their antioxidant activity, flavonoids inhibit platelet lipoxygenase or reduce phospholipase C activity [150].

Most clinical studies were conducted with cocoa because cocoa products contain more flavonoids than teas and wines [151,152]. Wright et al. [153] demonstrated that functional groups of the flavonoid skeleton regulated the polyphenol inhibition of collagen-induced aggregation. The flavonoid aglycone increases the hydroxyl groups on the A and B rings, decreasing flavonoid activity. In contrast, the presence of O-methyl groups can increase activity. On the other hand, a hydroxyl group at position C3 can increase flavonoid activity [154]. In a study of 30 healthy adults, Rein et al. (2000) demonstrated that a cocoa beverage containing 18.75 g procyanidin and a total epicatechin content of 897 mg inhibited platelet aggregation and suppressed membrane GPIIa/IIIb expression and reduced the shedding of platelet microparticles. Platelet microparticles are hemostatically active, phospholipid-rich microvesicles formed by activated platelets [155]. Using the same level of flavonoids in another study of sixteen healthy young men, Pearson and coworkers (2002) showed no effect on GPIIa/IIIb activity or P-selectin expression. Heptinstall et al. (2006) evaluated the impact of different amounts of cocoa-containing flavonoids in twelve healthy volunteers [147]. Study participants consumed 80 mg, 300 mg, 600 mg, or 900 mg cocoa flavanols. Cocoa drinks containing 600 or 900 mg of cocoa flavanols significantly inhibited platelet aggregation [147]. Tomato extract, Fruitflow®, is also a good source of polyphenols [156], which is discussed in a later section.

Flavonols are present in red wine, tea, grapes, grape juice, cocoa, and chocolates. Hermann and colleagues (2006) showed 40 gm of dark chocolate consumption by 20 healthy adult male smokers significantly improved flow-mediated dilation and decreased platelet adhesion [152]. Hamed and coworkers also evaluated the benefits of cocoa flavanols through dark chocolate consumption [149]. Consumption of dark chocolate (100 g) for one week (~70% cocoa; 700 mg flavonoids) significantly decreased GPIIa/IIIb expression [149]. Both the studies mentioned here are consistent with the findings of Innes et al. (2003) [157]. Consuming cocoa-related products in moderate amounts inhibited platelet aggregation [158].

Several reviews documented the impact of polyphenols on platelet function. Using different agonists, polyphenols' antithrombotic properties are determined by measuring their inhibitory effect on whole blood or platelet-rich plasma aggregation [29,32,159–161]. Table 1 summarizes the impact of the consumption of polyphenols on platelet aggregation ex vivo. Cocoa is a rich flavonoid source that modulates platelet activity, including catechins, proanthocyanins, anthocyanins, and flavonol glycosides [162]. Cocoa supplementation inhibited platelet aggregation when consumed acutely or chronically [163].

Table 1. Ex vivo effects of polyphenols on platelet aggregation in animals and human trials.

Source	Models	Experimental Conditions	Conclusions
Chlorogenic acid	Mice (n = 18)	Inhibition of in vivo thrombus formation	Inhibited thrombus formation [164].
Anthocyanin cyanidin-3-glucoside from purified black rice	Mice (n = 60)	Mice randomly assigned to 3 groups (n = 20): control group, high-fat diet, or a high-fat diet + Anthocyanin cyanidin-3-glucoside	Decreased platelet activation, and inhibited platelet ATP release [165].
Red wine polyphenols (Provinols™)	Rats (n = 149)	Rats were randomly grouped as treated with or without aldosterone–salt, with or without Provinols (20 mg/kg/day) or spironolactone (30 mg/kg/day) for 4 weeks	Provinols decreased circulating levels microparticles [166].
Cocoa	Healthy males (n = 16)	Double-blind, crossover study. Placebo-controlled. Eight subjects in two groups (trained and untrained) randomly received placebo or cocoa polyphenol (236 mg/day) for a week and then afterwards were subjected to one hour of exercise	No change in collagen induced platelet aggregation post-exercise. ATP release higher post-exercise in both groups. Cocoa supplementation did not normalize platelet activity after exercise [167].
Chicory coffee	Healthy subjects (n = 27)	Chicory coffee (300 mL) consumed every day for 1 week	Effect on platelet aggregation is variable depending on the agonists used [168].
High polyphenol beverage	Healthy Athletes (n = 103)	Group 1 received a polyphenol-rich beverage, Group 2 a placebo in a randomized, double-blind study. Samples were collected three weeks before, one day before, immediately, and 24 h and 72 h after a marathon run	Control group demonstrated a 2.2-fold increase in platelet aggregation after marathon completion. But there was no increase in platelet aggregation in polyphenol-rich beverage group [169].
Polyphenol-rich grape wine	Untreated, mildly hypertensive subjects (n = 60)	Grape juice extract; grape and wine extract each for 4 weeks including a 2-week run-in period in a double-blind placebo-controlled crossover study	There was no effect on ADP, collagen, or epinephrine induced platelet aggregation [170].
Polyphenol-rich grape seed extract	Untreated subjects with pre- and stage 1 hypertension (n = 35)	Double-blind, placebo-controlled, randomized, parallel-group intervention with 300 mg/day grape seed extract capsule. Eight-week duration study	Platelet aggregation was not affected [171].
Flavanol-rich chocolate	Patients with congestive heart failure (n = 20)	A total of 2 h after consumption of a chocolate bar and 4 weeks of consumption (two chocolate bars/day) in a double-blind, randomized placebo-controlled trial	Platelet adhesion significantly decreased 2 h after flavanol-rich chocolate ingestion. But no effect after 2- and 4-week supplementation [172].
Chokeberry (*Aronia mitschurinii*) products	Patients with untreated mild hypertension (n = 38)	Cold-pressed 100% chokeberry juice (300 mL/day) and oven-dried chokeberry powder (3 g/day), or placebo for 8 weeks without washout in a single-blinded crossover trial for 16 weeks	No change in platelet aggregation response [173].
Oats	Type 2 diabetes subjects (n = 22)	Randomized crossover involving 8-week intervention with either oat-enriched diet or a standard dietary advised diet. Pre-intervention habitual intakes were used to compare responses	Decreased in tissue factor-activated platelets (CD142) after oat-rich diet than habitual or standard advised diet. Decreased in tissue factor-positive platelet microparticles and fibrinogen-positive platelet microparticles with oat-enriched diet intervention [174].
Anthocyanin-rich beverage	Sedentary subjects (n = 21)	Queen garnet plum juice (200 mL/day) were consumed for 28 days in a double-blind placebo-controlled study	Reduced ADP-, collagen-, and ARA-induced platelet aggregation. Reduced P-selectin expression.

Olive leaf extract contains various polyphenols and flavones that inhibit platelet aggregation and ATP release 176 The olive leaf polyphenols inhibit oxidative stress-induced platelet activation via antioxidant activity [167]. Polyphenol reduces degranulation by scavenging H_2O_2, a substrate involved in COX-1 activation. Nevertheless, polyphenols can inhibit aggregation and secretion by inhibiting intracellular pathways in platelets.

Chlorogenic acid present in fruits inhibits collagen- and ADP-induced platelet aggregation [164]. Polyphenols dose-dependently inhibit platelet aggregation and ATP release mediated via the purinergic receptor and GPVI pathways [164]. In vitro studies showed that ellagic acid modulates platelet intracellular signaling pathways involving PLC/PKC pathways.

Zhou et al. [165] reported that anthocyanin cyanidin-3-glucoside (C3G) significantly attenuated thrombin-induced platelet activation and ATP secretion in mice fed with high-fat diets. C3G also inhibited thrombin and collagen-induced platelet aggregation [175]. Other low bioavailable polyphenols also had antiplatelet activity [176].

Hydroxytyrosol (HT) acetate and aspirin have similar antiaggregatory activity [170]. However, HT acetate had higher antiaggregation activity than HT. A more significant antiaggregation impact of aspirin and HT acetate was observed in whole blood aggregation induced by ADP or collagen compared with aggregation in platelet-rich plasma, indicating an alternative aggregation pathway involving leucocytes, erythrocytes, platelets, and other plasma proteins. Aspirin and the two phenolic compounds increase NO production in leucocytes, thus contributing to the antiaggregation effect. NO can also affect platelet aggregation by modulating cAMP, cGMP, and TxA_2 synthesis. Propolis inhibited ADP-induced platelet aggregation via the P2Y12 pathway [171] by decreasing the expression of the fibrinogen receptor (GPIIb/IIIa) [172].

Gallic acid inhibits ADP-induced platelet aggregation via decreasing intracellular Ca^{2+} levels, reducing phosphorylation and P-selectin secretion [173]. Olas et al. [174] demonstrated that grape seed extracts (gallic acid, falvan-3-ols, and proanthocyanins) inhibited thrombin- and thrombin receptor-activation peptide (TRAP)-induced platelet activation and platelet microparticle formation more than resveratrol [177]. Furthermore, resveratrol and its analog isorhapontigenin inhibited ADP-induced platelet aggregation [175]. Polyphenols inhibit the COX-1 and $P2Y_{12}$ pathways and may also attenuate platelet microparticles generation in activated platelets [176]. Several polyphenols in grape seed extracts may interact with different pathways involved in platelet function. Table 1 shows the ex vivo effects of polyphenols on platelet aggregation in animal and human trials.

Trimethyl-N-oxide (TMAO) is involved in the pathology of various diseases, including cancer and CVD [178]. TMA is synthesized by the gut microbiota using dietary choline and L-carnitine as substrate; then, it is carried into the liver and converted to TMAO by flavin-containing monooxygenase 3 [178]. The conversion of choline and carnitine to TMA depends on gut microbiota diversity [178]. Therefore, gut dysbiosis increases high plasma TMAO levels and thus may ultimately result in atherosclerosis and CVD. TMAO induces platelet hyperreactivity and dyslipidemia and enhances platelet-mediated diseases such as atherosclerosis, insulin resistance, CVD, and other diseases [179,180]. TMAO enhances sub-maximal stimulus-dependent platelet activation by agonists through increased Ca^{2+} release [179]. Gut dysbiosis promotes atherosclerosis by increasing the production of TMAO [181–183]. Gut metagenome analysis showed a relatively lower abundance of *Roseburia* and *Eubacterium*, while TMA-producing *Collinsella* was higher in CVD patients [184]. Targeting the gut microbiota and its metabolites can effectively treat and prevent CVD by modulating TMAO levels [185,186]. Several polyphenol-rich products lower plasma TMAO levels both in animals and humans [187–189]. Chen et al. [187] first showed that resveratrol decreases atherosclerosis via reduced production of TMAO synthesis via remodeling gut microbiota. This observation was corroborated in rodents [188]. A study involving 20 normal-weight subjects showed a significant decrease in serum TMAO after four weeks of supplementation with 300 mg of polyphenol-rich grape pomace [189]. The polyphenol-rich extract tomato extracts lowered plasma TMAO in obese adults via modulation of gut microbiota [156].

6. Water-Soluble Extracts from Tomato and Kiwifruit: The Latest Dietary Antiplatelet Regimes

Hyperlipzidemia, hypertension, and hyperactivity of blood platelets are critical contributors to the pathogenesis of CVD [190]. Hyperactive platelets, as observed in diabetes mellitus, insulin resistance, obesity, sedentary life, and smoking, contribute to the development of CVD [191–196]. Hyperactivity of platelets contributes to the progression of atherosclerotic plaque and other diseases [108,197]. Therefore, there is a need to decrease platelet hyperactivity through safe, effective, and practical approaches to prevent the risk of CVD and other platelet-mediated diseases. Consumption of fruits and vegetables protects against CVD [198–200]. The phytochemicals in fruits and vegetables may protect the cardiovascular system via different mechanisms, such as favorably modulating oxidative stress, plasma lipid levels, hypertension, normalizing platelet hyperactivity, and other CVD risk factors [31,201]. For example, plant flavonoids inhibit cyclic nucleotide phosphodiesterase enzyme and platelet TxA_2 synthesis, the main mechanisms responsible for inhibiting platelet activation.

Consequently, these phytochemicals in fruits may reduce more than one CVD risk factor, such as platelet hyperactivity [29,202]. Such nutritional antiplatelet regimes were identified in the water-soluble extract in tomatoes and kiwifruits [33,203,204]. The aqueous extract of tomatoes, also known as Fruitflow®, has undergone the most extensive preclinical and clinical testing to demonstrate its efficacy in inhibiting platelet hyperactivity. Recent studies showed that tamarillo, horned melon (kiwano), and raspberry extracts inhibited ADP-induced platelet aggregation [205].

7. Tomato

Epidemiological studies demonstrated that consumption of tomato and tomato products is associated with a reduced risk of CVD [206–208]. Tomatoes contain several compounds that might affect plasma lipids and platelet aggregation. During the last two decades, numerous studies have demonstrated that tomato's water-soluble components inhibit blood platelet aggregation both in vitro and in vivo [30,33,204,209]. This water-soluble tomato extract (trade name Fruitflow®) was the first food ingredient to be given a European Commission-authorized health claim under the "emerging science" category after evaluation by EFSA in 2009 (EFSA Journal 2010). The approved claim was "Helps to maintain normal platelet aggregation, which contributes to healthy blood flow". Fruitflow® is now an established naturally derived functional food ingredient marketed globally. Multiple human studies have shown that consumption of Fruitflow® causes a platelet suppression of up to 25% relative to baseline status [30].

Among all the fruits tested, the aqueous extract of tomato and kiwifruit inhibited platelet aggregation by 75–80%, whereas apple and pear had very little activity (2–5%) [31,201,203]. These tomato antiplatelet compounds had a molecular mass of less than 1000 Da and were highly water soluble and stable to boiling [33]. After removing sugars, the isolated active tomato extract accounted for 4% of the aqueous tomato extract dry matter, later named Fruitflow®. Sugar-free aqueous tomato (later named Fruitflow® extract) showed potent inhibition of platelet aggregation in vitro [210]. Fruitflow® extract had three categories of compounds: nucleosides, simple phenolic derivatives, and flavonoid derivatives.

Though the mechanisms are not yet well known, Fruitflow® inhibits the GPIIb/IIIa activation step [210]. Fruitflow® unaltered basal platelet cyclic AMP levels in vitro studies. In addition, Fruitflow® decreased the expression of P-selectin in the platelet membranes in response to ADP in whole blood [204,210]. Fruitflow® can strongly affect the size and longevity of platelet aggregates. Fruitflow® was also found to affect tissue factor (TF) binding to activated platelets, at least in part due to effects on P-selectin. These results demonstrate that the actions of Fruitflow® were consistent and mediated partly through polyphenols [201,211]. Effects on TF binding suggested that sugar-free aqueous tomato extract components could significantly impact some aspects of coagulation, such as thrombin generation. Fruitflow® inhibits platelet granule secretion by suppressing the Src-PLCγ2-PKC-mediated granule secretory pathway. Platelet granule secretion occurs when collagen and thrombin bind to their receptors, GPVI and PARS, which causes activation of the downstream signaling pathway [212]. In this pathway, sarcoma, a tyrosine-protein kinase (Src) family member such as Lyn, Fyn, and Src, is first activated by phosphorylation, activated Syk, then phosphorylate and activated LAT, which in turn causes the phosphorylation of the adaptor protein PLCγ2 in which protein kinase C (PKC) bind leads to the activation of downstream effector, which induces platelet granule secretion. One study reported that Fruitflow® has the ability to alter the generation of different interleukins such as IL-1β, IL-6, IL-10, and IL-12 and chemokines such as CCL2/MCP-1, CCL3/MIP-1α, CCL5/RANTES, CXCL8/IL-8, and CXCL10/IP-10 of blood leukocytes [212]. Fruitflow® interacts with immune cells and endothelial cells [213]. It distinctly modulates the production of inflammatory modulators in a context-specific way and in extenso presumably in different body compartments.

Consequently, Fruitflow® may beneficially enhance and attenuate inflammatory processes during acute and chronic inflammation. Fruitflow® modulates cytokines, chemokines, and adhesion molecules that produce cell trafficking, activation, and differentiation in different immune system compartments. However, the modulatory roles of Fruitflow® in immune and inflammation responses in platelets are yet to be known. Fruitflow® is expected to have similar effects in platelets as those observed in different immune cells.

Fruitflow® prevents the activation of integrin αIIbß3 (GPIIb/IIIa) [204]. Fruitflow® also inhibited platelet aggregation and P-selectin expression in collagen-stimulated human platelets [214]. A proteomics study demonstrated that compared with the Fruitflow®-treated collagen-stimulated platelets, only collagen-stimulated platelets, 60 proteins, were upregulated, and 10 proteins were downregulated. Additionally, 66 phosphorylated peptides were upregulated, whereas 37 were downregulated. Proteomic studies also demonstrated that Fruitflow® also strongly affected protein disulfide isomerase (PDI), an oxidoreductase that catalyzes disulfide bond formation and isomerization. In platelets, blocking PDI with inhibitory antibodies inhibits several platelet activation pathways, including aggregation, secretion, and fibrinogen binding [215,216]. Glycosides related to quercetin in Fruitflow® demonstrated that they interact with PDI in this way [217,218]. The interaction of polyphenols with PDI suggested a possible mechanism by which Fruitflow® ingredients inhibit different platelet activation pathways.

Fruitflow® inhibited platelet function, possibly via suppression of Akt, GSK3β, p38 MAPK, and Hsp27 phosphorylation in collagen-induced platelet aggregation. The inhibition of platelet aggregation and modification of platelet proteins in collagen-stimulated platelets by Fruitflow® suggest that it can provide health benefits for people at risk of platelet hyperactivity-related thrombosis.

8. Human Trials and Animal Experiments Using Fruitflow®

Several human trials were conducted using Fruitflow® to determine the ex vivo and the onset time of an acute antiplatelet effect after consumption [30,210]. An acute lowering of the platelet aggregation response to ADP and collagen was observed three hours after consuming Fruitflow®. The range of onset times was from one and a half hours to three hours after Fruitflow® consumption. On average, these studies have shown an inhibition of the platelet response to ADP of approximately 17–25%, and platelet aggregability returned to baseline level 18 h after consumption of a single dose (150 mg) of Fruitflow® [209]. A study involving 93 men and women showed that men responded more than women, and people with higher risk factors for CVD were more responsive than others [219]. Fruitflow® ingredients affect many aspects of platelet function, including thrombin generation. However, clotting time showed no significant increases from baseline levels in all intervention studies [30].

A human trial demonstrated that the efficacious range for Fruitflow® lies between 75 mg and 300 mg [220]. A single dose of Fruitflow® was compared with 75 mg aspirin, either as a single dose or taken continuously for one week, and the platelet aggregability response was measured ex vivo [221]. The effects of a single dose of Fruitflow® were similar to a 75 mg dose of aspirin in terms of antiplatelet action, effects on thromboxane synthesis, and time to form a primary hemostatic clot in a study involving 47 healthy subjects [221]. Unlike aspirin, Fruitflow®'s effects were not cumulative as its effects did not irreversibly disable platelet signaling pathways [221]. The antiplatelet effects of aspirin in healthy subjects are incredibly heterogeneous, with some subjects experiencing a massive increase in time to form a primary hemostatic clot while others respond poorly. The more moderate effects of Fruitflow® were related to the reversibility of its antiplatelet action, rendering its use for the primary prevention of CVD, in contrast to aspirin at any dosage.

Both Fruitflow® and aspirin affected 26 platelet proteins involved in platelet structure and function, coagulation, platelet secretory proteins, fibrinogen beta chain 5, Ras-related proteins, redox system proteins, and HSP70s. As described earlier, the platelet protein disulfide isomerase was affected by Fruitflow®, which regulates $\alpha_{IIb}\beta_3$ integrin activation.

Four weeks of supplementation with Fruitflow® decreased platelet aggregation and granule secretion in healthy Chinese middle-aged and older individuals [222]. After a 2-week washout period, the platelet suppressive effect of Fruitflow® had disappeared. After four weeks of Fruitflow® treatment in the obese subgroup (n = 14), significant declines in aspirin reaction units by 8.6% and in P2Y12 reaction units (PRU) by 7.5% were observed [223]. Patients with arterial hypertension and obesity may potentially benefit from consuming Fruitflow® [223].

The supplementation of Fruitflow® for four weeks in strenuous exercise rats reduced platelet hyperreactivity [224]. Fruitflow® treatment also reduced black tail length, blood flow pulse index, and vascular resistance index, ameliorating microcirculation perfusion in a rat thrombosis model. Fruitflow® inhibited platelet aggregation induced by shear flow and alleviated the blood flow and microcirculation abnormities.

The EFSA authorized Fruitflow® for daily consumption in 2009 [30]. The first Article 13 claim based on newly developed evidence or proprietary data (a particular category under Article 13(5)) was approved for Fruitflow® in 2009 [30]. The approved claim was based on the eight human studies (seven proprietaries) and seven non-human studies (three proprietaries) conducted with Fruitflow®.

Fruitflow® differs fundamentally from aspirin or other antiplatelet drugs in that its effects are reversible. This very significant property of Fruitflow® makes it suitable for use by the general population as a dietary functional ingredient, while antiplatelet drugs cannot be used.

9. Kiwifruit and Its Antiplatelet Factors

Kiwifruit contains substantial quantities of several bioactive polyphenols [220]. Kiwifruits contain significant amounts of vitamin C, E, folic acid, and various phytochemicals, such as anthocyanidins and flavonols. Some of these polyphenols in this fruit are known for their antiplatelet activity [4,220]. The familiar green kiwifruit, *Actinidia deliciosa*, has been investigated for bioactivity, especially its effects on the risk of CVD [31,225–227]. As in tomato extract, the aqueous extract of kiwifruits has maximum antiplatelet factors, which was unrelated to the fruits' antioxidant potential [201]. Daily consumption of two or three kiwifruits reduced ex vivo platelet aggregation response, blood pressure, and plasma lipids [31,225–227]. The diverse activities of the aqueous extract of kiwifruit, such as the lowering of antiplatelet, plasma triglycerides and the converting of enzyme (ACE) activity by anti-angiotensin, have been shown [31,228]. The aqueous kiwifruit extract (KFE) inhibited ADP- and collagen-induced platelet aggregation.

In contrast, KFE was not that effective against ARA-induced platelet aggregation. KFE-mediated inhibition of platelet aggregation may not involve the TxA_2 pathway. The antiplatelet compounds in kiwifruit are water soluble and heat stable, and their molecular mass is less than 1000 Da [31]. KFE had glucose (8.9 ± 0.4 mg/mL), fructose (9.9 ± 0.5 mg/mL), and sucrose (2.3 ± 0.2 mg/mL) [203]. The inhibition of platelet aggregation by sugar-free KFE was concomitantly associated with the inhibition of TxB_2 synthesis and inhibited PF4 release in a dose-dependent manner. KFE at 1.68 mg/mL inhibited ADP- and collagen-induced TxB_2 synthesis by 91% and 81% [229].

10. Human Trials

Several human intervention trials were conducted to investigate the ex vivo effects of whole kiwifruits and KFE on platelet aggregation, ACE, and blood pressure [31,230–232]. In one human trial involving 30 healthy volunteers aged 20–51 years [31], consuming two or three kiwifruits daily for 28 days reduced platelet aggregation ex vivo. Consuming two kiwifruit daily inhibited platelet aggregation induced by ADP significantly (18% in case of 4 μM ADP and 15% in case of 8 μM ADP) compared with those at day 0 ($p < 0.05$). A similar reduction in platelet aggregation was observed in response to collagen. Plasma triglyceride levels were significantly lowered on day 28. The total plasma cholesterol, LDL, and HDL levels were unchanged from days 0 to 28 in both groups [31].

Another human trial showed that consuming one kiwifruit daily for four weeks reduced whole-blood platelet aggregation in healthy volunteers [230]. The effects of consumption of three kiwifruit for eight weeks on blood pressure, plasma lipids, and whole-blood aggregation were investigated in a randomized, controlled trial in male smokers (aged 44–74 years) [232]. In the kiwifruit group, reductions of 10 mm Hg in systolic blood pressure and 9 mm Hg in diastolic blood pressure were observed [232]. Additionally, a 15% reduction in whole-blood aggregation and an 11% reduction in ACE activity were observed in the kiwifruit group [232]. Although only blood pressure was decreased in hypertensives, no effects on other parameters were observed in the antioxidant-rich diet group. These diverse activities of kiwifruits, such as antiplatelet and anti-ACE, were also demonstrated in differently processed aqueous extracts of kiwifruits [31,228]. These results bear on not only green kiwifruits: consuming one gold kiwifruit daily for four weeks also reduced whole-blood platelet aggregation and plasma triglycerides in healthy volunteers [230]. Consuming 2 mg of KFE in 10 g margarine inhibited ex vivo platelet aggregation by 12.7% two hours after consumption by healthy volunteers (n = 9) [203].

11. Conclusions

Many studies have explored the relationship between dietary components, platelet function, and CVD risk factors. Several antiplatelet regimes, such as polyphenols, omega-3 fatty acids, and fruits and vegetables, have been developed. The overall data are positive for nutritional antiplatelets (such as fish and fish oil, polyphenols, Fruitflow, and KFE) to prevent CVD. However, platelet hyperactivity is also associated with many non-hemostatic diseases. Therefore, the impacts of these antiplatelet dietary factors on these diseases must be further investigated. The next question is, which of these nutritional antiplatelets is superior in its efficacy as an antiplatelet ingredient? At present, Fruitflow® is the most studied potent antiplatelet functional food. Fruitflow®, developed from tomato-containing bioavailable cardioprotective compounds, can benefit people vulnerable to developing CVD.

Beyond efficacy, one must also consider the practical aspects of consuming such dietary antiplatelets daily. For example, dosing, product form, commercial viability, and cost should also be considered. Finally, reliable markers of platelet activity and blood flow and the techniques thereof need to be further studied. Platelets become hyperactive in obesity, diabetes, a sedentary lifestyle, or hypertension, and in people who smoke. Platelet hyperreactivity is not merely an inevitable adverse effect of conditions but also a substantial contributing factor that exacerbates most human pathologies [29,194,233]. Recent studies indicate that platelet hyperactivity is not just a biomarker of adverse effects but a condition that requires management. Modulating platelet reactivity towards collagen,

ADP, and plasma triglyceride levels by functional foods could be of potential prophylactic and therapeutic benefit in preventing and halting pathologic processes.

An array of extensive basic, mechanistic, compositional, and several human trials testify to the cardio-protective benefits of Fruitflow® [31,201,211,234]. In addition to Fruitflow®, Kiwifruits have great potential for maintaining normal platelet activity.

It is now recognized that 20–30% of persons experience so-called aspirin-resistance syndrome, in which the expected antiplatelet effects are not observed [235]. This finding indicates an advantage of functional foods' broad antiplatelet activity profile over single-target drugs such as aspirin. Dietary antiplatelet functional foods help provide suitably gentle and safe yet efficacious therapies to improve public health in response to various health challenges involving platelet hyperactivity. Evidence from interventional trials have shown that consuming certain functional foods may improve cardiovascular health through their antiplatelet properties. However, further work is required on the beneficial effects of other platelet-mediated diseases such as cancer metastasis, immune disorders, hypertension, diabetes, inflammatory diseases, rheumatoid arthritis, myeloproliferative disease, and Alzheimer's disease. Well-controlled studies on food sources and their impacts on these diseases will help improve our understanding of potential antiplatelet effects on health and disease.

Funding: This research received no external funding.

Acknowledgments: The author is grateful to the Faculty of Medicine, University of Oslo.

Conflicts of Interest: The author has patented antiplatelet and antihypertensive factors in tomatoes (Fruitflow®) and Kiwifruit extract.

Abbreviations

CVD: cardiovascular disease; EPA, eicosapentaenoic acid, 20:5n-3; ARA, arachidonic acid, 20:4n-6; DHA, docosahexaenoic, 22:6n-3; EFSA, European Food Safety Authority; PDI, protein disulphide isomerase; TF; tissue factor, PRP, platelet-rich plasma; TxA_2, thromboxane A_2.

References

1. Ho-Tin-Noe, B.; Boulaftali, Y.; Camerer, E. Platelets and vascular integrity: How platelets prevent bleeding in inflammation. *Blood* **2018**, *131*, 277–288. [CrossRef] [PubMed]
2. Davi, G.; Patrono, C. Platelet activation and atherothrombosis. *N. Engl. J. Med.* **2007**, *357*, 2482–2494. [CrossRef] [PubMed]
3. Xu, X.R.; Zhang, D.; Oswald, B.E.; Carrim, N.; Wang, X.; Hou, Y.; Zhang, Q.; Lavalle, C.; McKeown, T.; Marshall, A.H.; et al. Platelets are versatile cells: New discoveries in hemostasis, thrombosis, immune responses, tumor metastasis and beyond. *Crit. Rev. Clin. Lab. Sci.* **2016**, *53*, 409–430. [CrossRef] [PubMed]
4. Das, D.; Adhikary, S.; Das, R.K.; Banerjee, A.; Radhakrishnan, A.K.; Paul, S.; Pathak, S.; Duttaroy, A.K. Bioactive food components and their inhibitory actions in multiple platelet pathways. *J. Food Biochem.* **2022**, *46*, e14476. [CrossRef] [PubMed]
5. O'Kennedy, N.; Duss, R.; Duttaroy, A.K. Dietary Antiplatelets: A New Perspective on the Health Benefits of the Water-Soluble Tomato Concentrate Fruitflow®. *Nutrients* **2021**, *13*, 2184. [CrossRef]
6. Das, D.; Shruthi, N.R.; Banerjee, A.; Jothimani, G.; Duttaroy, A.K.; Pathak, S. Endothelial dysfunction, platelet hyperactivity, hypertension, and the metabolic syndrome: Molecular insights and combating strategies. *Front. Nutr.* **2023**, *10*, 1221438. [CrossRef]
7. Xu, X.R.; Yousef, G.M.; Ni, H. Cancer and platelet crosstalk: Opportunities and challenges for aspirin and other antiplatelet agents. *Blood* **2018**, *131*, 1777–1789. [CrossRef]
8. Koupenova, M.; Corkrey, H.A.; Vitseva, O.; Manni, G.; Pang, C.J.; Clancy, L.; Yao, C.; Rade, J.; Levy, D.; Wang, J.P.; et al. The role of platelets in mediating a response to human influenza infection. *Nat. Commun.* **2019**, *10*, 1780. [CrossRef] [PubMed]
9. Puurunen, M.K.; Hwang, S.J.; Larson, M.G.; Vasan, R.S.; O'Donnell, C.J.; Tofler, G.; Johnson, A.D. ADP Platelet Hyperreactivity Predicts Cardiovascular Disease in the FHS (Framingham Heart Study). *J. Am. Heart Assoc.* **2018**, *7*, e008522. [CrossRef]
10. Natarajan, A.; Zaman, A.G.; Marshall, S.M. Platelet hyperactivity in type 2 diabetes: Role of antiplatelet agents. *Diab. Vasc. Dis. Res.* **2008**, *5*, 138–144. [CrossRef]
11. Massberg, S.; Brand, K.; Gruner, S.; Page, S.; Muller, E.; Muller, I.; Bergmeier, W.; Richter, T.; Lorenz, M.; Konrad, I.; et al. A critical role of platelet adhesion in the initiation of atherosclerotic lesion formation. *J. Exp. Med.* **2002**, *196*, 887–896. [CrossRef] [PubMed]
12. Kaplan, Z.S.; Jackson, S.P. The role of platelets in atherothrombosis. *Hematol. Am. Soc. Hematol. Educ. Program* **2011**, *2011*, 51–61. [CrossRef]

13. Lagadinou, M.; Onisor, M.O.; Rigas, A.; Musetescu, D.V.; Gkentzi, D.; Assimakopoulos, S.F.; Panos, G.; Marangos, M. Antimicrobial Properties on Non-Antibiotic Drugs in the Era of Increased Bacterial Resistance. *Antibiotics* **2020**, *9*, 107. [CrossRef]
14. McDonald, B.; Dunbar, M. Platelets and Intravascular Immunity: Guardians of the Vascular Space During Bloodstream Infections and Sepsis. *Front. Immunol.* **2019**, *10*, 2400. [CrossRef]
15. Koupenova, M.; Clancy, L.; Corkrey, H.A.; Freedman, J.E. Circulating Platelets as Mediators of Immunity, Inflammation, and Thrombosis. *Circ. Res.* **2018**, *122*, 337–351. [CrossRef]
16. Thomas, M.R.; Storey, R.F. The role of platelets in inflammation. *Thromb. Haemost.* **2015**, *114*, 449–458. [CrossRef] [PubMed]
17. Varon, D.; Shai, E. Platelets and their microparticles as key players in pathophysiological responses. *J. Thromb. Haemost.* **2015**, *13* (Suppl. 1), S40–S46. [CrossRef] [PubMed]
18. Le Blanc, J.; Lordkipanidze, M. Platelet Function in Aging. *Front. Cardiovasc. Med.* **2019**, *6*, 109. [CrossRef]
19. Eisenhardt, S.U.; Habersberger, J.; Peter, K. Monomeric C-reactive protein generation on activated platelets: The missing link between inflammation and atherothrombotic risk. *Trends Cardiovasc. Med.* **2009**, *19*, 232–237. [CrossRef]
20. Muller, I.; Massberg, S.; Zierhut, W.; Binz, C.; Schuster, A.; Rudiger-von Hoch, S.; Braun, S.; Gawaz, M. Effects of aspirin and clopidogrel versus oral anticoagulation on platelet function and on coagulation in patients with nonvalvular atrial fibrillation (CLAFIB). *Pathophysiol. Haemost. Thromb.* **2002**, *32*, 16–24. [CrossRef]
21. Cai, G.; Zhou, W.; Lu, Y.; Chen, P.; Lu, Z.; Fu, Y. Aspirin resistance and other aspirin-related concerns. *Neurol. Sci.* **2016**, *37*, 181–189. [CrossRef] [PubMed]
22. Piepoli, M.F.; Hoes, A.W.; Agewall, S.; Albus, C.; Brotons, C.; Catapano, A.L.; Cooney, M.T.; Corra, U.; Cosyns, B.; Deaton, C.; et al. 2016 European Guidelines on cardiovascular disease prevention in clinical practice: The Sixth Joint Task Force of the European Society of Cardiology and Other Societies on Cardiovascular Disease Prevention in Clinical Practice (constituted by representatives of 10 societies and by invited experts)Developed with the special contribution of the European Association for Cardiovascular Prevention & Rehabilitation (EACPR). *Eur. Heart J.* **2016**, *37*, 2315–2381. [CrossRef] [PubMed]
23. Tomczynska, M.; Salata, I.; Bijak, M.; Saluk-Bijak, J. The potential contribution and role of a blood platelets in autoimmune thyroid diseases. *J. Cell Mol. Med.* **2018**, *22*, 6386–6390. [CrossRef] [PubMed]
24. Garcia-Leon, M.J.; Liboni, C.; Mittelheisser, V.; Bochler, L.; Follain, G.; Mouriaux, C.; Busnelli, I.; Larnicol, A.; Colin, F.; Peralta, M.; et al. Platelets favor the outgrowth of established metastases. *Nat. Commun.* **2024**, *15*, 3297. [CrossRef] [PubMed]
25. El Haouari, M.; Rosado, J.A. Platelet function in hypertension. *Blood Cells Mol. Dis.* **2009**, *42*, 38–43. [CrossRef] [PubMed]
26. Xu, C.; Song, Z.; Hu, L.T.; Tong, Y.H.; Hu, J.Y.; Shen, H. Abnormal platelet parameters in inflammatory bowel disease: A systematic review and meta-analysis. *BMC Gastroenterol.* **2024**, *24*, 214. [CrossRef]
27. Harifi, G.; Sibilia, J. Pathogenic role of platelets in rheumatoid arthritis and systemic autoimmune diseases. Perspectives and therapeutic aspects. *Saudi Med. J.* **2016**, *37*, 354–360. [CrossRef]
28. Ross, D.M.; Liang, H.P.H.; Iqra, Z.; Whittaker, S.; Tan, C.W.; Dale, B.J.; Chen, V.M. Platelets from patients with myeloproliferative neoplasms have increased numbers of mitochondria that are hypersensitive to depolarization by thrombin. *Sci. Rep.* **2023**, *13*, 9172. [CrossRef]
29. Dutta-Roy, A.K. Dietary components and human platelet activity. *Platelets* **2002**, *13*, 67–75. [CrossRef]
30. O'Kennedy, N.; Raederstorff, D.; Duttaroy, A.K. Fruitflow®: The first European Food Safety Authority-approved natural cardio-protective functional ingredient. *Eur. J. Nutr.* **2017**, *56*, 461–482. [CrossRef]
31. Duttaroy, A.K.; Jorgensen, A. Effects of kiwi fruit consumption on platelet aggregation and plasma lipids in healthy human volunteers. *Platelets* **2004**, *15*, 287–292. [CrossRef] [PubMed]
32. Dutta-Roy, A.K.; Gordon, M.J.; Kelly, C.; Hunter, K.; Crosbie, L.; Knight-Carpentar, T.; Williams, B.C. Inhibitory effect of Ginkgo biloba extract on human platelet aggregation. *Platelets* **1999**, *10*, 298–305. [CrossRef] [PubMed]
33. Dutta-Roy, A.K.; Crosbie, L.; Gordon, M.J. Effects of tomato extract on human platelet aggregation in vitro. *Platelets* **2001**, *12*, 218–227. [PubMed]
34. Lowery, C.L., 3rd; Elliott, C.; Cooper, A.; Hadden, C.; Sonon, R.N.; Azadi, P.; Williams, D.K.; Marsh, J.D.; Woulfe, D.S.; Kilic, F. Cigarette Smoking-Associated Alterations in Serotonin/Adrenalin Signaling Pathways of Platelets. *J. Am. Heart Assoc.* **2017**, *6*, e005465. [CrossRef]
35. Ishida, M.; Sakai, C.; Kobayashi, Y.; Ishida, T. Cigarette Smoking and Atherosclerotic Cardiovascular Disease. *J. Atheroscler. Thromb.* **2024**, *31*, 189–200. [CrossRef]
36. Robertson, S.; Miller, M.R. Ambient air pollution and thrombosis. *Part Fibre Toxicol.* **2018**, *15*, 1. [CrossRef]
37. Zhang, X.; McGeoch, S.C.; Johnstone, A.M.; Holtrop, G.; Sneddon, A.A.; MacRury, S.M.; Megson, I.L.; Pearson, D.W.; Abraham, P.; De Roos, B.; et al. Platelet-derived microparticle count and surface molecule expression differ between subjects with and without type 2 diabetes, independently of obesity status. *J. Thromb. Thrombolysis* **2014**, *37*, 455–463. [CrossRef]
38. Huskens, D.; Roest, M.; Remijn, J.A.; Konings, J.; Kremers, R.M.; Bloemen, S.; Schurgers, E.; Selmeczi, A.; Kelchtermans, H.; van Meel, R.; et al. Strenuous exercise induces a hyperreactive rebalanced haemostatic state that is more pronounced in men. *Thromb. Haemost.* **2016**, *115*, 1109–1119. [CrossRef]
39. Chaudhary, P.K.; Kim, S.; Kim, S. An Insight into Recent Advances on Platelet Function in Health and Disease. *Int. J. Mol. Sci.* **2022**, *23*, 6022. [CrossRef]
40. O'Kennedy, N.; Duttaroy, A.K. Platelet hyperactivity in COVID-19: Can the tomato extract Fruitflow(R) be used as an antiplatelet regime? *Med. Hypotheses* **2021**, *147*, 110480. [CrossRef]

41. Alberio, L.; Safa, O.; Clemetson, K.J.; Esmon, C.T.; Dale, G.L. Surface expression and functional characterization of alpha-granule factor V in human platelets: Effects of ionophore A23187, thrombin, collagen, and convulxin. *Blood* **2000**, *95*, 1694–1702. [CrossRef] [PubMed]
42. Podrez, E.A.; Byzova, T.V.; Febbraio, M.; Salomon, R.G.; Ma, Y.; Valiyaveettil, M.; Poliakov, E.; Sun, M.; Finton, P.J.; Curtis, B.R.; et al. Platelet CD36 links hyperlipidemia, oxidant stress and a prothrombotic phenotype. *Nat. Med.* **2007**, *13*, 1086–1095. [CrossRef] [PubMed]
43. Chen, K.; Febbraio, M.; Li, W.; Silverstein, R.L. A specific CD36-dependent signaling pathway is required for platelet activation by oxidized low-density lipoprotein. *Circ. Res.* **2008**, *102*, 1512–1519. [CrossRef]
44. Jennings, L.K. Mechanisms of platelet activation: Need for new strategies to protect against platelet-mediated atherothrombosis. *Thromb. Haemost.* **2009**, *102*, 248–257. [CrossRef]
45. Dutta-Roy, A.K.; Ray, T.K.; Sinha, A.K. Prostacyclin stimulation of the activation of blood coagulation factor X by platelets. *Science* **1986**, *231*, 385–388. [CrossRef]
46. Weyrich, A.S.; Zimmerman, G.A. Platelets in lung biology. *Annu. Rev. Physiol.* **2013**, *75*, 569–591. [CrossRef]
47. Yeung, J.; Li, W.; Holinstat, M. Platelet Signaling and Disease: Targeted Therapy for Thrombosis and Other Related Diseases. *Pharmacol. Rev.* **2018**, *70*, 526–548. [CrossRef]
48. Leiter, O.; Walker, T.L. Platelets in Neurodegenerative Conditions-Friend or Foe? *Front. Immunol.* **2020**, *11*, 747. [CrossRef] [PubMed]
49. Rendu, F.; Brohard-Bohn, B. The platelet release reaction: Granules' constituents, secretion and functions. *Platelets* **2001**, *12*, 261–273. [CrossRef]
50. Janowska-Wieczorek, A.; Majka, M.; Kijowski, J.; Baj-Krzyworzeka, M.; Reca, R.; Turner, A.R.; Ratajczak, J.; Emerson, S.G.; Kowalska, M.A.; Ratajczak, M.Z. Platelet-derived microparticles bind to hematopoietic stem/progenitor cells and enhance their engraftment. *Blood* **2001**, *98*, 3143–3149. [CrossRef]
51. Heijnen, H.F.; Schiel, A.E.; Fijnheer, R.; Geuze, H.J.; Sixma, J.J. Activated platelets release two types of membrane vesicles: Microvesicles by surface shedding and exosomes derived from exocytosis of multivesicular bodies and alpha-granules. *Blood* **1999**, *94*, 3791–3799. [CrossRef] [PubMed]
52. Lazar, S.; Goldfinger, L.E. Platelets and extracellular vesicles and their cross talk with cancer. *Blood* **2021**, *137*, 3192–3200. [CrossRef] [PubMed]
53. Haemmerle, M.; Stone, R.L.; Menter, D.G.; Afshar-Kharghan, V.; Sood, A.K. The Platelet Lifeline to Cancer: Challenges and Opportunities. *Cancer Cell* **2018**, *33*, 965–983. [CrossRef] [PubMed]
54. Chew, H.K.; Wun, T.; Harvey, D.; Zhou, H.; White, R.H. Incidence of venous thromboembolism and its effect on survival among patients with common cancers. *Arch. Intern. Med.* **2006**, *166*, 458–464. [CrossRef]
55. Frossard, M.; Fuchs, I.; Leitner, J.M.; Hsieh, K.; Vlcek, M.; Losert, H.; Domanovits, H.; Schreiber, W.; Laggner, A.N.; Jilma, B. Platelet function predicts myocardial damage in patients with acute myocardial infarction. *Circulation* **2004**, *110*, 1392–1397. [CrossRef]
56. Tantry, U.S.; Bonello, L.; Aradi, D.; Price, M.J.; Jeong, Y.H.; Angiolillo, D.J.; Stone, G.W.; Curzen, N.; Geisler, T.; Ten Berg, J.; et al. Consensus and update on the definition of on-treatment platelet reactivity to adenosine diphosphate associated with ischemia and bleeding. *J. Am. Coll. Cardiol.* **2013**, *62*, 2261–2273. [CrossRef]
57. Tran, H.; Anand, S.S. Oral antiplatelet therapy in cerebrovascular disease, coronary artery disease, and peripheral arterial disease. *JAMA* **2004**, *292*, 1867–1874. [CrossRef]
58. Dentali, F.; Squizzato, A.; Ageno, W. The metabolic syndrome as a risk factor for venous and arterial thrombosis. *Semin. Thromb. Hemost.* **2009**, *35*, 451–457. [CrossRef]
59. Thomas, D.P. Effect of catecholamines on platelet aggregation caused by thrombin. *Nature* **1967**, *215*, 298–299. [CrossRef]
60. Arnoldussen, I.A.C.; Witkamp, R.F. Effects of Nutrients on Platelet Function: A Modifiable Link between Metabolic Syndrome and Neurodegeneration? *Biomolecules* **2021**, *11*, 1455. [CrossRef]
61. Barale, C.; Russo, I. Influence of Cardiometabolic Risk Factors on Platelet Function. *Int. J. Mol. Sci.* **2020**, *21*, 623. [CrossRef] [PubMed]
62. Russo, I. The prothrombotic tendency in metabolic syndrome: Focus on the potential mechanisms involved in impaired haemostasis and fibrinolytic balance. *Scientifica* **2012**, *2012*, 525374. [CrossRef]
63. Yang, M.; Kholmukhamedov, A. Platelet reactivity in dyslipidemia: Atherothrombotic signaling and therapeutic implications. *Rev. Cardiovasc. Med.* **2021**, *22*, 67–81. [CrossRef] [PubMed]
64. Dutta-Roy, A.K.; Gordon, M.J.; Campbell, F.M.; Crosbie, L.C. Arachidonic acid uptake by human platelets is mediated by CD36. *Platelets* **1996**, *7*, 291–295. [CrossRef]
65. Li, N. Platelets as an inter-player between hyperlipidaemia and atherosclerosis. *J. Intern. Med.* **2024**, *296*, 39–52. [CrossRef] [PubMed]
66. Elbatarny, H.S.; Maurice, D.H. Leptin-mediated activation of human platelets: Involvement of a leptin receptor and phosphodiesterase 3A-containing cellular signaling complex. *Am. J. Physiol. Endocrinol. Metab.* **2005**, *289*, E695–E702. [CrossRef]
67. Konstantinides, S.; Schafer, K.; Koschnick, S.; Loskutoff, D.J. Leptin-dependent platelet aggregation and arterial thrombosis suggests a mechanism for atherothrombotic disease in obesity. *J. Clin. Investig.* **2001**, *108*, 1533–1540. [CrossRef]

68. Bladowski, M.; Gawrys, J.; Gajecki, D.; Szahidewicz-Krupska, E.; Sawicz-Bladowska, A.; Doroszko, A. Role of the Platelets and Nitric Oxide Biotransformation in Ischemic Stroke: A Translative Review from Bench to Bedside. *Oxid. Med. Cell Longev.* **2020**, *2020*, 2979260. [CrossRef]
69. Wang, Q.; Zennadi, R. Oxidative Stress and Thrombosis during Aging: The Roles of Oxidative Stress in RBCs in Venous Thrombosis. *Int. J. Mol. Sci.* **2020**, *21*, 4259. [CrossRef]
70. Freedman, J.E. Oxidative stress and platelets. *Arter. Thromb. Vasc. Biol.* **2008**, *28*, s11–s16. [CrossRef]
71. Ceriello, A. Postprandial hyperglycemia and diabetes complications: Is it time to treat? *Diabetes* **2005**, *54*, 1–7. [CrossRef] [PubMed]
72. Andre, P.; Nannizzi-Alaimo, L.; Prasad, S.K.; Phillips, D.R. Platelet-derived CD40L: The switch-hitting player of cardiovascular disease. *Circulation* **2002**, *106*, 896–899. [CrossRef] [PubMed]
73. Henn, V.; Steinbach, S.; Buchner, K.; Presek, P.; Kroczek, R.A. The inflammatory action of CD40 ligand (CD154) expressed on activated human platelets is temporally limited by coexpressed CD40. *Blood* **2001**, *98*, 1047–1054. [CrossRef] [PubMed]
74. Miceli, G.; Basso, M.G.; Rizzo, G.; Pintus, C.; Tuttolomondo, A. The Role of the Coagulation System in Peripheral Arterial Disease: Interactions with the Arterial Wall and Its Vascular Microenvironment and Implications for Rational Therapies. *Int. J. Mol. Sci.* **2022**, *23*, 4914. [CrossRef]
75. Azimova, K.; San Juan, Z.; Mukherjee, D. Cardiovascular safety profile of currently available diabetic drugs. *Ochsner J.* **2014**, *14*, 616–632.
76. Johnson, M.; Harrison, H.E.; Raftery, A.T.; Elder, J.B. Vascular prostacyclin may be reduced in diabetes in man. *Lancet* **1979**, *1*, 325–326. [CrossRef]
77. Rabini, R.A.; Staffolani, R.; Fumelli, P.; Mutus, B.; Curatola, G.; Mazzanti, L. Decreased nitric oxide synthase activity in platelets from IDDM and NIDDM patients. *Diabetologia* **1998**, *41*, 101–104. [CrossRef]
78. Blann, A.D.; Nadar, S.; Lip, G.Y. Pharmacological modulation of platelet function in hypertension. *Hypertension* **2003**, *42*, 1–7. [CrossRef]
79. Pravenec, M.; Kunes, J.; Zicha, J.; Kren, V.; Klir, P. Platelet aggregation in spontaneous hypertension: Genetic determination and correlation analysis. *J. Hypertens.* **1992**, *10*, 1453–1456. [CrossRef]
80. Breddin, H.K.; Lippold, R.; Bittner, M.; Kirchmaier, C.M.; Krzywanek, H.J.; Michaelis, J. Spontaneous platelet aggregation as a predictive risk factor for vascular occlusions in healthy volunteers? Results of the HAPARG Study. Haemostatic parameters as risk factors in healthy volunteers. *Atherosclerosis* **1999**, *144*, 211–219. [CrossRef]
81. Torsellini, A.; Becucci, A.; Citi, S.; Cozzolino, F.; Guidi, G.; Lombardi, V.; Vercelli, D.; Veloci, M. Effects of pressure excursions on human platelets. In vitro studies on betathromboglobulin (beta-TG) and platelet factor 4 (PF4) release and on platelet sensitivity to ADP-aggregation. *Haematologica* **1982**, *67*, 860–866. [PubMed]
82. Lip, G.Y.; Blann, A.D.; Farooqi, I.S.; Zarifis, J.; Sagar, G.; Beevers, D.G. Sequential alterations in haemorheology, endothelial dysfunction, platelet activation and thrombogenesis in relation to prognosis following acute stroke: The West Birmingham Stroke Project. *Blood Coagul. Fibrinolysis* **2002**, *13*, 339–347. [CrossRef] [PubMed]
83. Blann, A.D.; Naqvi, T.; Waite, M.; McCollum, C.N. von Willebrand factor and endothelial damage in essential hypertension. *J. Hum. Hypertens.* **1993**, *7*, 107–111.
84. Nityanand, S.; Pande, I.; Bajpai, V.K.; Singh, L.; Chandra, M.; Singh, B.N. Platelets in essential hypertension. *Thromb. Res.* **1993**, *72*, 447–454. [CrossRef]
85. Kjeldsen, S.E.; Gjesdal, K.; Eide, I.; Aakesson, I.; Amundsen, R.; Foss, O.P.; Leren, P. Increased beta-thromboglobulin in essential hypertension: Interactions between arterial plasma adrenaline, platelet function and blood lipids. *Acta Med. Scand.* **1983**, *213*, 369–373. [CrossRef]
86. Spencer, C.G.; Gurney, D.; Blann, A.D.; Beevers, D.G.; Lip, G.Y.; Ascot Steering Committee, A.-S.C.O.T. Von Willebrand factor, soluble P-selectin, and target organ damage in hypertension: A substudy of the Anglo-Scandinavian Cardiac Outcomes Trial (ASCOT). *Hypertension* **2002**, *40*, 61–66. [CrossRef]
87. Lechi, C.; Sinigaglia, D.; Delva, P.; Guzzo, P.; Arosio, E.; Steele, A.; Lechi, A. Platelet intracellular free Ca^{2+} after incubation with plasma from hypertensive patients. *J. Hum. Hypertens.* **1989**, *3*, 45–48. [PubMed]
88. Yamanishi, J.; Sano, H.; Saito, K.; Furuta, Y.; Fukuzaki, H. Plasma concentrations of platelet-specific proteins in different stages of essential hypertension: Interactions between platelet aggregation, blood lipids and age. *Thromb. Haemost.* **1985**, *54*, 539–543. [CrossRef]
89. Duhamel, T.A.; Xu, Y.J.; Arneja, A.S.; Dhalla, N.S. Targeting platelets for prevention and treatment of cardiovascular disease. *Expert Opin. Ther. Targets* **2007**, *11*, 1523–1533. [CrossRef]
90. Holmsen, H. Platelet metabolism and activation. *Semin. Hematol.* **1985**, *22*, 219–240.
91. Touyz, R.M.; Schiffrin, E.L. Effects of angiotensin II and endothelin-1 on platelet aggregation and cytosolic pH and free Ca^{2+} concentrations in essential hypertension. *Hypertension* **1993**, *22*, 853–862. [CrossRef] [PubMed]
92. Pechan, J.; Okrucka, A. Diltiazem inhibits the spontaneous platelet aggregation in essential hypertension. *Cardiology* **1991**, *79*, 116–119. [CrossRef] [PubMed]
93. Andrioli, G.; Ortolani, R.; Fontana, L.; Gaino, S.; Bellavite, P.; Lechi, C.; Minuz, P.; Manzato, F.; Tridente, G.; Lechi, A. Study of platelet adhesion in patients with uncomplicated hypertension. *J. Hypertens.* **1996**, *14*, 1215–1221. [CrossRef]

94. Forte, P.; Copland, M.; Smith, L.M.; Milne, E.; Sutherland, J.; Benjamin, N. Basal nitric oxide synthesis in essential hypertension. *Lancet* **1997**, *349*, 837–842. [CrossRef]
95. Camilletti, A.; Moretti, N.; Giacchetti, G.; Faloia, E.; Martarelli, D.; Mantero, F.; Mazzanti, L. Decreased nitric oxide levels and increased calcium content in platelets of hypertensive patients. *Am. J. Hypertens.* **2001**, *14*, 382–386. [CrossRef] [PubMed]
96. Dockrell, M.E.; Walker, B.R.; Noon, J.P.; Watt, G.C.; Williams, B.C.; Webb, D.J. Platelet aggregation in young men with contrasting predisposition to high blood pressure. *Am. J. Hypertens.* **1999**, *12*, 115–119. [CrossRef]
97. Li, B.; Lu, Z.; Yang, Z.; Zhang, X.; Wang, M.; Chu, T.; Wang, P.; Qi, F.; Anderson, G.J.; Jiang, E.; et al. Monitoring circulating platelet activity to predict cancer-associated thrombosis. *Cell Rep. Methods* **2023**, *3*, 100513. [CrossRef]
98. Gussoni, G.; Frasson, S.; La Regina, M.; Di Micco, P.; Monreal, M.; Investigators, R. Three-month mortality rate and clinical predictors in patients with venous thromboembolism and cancer. Findings from the RIETE registry. *Thromb. Res.* **2013**, *131*, 24–30. [CrossRef]
99. Huang, C.; Wang, Y.; Li, X.; Ren, L.; Zhao, J.; Hu, Y.; Zhang, L.; Fan, G.; Xu, J.; Gu, X.; et al. Clinical features of patients infected with 2019 novel coronavirus in Wuhan, China. *Lancet* **2020**, *395*, 497–506. [CrossRef]
100. Ried, K.; Frank, O.R.; Stocks, N.P. Dark chocolate or tomato extract for prehypertension: A randomised controlled trial. *BMC Complement Altern. Med.* **2009**, *9*, 22. [CrossRef]
101. Ludovici, V.; Barthelmes, J.; Nagele, M.P.; Flammer, A.J.; Sudano, I. Polyphenols: Anti-Platelet Nutraceutical? *Curr. Pharm. Des.* **2018**, *24*, 146–157. [CrossRef]
102. Olas, B. Biochemistry of blood platelet activation and the beneficial role of plant oils in cardiovascular diseases. *Adv. Clin. Chem.* **2020**, *95*, 219–243. [CrossRef]
103. Zaragoza, C.; Monserrat, J.; Mantecon, C.; Villaescusa, L.; Zaragoza, F.; Alvarez-Mon, M. Antiplatelet activity of flavonoid and coumarin drugs. *Vasc. Pharmacol.* **2016**, *87*, 139–149. [CrossRef]
104. Wang, C.; Harris, W.S.; Chung, M.; Lichtenstein, A.H.; Balk, E.M.; Kupelnick, B.; Jordan, H.S.; Lau, J. n-3 Fatty acids from fish or fish-oil supplements, but not alpha-linolenic acid, benefit cardiovascular disease outcomes in primary- and secondary-prevention studies: A systematic review. *Am. J. Clin. Nutr.* **2006**, *84*, 5–17. [CrossRef]
105. Andrioli, G.; Carletto, A.; Guarini, P.; Galvani, S.; Biasi, D.; Bellavite, P.; Corrocher, R. Differential effects of dietary supplementation with fish oil or soy lecithin on human platelet adhesion. *Thromb. Haemost.* **1999**, *82*, 1522–1527.
106. Golanski, J.; Szymanska, P.; Rozalski, M. Effects of Omega-3 Polyunsaturated Fatty Acids and Their Metabolites on Haemostasis-Current Perspectives in Cardiovascular Disease. *Int. J. Mol. Sci.* **2021**, *22*, 2394. [CrossRef]
107. Parent, C.A.; Lagarde, M.; Venton, D.L.; Le Breton, G.C. Selective modulation of the human platelet thromboxane A2/prostaglandin H2 receptor by eicosapentaenoic and docosahexaenoic acids in intact platelets and solubilized platelet membranes. *J. Biol. Chem.* **1992**, *267*, 6541–6547. [CrossRef]
108. Dutta-Roy, A.K. Insulin mediated processes in platelets, erythrocytes and monocytes/macrophages: Effects of essential fatty acid metabolism. *Prostaglandins Leukot. Essent. Fat. Acids* **1994**, *51*, 385–399. [CrossRef]
109. von Schacky, C. Prophylaxis of atherosclerosis with marine omega-3 fatty acids. A comprehensive strategy. *Ann. Intern. Med.* **1987**, *107*, 890–899. [CrossRef]
110. Gao, L.G.; Cao, J.; Mao, Q.X.; Lu, X.C.; Zhou, X.L.; Fan, L. Influence of omega-3 polyunsaturated fatty acid-supplementation on platelet aggregation in humans: A meta-analysis of randomized controlled trials. *Atherosclerosis* **2013**, *226*, 328–334. [CrossRef]
111. Hashimoto, M.; Hossain, S.; Shido, O. Docosahexaenoic acid but not eicosapentaenoic acid withstands dietary cholesterol-induced decreases in platelet membrane fluidity. *Mol. Cell Biochem.* **2006**, *293*, 1–8. [CrossRef]
112. Larson, M.K.; Tormoen, G.W.; Weaver, L.J.; Luepke, K.J.; Patel, I.A.; Hjelmen, C.E.; Ensz, N.M.; McComas, L.S.; McCarty, O.J. Exogenous modification of platelet membranes with the omega-3 fatty acids EPA and DHA reduces platelet procoagulant activity and thrombus formation. *Am. J. Physiol. Cell Physiol.* **2013**, *304*, C273–C279. [CrossRef]
113. McEwen, B.J.; Morel-Kopp, M.C.; Tofler, G.H.; Ward, C.M. The effect of omega-3 polyunsaturated fatty acids on fibrin and thrombin generation in healthy subjects and subjects with cardiovascular disease. *Semin. Thromb. Hemost.* **2015**, *41*, 315–322. [CrossRef]
114. Dona, M.; Fredman, G.; Schwab, J.M.; Chiang, N.; Arita, M.; Goodarzi, A.; Cheng, G.; von Andrian, U.H.; Serhan, C.N. Resolvin E1, an EPA-derived mediator in whole blood, selectively counterregulates leukocytes and platelets. *Blood* **2008**, *112*, 848–855. [CrossRef]
115. Yamaguchi, A.; Stanger, L.; Freedman, C.J.; Standley, M.; Hoang, T.; Adili, R.; Tsai, W.C.; van Hoorebeke, C.; Holman, T.R.; Holinstat, M. DHA 12-LOX-derived oxylipins regulate platelet activation and thrombus formation through a PKA-dependent signaling pathway. *J. Thromb. Haemost.* **2021**, *19*, 839–851. [CrossRef]
116. Fischer, S.; Weber, P.C. Thromboxane A3 (TXA3) is formed in human platelets after dietary eicosapentaenoic acid (C20:5 omega 3). *Biochem. Biophys. Res. Commun.* **1983**, *116*, 1091–1099. [CrossRef]
117. Gibney, M.J.; Bolton-Smith, C. The effect of a dietary supplement of n-3 polyunsaturated fat on platelet lipid composition, platelet function and platelet plasma membrane fluidity in healthy volunteers. *Br. J. Nutr.* **1988**, *60*, 5–12. [CrossRef]
118. Li, X.L.; Steiner, M. Dose response of dietary fish oil supplementations on platelet adhesion. *Arter. Thromb.* **1991**, *11*, 39–46. [CrossRef]
119. Pirich, C.; Gaszo, A.; Granegger, S.; Sinzinger, H. Effects of fish oil supplementation on platelet survival and ex vivo platelet function in hypercholesterolemic patients. *Thromb. Res.* **1999**, *96*, 219–227. [CrossRef]

120. Svaneborg, N.; Kristensen, S.D.; Hansen, L.M.; Bullow, I.; Husted, S.E.; Schmidt, E.B. The acute and short-time effect of supplementation with the combination of n-3 fatty acids and acetylsalicylic acid on platelet function and plasma lipids. *Thromb. Res.* **2002**, *105*, 311–316. [CrossRef]
121. Eschen, O.; Christensen, J.H.; De Caterina, R.; Schmidt, E.B. Soluble adhesion molecules in healthy subjects: A dose-response study using n-3 fatty acids. *Nutr. Metab. Cardiovasc. Dis.* **2004**, *14*, 180–185. [CrossRef]
122. Vanschoonbeek, K.; Feijge, M.A.; Paquay, M.; Rosing, J.; Saris, W.; Kluft, C.; Giesen, P.L.; de Maat, M.P.; Heemskerk, J.W. Variable hypocoagulant effect of fish oil intake in humans: Modulation of fibrinogen level and thrombin generation. *Arter. Thromb. Vasc. Biol.* **2004**, *24*, 1734–1740. [CrossRef]
123. Din, J.N.; Harding, S.A.; Valerio, C.J.; Sarma, J.; Lyall, K.; Riemersma, R.A.; Newby, D.E.; Flapan, A.D. Dietary intervention with oil rich fish reduces platelet-monocyte aggregation in man. *Atherosclerosis* **2008**, *197*, 290–296. [CrossRef]
124. Larson, M.K.; Shearer, G.C.; Ashmore, J.H.; Anderson-Daniels, J.M.; Graslie, E.L.; Tholen, J.T.; Vogelaar, J.L.; Korth, A.J.; Nareddy, V.; Sprehe, M.; et al. Omega-3 fatty acids modulate collagen signaling in human platelets. *Prostaglandins Leukot. Essent. Fat. Acids* **2011**, *84*, 93–98. [CrossRef]
125. Vericel, E.; Calzada, C.; Chapuy, P.; Lagarde, M. The influence of low intake of n-3 fatty acids on platelets in elderly people. *Atherosclerosis* **1999**, *147*, 187–192. [CrossRef]
126. Croset, M.; Vericel, E.; Rigaud, M.; Hanss, M.; Courpron, P.; Dechavanne, M.; Lagarde, M. Functions and tocopherol content of blood platelets from elderly people after low intake of purified eicosapentaenoic acid. *Thromb. Res.* **1990**, *57*, 1–12. [CrossRef]
127. Driss, F.; Vericel, E.; Lagarde, M.; Dechavanne, M.; Darcet, P. Inhibition of platelet aggregation and thromboxane synthesis after intake of small amount of icosapentaenoic acid. *Thromb. Res.* **1984**, *36*, 389–396. [CrossRef]
128. Guillot, N.; Caillet, E.; Laville, M.; Calzada, C.; Lagarde, M.; Vericel, E. Increasing intakes of the long-chain omega-3 docosahexaenoic acid: Effects on platelet functions and redox status in healthy men. *FASEB J.* **2009**, *23*, 2909–2916. [CrossRef]
129. Nomura, S.; Kanazawa, S.; Fukuhara, S. Effects of eicosapentaenoic acid on platelet activation markers and cell adhesion molecules in hyperlipidemic patients with Type 2 diabetes mellitus. *J. Diabetes Complicat.* **2003**, *17*, 153–159. [CrossRef]
130. Chen, G.; Qian, Z.M.; Zhang, J.; Zhang, S.; Zhang, Z.; Vaughn, M.G.; Aaron, H.E.; Wang, C.; Lip, G.Y.; Lin, H. Regular use of fish oil supplements and course of cardiovascular diseases: Prospective cohort study. *BMJ Med.* **2024**, *3*, e000451. [CrossRef]
131. Van Dael, P. Role of n-3 long-chain polyunsaturated fatty acids in human nutrition and health: Review of recent studies and recommendations. *Nutr. Res. Pract.* **2021**, *15*, 137–159. [CrossRef]
132. Wen, Y.T.; Dai, J.H.; Gao, Q. Effects of Omega-3 fatty acid on major cardiovascular events and mortality in patients with coronary heart disease: A meta-analysis of randomized controlled trials. *Nutr. Metab. Cardiovasc. Dis.* **2014**, *24*, 470–475. [CrossRef]
133. Kwak, S.M.; Myung, S.K.; Lee, Y.J.; Seo, H.G.; Korean Meta-analysis Study, G. Efficacy of omega-3 fatty acid supplements (eicosapentaenoic acid and docosahexaenoic acid) in the secondary prevention of cardiovascular disease: A meta-analysis of randomized, double-blind, placebo-controlled trials. *Arch. Intern. Med.* **2012**, *172*, 686–694. [CrossRef]
134. Nestel, P.; Clifton, P.; Colquhoun, D.; Noakes, M.; Mori, T.A.; Sullivan, D.; Thomas, B. Indications for Omega-3 Long Chain Polyunsaturated Fatty Acid in the Prevention and Treatment of Cardiovascular Disease. *Heart Lung. Circ.* **2015**, *24*, 769–779. [CrossRef]
135. Meyer, B.J.; Groot, R.H.M. Effects of Omega-3 Long Chain Polyunsaturated Fatty Acid Supplementation on Cardiovascular Mortality: The Importance of the Dose of DHA. *Nutrients* **2017**, *9*, 1305. [CrossRef]
136. Mozaffarian, D.; Wu, J.H. Omega-3 fatty acids and cardiovascular disease: Effects on risk factors, molecular pathways, and clinical events. *J. Am. Coll. Cardiol.* **2011**, *58*, 2047–2067. [CrossRef]
137. Kris-Etherton, P.M.; Harris, W.S.; Appel, L.J.; American Heart Association; Nutrition Committee. Fish consumption, fish oil, omega-3 fatty acids, and cardiovascular disease. *Circulation* **2002**, *106*, 2747–2757. [CrossRef]
138. Siscovick, D.S.; Barringer, T.A.; Fretts, A.M.; Wu, J.H.; Lichtenstein, A.H.; Costello, R.B.; Kris-Etherton, P.M.; Jacobson, T.A.; Engler, M.B.; Alger, H.M.; et al. Omega-3 Polyunsaturated Fatty Acid (Fish Oil) Supplementation and the Prevention of Clinical Cardiovascular Disease: A Science Advisory from the American Heart Association. *Circulation* **2017**, *135*, e867–e884. [CrossRef]
139. Skulas-Ray, A.C.; Wilson, P.W.F.; Harris, W.S.; Brinton, E.A.; Kris-Etherton, P.M.; Richter, C.K.; Jacobson, T.A.; Engler, M.B.; Miller, M.; Robinson, J.G.; et al. Omega-3 Fatty Acids for the Management of Hypertriglyceridemia: A Science Advisory from the American Heart Association. *Circulation* **2019**, *140*, e673–e691. [CrossRef]
140. Aung, T.; Halsey, J.; Kromhout, D.; Gerstein, H.C.; Marchioli, R.; Tavazzi, L.; Geleijnse, J.M.; Rauch, B.; Ness, A.; Galan, P.; et al. Associations of Omega-3 Fatty Acid Supplement Use with Cardiovascular Disease Risks: Meta-analysis of 10 Trials Involving 77 917 Individuals. *JAMA Cardiol.* **2018**, *3*, 225–234. [CrossRef]
141. Abdelhamid, A.S.; Brown, T.J.; Brainard, J.S.; Biswas, P.; Thorpe, G.C.; Moore, H.J.; Deane, K.H.; AlAbdulghafoor, F.K.; Summerbell, C.D.; Worthington, H.V.; et al. Omega-3 fatty acids for the primary and secondary prevention of cardiovascular disease. *Cochrane Database Syst. Rev.* **2018**, *7*, CD003177. [CrossRef]
142. Rimm, E.B.; Appel, L.J.; Chiuve, S.E.; Djousse, L.; Engler, M.B.; Kris-Etherton, P.M.; Mozaffarian, D.; Siscovick, D.S.; Lichtenstein, A.H.; American Heart Association Nutrition Committee of the Council on Lifestyle; et al. Seafood Long-Chain n-3 Polyunsaturated Fatty Acids and Cardiovascular Disease: A Science Advisory from the American Heart Association. *Circulation* **2018**, *138*, e35–e47. [CrossRef]
143. Ed Nignpense, B.; Chinkwo, K.A.; Blanchard, C.L.; Santhakumar, A.B. Polyphenols: Modulators of Platelet Function and Platelet Microparticle Generation? *Int. J. Mol. Sci.* **2019**, *21*, 146. [CrossRef]

144. Goszcz, K.; Duthie, G.G.; Stewart, D.; Leslie, S.J.; Megson, I.L. Bioactive polyphenols and cardiovascular disease: Chemical antagonists, pharmacological agents or xenobiotics that drive an adaptive response? *Br. J. Pharmacol.* **2017**, *174*, 1209–1225. [CrossRef]
145. Arts, I.C.; Hollman, P.C. Polyphenols and disease risk in epidemiologic studies. *Am. J. Clin. Nutr.* **2005**, *81*, 317S–325S. [CrossRef]
146. Khan, H.; Jawad, M.; Kamal, M.A.; Baldi, A.; Xiao, J.; Nabavi, S.M.; Daglia, M. Evidence and prospective of plant derived flavonoids as antiplatelet agents: Strong candidates to be drugs of future. *Food Chem. Toxicol.* **2018**, *119*, 355–367. [CrossRef]
147. Heptinstall, S.; May, J.; Fox, S.; Kwik-Uribe, C.; Zhao, L. Cocoa flavanols and platelet and leukocyte function: Recent in vitro and ex vivo studies in healthy adults. *J. Cardiovasc. Pharmacol.* **2006**, *47* (Suppl. 2), S197–S205; discussion S199–S206. [CrossRef]
148. Holt, R.R.; Actis-Goretta, L.; Momma, T.Y.; Keen, C.L. Dietary flavanols and platelet reactivity. *J. Cardiovasc. Pharmacol.* **2006**, *47* (Suppl. 2), S187–S196; discussion S189–S206. [CrossRef]
149. Hamed, M.S.; Gambert, S.; Bliden, K.P.; Bailon, O.; Singla, A.; Antonino, M.J.; Hamed, F.; Tantry, U.S.; Gurbel, P.A. Dark chocolate effect on platelet activity, C-reactive protein and lipid profile: A pilot study. *South Med. J.* **2008**, *101*, 1203–1208. [CrossRef]
150. Pearson, D.A.; Holt, R.R.; Rein, D.; Paglieroni, T.; Schmitz, H.H.; Keen, C.L. Flavanols and platelet reactivity. *Clin. Dev. Immunol.* **2005**, *12*, 1–9. [CrossRef]
151. Ding, E.L.; Hutfless, S.M.; Ding, X.; Girotra, S. Chocolate and prevention of cardiovascular disease: A systematic review. *Nutr. Metab.* **2006**, *3*, 2. [CrossRef] [PubMed]
152. Hermann, F.; Spieker, L.E.; Ruschitzka, F.; Sudano, I.; Hermann, M.; Binggeli, C.; Luscher, T.F.; Riesen, W.; Noll, G.; Corti, R. Dark chocolate improves endothelial and platelet function. *Heart* **2006**, *92*, 119–120. [CrossRef] [PubMed]
153. Wright, B.; Moraes, L.A.; Kemp, C.F.; Mullen, W.; Crozier, A.; Lovegrove, J.A.; Gibbins, J.M. A structural basis for the inhibition of collagen-stimulated platelet function by quercetin and structurally related flavonoids. *Br. J. Pharmacol.* **2010**, *159*, 1312–1325. [CrossRef] [PubMed]
154. Bojic, M.; Debeljak, Z.; Tomicic, M.; Medic-Saric, M.; Tomic, S. Evaluation of antiaggregatory activity of flavonoid aglycone series. *Nutr. J.* **2011**, *10*, 73. [CrossRef]
155. Rein, D.; Paglieroni, T.G.; Pearson, D.A.; Wun, T.; Schmitz, H.H.; Gosselin, R.; Keen, C.L. Cocoa and wine polyphenols modulate platelet activation and function. *J. Nutr.* **2000**, *130*, 2120S–2126S. [CrossRef]
156. Rehman, A.; Tyree, S.M.; Fehlbaum, S.; DunnGalvin, G.; Panagos, C.G.; Guy, B.; Patel, S.; Dinan, T.G.; Duttaroy, A.K.; Duss, R.; et al. A water-soluble tomato extract rich in secondary plant metabolites lowers trimethylamine-n-oxide and modulates gut microbiota: A randomized, double-blind, placebo-controlled cross-over study in overweight and obese adults. *J. Nutr.* **2023**, *153*, 96–105. [CrossRef]
157. Innes, A.J.; Kennedy, G.; McLaren, M.; Bancroft, A.J.; Belch, J.J. Dark chocolate inhibits platelet aggregation in healthy volunteers. *Platelets* **2003**, *14*, 325–327. [CrossRef]
158. Manach, C.; Williamson, G.; Morand, C.; Scalbert, A.; Remesy, C. Bioavailability and bioefficacy of polyphenols in humans. I. Review of 97 bioavailability studies. *Am. J. Clin. Nutr.* **2005**, *81*, 230S–242S. [CrossRef]
159. Dutta-Roy, A.K.; Crosbie, L.C.; Gordon, M.J.; Campbell, F.M. Platelet membrane glycoprotein IV (CD36) is involved in arachidonic acid induced-platelet aggregation. *Biochem. Soc. Trans.* **1996**, *24*, 167S. [CrossRef]
160. Pierre, S.; Crosbie, L.; Duttaroy, A.K. Inhibitory effect of aqueous extracts of some herbs on human platelet aggregation in vitro. *Platelets* **2005**, *16*, 469–473. [CrossRef]
161. Rimbach, G.; Melchin, M.; Moehring, J.; Wagner, A.E. Polyphenols from cocoa and vascular health—A critical review. *Int. J. Mol. Sci.* **2009**, *10*, 4290–4309. [CrossRef] [PubMed]
162. Ostertag, L.M.; O'Kennedy, N.; Kroon, P.A.; Duthie, G.G.; de Roos, B. Impact of dietary polyphenols on human platelet function—A critical review of controlled dietary intervention studies. *Mol. Nutr. Food Res.* **2010**, *54*, 60–81. [CrossRef] [PubMed]
163. Singh, I.; Mok, M.; Christensen, A.M.; Turner, A.H.; Hawley, J.A. The effects of polyphenols in olive leaves on platelet function. *Nutr. Metab. Cardiovasc. Dis.* **2008**, *18*, 127–132. [CrossRef] [PubMed]
164. Singh, I.; Quinn, H.; Mok, M.; Southgate, R.J.; Turner, A.H.; Li, D.; Sinclair, A.J.; Hawley, J.A. The effect of exercise and training status on platelet activation: Do cocoa polyphenols play a role? *Platelets* **2006**, *17*, 361–367. [CrossRef] [PubMed]
165. Fuentes, E.; Caballero, J.; Alarcon, M.; Rojas, A.; Palomo, I. Chlorogenic acid inhibits human platelet activation and thrombus formation. *PLoS ONE* **2014**, *9*, e90699. [CrossRef]
166. Zhou, F.H.; Deng, X.J.; Chen, Y.Q.; Ya, F.L.; Zhang, X.D.; Song, F.; Li, D.; Yang, Y. Anthocyanin Cyanidin-3-Glucoside Attenuates Platelet Granule Release in Mice Fed High-Fat Diets. *J. Nutr. Sci. Vitaminol.* **2017**, *63*, 237–243. [CrossRef]
167. Yao, Y.; Chen, Y.; Adili, R.; McKeown, T.; Chen, P.; Zhu, G.; Li, D.; Ling, W.; Ni, H.; Yang, Y. Plant-based Food Cyanidin-3-Glucoside Modulates Human Platelet Glycoprotein VI Signaling and Inhibits Platelet Activation and Thrombus Formation. *J. Nutr.* **2017**, *147*, 1917–1925. [CrossRef]
168. de la Torre, R. Bioavailability of olive oil phenolic compounds in humans. *Inflammopharmacology* **2008**, *16*, 245–247. [CrossRef]
169. Correa, J.A.; Lopez-Villodres, J.A.; Asensi, R.; Espartero, J.L.; Rodriguez-Gutierez, G.; De La Cruz, J.P. Virgin olive oil polyphenol hydroxytyrosol acetate inhibits in vitro platelet aggregation in human whole blood: Comparison with hydroxytyrosol and acetylsalicylic acid. *Br. J. Nutr.* **2009**, *101*, 1157–1164. [CrossRef]
170. Bojic, M.; Antolic, A.; Tomicic, M.; Debeljak, Z.; Males, Z. Propolis ethanolic extracts reduce adenosine diphosphate induced platelet aggregation determined on whole blood. *Nutr. J.* **2018**, *17*, 52. [CrossRef]

171. Faggio, C.; Sureda, A.; Morabito, S.; Sanches-Silva, A.; Mocan, A.; Nabavi, S.F.; Nabavi, S.M. Flavonoids and platelet aggregation: A brief review. *Eur. J. Pharmacol.* **2017**, *807*, 91–101. [CrossRef] [PubMed]
172. Chang, S.S.; Lee, V.S.; Tseng, Y.L.; Chang, K.C.; Chen, K.B.; Chen, Y.L.; Li, C.Y. Gallic Acid Attenuates Platelet Activation and Platelet-Leukocyte Aggregation: Involving Pathways of Akt and GSK3beta. *Evid. Based Complement. Altern. Med.* **2012**, *2012*, 683872. [CrossRef] [PubMed]
173. Olas, B.; Wachowicz, B.; Stochmal, A.; Oleszek, W. The polyphenol-rich extract from grape seeds inhibits platelet signaling pathways triggered by both proteolytic and non-proteolytic agonists. *Platelets* **2012**, *23*, 282–289. [CrossRef] [PubMed]
174. Shi, J.; Yu, J.; Pohorly, J.E.; Kakuda, Y. Polyphenolics in grape seeds-biochemistry and functionality. *J. Med. Food* **2003**, *6*, 291–299. [CrossRef]
175. Bijak, M.; Saluk-Bijak, J. Flavonolignans inhibit the arachidonic acid pathway in blood platelets. *BMC Complement. Altern. Med.* **2017**, *17*, 396. [CrossRef]
176. Duttaroy, A.K. Role of Gut Microbiota and Their Metabolites on Atherosclerosis, Hypertension and Human Blood Platelet Function: A Review. *Nutrients* **2021**, *13*, 144. [CrossRef]
177. Wang, Z.; Huang, Y.; Zou, J.; Cao, K.; Xu, Y.; Wu, J.M. Effects of red wine and wine polyphenol resveratrol on platelet aggregation in vivo and in vitro. *Int. J. Mol. Med.* **2002**, *9*, 77–79. [CrossRef]
178. Zhu, W.; Gregory, J.C.; Org, E.; Buffa, J.A.; Gupta, N.; Wang, Z.; Li, L.; Fu, X.; Wu, Y.; Mehrabian, M.; et al. Gut Microbial Metabolite TMAO Enhances Platelet Hyperreactivity and Thrombosis Risk. *Cell* **2016**, *165*, 111–124. [CrossRef] [PubMed]
179. Wang, Z.; Klipfell, E.; Bennett, B.J.; Koeth, R.; Levison, B.S.; Dugar, B.; Feldstein, A.E.; Britt, E.B.; Fu, X.; Chung, Y.M.; et al. Gut flora metabolism of phosphatidylcholine promotes cardiovascular disease. *Nature* **2011**, *472*, 57–63. [CrossRef]
180. Drosos, I.; Tavridou, A.; Kolios, G. New aspects on the metabolic role of intestinal microbiota in the development of atherosclerosis. *Metabolism* **2015**, *64*, 476–481. [CrossRef]
181. Gregory, J.C.; Buffa, J.A.; Org, E.; Wang, Z.; Levison, B.S.; Zhu, W.; Wagner, M.A.; Bennett, B.J.; Li, L.; DiDonato, J.A.; et al. Transmission of atherosclerosis susceptibility with gut microbial transplantation. *J. Biol. Chem.* **2015**, *290*, 5647–5660. [CrossRef] [PubMed]
182. Jie, Z.; Xia, H.; Zhong, S.L.; Feng, Q.; Li, S.; Liang, S.; Zhong, H.; Liu, Z.; Gao, Y.; Zhao, H.; et al. The gut microbiome in atherosclerotic cardiovascular disease. *Nat. Commun.* **2017**, *8*, 845. [CrossRef]
183. Karlsson, F.H.; Fak, F.; Nookaew, I.; Tremaroli, V.; Fagerberg, B.; Petranovic, D.; Backhed, F.; Nielsen, J. Symptomatic atherosclerosis is associated with an altered gut metagenome. *Nat. Commun.* **2012**, *3*, 1245. [CrossRef] [PubMed]
184. Lau, K.; Srivatsav, V.; Rizwan, A.; Nashed, A.; Liu, R.; Shen, R.; Akhtar, M. Bridging the Gap between Gut Microbial Dysbiosis and Cardiovascular Diseases. *Nutrients* **2017**, *9*, 859. [CrossRef]
185. Santisteban, M.M.; Qi, Y.; Zubcevic, J.; Kim, S.; Yang, T.; Shenoy, V.; Cole-Jeffrey, C.T.; Lobaton, G.O.; Stewart, D.C.; Rubiano, A.; et al. Hypertension-Linked Pathophysiological Alterations in the Gut. *Circ. Res.* **2017**, *120*, 312–323. [CrossRef]
186. Chen, M.L.; Yi, L.; Zhang, Y.; Zhou, X.; Ran, L.; Yang, J.; Zhu, J.D.; Zhang, Q.Y.; Mi, M.T. Resveratrol Attenuates Trimethylamine-N-Oxide (TMAO)-Induced Atherosclerosis by Regulating TMAO Synthesis and Bile Acid Metabolism via Remodeling of the Gut Microbiota. *mBio* **2016**, *7*, e02210–e02215. [CrossRef] [PubMed]
187. Lim, T.; Ryu, J.; Lee, K.; Park, S.Y.; Hwang, K.T. Protective Effects of Black Raspberry (*Rubus occidentalis*) Extract against Hypercholesterolemia and Hepatic Inflammation in Rats Fed High-Fat and High-Choline Diets. *Nutrients* **2020**, *12*, 2448. [CrossRef]
188. Annunziata, G.; Maisto, M.; Schisano, C.; Ciampaglia, R.; Narciso, V.; Tenore, G.C.; Novellino, E. Effects of Grape Pomace Polyphenolic Extract (Taurisolo®) in Reducing TMAO Serum Levels in Humans: Preliminary Results from a Randomized, Placebo-Controlled, Cross-Over Study. *Nutrients* **2019**, *11*, 139. [CrossRef] [PubMed]
189. Grundy, S.M.; Cleeman, J.I.; Daniels, S.R.; Donato, K.A.; Eckel, R.H.; Franklin, B.A.; Gordon, D.J.; Krauss, R.M.; Savage, P.J.; Smith, S.C., Jr.; et al. Diagnosis and management of the metabolic syndrome: An American Heart Association/National Heart, Lung, and Blood Institute Scientific Statement. *Circulation* **2005**, *112*, 2735–2752. [CrossRef]
190. Shimodaira, M.; Niwa, T.; Nakajima, K.; Kobayashi, M.; Hanyu, N.; Nakayama, T. Correlation between mean platelet volume and fasting plasma glucose levels in prediabetic and normoglycemic individuals. *Cardiovasc. Diabetol.* **2013**, *12*, 14. [CrossRef]
191. Pamukcu, B.; Lip, G.Y.; Snezhitskiy, V.; Shantsila, E. The CD40-CD40L system in cardiovascular disease. *Ann. Med.* **2011**, *43*, 331–340. [CrossRef] [PubMed]
192. Ferroni, P.; Basili, S.; Falco, A.; Davi, G. Platelet activation in type 2 diabetes mellitus. *J. Thromb. Haemost. JTH* **2004**, *2*, 1282–1291. [CrossRef] [PubMed]
193. Ferroni, P.; Martini, F.; D'Alessandro, R.; Magnapera, A.; Raparelli, V.; Scarno, A.; Davi, G.; Basili, S.; Guadagni, F. In vivo platelet activation is responsible for enhanced vascular endothelial growth factor levels in hypertensive patients. *Clin. Chim. Acta* **2008**, *388*, 33–37. [CrossRef]
194. Huang, Y.; Yang, Z.; Ye, Z.; Li, Q.; Wen, J.; Tao, X.; Chen, L.; He, M.; Wang, X.; Lu, B.; et al. Lipocalin-2, glucose metabolism and chronic low-grade systemic inflammation in Chinese people. *Cardiovasc. Diabetol.* **2012**, *11*, 11. [CrossRef]
195. Slavin, J.L.; Lloyd, B. Health benefits of fruits and vegetables. *Adv. Nutr.* **2012**, *3*, 506–516. [CrossRef]
196. Gaziano, J.M.; Manson, J.E.; Branch, L.G.; Colditz, G.A.; Willett, W.C.; Buring, J.E. A prospective study of consumption of carotenoids in fruits and vegetables and decreased cardiovascular mortality in the elderly. *Ann. Epidemiol.* **1995**, *5*, 255–260. [CrossRef]

197. Joshipura, K.J.; Ascherio, A.; Manson, J.E.; Stampfer, M.J.; Rimm, E.B.; Speizer, F.E.; Hennekens, C.H.; Spiegelman, D.; Willett, W.C. Fruit and vegetable intake in relation to risk of ischemic stroke. *JAMA* **1999**, *282*, 1233–1239. [CrossRef]
198. Obarzanek, E.; Sacks, F.M.; Vollmer, W.M.; Bray, G.A.; Miller, E.R., 3rd; Lin, P.H.; Karanja, N.M.; Most-Windhauser, M.M.; Moore, T.J.; Swain, J.F.; et al. Effects on blood lipids of a blood pressure-lowering diet: The Dietary Approaches to Stop Hypertension (DASH) Trial. *Am. J. Clin. Nutr.* **2001**, *74*, 80–89. [CrossRef] [PubMed]
199. Dizdarevic, L.L.; Biswas, D.; Uddin, M.D.; Jorgenesen, A.; Falch, E.; Bastani, N.E.; Duttaroy, A.K. Inhibitory effects of kiwifruit extract on human platelet aggregation and plasma angiotensin-converting enzyme activity. *Platelets* **2014**, *25*, 567–575. [CrossRef]
200. O'Kennedy, N.; Crosbie, L.; van Lieshout, M.; Broom, J.I.; Webb, D.J.; Duttaroy, A.K. Effects of antiplatelet components of tomato extract on platelet function in vitro and ex vivo: A time-course cannulation study in healthy humans. *Am. J. Clin. Nutr.* **2006**, *84*, 570–579. [CrossRef]
201. Barin, A.; Das, R.K.; Bastani, N.E.; Iversen, P.O.; Duttaroy, A.K. Extracts of tamarillo, horned melon, and raspberry, but not extract of pear, inhibit human blood platelet aggregation: Investigating the underlying factors for their differential mechanisms. *J. Funct. Foods* **2023**, *110*, 105847. [CrossRef]
202. Giovannucci, E. Tomatoes, tomato-based products, lycopene, and cancer: Review of the epidemiologic literature. *J. Natl. Cancer Inst.* **1999**, *91*, 317–331. [CrossRef]
203. Giovannucci, E. A review of epidemiologic studies of tomatoes, lycopene, and prostate cancer. *Exp. Biol. Med.* **2002**, *227*, 852–859. [CrossRef]
204. Giovannucci, E.; Rimm, E.B.; Liu, Y.; Stampfer, M.J.; Willett, W.C. A prospective study of tomato products, lycopene, and prostate cancer risk. *J. Natl. Cancer Inst.* **2002**, *94*, 391–398. [CrossRef] [PubMed]
205. O'Kennedy, N.; Crosbie, L.; Whelan, S.; Luther, V.; Horgan, G.; Broom, J.I.; Webb, D.J.; Duttaroy, A.K. Effects of tomato extract on platelet function: A double-blinded crossover study in healthy humans. *Am. J. Clin. Nutr.* **2006**, *84*, 561–569. [CrossRef]
206. Fuentes, E.; Castro, R.; Astudillo, L.; Carrasco, G.; Alarcon, M.; Gutierrez, M.; Palomo, I. Bioassay-Guided Isolation and HPLC Determination of Bioactive Compound That Relate to the Antiplatelet Activity (Adhesion, Secretion, and Aggregation) from *Solanum lycopersicum*. *Evid. Based Complement. Altern. Med.* **2012**, *2012*, 147031. [CrossRef]
207. Chen, H.; Zhang, S.; Wang, H.; Bao, L.; Wu, W.; Qi, R. Fruitflow inhibits platelet function by suppressing Akt/GSK3beta, Syk/PLCgamma2 and p38 MAPK phosphorylation in collagen-stimulated platelets. *BMC Complement. Med. Ther.* **2022**, *22*, 75. [CrossRef] [PubMed]
208. Schwager, J.; Richard, N.; Mussler, B.; Raederstorff, D. Tomato Aqueous Extract Modulates the Inflammatory Profile of Immune Cells and Endothelial Cells. *Molecules* **2016**, *21*, 168. [CrossRef]
209. Zhang, S.; Chen, H.; Li, C.; Chen, B.; Gong, H.; Zhao, Y.; Qi, R. Water-Soluble Tomato Extract Fruitflow Alters the Phosphoproteomic Profile of Collagen-Stimulated Platelets. *Front. Pharmacol.* **2021**, *12*, 746107. [CrossRef]
210. Cho, J. Protein disulfide isomerase in thrombosis and vascular inflammation. *J. Thromb. Haemost.* **2013**, *11*, 2084–2091. [CrossRef]
211. Manickam, N.; Sun, X.; Li, M.; Gazitt, Y.; Essex, D.W. Protein disulphide isomerase in platelet function. *Br. J. Haematol.* **2008**, *140*, 223–229. [CrossRef] [PubMed]
212. Jasuja, R.; Passam, F.H.; Kennedy, D.R.; Kim, S.H.; van Hessem, L.; Lin, L.; Bowley, S.R.; Joshi, S.S.; Dilks, J.R.; Furie, B.; et al. Protein disulfide isomerase inhibitors constitute a new class of antithrombotic agents. *J. Clin. Investig.* **2012**, *122*, 2104–2113. [CrossRef] [PubMed]
213. Sheu, J.R.; Hsiao, G.; Chou, P.H.; Shen, M.Y.; Chou, D.S. Mechanisms involved in the antiplatelet activity of rutin, a glycoside of the flavonol quercetin, in human platelets. *J. Agric. Food Chem.* **2004**, *52*, 4414–4418. [CrossRef] [PubMed]
214. Das, R.K.; Datta, T.; Biswas, D.; Duss, R.; O'Kennedy, N.; Duttaroy, A.K. Evaluation of the equivalence of different intakes of Fruitflow in affecting platelet aggregation and thrombin generation capacity in a randomized, double-blinded pilot study in male subjects. *BMC Nutr.* **2021**, *7*, 80. [CrossRef] [PubMed]
215. O'Kennedy, N.; Crosbie, L.; Song, H.J.; Zhang, X.; Horgan, G.; Duttaroy, A.K. A randomised controlled trial comparing a dietary antiplatelet, the water-soluble tomato extract Fruitflow, with 75 mg aspirin in healthy subjects. *Eur. J. Clin. Nutr.* **2017**, *71*, 723–730. [CrossRef]
216. Tian, Z.; Fan, D.; Li, K.; Zhao, D.; Liang, Y.; Ji, Q.; Gao, X.; Ma, X.; Zhao, Y.; Mao, Y.; et al. Four-Week Supplementation of Water-Soluble Tomato Extract Attenuates Platelet Function in Chinese Healthy Middle-Aged and Older Individuals: A Randomized, Double-Blinded, and Crossover Clinical Trial. *Front. Nutr.* **2022**, *9*, 891241. [CrossRef]
217. Krasinska, B.; Osinska, A.; Osinski, M.; Krasinska, A.; Rzymski, P.; Tykarski, A.; Krasinski, Z. Standardised tomato extract as an alternative to acetylsalicylic acid in patients with primary hypertension and high cardiovascular risk—A randomised, controlled trial. *Arch. Med. Sci.* **2018**, *14*, 773–780. [CrossRef]
218. Liu, L.; Xiao, S.; Wang, Y.; Wang, Y.; Liu, L.; Sun, Z.; Zhang, Q.; Yin, X.; Liao, F.; You, Y.; et al. Water-soluble tomato concentrate modulates shear-induced platelet aggregation and blood flow in vitro and in vivo. *Front. Nutr.* **2022**, *9*, 961301. [CrossRef]
219. Fiorentino, A.; D'Abrosca, B.; Pacifico, S.; Mastellone, C.; Scognamiglio, M.; Monaco, P. Identification and assessment of antioxidant capacity of phytochemicals from kiwi fruits. *J. Agric. Food Chem.* **2009**, *57*, 4148–4155. [CrossRef]
220. Karlsen, A.; Svendsen, M.; Seljeflot, I.; Laake, P.; Duttaroy, A.K.; Drevon, C.A.; Arnesen, H.; Tonstad, S.; Blomhoff, R. Kiwifruit decreases blood pressure and whole-blood platelet aggregation in male smokers. *J. Hum. Hypertens.* **2012**, *27*, 126–130. [CrossRef]

221. Brevik, A.; Gaivao, I.; Medin, T.; Jorgenesen, A.; Piasek, A.; Elilasson, J.; Karlsen, A.; Blomhoff, R.; Veggan, T.; Duttaroy, A.K.; et al. Supplementation of a western diet with golden kiwifruits (*Actinidia chinensis* var.'Hort 16A'.) effects on biomarkers of oxidation damage and antioxidant protection. *Nutr. J.* **2011**, *10*, 54. [CrossRef] [PubMed]
222. Chang, W.H.; Liu, J.F. Effects of kiwifruit consumption on serum lipid profiles and antioxidative status in hyperlipidemic subjects. *Int. J. Food Sci. Nutr.* **2009**, *60*, 709–716. [CrossRef] [PubMed]
223. Jung, K.A.; Song, T.C.; Han, D.; Kim, I.H.; Kim, Y.E.; Lee, C.H. Cardiovascular protective properties of kiwifruit extracts in vitro. *Biol. Pharm. Bull.* **2005**, *28*, 1782–1785. [CrossRef] [PubMed]
224. Kroll, M.H.; Schafer, A.I. Biochemical mechanisms of platelet activation. *Blood* **1989**, *74*, 1181–1195. [CrossRef] [PubMed]
225. Ferroni, P.; Santilli, F.; Guadagni, F.; Basili, S.; Davi, G. Contribution of platelet-derived CD40 ligand to inflammation, thrombosis and neoangiogenesis. *Curr. Med. Chem.* **2007**, *14*, 2170–2180. [CrossRef]
226. Fuentes, E.J.; Astudillo, L.A.; Gutierrez, M.I.; Contreras, S.O.; Bustamante, L.O.; Rubio, P.I.; Moore-Carrasco, R.; Alarcon, M.A.; Fuentes, J.A.; Gonzalez, D.E.; et al. Fractions of aqueous and methanolic extracts from tomato (*Solanum lycopersicum* L.) present platelet antiaggregant activity. *Blood Coagul. Fibrinolysis Int. J. Haemost. Thromb.* **2012**, *23*, 109–117. [CrossRef]
227. Hankey, G.J.; Eikelboom, J.W. Aspirin resistance. *Lancet* **2006**, *367*, 606–617. [CrossRef]
228. Ravishankar, D.; Albadawi, D.A.I.; Chaggar, V.; Patra, P.H.; Williams, H.F.; Salamah, M.; Vaiyapuri, R.; Dash, P.R.; Patel, K.; Watson, K.A.; et al. Isorhapontigenin, a resveratrol analogue selectively inhibits ADP-stimulated platelet activation. *Eur. J. Pharmacol.* **2019**, *862*, 172627. [CrossRef]
229. Schumacher, E.; Vigh, E.; Molnar, V.; Kenyeres, P.; Feher, G.; Kesmarky, G.; Toth, K.; Garai, J. Thrombosis preventive potential of chicory coffee consumption: A clinical study. *Phytother. Res.* **2011**, *25*, 744–748. [CrossRef]
230. Nickel, T.; Lackermair, K.; Scherr, J.; Calatzis, A.; Vogeser, M.; Hanssen, H.; Waidhauser, G.; Schonermark, U.; Methe, H.; Horster, S.; et al. Influence of High Polyphenol Beverage on Stress-Induced Platelet Activation. *J. Nutr. Health Aging* **2016**, *20*, 586–593. [CrossRef]
231. Draijer, R.; de Graaf, Y.; Slettenaar, M.; de Groot, E.; Wright, C.I. Consumption of a polyphenol-rich grape-wine extract lowers ambulatory blood pressure in mildly hypertensive subjects. *Nutrients* **2015**, *7*, 3138–3153. [CrossRef] [PubMed]
232. Ras, R.T.; Zock, P.L.; Zebregs, Y.E.; Johnston, N.R.; Webb, D.J.; Draijer, R. Effect of polyphenol-rich grape seed extract on ambulatory blood pressure in subjects with pre- and stage I hypertension. *Br. J. Nutr.* **2013**, *110*, 2234–2241. [CrossRef] [PubMed]
233. Flammer, A.J.; Sudano, I.; Wolfrum, M.; Thomas, R.; Enseleit, F.; Periat, D.; Kaiser, P.; Hirt, A.; Hermann, M.; Serafini, M.; et al. Cardiovascular effects of flavanol-rich chocolate in patients with heart failure. *Eur. Heart J.* **2012**, *33*, 2172–2180. [CrossRef] [PubMed]
234. Loo, B.M.; Erlund, I.; Koli, R.; Puukka, P.; Hellstrom, J.; Wahala, K.; Mattila, P.; Jula, A. Consumption of chokeberry (*Aronia mitschurinii*) products modestly lowered blood pressure and reduced low-grade inflammation in patients with mildly elevated blood pressure. *Nutr. Res.* **2016**, *36*, 1222–1230. [CrossRef]
235. Zhang, X.; McGeoch, S.C.; Megson, I.L.; MacRury, S.M.; Johnstone, A.M.; Abraham, P.; Pearson, D.W.; de Roos, B.; Holtrop, G.; O'Kennedy, N.; et al. Oat-enriched diet reduces inflammatory status assessed by circulating cell-derived microparticle concentrations in type 2 diabetes. *Mol. Nutr. Food Res.* **2014**, *58*, 1322–1332. [CrossRef]

nutrients

MDPI

Review

Exploring the Phytochemical, Pharmacological and Nutritional Properties of *Moringa oleifera*: A Comprehensive Review

Surisetti Divya [1], Vinay Kumar Pandey [2,*], Ritik Dixit [3], Sarvesh Rustagi [4], Tejas Suthar [5], David Atuahene [6], Vivien Nagy [7,8], Diána Ungai [8], Abdelhakam Esmaeil Mohamed Ahmed [8,9,10], Béla Kovács [8,11] and Ayaz Mukarram Shaikh [8,10,11,*]

1 Department of Pharmacology, Kanpur Institute of Technology and Pharmacy, Kanpur 208001, Uttar Pradesh, India; divya.pharmacy.50@gmail.com
2 Research & Development Cell, Biotechnology Department, Manav Rachna International Institute of Research and Studies (Deemed to Be University), Faridabad 121004, Haryana, India
3 Department of Pharmaceutical Chemistry, Advance Institute of Biotech & Paramedical Sciences, Kanpur 209217, Uttar Pradesh, India; ritikdixit045@gmail.com
4 Department of Food Technology, School of Applied & Life Sciences, Uttaranchal University, Dehradun 248007, Uttarakhand, India; sarveshrustagi@gmail.com
5 Independent Researcher, Chicago, IL 60616, USA; suthartejas2525@gmail.com
6 Department of Veterinary Sciences, School of Agriculture and Veterinary Medicine, University of Turin, Grugliasco, I-10095 Turin, Italy; david.atuahene@unito.it
7 Faculty of Agriculture, Food Science, and Environmental Management, Institute of Food Technology, University of Debrecen, Böszörményi út 138, 4032 Debrecen, Hungary; nagy.vivien@agr.unideb.hu
8 Doctoral School of Nutrition and Food Sciences, University of Debrecen, Böszörményi út 138, 4032 Debrecen, Hungary; ungai@agr.unideb.hu (D.U.); ahmed.abdelhakam@agr.unideb.hu (A.E.M.A.); kovacsb@agr.unideb.hu (B.K.)
9 Faculty of Forestry, University of Khartoum, Khartoum North 13314, Sudan
10 Faculty of Agriculture, Food Science and Environmental Management, Institute of Food Science, University of Debrecen, 4032 Debrecen, Hungary
11 World Food Forum, I-00100 Rome, Italy
* Correspondence: v.k.pandey30@gmail.com (V.K.P.); ayaz.shaikh@agr.unideb.hu (A.M.S.)

Abstract: Background: *Moringa oleifera* is one of the most nutrient-packed species, commonly known as the drumstick tree or miracle tree, and has garnered substantial popularity for its health benefits, phytochemical profile, and therapeutic potential. *Moringa oleifera* is a plant that is native to the Indian subcontinent and has been used in traditional medicine for thousands of years owing to its nutritional and therapeutic properties. **Methods:** The leaves, seeds, pods, roots, and flowers of this plant are enriched with a wide range of bioactive compounds such as flavonoids, alkaloids, vitamins, minerals, and essential amino acids. Therefore, it is considered a reservoir crop for both nutritional and medicinal applications. **Result:** The recent rediscovery of the plant is at the forefront of changes in nutrition, medicine, and public health. Owing to its varied clinical applications, the plant is a potential candidate for research in new drug development and functional foods. **Conclusions:** Potential applications of *Moringa* compounds in the treatment of chronic diseases include antioxidant, anti-inflammatory, antimicrobial (bacterial or fungal), and anticancerous effects. In this review, various phytochemical extraction techniques, therapeutic properties, and applications are discussed.

Keywords: *Moringa oleifera*; pharmaceutical properties; health benefits; nutrition; bioactive compounds

1. Introduction

From the sub-Himalayan regions of India, Pakistan, Afghanistan, and Bangladesh, *Moringa oleifera* is the predominant pantropical species within the Monogeneric Moringaceae family. It is an all-purpose tree that is a lifeline for many communities [1]. It is commercially grown across several continents, regions, and countries including Africa, Hawaii, South and Central America, Mexico, and Asia. It is also known as the "horseradish tree" for its ground root taste, or the "drumstick tree" because its pods look like drumsticks when the seeds are not fully mature. Due to the oil made from the seeds of this plant, it has also been referred to as a "ben oil tree" [2]. In some areas, people consume the tender seed pods; fresh leaves are common ingredients in their food because they are rich in nutrients. This plant is commonly referred to as *Moringa oleifera* but is also known by other synonyms such as the "miracle tree" due to its numerous bioactive compounds that attract attention in traditional medicine/nutritional circles [3]. Deciduous trees or shrubs can grow up to approximately 12 m with rapid growth and the ability to survive drought. Among the various species are *M. arborea, M. arivae, M. concanensis, M. drouhardii, M. ruspolian, M. longituba, M. stenoprtala, M. peregrina, M. pygmaea, M. borziana, M. hildebrandtii,* and *M. ovalifolia*. These plants have medicinal value owing to the presence of natural compounds that can be used for treatment. In this area, one tree known as *Moringa oleifera* stands out because it has a variety of health-related positives. Normally growing between 10 and 12 m tall, *Moringa oleifera* is a small but fast-growing evergreen and deciduous tree. Leaves, which are tripinnate in nature, have a spreading crown characterized by delicate drooping branches and dense corky whitish bark [4].

All parts of the plant contain proteins, vitamins, minerals, and carotenoids, which make up the overall nutritional profile worldwide. Poor nutrition among infants and lactating mothers has been addressed with the use of *Moringa* trees [5]. Essential nutrients, such as proteins and minerals (including vitamins A and C), are abundant in leaves. Additionally, *Moringa* is equipped with approximately 46 antioxidants; hence, it is one of the most potent natural sources of these substances. Antioxidants play a key role in destroying the negative effects of free radicals on the human body. Flavonoids, tannins, saponins, alkaloids, phenolics, and triterpenoids are active constituents of *M. oleifera,* with antibacterial properties acting as antioxidants [6]. These plant leaves can be eaten fresh, roasted, or dried, and they retain their nutritional value for several months according to reports. Other foods are scarce during the dry season. *M. oleifera* blooms towards the end of a long dry period when it can flourish into lush foliage, which means that other food sources have disappeared or diminished greatly, meaning that this plant is a possible food crop for human use [7].

The native drugs are said to be derived from a particular plant with many different types that have been used for the treatment of various diseases for generations. Furthermore, this plant is all-purpose: the leaf bark, sap flower seed oil, or root can be used medicinally throughout [8,9]. Aiding hypertension, anxiety, and diarrhea, and being a natural diuretic are some of the conditions that give *Moringa oleifera* healing properties [10,11]. It also has an effect against dysentery and colitis [12,13]. *Moringa* leaves can be used topically to treat inflammatory problems, such as glandular swelling, headaches, and bronchitis [14]. The pods are good for the liver while relieving joint pain [15]. In herbal medicine, the roots cure kidney stones [16], liver ailments [17], inflammation [18], ulcers [19], and earache/toothache [20]. The gum taken from this plant is used by Indians to induce abortions and treat fever [21,22]. The seeds of this plant have laxative potential and are used to treat ailments of the bladder and prostate, and cancer [23]. Because the seeds alter oxidative stress and reduce inflammation, they have the potential to treat arthritis [24]. Preparations made from the leaves of the plant enhance overall population health and help nursing mothers and undernourished babies. These substances increase the synthesis of estrogen, which in turn provokes the growth of mammalian tissue, resulting in the secretion of milk. They are instrumental in addressing malnutrition in children under three years of age. The leaves are also valuable for individuals with insomnia [25] and wound care [26]. *Moringa* has gained widespread use in the cosmetic industry today. Historically, it was similarly employed in ancient Egypt to make skin ointments [27]. The capacity of *M. oleifera* plants to purify aquaculture wastewater has been evaluated. Studies have demonstrated its ability to concurrently remove water cloudiness, suspended solids, and microorganisms, potentially replacing or supplementing traditional coagulants and thus offering economic, health, and environmental benefits [28].

Moringa is renowned for its exceptional nutritional profile, offering a multitude of vitamins and minerals that far exceed those found in many common foods. It boasts seven times the ascorbic acid (vit C) found in oranges, 10 times the retinol (vit A) of carrots, 17 times the calcium of milk, nine times the protein of yogurt, 15 times the potassium of bananas, and 25 times the iron of spinach [29]. This plant is a powerhouse for essential minerals, with calcium being a standout for human development. For instance, while eight ounces of milk provide 300 to 400 mg of calcium (an important element of bone density), this plant's leaves offer 1000 mg, and *Moringa* powder can deliver over 4000 mg of bone density. Anemia can be treated using *Moringa* powder as an alternative to iron pills. The iron content in beef is only 2 mg, whereas powdered *Moringa* leaves contain 28 mg. One of the essential elements of zinc is obtained through nutrition for sperm cell synthesis and growth and for nucleic acid synthesis. The amount of this element found in *M. oleifera* leaves constitutes about 25.5–31.03 mg/kg, which is the recommended everyday allowance for zinc in a healthy diet [30]. Tree bark is thought to be highly helpful in treating a variety of conditions including ulcers, toothaches, and high blood pressure. In addition, it has been discovered that the roots can help treat paralysis, helminthiasis, and toothaches. The flowers are used to produce aphrodisiac compounds, cure ulcers, and enlarge the spleen [14,31,32]. Temperatures between 25 and 35 °C are ideal for growing *M. oleifera* in all semi-tropical and tropical parts of the planet. It requires loamy or sandy soil with a pH range of mildly acidic to moderately alkaline and 250–3000 mm net precipitation [33,34]. *M. oleifera* differs in the distribution of nutrients at various sites. The nutritional components of plants cultivated in Nigeria and India differ slightly [35]. Recent pharmacological research has uncovered a variety of therapeutic properties of different extracts of *Moringa*, including antimicrobial, antifungal, anti-inflammatory, antioxidant, anticancer, fertility-enhancing, and wound-healing effects. This review aims to consolidate the latest findings on the pharmacological actions, global research, toxicology, phytochemistry, and overall attributes of *M. oleifera*.

Traditional Uses of Moringa oleifera in Herbal Medicine

In accordance with the tenets of Traditional Ayurvedic Medicine, the physiological characteristics and therapeutic utility of various components of *Moringa oleifera* are projected to elicit a diverse array of effects contingent on the individual's bodily constitution and their alignment with Vata or Kapha doshas. *Moringa oleifera* manifests bitterness and acridity, is imbued with thermogenic properties, fosters digestion, functions as a carminative and anthelmintic as well as a constipating agent, mitigates pain, and exhibits anti-inflammatory effects. Moreover, it facilitates menstruation, induces sweating, enhances urine production, promotes ocular health, engenders local warmth, aids expectoration, elevates hemoglobin levels, dissolves urinary stones, serves as an antidote, stimulates physiological functions, and evokes blistering. It rectifies imbalances associated with the Vata and Kapha constitutions, including dyspepsia, anorexia, helminthiasis, diarrhea, colic, bloating, otalgia, paralysis, inflammation, menstrual irregularities, dysmenorrhea, fever, dysuria, urolithiasis, ascites, ophthalmic ailments, cough, bronchial asthma, cardiac disorders, abscesses, and otolaryngological infections. It possesses acrid and bitter flavors, is endowed with thermogenic properties, exerts abortifacient effects, combats fungal infections, and stimulates cardiovascular and circulatory functions. Mitigating Vata–Kapha imbalances and dermatophyte afflictions is recommended to address ascites [36,37]. The nutritional and therapeutic values of *Moringa oleifera* are shown in Figure 1.

Moringa oleifera is distinguished by its bitter taste and cooling potency, exhibiting anti-inflammatory and analgesic effects, acting as anthelmintics, promoting ocular health, and serving as rich reservoirs of vitamins A and C. It is valuable in the management of scurvy, Vata–Kapha imbalances, wounds, tumors, inflammations, and helminthic infestations. It possesses acrid and bitter tastes, imparting a cooling sensation, exerting analgesic and anti-inflammatory effects, functioning as a purgative, reducing fever, and enhancing ocular health. It is recommended for assuaging neuralgic pain, inflammation, intermittent fever, and ophthalmic disorders [24]. *Moringa oleifera*, hailing from the Himalayas, is delineated in the Chinese herbal medicine compendium, although it remains absent from classical texts of Traditional Chinese Medicine (TCM) and lacks widespread recognition as a conventional Chinese herb. Nevertheless, a variant with wingless seeds has been identified in Southern Yunnan. Imported to China from India during the 1960s, *M. oleifera* was extensively cultivated for ornamental purposes and disseminated across provinces such as Guangdong, Taiwan, and Yunnan, where it is denoted as "lamu" in Mandarin. While its nutritional significance is duly recognized, TCM principles accentuate the thermal and gustatory characteristics of herbs or foodstuffs to determine their appropriateness for individuals based on their constitutional predispositions and thermal tendencies. Predominantly ingested for its foliage, *M. oleifera* manifests both bitter and sweet flavor profiles, with a downward refrigerating impact. Given its refrigerant nature, circumspection is warranted for individuals exhibiting cold constitutions or yang deficiency, characterized by sensations of coldness, lethargy, and other manifestations associated with cold syndrome ailments [38].

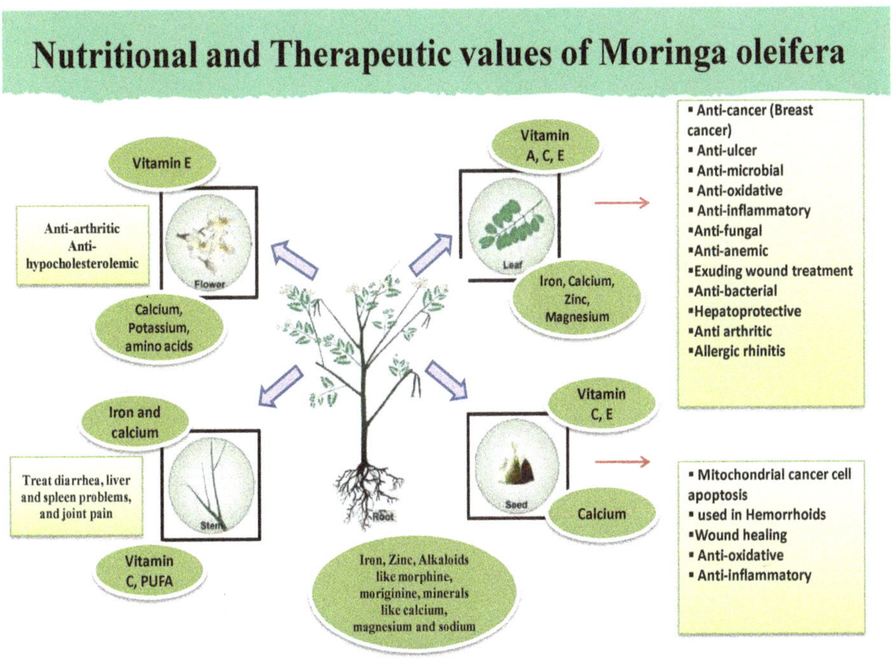

Figure 1. Nutritional and therapeutic values of *Moringa oleifera* whole plant.

2. Phytochemical Composition of *Moringa oleifera*

Research on *M. oleifera* and its derivatives has delved deeply into the understanding of its many facets. More than 90 distinct compounds have been identified in the genus *Moringa*, showing potential therapeutic benefits. Proteins, amino acids [39], phenolic acids [40], carotenoids [41], alkaloids [42], glucosinolates [43], flavonoids [3], sterols [44], terpenes [45], tannins and saponins [46], fatty acids [47], glycosides, and polysaccharides [48] are only a few examples of the diverse substances that are included in this classification. Examination of the chemical composition of *M. oleifera*'s many constituents has yielded a multitude of bioactive compounds, primarily secondary metabolites. Notable among them are glucosinolates; flavonoids such as kaempferol, vanillin, and quercetin; and phenolic acids such as gallic, ellagic, chlorogenic, and ferulic acids. These materials have rich nutritional, therapeutic, and anti-microbial properties. However, the amount of these compounds in *M. oleifera* isolates can vary depending on factors such as temperature, sun exposure, soil composition, and geographic location.

2.1. Amino Acids

M. oleifera contains more than 90 nutritious chemical components, such as proteins, lipids, carbohydrates, and dietary fibers. Of the several nutrients present in various sections of *M. oleifera*, proteins are the most prevalent, accounting for approximately 25% of the plant's dry weight [49]. This plant is known to contain at least 19 distinct amino acids, including both essential and non-essential amino acids. Approximately 30% of the dry weight of seeds is composed of lipids, primarily stearic acid, saturated palmitic acid, and oleic acid [50]. The primary components of *M. oleifera* leaves are lipid molecules, palmitic acid, and linolenic acid. Furthermore, the high nutritional value of dried leaves indicates that the plant is a valuable food source [51].

2.2. Vitamins and Minerals

The entire *M. oleifera* plant contains several vitamins and minerals. Among the many minerals found in *Moringa* that are essential for human growth and development, calcium is thought to be one of the most vital minerals. Fresh *M. oleifera* leaves are thought to provide around 11,300 to 23,000 International Units of vitamin A. Vitamin A is necessary for many physiological activities, including vision, development, prenatal growth and development, immunologic competency, cell division, proliferation of cells and a process called apoptosis, maintenance of epidermal tissue, and cognitive function [52]. Nutritional information for *M. oleifera* is presented in Table 1.

Table 1. Phytoconstituents of *M. oleifera* leaves per 1 g net quantity.

Phytoconstituents	Concentration	Category	Reference
Isoquercetin	1575.28 g/g (*w*/*w*)	Flavonoids	
Astragalin	0.153 g/g (*w*/*w*)	Flavonoids	
Isorhamnetin	2.9 mg/g (*w*/*w*)	Flavonoids	
4-(_-L-rhamnopyranosyloxy) benzyl glucosinolate	33.9 mg/g	Glucosinolates	
4-[(20-O-acetyl-_-L-rhamnosyloxy) benzyl] Glucosinolate	21.84 to 59.4 mg/g	Glucosinolates	
Epicatechin	5.68 mg/g	Flavonoid	[51,52]
Ferulic acid	0.078 mg/g	Phenolic acid	
Caffeic acid	0.409 mg/g	Phenolic acid	
Ellagic acid	0.018 mg/g	Phenolic acid	
Sinalbin	2.36 mg/g	Glucosinolates	
Chlorogenic acid	0.018 mg/g	Phenolic acid	
Gallic acid	1.034 mg/g	Phenolic acid	
Salicylic acid	0.14 μg/g	Phenolic acid	
4-[(40-O-Acetyl-_-Lrhamnosyloxy) benzyl]	2.16 to 5.0 mg/g	Glucosinolates	

2.3. Flavonoids

The wide variety of bioactive compounds found in *Moringa oleifera* seeds and leaves are highlighted in this text as having possible medical benefits. The leaves and seeds of *M. oleifera* are rich in flavonoids such as myricetin, rutin, kaempferol, quercetin, isorhamnetin, procyanidin, and catechin. In addition, there are noticeable amounts of lutein pigments in leaves [3]. The claimed therapeutic advantages of *M. oleifera* are attributed mainly to its active components. Gas chromatography–mass spectrometry examination revealed over 35 chemicals in the leaves, including β-sitosterol, pregna-7-dien-3-ol-20-one, palmitoyl chloride, cis-vaccenic acid, 5-O-acetyl-thio-octyl, tetradecanoic acid, and α-l-rhamnofuranoside [47,48,53].

2.4. Phenolic Acids

Sinapic, syringic, cinnamic, gentisic, and ferulic acids, along with gallic, protocatechuic, caffeic, epicatechin, p-coumaric, o-coumaric, and vanillin are found in *M. oleifera*. These compounds belong to a larger group of phenolic chemicals, obtained mainly from the naturally occurring hydroxycinnamic acid and hydroxybenzoic acid found in plants. Phenolic acids present in food have garnered increasing attention owing to their impact on individual health. These substances have been extensively studied for their beneficial effects, including anti-mutagenic, anti-inflammatory, anti-cancer, and antioxidant properties. They are abundant in fruits and vegetables and have also been present in notable amounts in the leaves of *M. oleifera*, a plant known for its nutritional value [54]. Among these phenolic acids, gallic acid was the most prevalent in dried *M. oleifera* leaves, with a mass of approximately 1.034 mg/g of dry weight. Interestingly, previous studies have reported only minimal levels of gallic acid. Additionally, chlorogenic acid and caffeic acid were found in varying concentrations, from 0.018 to 0.489 mg/g and 0.409 mg/g, respectively [44].

2.5. Alkaloids

Alkaloids are a group of basic nitrogenous compounds. These nitrogen atoms form amines that can be categorized as primary, secondary, and tertiary. Their therapeutic properties make them highly attractive. Alkaloids have been identified in *M. oleifera* leaves, including two newly discovered alkaloids, marumoside A and B, and aurnatiamide acetate isolated from the roots [42,46]. In addition, the stem of the plant contains moringinine and moringin-type alkaloids [47]. Glucosinolates are abundant in *M. oleifera*, and 4-O-(L-rhamnopyranosyloxy)-benzyl glucosinolate, or glucomoringin, is the most prevalent glucosinolate in the species [43]. The seeds and leaves contain the sterol isolate sitosterol, whereas the bark contains -sitosterol-3-O-D-galactopyranoside, another sterol glycoside [3,43]. Furthermore, the leaves contain an array of diterpenes and terpenes, with phytol being a notable diterpene alcohol found abundantly owing to its association with chlorophyll. Trace amounts of terpenes and their derivatives, such as farnsylacetone, linalool oxide, isolongifolene, ionone, and ionene, are present, with hexahydro-farnesyl acetone being more abundant [44].

2.6. Tannins, Fatty Acids, and Sterols

Natural polyphenols called tannins are found in a wide variety of plants, including fruits, vegetables, and seeds. Tannins are commonly employed in the wine industry as wine fining agents and color stabilizers, and to balance the complexity of wines by inhibiting enzymes in infested fruits. The concentration of tannins in the *Moringa* tree varies, with dried leaves having the maximum concentration (20.7 mg/g). Seeds also contain a small quantity of tannins. Out of the total antioxidant content, the proportion of total tannin content in the seeds amounts to 0.890 ± 0.020 mg GAE/g of dry matter. *M. oleifera* seeds include major fatty acids such as arachidic acid, octacosanoic acid, oleic acid, and palmitic acids. This plant also contains other fatty acids such as stearic acid, linolenic acid, behenic acid, and paullinic acid. *M. oleifera* seeds and leaves contain the sterol isolate β-sitosterol. Bark from *M. oleifera* has been used to extract β-sitosterol-3-O-β-D-galactopyranoside, another form of sterol glycoside. These tannins and sterols are responsible for various pharmacological actions [44]. Further nutritional information has been presented in Table 2.

Table 3 displays the structures of some of the major phytoconstituents separated from *M. oleifera*.

Table 2. Nutritional information for *Moringa oleifera*.

Category	Subcategory	Details	Reference
Comparison of Nutrient Content	Milk	Provides 300–400 mg of certain nutrients	[48]
	Moringa Leaves	Offers significantly higher amounts, around 1000 mg	[55]
	Moringa (whole plant) Powder	Surpasses with more than 4000 mg of essential nutrients	[49]
Anemia Treatment		*Moringa* powder serves as a substitute for iron tablets, can be utilized in the treatment of anemia	[48]
Micronutrient Composition of *M. oleifera* (mg/100 g)	Calcium	440–3650 mg	[15]
	Magnesium	24–1050 mg	
	Sulfur	137–925 mg	
	Sodium	164.0–272 mg	
	Potassium	259–2061 mg	
	Phosphorus	70–300 mg	
	Iron	0.85–126 mg	
	Zinc	0.16–3.30 mg	
	Copper	0.6–1.1 mg	
Vitamin Content	Vit A	6.78–18.90 mg	
	Vit B2	0.05–20.50 mg	
	Vit B3	0.8–8.2 mg	
	Vit B7	423 mg	
	Vit B12	0.06–2.64 mg	
	Vit C	17.3–220.0 mg	
	Vit E	77 mg	

M. oleifera seed oil extract typically includes tannins and saponins, which oversee a variety of pharmacological actions [45]. *M. oleifera* seeds contain a variety of fatty acids, including arachidic, stearic, octacosanoic, palmitic, oleic, linolenic, behenic, and paullinic acid [46]. Two glycosides, niazirin and niazirinin, were isolated from *M. oleifera*'s ethanolic extract of *M. oleifera* [47]. Numerous polysaccharides, including D-xylose, D-galactose, L-rhamnose, L-arabinose, D-mannose, and glucuronic acid, are present in gum exudates [48].

Table 3. Chemical constituents of *Moringa oleifera*.

Plant Part	Phytoconstituent	Type	Chemical Structure	Therapeutic Potential	Reference
Leaves	Rutin (555.6 µg/g)	Flavonoid	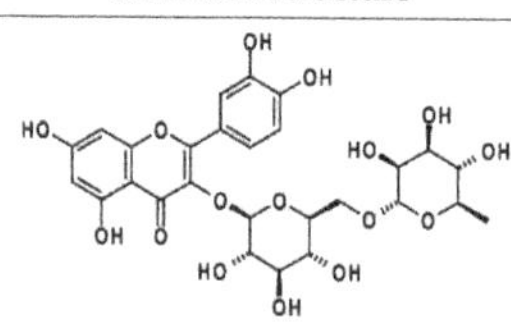	Maximum affinity towards BRAC-1 genes.	[52,56]
	Quercetin (2030.9 µmol/100 g)	Flavonoid	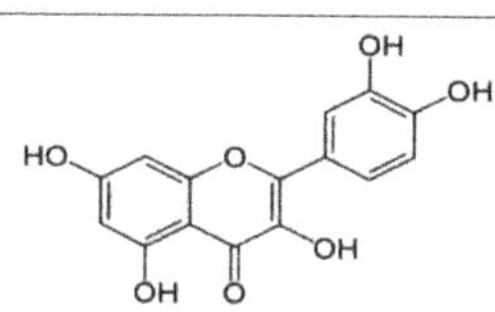	Anti-diabetic agent	[57]

Table 3. *Cont.*

Plant Part	Phytoconstituent	Type	Chemical Structure	Therapeutic Potential	Reference
	Kaempherol (197.6 μg/g)	Flavonoid	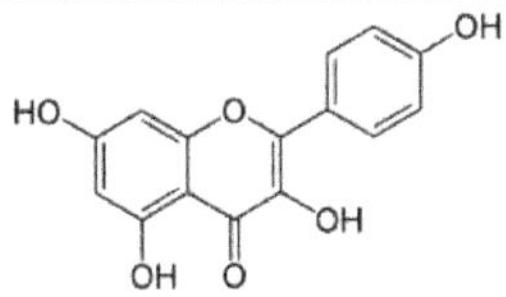	Oxidative damage protective activity.	[58]
	Isorhamnetin (0.118 mg/g)	Flavonoid	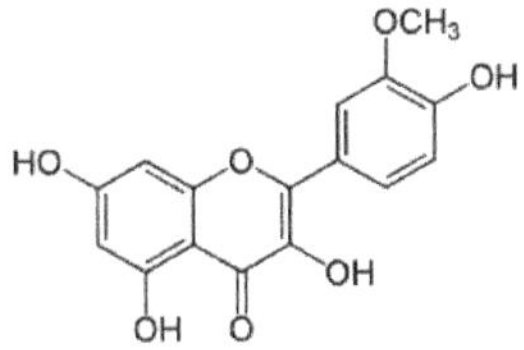	Antioxidant	[59]
	O coumaric acid (0.536 mg/g)	Phenolic acid	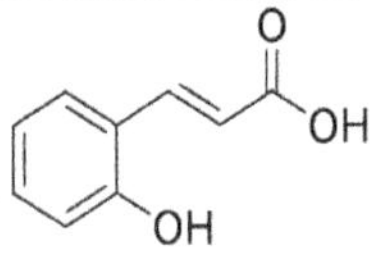	Antioxidant and antimicrobial	[60]
	Syringic acid (trace amount)	Phenol	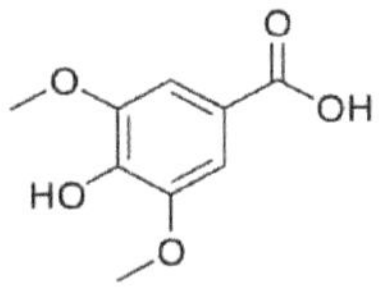	Antioxidant and antimicrobial	[60]
	Gallic acid (1.034 mg/g)	Phenol	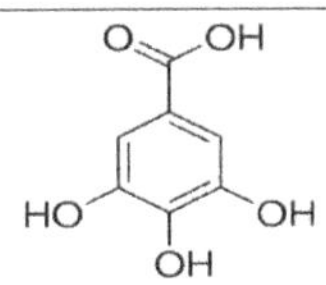	Anti-inflammatory, anti-neoplastic, antioxidant	[60]
	Sinapic acid (trace amount)	Phenol	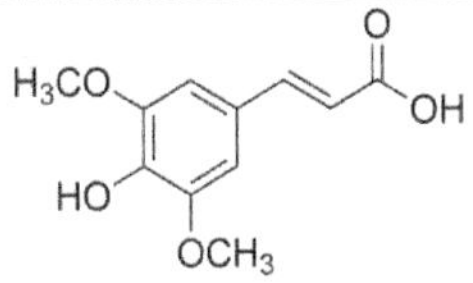	Cardioprotective, renoprotective, neuroprotective, anxiolytic	[60]
	Caffeic acid (0.409 mg/g)	Phenol	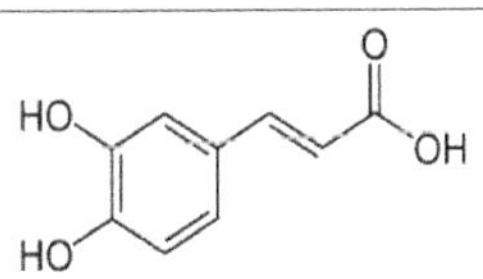	enhances athletic performance, reduces fatigue, helps weight management, protects against HIV, herpes, and cancer.	[60]
	Ellagic acid (0.078 to 0.128 mg/g)	Polyphenol	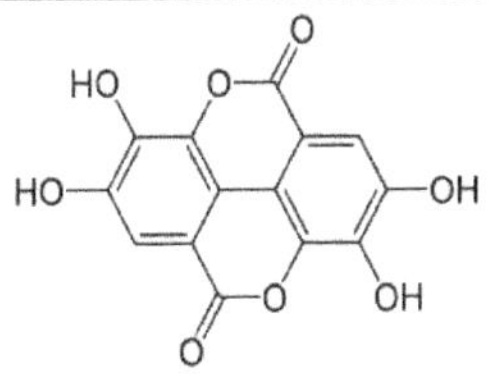	Antiviral, antibacterial and antioxidant	[60]

Table 3. *Cont.*

Plant Part	Phytoconstituent	Type	Chemical Structure	Therapeutic Potential	Reference
Leaves and Seeds	Myricetin (5.804 mg/g)	Flavonoid	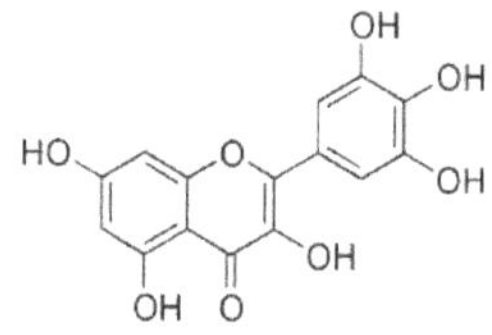	Prevention of diabetes and its complications.	[60]
Seeds	Arachidic acid	Fatty acid	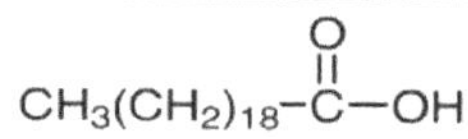	Increases mothers' milk production	[61]
	Oleic acid	Fatty acid	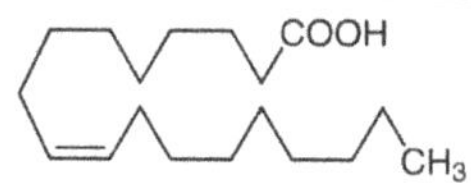	Reduces blood pressure, antioxidant	[62]
	Myristic acid	Fatty acid	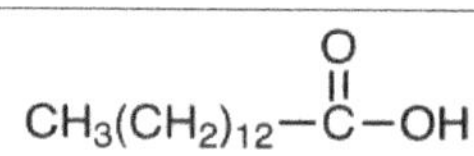	Anxiolytic	[63]
	Palmitic acid	Fatty acid	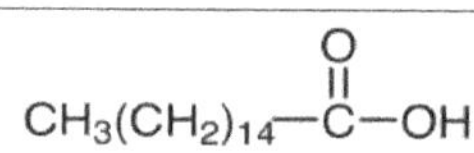	Anti-leukemic effect	[64]

3. Extraction Methods and Analytical Techniques for Phytochemical Analysis

The utilization of natural substances continues to garner significant attention, owing to their numerous advantages. *Moringa oleifera* has demonstrated diverse applications in the pharmaceutical, food, cosmetic, and other sectors. This review examines the constituents of *Moringa oleifera*, such as seed extract, seed oil, and leaf extract, and details their isolation methods, processing techniques, phytochemical compositions, and modern uses. *Moringa oleifera* contains notable levels of phytochemicals, including flavonoids, carotenoids, phenolics, tannins, chlorophylls, saponins, tocopherols, and sterols [65]. The pronounced antioxidant activity of *Moringa oleifera* confers various pharmaceutical benefits across different parts of the plant, including anti-obesity, antihypertensive, anti-cancer, anti-diabetic, anti-arthritic, anti-inflammatory, and wound healing properties. Moreover, the substantial nutritional value and antimicrobial properties of the various components of *Moringa oleifera* render it suitable for diverse applications in the development of functional food products, skincare ingredients, the biodiesel industry, water treatment processes, and pharmaceuticals.

3.1. Extraction and Processing

3.1.1. Conventional Methods

The simplest way to extract chemicals is through solid–liquid extraction, which involves transferring solutes from a solid substance into a solvent and then separating the solvent to obtain the desired extract. In one extraction method, *Moringa* leaf powder was mixed in a 70% ethanol solution for 48 h at room temperature, and the mixture was stirred every so often to aid in extraction. In contrast, others used a cold maceration method in which *Moringa* leaves were soaked for five days at ambient temperature in 70% ethanol. Another extraction process using methanol as a solvent with a solid-to-solvent ratio of 1:15 and shaking at 500 rpm for five hours at 30 °C produced a much greater yield of 14%, demonstrating the effectiveness and affordability of the maceration technique [64].

Other solvent combinations were also investigated, such as macerating *Moringa* leaves for two days at ambient temperature in an ethanol–water mixture (7:3) and extracting the leaves for 72 h in an ethanol–water solution (80:20%). After extraction, the solvent needs to be filtered and evaporated under low pressure; alternatively,, the extract can be dried in an oven or in air to produce the finished product. The percentages of extract yields observed were 14.30% for acetone, 14.50% for ethanol, 5.50% for water, and 17.50% for ethanol and water. Interestingly, clean water did not remove *Moringa* leaves as well as it could have. Therefore, a mixture of solvents might work better to make it easier to extract the various polar chemicals found in the leaves. In another method, Soxhlet extraction was performed using *n*-hexane solvent for nine hours at 70 °C and a solid-to-solvent ratio of 1:10. An effective method for extracting *Moringa* leaves with an organic solvent is the Soxhlet device. Using Soxhlet extraction apparatus with 95% ethanol over an 8-h period produced a 10.7% yield of *M. oleifera* leaf extract. Other researchers have used methanol as the solvent of choice for Soxhlet extraction and obtained a greater yield (18.56%). To achieve the final extract, the solvent is usually removed by partial vacuum drying; nevertheless, the high temperature of the extraction process may damage the delicate bioactive components [66].

3.1.2. Non-Conventional Methods of Extraction

Ultrasonic-assisted extraction (UAE) is a particularly successful extraction technique that includes sonication of *Moringa* leaves with water and 0.1% formic acid at room temperature for 15 min. Conversely, 100% ethanol was used to sonicate *Moringa* leaves at a solid-to-solvent ratio of 1:10 for 30 min. Other researchers studied the effect of UAE at different temperatures (30, 35, 40, and 45 °C) and durations (15, 20, 25, and 30 min) on *Moringa* leaves with a solid-to-solvent ratio of 1:50 (g/mL). In another method, it was found that 45 °C and 30 min were the optimal conditions, as higher temperatures increased the phytochemical solubility and mass transfer rate into the solvent. UAE at 50 °C with pure water, 50% ethanol, and 20% ethanol, a constant frequency of 20 kHz, and an amplitude of 79 mm, showed that water might increase the initially determined extraction rate as well as phenolic content in *M. oleifera* leaf extract. Ultrasound waves may pass through the extraction liquid and cause cavitation, which aids in breaking the leaf cell wall and facilitates phytochemical release during extraction. Furthermore, this study focuses on the phytochemicals found in *Moringa* leaves, such as alkaloids, saponins, tannins, steroids, phenolic acids, flavonoids, glucosinolates, and anthocyanins. These chemicals provide medical benefits and can be used in the pharmaceutical, cosmetic, and food industries. The concentrations of phytonutrients in *M. oleifera* leaf extract depend on the extraction process, solvent type, solvent-to-solid ratio, ambient temperature, stirring rate, and particle size. The petroleum ether and dichloromethane samples of *M. oleifera* roots, which shown encouraging biological activity, were subjected to GC-MS (Gas chromatography and Mass Spectroscopy) analysis, which identified 102 constituents. These ingredients are classified into 13 different types of compounds, which include halo compounds, aromatics, alkamides, cyanides, fatty acids, alcohols, pyrazine, hydrocarbons, urea and *N*-hydroxyimine derivatives, unsaturated alkenamides, alkyne, and indole. A total of 39 chemicals from nine classes were found in the petroleum ether extract of the roots, according to GC/GC-MS analyses [66].

4. Pharmacological Activities

4.1. Antioxidant Properties and Mechanisms

Moringa oleifera leaves have a powerful array of antioxidants because of the presence of a wide range of natural bioactive compounds, such as phenolics, vitamins A, E, and ascorbic acid, as well as flavonoids. The aqueous, methanolic, and ethanolic extracts produced from both leaves and roots have demonstrated exceptional in vitro antioxidant capabilities, highlighting their quantity of antioxidant components and potential for treating oxidative stress-related diseases in animal models. The administration of *Moringa oleifera* leaf extract has demonstrated a discernible capacity to ameliorate oxidative damage induced by a high-fat diet. Particularly noteworthy is the significant augmentation in the activity of pivotal antioxidant enzymes, such as superoxide dismutase, catalase, and glutathione S-transferase elicited by aqueous leaf extracts, concomitant with a reduction in lipid peroxidation levels observed in both normoglycemic and diabetic rodent models. Accumulating evidence suggests that the elevated phenolic and flavonoid content of the extract may shield against oxidative injury, conferring benefits to both individuals with normoglycemia and those with diabetes [4]. Moreover, an investigation encompassing 60 postmenopausal women showed that supplementation with *Moringa oleifera* leaf powder over a span of three months resulted in notable decreases in serum malondialdehyde levels, an indicator of lipid peroxidation, coupled with elevations in levels of ascorbic acid, superoxide dismutase, and glutathione peroxidase, underscoring the formidable antioxidant capacity of this botanical specimen [67]. Figure 2 shows hepatoprotective, antioxidant and anti-inflammatory mechanisms of *M. olifera*.

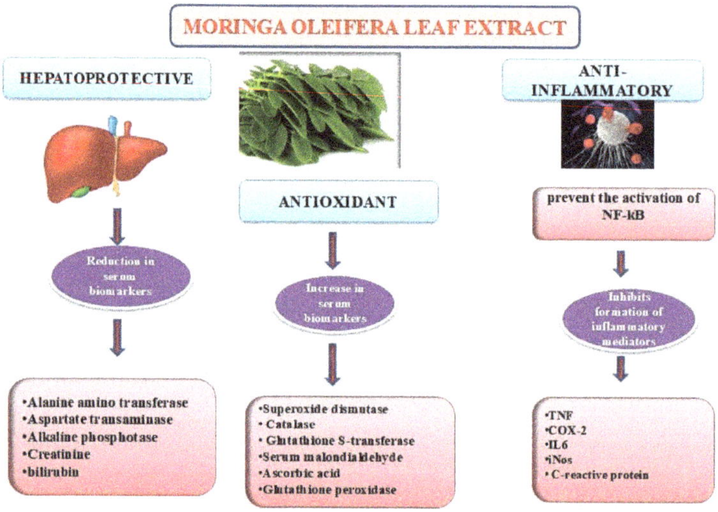

Figure 2. Hepatoprotective, antioxidant, and anti-inflammatory mechanisms of *M. oleifera*.

4.2. Anti-Inflammatory Effects

The anti-inflammatory potency of *Moringa oleifera* has been substantiated by the application of extracts from diverse plant components, including roots, stems, leaves, flowers, pods, and seeds. In a mouse study, the root extract of *M. oleifera* significantly decreased the progression of paw edema, similar to phenylbutazone, a nonsteroidal anti-inflammatory medication known for its analgesic and antipyretic properties [68]. In addition, acetylcholine-induced bronchospasms were diminished and airway inflammation in guinea pigs was alleviated by Th1/Th2 cytokine modulation using *Moringa oleifera* seed butanol extract. In addition, a clinical trial involving subjects with mild to moderate asthma demonstrated a significant increase in Forced Vital Capacity (FVC), forced expiratory volume (FEV), and peak expiratory flow rate (PEFR) following the consumption of *Moringa oleifera* dry seed powder without any adverse effects [69]. The anti-inflammatory nature of *Moringa oleifera* is attributed to the abundance of its bioactive compounds, such as quercetin. Quercetin has an astonishing capability to inhibit NF-kB activity, which is important for the swelling process. Additionally, the greater quantities of flavonoids and phenolic acids found in *M. oleifera* leaves enhance their anti-inflammatory properties. In addition, *M. oleifera* leaf extract and quercetin have been shown to control some key signs of inflammation, including iNOS, IFN-gamma, and C-reactive protein, while reducing TNF-α and IL-6 secretion in mouse models [70]. Likewise, macromolecules such as IL-1β, iNOS, TNF-α, and NO are tremendously reduced by isothiocyanates generated from *M. oleifera* leaves, thereby displaying a profound inhibitory effect on the production of pro-inflammatory substances by RAW macrophages, apart from their anti-inflammatory properties [71].

4.3. Antimicrobial and Antiviral Activities

N-benzylethylthioformate, the aglycone derivative of deoxyniazimincin, is a bioactive molecule found in the alcoholic root extract of *Moringa oleifera*. It exhibits broad-spectrum antimicrobial and antifungal activities against numerous microbes and fungi. This potential to limit microbial development and impede fungal proliferation makes it a viable option for treating infectious diseases and fighting microbial resistance [72]. Additionally, methanolic extracts from *Moringa oleifera* leaves have been found to be effective in treating urinary tract infections caused by many different types of bacteria, including gram-negative and gram-positive bacteria. Similarly, it also exhibits antibacterial effects against common infections caused by *Klebsiella pneumoniae*, *Staphylococcus aureus*, *Escherichia coli*, and *Staphylococcus saprophyticus* [73]. The inhibitory potential of *Moringa oleifera* extracts derived from its leaves, seeds, and stems is investigated across a spectrum of fungal strains, encompassing notable species such as *Aspergillus flavus*, *Aspergillus terreus*, *Aspergillus nidulans*, *Rhizoctonia solani*, *Aspergillus niger*, *Aspergillus oryzae*, *Fusarium solani*, *Penicillium sclerotigenum*, *Cladosporium cladosporioides*, *Trichophyton mentagrophytes*, *various Penicillium* species, and *Pullarium* species. The aim of this study was to elucidate the efficacy of *M. oleifera* isolates as prospective antifungal agents against a wide array of pathogenic fungi, thus enabling the design of novel preventive strategies against fungal diseases [72]. The anti-bacterial potential of *Moringa oleifera* seeds is recognized to be associated with its special bioactive constituents, including 4-(α-l-rhamnosyloxy) benzyl isothiocyanates. Additionally, juice from the leaves of *Moringa* has an excellent anti-pathogenic capacity against microbial organisms that negatively affect human lives. Surprisingly, the result achieved by methanolic leaf extract completely suppressed (99%) *Botrytis cinerea*, a necrotrophic disease that mostly affects plants [73].

Alkaloids, flavonoids, and steroids are the only bioactive substances found in *Moringa oleifera* fruits. Because of the special makeup of their steroid rings, these components impede the growth of *Candida albicans* cells through mechanisms such as protein denaturation and spore germination suppression. This intricate interaction of phytochemicals highlights *M. oleifera*'s viability as a natural treatment for Candida infections and highlights the diverse nature of its antifungal qualities [74]. *Moringa* seed kernel extract is particularly effective against different types of *Aspergillus* and Mucor, as well as *Bacillus cereus* and *Staphylococcus aureus*. However, it seems to be less effective against *Pseudomonas aeruginosa* and *Escherichia coli*, suggesting that it could be useful in treating infections caused by these bacterial strains. Recent analysis highlights the fact that only the apolar extract derived from *Moringa oleifera* seeds exhibits antibacterial activity that is selectively directed towards gram-positive bacterial strains [75].

4.4. Anticancer Potential

Moringa plant foliage has promising anticancer properties. Through advanced scientific analysis, the compound O-Ethyl-4-(α-L-rhamnosyloxy) benzyl carbamate, in synergy with 4-(α-L-rhamnosyloxy)-benzyl isothiocyanate, niazimicin, and 3-O-(6′-O-oleoyl-β-D-glucopyranosyl)-sitosterol, was subjected to rigorous assessment of their potential as antitumor agents using an in vitro assay. The extracts were made employing different solvents like chloroform, *n*-butanol, dichloromethane, and hexane by distilling the crude 80% methanol extract of the tree's leaves. The CellTiter 96® Aqueous One Solution Cell Proliferation (MTS) assay was used to assess the extracts' cytotoxic effect on MCF7 cells. The apoptosis investigation was carried out with Annexin V-FITC analysis and validated by Western blotting with specific proteins, namely caspase 8, p53, Bax, and cytochrome c. The outcomes demonstrated that MCF7 cells (5 μg/mL) were specifically cytotoxic to the dichloromethane extract, but MCF 10A (non-cancerous breast) cells were not considerably inhibited. Out of all the studied extracts, it had the highest possible selectivity index

(SI) value, at 9.5. Additionally, it caused early apoptosis and elevated the expression of caspase 8, p53, and the pro-apoptotic proteins Bax in MCF7 cells. Apoptosis induction was found to be the action mechanism through which the active principles of this plant are likely to be responsible for anticancer activity.

Remarkably, they demonstrated significant inhibition of the Epstein–Barr virus early antigen 36, indicating their capacity as potent antitumor promoters. Niazimicin is speculated to exert profound chemo preventive effects against carcinogenesis. Moreover, seed extracts have exhibited beneficial effects on various fronts, including antioxidant parameters, cutaneous papillomagenesis in murine models, and the modulation of hepatic carcinogen-metabolizing enzymes. These results highlight the diverse range of applications of *Moringa* chemicals in cancer research and treatment [76]. Mice with *Staphylococcus aureus* pyoderma were successfully treated with neomycin and an ointment derived from the seeds. It has been shown that niaziminin, a thiocarbamate present in *M. oleifera* leaves, inhibits Epstein–Barr virus activation brought on by tumor promoters. In contrast, tumor-promoter-driven Epstein–Barr virus activation was effectively repressed by the naturally found 4-[(4′-O-acetyl-α-L-rhamnosyloxy) benzyl] isothiocyanate, indicating the critical involvement of the isothiocyanate group in its action [76]. A crude ethanol extract prepared from dried seeds was administered to mice to reduce the inflammatory response caused by carrageenan in their hind paws. Moreover, various fractions of this crude ethanol concentrate, such as butanol, water, and hexane, showed anti-inflammatory characteristics. Remarkably, the portion containing ethyl acetate paradoxically increased inflammation and demonstrated toxicity in mice following oral consumption. Furthermore, the manufacture of Epstein–Barr virus-early antigen (EBV-EA) generated by 12-O-tetradecanoylphorbol-13-acetate (TPA) was successfully suppressed by the crude ethanol extract, indicating that it may be a promising agent against tumor promotion. A correlation between elevated levels of inflammatory mediators and reactive oxygen species (ROS) and many illnesses has been demonstrated. Therefore, it is crucial to specifically intervene in these pathways to manage the conditions associated with inflammation and oxidative stress. There is increasing interest in investigating alternative therapeutic options because of the inherent health concerns associated with standard anti-inflammatory medications. *M. oleifera* seeds have been shown to contain a variety of bioactive compounds, including nitriles, glycosidic glucosinolates, isothiocyanates, carbamates, and thiocarbamates. It has been demonstrated that these substances possess strong anti-inflammatory and antioxidant properties [77]. The mechanism of anticancer potential of *M. olifera* has been shown in Figure 3.

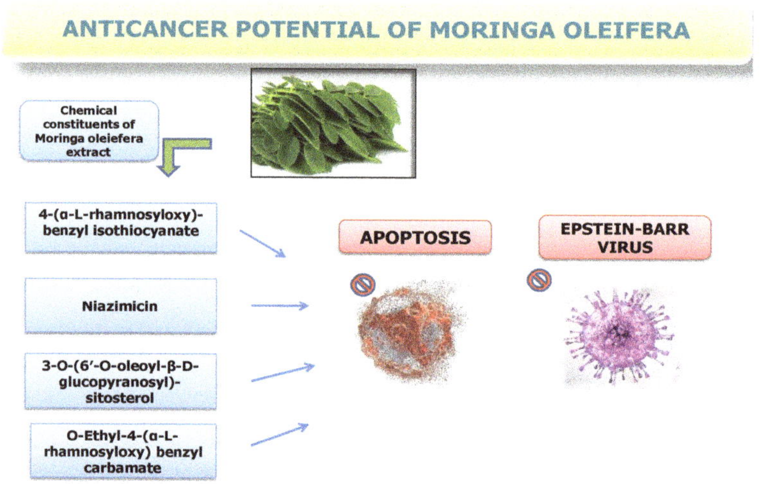

Figure 3. Anticancer potential of *Moringa oleifera*.

4.5. Immunomodulatory Effects

The plant extract prepared using methanol was found to contain strong active ingredients, including cyanogenic glycosides and isothiocyanates, which have shown strong immunostimulatory activities and thus greatly improve the host's immunological response. A recent comprehensive analysis explains the deliberate application of numerous bioactive substances for the treatment of a variety of immune-mediated diseases, including cancers, hypertension, and diabetes, to boost the immune system of their hosts [77]. *Moringa oleifera* is an important research area for neuroprotection. It can improve cognitive abilities and serve as a neuroprotectant in addition to being an antioxidant in mice with dementia following amyloid beta peptide injection [78,79]. It has been demonstrated that using both aqueous and hydroalcoholic extracts from *Moringa oleifera* leaves dramatically reduces cerebral lipid peroxidation while concurrently raising brain activity levels of catalase and superoxide dismutase [78]. Additionally, a thorough analysis of the neuroprotective properties of an ethanolic extract derived from *Moringa oleifera* leaves showed significant stimulation of neurite outgrowth when primary hippocampal neuron cells were incubated with the extract. This facilitation was demonstrated by significant increases in dendritic and axonal branching as well as in length. Owing to *M. oleifera's* capacity to lessen oxidative stress, our results unequivocally demonstrate the potential of the plant as a neuroprotective adjuvant [80].

4.6. Hepatoprotective and Nephroprotective Activities

Scientific data support the remarkable potential of *Moringa oleifera* leaves in mitigating drug-induced damage to the liver and kidneys in animal models. The hepatorenal protective potential of *M. oleifera* against a variety of pharmaceutical medications such as acetaminophen, gentamicin, pyrazinamide, rifampicin, and isoniazid has been elucidated in several studies. Its leaves are primarily responsible for its quality protection. More specifically, *M. oleifera* leaf extract was administered to treated rats, and the blood levels of key markers such as urea, creatinine, alkaline phosphatase, aspartate aminotransferase, and alanine aminotransferase were decreased consequently. Histological analyses corroborated these findings by showing that individuals treated with *M. oleifera* exhibited a significant reduction in drug-induced damage to the renal and hepatic systems. Furthermore, both aqueous and alcoholic extracts derived from *M. oleifera* roots and flowers exhibit notable hepatoprotective properties against acetaminophen-induced hepatotoxicity. This is evidenced by diminished levels of serum transaminases (alanine aminotransferase and aspartate aminotransferase), alkaline phosphatase, and bilirubin, suggesting a multifaceted protective mechanism conferred by *M. oleifera* [81,82].

4.7. Antifungal Activity

In a variety of fungal strains, including *Aspergillus flavus*, *A. terreus*, *A. nidulans*, *A. niger*, *A. oryzae*, *Rhizoctonia solani*, *Fusarium solani*, *Penicillium sclerotigenum*, *Trichophyton mentagrophytes*, *Cladosporium cladosporioides*, and *Penicillium* species, the inhibitory effect of extracts from leaves, seeds, and stems of *M. oleifera* has been identified [72]. The active ingredients in *M. oleifera* seeds, 4-(alpha-L-rhamanosyloxy) benzyl isothiocyanates, are thought to be the cause of their antibacterial activity [83]. Additionally, the juice from *Moringa* leaves demonstrated potential against harmful microbes to humans. *Botrytis cinerea*, a necrotrophic plant fungus, is nearly 99% inhibited by the methanolic extract of leaves [74]. Alkaloids, flavonoids, and steroids found in *M. oleifera* fruit have an inhibitory effect on *Candida albicans* culture by either weakening the protein or preventing spore germination due to the presence of a steroid ring [75]. *Moringa* seed kernel extract was found to have potent inhibitory effects on *Aspergillus* species, *Bacillus cereus*, *Staphylococcus aureus*, and *Mucor* species. However, its efficacy against *E. coli* and *P. aeruginosa* was reduced. This suggested that *Moringa* seed kernel concentrate might be used to treat infections that arise from all species but not *P. aeruginosa* and *E. coli* [84].

4.8. Cardioprotective Activity

Animals with myocardial infarction caused by isoproterenol had a cardioprotective effect in response to the freeze-dried alcoholic and aqueous extract of *M. oleifera*. Chronic *M. oleifera* treatment enhanced the levels of enzymes such SOD, catalase, lactase dehydrogenase, glutathione peroxidase, and creatine kinase and effectively treated the hemodynamic effects of isoproterenol. It has been demonstrated that in rats with isoproterenol-induced cardiac necrosis, butanolic extract is a significant source of antioxidants [85]. Moreover, because *N*-α-rhamnopyranosyl vincosamide is present, it was discovered to considerably lower inflammatory responses and myocardial necrosis [86]. *Moringa* leaves protected hypertensive rats from hypertension, resulting in markedly reduced cholesterol levels. The active ingredients niazirimin A, niazirimin B, and niazimincin were found to be the ones thought to oversee this activity [22].

Niazimin-A, niazicin-A, and niaziminin-B are among the compounds that are allegedly found in the *M. oleifera* plant extract. When these substances were directed towards (ACE), a crucial renin-angiotensin system enzyme, they were shown to have strong antihypertensive effects. By using protein–ligand docking to monitor this activity, researchers discovered that the compounds had a higher affinity for the angiotensin-converting enzyme than captopril and enalapril [87]. Rennin, an angiotensin enzyme, is a major contributor to blood pressure regulation and the development of conditions like hypertension, renal disease, and other cardiovascular disorders. In comparison to typical medications (captopril and enalapril), the study discovered that *M. oleifera*, along with two other plants (*Azadirachta indica* and *Hibiscus sabdariffa*), inhibited the enzyme with percentage inhibitions (71.8%, 74%, and 73.4%). The substance identified as β-sitosterol is what gives *Moringa* its action [88].

4.9. Hypocholesterolaemic and Hypolipidemic Activities

Indians employ the leaves of *M. oleifera* as a hypocholesterolemic drug in their herbal treatment for patients who are obese. Thus, the scientific rationale behind their application in hypercholesterolemia was investigated. The study revealed that the consumption of *Moringa oleifera*'s crude leaf extract in conjunction with a high-fat diet reduced the elevations in serum, liver, and kidney cholesterol levels caused by the diet by 14.35% (115–103.2 mg/100 mL of serum), 6.40% (9.4–8.8 mg/g wet weight), and 11.09% (1.09–0.97 mg/g wet weight), in that order. The impact on the blood cholesterol was statistically noteworthy. There was no discernible change in serum total protein levels. On the other hand, serum albumin rose by 15.22% (46–53 g/L) due to the crude extract. It was also discovered that this value was statistically significant. The study concluded that *Moringa oleifera* leaves possess a distinct hypocholesterolemic effect and that there is a sound pharmacological foundation for its use in India. It is also effective in reducing serum concentrations of VLDL (called very-low-density lipoprotein) and LDL (called low-density lipoprotein) by consuming fruit from *M. oleifera*. In addition to these advantages, *M. oleifera* leaf extract is also known to reduce the progression of atherosclerotic plaques. Although few human trials have been done, some research has indicated that *M. oleifera* may be helpful in treating dyslipidemia and diabetes [17].

5. Health Benefits and Therapeutic Applications

Modern Therapeutic Applications Based on Scientific Evidence

The definitive findings of this investigation underscore the promising efficacy of traditional methodology in evaluating the efficiency of formulating cosmetic and natural health products. The detrimental effects of neem oil, deployed in aquaculture as an insecticide to counteract the risks posed by predators and parasites to juvenile fish, were proficiently counteracted by the application of *Moringa oleifera* leaf extract. According to the researcher's concluding observations, *Moringa* emerges as a noteworthy dietary adjunct owing to its abundant reservoir of proteins, lipids, and amino acids, notably sulphur, alongside its minimal concentration of deleterious constituents [89]. Palmitic acid, an active constituent derived from *Moringa* leaf extract, shows a multifaceted spectrum of therapeutic attributes.

A collaborative endeavor by a team of researchers delved into its pharmacological prowess, subjecting it to rigorous evaluation against an array of microbial and fungal strains. As illustrated by the accomplishment of the largest inhibitory zone among its fungal and microbial rivals, the results showed extraordinary efficiency. Extending the boundaries of innovation, *Moringa* extract was seamlessly blended into nanoparticle technology, acting as a novel drug delivery vehicle. This strategic integration not only improves drug bioavailability, but also supports a shift towards precision medicine. The use of *Moringa* is not confined only to pharmaceuticals; it is also widely used in other sectors such as poultry farming. Its huge armory includes protection from viruses such as Newcastle Disease Virus (NCDV), bacteria, and parasites, all contributing to keeping animals on earth from becoming extinct [24].

Additionally, *Moringa* serves as a noteworthy instance of an agricultural breakthrough by controlling the growth of crops in their initial stages, such as maize, tomatoes, peanuts, and cereals. This relationship promotes resilience and vigor, which enhances production volume and agricultural viability. It is also a pioneer in sustainable pest management, among other uses in agriculture. The use of naturally occurring bioactive compounds from *Moringa* to produce biopesticides not only provides a cheaper alternative but is also a shift towards sustainable agriculture. This concept democratizes pest control practices while increasing accessibility and improving resilience to different ecological settings through reduced environmental footprint [90]. Various nutrients and growth promoters, including gibberellins, cytokinins, and indoleacetic acid, are present in the aqueous extract of *Moringa oleifera*. It then becomes an effective plant bio-stimulant, convincingly safer, and thus better than conventional chemical fertilizers and pesticides used in modern farming techniques. Zeatin is an important plant hormone responsible for high drought tolerance in plants; it plays a crucial role in the ability of plants to withstand dry conditions. Consequently, compared to plants produced with proper watering, the growth properties of plants infused with methanol-based extracts of *Moringa* are greatly enhanced when they are cultivated under dry conditions. *Moringa* is used by many African tribes because it has a very low cost and can be used to enhance water quality. This can help in dealing with issues such as turbidity, alkalinity, and dissolved organic carbon. Alternatively, turbidity within water could also be reduced using *Moringa* instead of alum, indicating that it can be applied in eco-friendly water treatment techniques [4]. This makes it a better option for biopesticide applications, because it is resistant to plant diseases. *Moringa* leaves mixed with soil were found to facilitate the recovery of several plants from *Pythium debaryanum*-induced damping-off disease [1]. Incredibly, *Moringa* is said to have fruit, flowers, leaves, seeds, and roots that are useful for mental health and spiritual well-being. A range of these plants may be helpful in developing holistic healing methods that agree with both traditional knowledge and modern scientific findings [24].

6. Safety and Toxicity Considerations

The inquiry was a complete one that combined various experimental approaches to explore the safety limits of *Moringa oleifera*, a plant widely known for its nutritional and medicinal use. A multidisciplinary approach involved a detailed investigation of different parts of the plant with animals through leaves, seeds, and stem bark, with the aim of ascertaining possible toxicity. One aspect of this study used non-pregnant female albino Wistar rats that were exposed to aqueous methanol extract of *M. oleifera*. Following the oral administration of the extract at a dose of 2000 mg/kg to a randomly selected cohort, blood samples were obtained for analysis. Aspartate aminotransferase (AST), alanine aminotransferase (ALT), and total bilirubin levels were important parameters that were closely monitored. From the experiments, it was noted that the lethal dose in female Wistar rats exceeded 2000 mg/kg by aqueous extract, indicating a good safety rating for the administered dose [91]. The aim of this study was to determine the safety of *Moringa* leaf powder in Sprague-Dawley rats. The research was very broad to check for possible dangers or death caused by oral administration of sun-dried leaves at various doses of up to

2000 mg/kg. Its safety has been confirmed in several extensive tests, which clearly showed that no adverse effects occurred and therefore renders *Moringa* leaf extract safe within the stipulated dosage limit. The toxicological profile of *M. oleifera* seeds is an important field that needs much scrutiny. Methanolic extracts were used by scholars in their study, which involved acute and sub-acute toxicity assessments in animals aimed at establishing their health effects. Symptoms of acute poisoning were observed when the threshold dose reached 4000 mg/kg. Unfortunately, deaths have been recorded at high doses, especially above 5000 mg/kg, which is also known as the fatal dose. No negative effects were noted at values lower than 3000 mg/kg. When the seed extract was administered sub-acutely, the weight of the experimental rats decreased significantly ($p < 0.05$) and the concentrations of ALT and AST (alanine and aspartate transferases) increased significantly ($p < 0.05$) at a dose of 1600 mg/kg. This analysis concludes that *M. oleifera* seed extract is safe for use in both nutrition and medicine [92]. Although short-term harmful effects have been observed, studies have shown promising prospects for utilizing *Moringa oleifera* seed extract for nutritional purposes. The acute manifestations observed in this study underscore the need for careful dosage considerations and more refined formulation strategies to reduce the risk of adverse events.

Nonetheless, despite this immediate impact, seed extract has great potential for use in functional foods and dietary supplements that need to be investigated further, as far as these nutritional advantages are concerned [92]. Furthermore, *Moringa oleifera* stem bark extract was evaluated through oral gavage dosing up to 2000 mg/kg/day, followed by acute and sub-acute toxicity studies, which were found to be non-toxic. These findings confirm the safety of *M. oleifera* stem bark upon oral intake and its potential for medicinal use with possible bioactive components. Additionally, a subacute toxicity trial conducted over 60 days provided informative data regarding the safety profile of the extract. There were also no noticeable changes in sperm parameters (quality), biochemical, or hematological parameters (control group), as shown by the lethal dose of 1585 mg/kg after various doses ranging between 250–1500 mg/kg administered. These findings emphasize the necessity for more thorough toxicity evaluations to fully understand the safety profile of plant extracts [93].

7. Future Perspectives and Research Directions

Bioactive compounds obtained from the leaves, roots, seeds, and oils of *Moringa oleifera* have the potential to provide a wide range of health benefits including strong antibacterial, anticancer, antiproliferative, antihypertensive, and anti-inflammatory effects. This potential has been carefully verified by extensive studies carried out in living organisms (in vivo) and controlled laboratory environments (in vitro). The bioactive compounds derived from *M. oleifera* Lam. into the human diet is a critical step in improving nutritional profiles, promoting human welfare, and advancing sustainability initiatives in the food production sector. The intrinsic bioactivity and stability of bioactive ingredients are two key factors that determine their efficacy. These characteristics are closely related to their molecular makeup and ability to retain their bioactive characteristics when incorporated into food matrices. Optimizing the utilization of these bioactive substances in food and beverage formulations can be greatly enhanced by combining traditional and cutting-edge approaches in the chemical, thermal, and biotechnological domains. In the food industry, encapsulation is emerging as a highly promising method that provides a sophisticated way to transport bioactive chemicals from *M. oleifera* into the gastrointestinal tract while guaranteeing the sensory appeal, safety, and affordability of the end products. Therefore, in contrast to typical food offerings, developing healthful meals supplemented with *M. oleifera* bioactive compounds requires careful tailoring while keeping an eye on environmental sustainability and cost-effectiveness. Spray drying is a versatile and affordable encapsulation technique, especially when utilizing specific biopolymers, such as proteins or their derivatives, as demonstrated by a thorough literature review. The long-term durability of the enclosed materials reflects the effectiveness of the process. Future studies should be conducted to assess the environmental sustainability concerns associated with different encapsulation processes, such as the acquisition of encapsulating matrices. Despite its potential to address socioeconomic challenges, such as poverty and malnutrition, several barriers hinder the large-scale cultivation of *Moringa* trees, particularly in regions like Nepal, due to ignorance about its importance. Two other issues are the lack of awareness about farming methods, product use, and volatile market conditions. If farmers in rural areas are encouraged to grow *Moringa* trees, nutrition and health outcomes might improve, rural communities may become empowered, and more generalized socio-economic development goals can be achieved. This could generate funding for rural development activities by reducing the dependence on imported artificial supplements and medications for locally produced nutrient-dense substances.

The benefit of extracts from the *Moringa* plant is that, at the quantities and volumes often used for medicinal efficacy, they seem to be extremely safe. In the field of research, *M. oleifera* has gained widespread acceptance, and scientists have developed a variety of formulations using a variety of techniques. Table 4 lists the many phytoformulations made with *M. oleifera*.

Table 4. Different Phytoformulations of *M. oleifera*.

Part of the Plant	Formulation	Application	Reference
Leaves	Polyherbal formulation	Anti-ulcer	[94]
	Polyherbal ointments	Edema	
	Lozenges	Anti-microbial activity	
	Film dressing	Wound healing	
	Effervescent tablets	Anti-anemia	
	Granules	Anti-inflammatory and anti-arthritic	
Seed	Micro-dispersion	Anti-inflammatory	
	Nano-micelle	Mitochondrial cancer cell apoptosis	
	Anti-inflammatory cream	Anti-inflammatory	

8. Conclusions

Several experiments have demonstrated the myriad undeniable healing and therapeutic properties of *Moringa oleifera*. This study aimed to examine its nutritional composition and how well it can combat microbial infections, inflammation, and fibrosis. The components and mechanisms of action of plants can be researched on a large scale to bring about drastic changes in medicine. *Moringa* has medicinal value as well as being pharmacological. It is also rich in bioactive compounds, in addition to providing basic nutrition that provides additional health benefits. This synthesis provides comprehensive information about *Moringa oleifera*, considering its global exploration, ethnopharmacological findings, drug efficacy profiles, phytochemical compositions, formulation as a phytopharmaceutical, clinical validations, and toxicological profiles. As for *Moringa oleifera*, it is a potent botanical antibacterial agent owing to many biomolecules including flavonoids, tannins, saponins, alkaloids, phenolics, and triterpenoids among others. The protein and mineral contents of *Moringa oleifera* leaf extract have traditionally helped manage soft tissue infections in the mouth. In addition, it might be possible to isolate the endophytic fungus further for the identification of specific enzymes or proteins that are responsible for anti- cancer and anti-diabetic activities of *M. oleifera*, leading to the discovery of new therapeutic modalities. Therefore, by considering the economic viability of *M. oleifera* as a bio-coagulant for water treatment, examining whether it is accessible would also be a good idea. Additionally, snacks enriched with *Moringa* can be both profitable and helpful for hunger alleviation because they are in high demand by members of the population looking to have nutritious diets. If industries and researchers investigate its nutritional benefits through long-term studies for proper affirmation after earlier claims, this Indian native plant (*Moringa*) possesses huge economic potential.

Author Contributions: Conceptualization, S.D., R.D. and V.K.P.; methodology, T.S., D.U., V.N., S.R. and A.E.M.A.; software, A.M.S. and V.K.P.; validation, D.A., D.U., B.K. and V.K.P.; formal analysis, S.D., V.K.P. and S.R.; investigation, S.D., V.K.P., T.S., D.U. and V.N.; resources, B.K.; data curation, A.M.S. and V.K.P.; writing—original draft preparation, S.D., V.K.P., S.R. and A.M.S.; writing—review and editing, T.S., D.A., V.N. and D.U.; visualization, A.M.S., V.K.P. and B.K.; supervision, B.K.; project administration, B.K; funding acquisition, B.K. All authors have read and agreed to the published version of the manuscript.

Funding: Project No. TKP2021-NKTA-32 was implemented with support from the National Research, Development, and Innovation Fund of Hungary, financed under the TKP2021-NKTA funding scheme, and supported by the University of Debrecen Program for Scientific Publication.

Data Availability Statement: No new data were created or analyzed in this study.

Acknowledgments: The authors would like to convey thanks and express gratitude to all the partner universities and University of Debrecen for collaborating on this project.

Conflicts of Interest: The authors declare no conflicts of interest.

References

1. Meena, R.; Prajapati, S.K.; Nagar, R.; Porwal, O.; Nagar, T.; Tilak, V.K.; Jayakumararaj, R.; Arya, R.K.K.; Dhakar, R.C. Application of *Moringa oleifera* in Dentistry. *Asian J. Dent. Health Sci.* **2021**, *1*, 10–13. [CrossRef]
2. Dixit, S.; Tripathi, A.; Kumar, P. Medicinal properties of *Moringa oleifera*: A review. *Int. J. Educ. Sci. Res. Rev.* **2016**, *3*, 173–185.
3. Abdull Razis, A.F.; Ibrahim, M.D.; Kntayya, S.B. Health benefits of *Moringa oleifera*. *Asian Pac. J. Cancer Prev.* **2014**, *15*, 8571–8576. [CrossRef] [PubMed]
4. Sarode, S.A.; Sonawane, Y.N.; Suralkar, R.K.; Kumbhar, D.D.; Warade, P.P.; Patil, P.R. *Moringa oleifera*: Phytochemistry, pharmacology. *GSC Biol. Pharm. Sci.* **2023**, *24*, 41–55. [CrossRef]
5. Ram, J. *Moringa* a highly nutritious vegetable tree, Tropical Rural and Island/Atoll Development Experimental Station (TRIADES). *Tech. Bull.* **1994**, *2*, 7–9.
6. Anwar, F.; Bhanger, M.I. Analytical characterization of *Moriga oleifera* seed oil growth in temperate region of Pakistan. *J. Agric. Food Chem.* **2003**, *51*, 6558–6563. [CrossRef] [PubMed]
7. Fahey, J.W. *Moringa oleifera*: A review of the medical evidence for its nutritional, therapeutic, and prophylactic properties. Part 1. *Trees Life J.* **2005**, *1*, 1–5.
8. Stohs, S.J.; Hartman, M.J. Review of the Safety and Efficacy of *Moringa oleifera*. *Phytother. Res.* **2015**, *29*, 796–804. [CrossRef]
9. Bhat, S.K.; Joy, A.E. Antianxiety effect of ethanolic extract of leaves of *Moringa oleifera* in Swiss albino mice. *Arch. Med. Health Sci.* **2014**, *2*, 5–7.
10. Misra, A.; Srivastava, S.; Srivastava, M. Evaluation of antidiarrheal potential of *Moringa oleifera* (Lam.) leaves. *J. Pharmacogn. Phytochem.* **2014**, *2*, 43–46.
11. Tahkur, R.S.; Soren, G.; Pathapati, R.M.; Buchineni, M. Diuretic activity of *Moringa oleifera* leaves extract in swiss albino rats. *J. Pharm. Innov.* **2016**, *5*, 8–10.
12. Woldeyohannes, M.G.; Eshete, G.T.; Abiye, A.A.; Hailu, A.E.; Huluka, S.A.; Tadesse, W.T. Antidiarrheal and Antisecretory Effect of 80% Hydromethanolic Leaf Extract of *Moringa stenopetala* Baker f. in Mice. *Biochem. Res. Int.* **2022**, *2022*, 2090–2247. [CrossRef]
13. Zhang, Y.; Peng, L.; Li, W.; Dai, T.; Nie, L.; Xie, J.; Ai, Y.; Li, L.; Tian, Y.; Sheng, J. Polyphenol Extract of *Moringa oleifera* Leaves Alleviates Colonic Inflammation in Dextran Sulfate Sodium-Treated Mice. *Evid. Based Complement. Altern. Med.* **2020**, *2020*, 6295402. [CrossRef]
14. Posmontier, B. The medicinal qualities of *Moringa oleifera*. *Holist. Nurs. Pr.* **2011**, *25*, 80–87. [CrossRef]
15. Gopalakrishnan, L.; Doriya, K.; Kumar, D.S. *Moringa oleifera*: A review on nutritive importance and its medicinal application. *Food Sci. Hum. Wellness* **2016**, *5*, 49–56. [CrossRef]
16. Karadi, R.V.; Gadge, N.B.; Alagawadi, K.R.; Savadi, R.V. Effect of *Moringa oleifera* Lam. root-wood on ethylene glycol induced urolithiasis in rats. *J. Ethnopharmacol.* **2006**, *105*, 306–311. [CrossRef] [PubMed]
17. Ghasi, S.; Nwobodo, E.; Ofili, J.O. Hypocholesterolemic effects of crude extract of leaf of *Moringa oleifera* Lam in high-fat diet fed wistar rats. *J. Ethnopharmacol.* **2000**, *69*, 21–25. [CrossRef] [PubMed]
18. Paliwal, R.; Sharma, V.; Pracheta, P. A Review on Horse Radish Tree (*Moringa oleifera*): A Multipurpose Tree with High Economic and Commercial Importance. *Asian J. Biotechnol.* **2011**, *3*, 317–328. [CrossRef]
19. Debnath, S.; Guha, D. Role of *Moringa oleifera* on enterochromaffin cell count and serotonin content of experimental ulcer model. *Indian. J. Exp. Biol.* **2007**, *45*, 726–731.
20. Mahajan, S.G.; Mali, R.G.; Mehta, A.A. Protective Effect of Ethanolic Extract of Seeds of *Moringa oleifera* Lam. Against Inflammation Associated with Development of Arthritis in Rats. *J. Immunotoxicol.* **2007**, *4*, 39–47. [CrossRef]
21. Rathi, B.S.; Bodhankar, S.L.; Baheti, A.M. Evaluation of aqueous leaves extract of *Moringa oleifera* Linn for wound healing in albino rats. *Indian J. Exp. Biol.* **2006**, *44*, 898–901. [PubMed]

22. Bhattacharya, A.; Tiwari, P.; Sahu, P.K.; Kumar, S. A review of the phytochemical and pharmacological characteristics of *Moringa oleifera*. *J. Pharm. Bioallied Sci.* **2018**, *10*, 181–191.
23. Pandey, A.; Pandey, R.D.; Tripathi, P.; Gupta, P.P.; Haider, J.; Bhatt, S.; Singh, A.V. *Moringa oleifera* Lam. (Sahijan)—A plant with a plethora of diverse therapeutic benefits: An Updated Retrospection. *Int. J. Med. Aromat.* **2012**, *1*, 1–8. [CrossRef]
24. Meireles, D.; Gomes, J.; Lopes, L. A review of properties, nutritional and pharmaceutical applications of *Moringa oleifera*: Integrative approach on conventional and traditional Asian medicine. *Adv. Tradit. Med.* **2020**, *20*, 495–515. [CrossRef]
25. Liu, W.L.; Wu, B.F.; Shang, J.H.; Wang, X.F.; Zhao, Y.L.; Huang, A.X. *Moringa oleifera* seed ethanol extract and its active component kaempferol potentiate pentobarbital-induced sleeping behaviours in mice via a GABAergic mechanism. *Pharm. Biol.* **2022**, *60*, 810–824. [CrossRef] [PubMed]
26. Gothai, S.; Arulselvan, P.; Tan, W.S.; Fakurazi, S. Wound healing properties of ethyl acetate fraction of *Moringa oleifera* in normal human dermal fibroblasts. *J. Intercult. Ethnopharmacol.* **2016**, *5*, 1–6. [CrossRef]
27. Toma, A.; Deyno, S. Phytochemistry and pharmacological activities of *Moringa oleifera*. *Indian. J. Pharmacol.* **2014**, *4*, 222–231.
28. Sanchez-Martín, J.; Ghebremichael, K.; Beltrán-Heredia, J. Comparison of single-step and two-step purified coagulants from *Moringa oleifera* seed for turbidity and DOC removal. *Bioresour. Technol.* **2010**, *101*, 6259–6261. [CrossRef]
29. Rockwood, J.L.; Anderson, B.G.; Casamatta, D.A. Potential uses of *Moringa oleifera* and an examination of antibiotic efficacy conferred by *M. oleifera* seed and leaf extracts using crude extraction techniques available to under-served indigenous populations. *Int. J. Phytothearpy* **2013**, *3*, 61–71.
30. Barminas, J.T.; Charles, M.; Emmanuel, D. Mineral composition of non-conventional leafy vegetables. *Plant Foods Hum. Nutr.* **1998**, *53*, 29–36. [CrossRef]
31. Choudhary, M.K.; Bodakhe, S.H.; Gupta, S.K. Assessment of the antiulcer potential of *Moringa oleifera* root-bark extract in rats. *J. Acupunct. Meridian Stud.* **2013**, *6*, 214–220. [CrossRef] [PubMed]
32. Aekthammarat, D.; Pannangpetch, P.; Tangsucharit, P. *Moringa oleifera* leaf extract lowers high blood pressure by alleviating vascular dysfunction and decreasing oxidative stress in L-NAME hypertensive rats. *Phytomedicine* **2019**, *54*, 9–16. [CrossRef] [PubMed]
33. Tayo, G.M.; Pone, G.W.; Komtangi, M.C.; Yondo, G.; Ngangout, A.M.; Mbida, M. Anthelminthic Activity of *Moringa oleifera* Leaf Extracts Evaluated in Vitro on Four Developmental Stages of Haemonchuscontortus from Goats. *AJPS* **2014**, *5*, 1702–1710. [CrossRef]
34. Thurber, M.D.; Fahey, J.W. Adoption of *Moringa oleifera* to combat under-nutrition viewed through the lens of the diffusion of innovations theory. *Ecol. Food Sci. Nutr.* **2010**, *48*, 1–13.
35. Aslam, M.F.; Anwar, R.; Nadeem, U.; Rashid, T.G.; Kazi, A.; Nadeem, M. Mineral composition of *Moringa oleifera* leaves and pods from differentregions of Punjab, Pakistan. *Asian J. Plant Sci.* **2005**, *4*, 417–421. [CrossRef]
36. Pop, O.L.; Kerezsi, A.D.; Ciont, C. A comprehensive review of *Moringa oleifera* bioactive compounds—Cytotoxicity evaluation and their encapsulation. *Foods* **2022**, *11*, 3787. [CrossRef]
37. Thapa, K.; Poudel, M.; Adhikari, P. *Moringa oleifera*: A review article on nutritional properties and its prospect in the context of Nepal. *Acta Sci. Agric.* **2019**, *3*, 47–54. [CrossRef]
38. Dong, X.; Guo, X.; Hu, Y. Summary of studies on traditional Chinese medicine properties of overseas plant medicine *Moringa* leaves. *Glob. Tradit. Chin. Med.* **2019**, *12*, 149–153.
39. Mahmood, K.T.; Mugal, T.; Haq, I.U. *Moringa oleifera*: A natural gift—A review. *J. Pharm. Sci. Res.* **2010**, *2*, 775–781.
40. López-Salazar, H.; Camacho-Díaz, B.H.; Ávila-Reyes, S.V.; Pérez-García, M.D.; Cortazar, M.G.; Ocampo, M.L.A.; Jiménez-Aparicio, A.R. Identification and Quantification of -Sitosterol-d-Glucoside of an Ethanolic Extract Obtained by Microwave-Assisted Extraction from Agave angustifolia Haw. *Molecules* **2019**, *24*, 3926. [CrossRef]
41. Saini, R.K.; Shetty, N.P.; Giridhar, P. Carotenoid content in vegetative and reproductive parts of commercially grown *Moringa oleifera* Lam. cultivars from India by LC–APCI–MS. *Eur. Food Res. Technol.* **2014**, *238*, 971–978. [CrossRef]
42. Sahakitpichan, P.; Mahidol, C.; Disadee, W.; Ruchirawat, S.; Kanchanapoom, T. Unusual glycosides of pyrrole alkaloid and 40-hydroxyphenylethanamide from leaves of *Moringa oleifera*. *Phytochemistry* **2011**, *72*, 791–795. [CrossRef]
43. Abd Rani, N.Z.; Husain, K.; Kumolosasi, E. *Moringa* Genus: A Review of Phytochemistry and Pharmacology. *Front. Pharmacol.* **2018**, *9*, 1–26. [CrossRef] [PubMed]
44. Anzano, A.; Ammar, M.; Papaianni, M.; Grauso, L.; Sabbah, M.; Capparelli, R.; Lanzotti, V. *Moringa oleifera* Lam.: A Phytochemical and Pharmacological Overview. *Horticulturae* **2021**, *7*, 409. [CrossRef]
45. Matic, I.; Guidi, A.; Kenzo, M.; Mattei, M.; Galgani, A. Investigation of medicinal plants traditionally used as dietary supplements: A review on *Moringa oleifera*. *J. Public Health Afr.* **2018**, *9*, 841. [CrossRef]
46. Bhattacharya, A.; Ghosh, G.; Agrawal, D.; Sahu, P.K.; Kumar, S.; Mishra, S.S. GC-MS profiling of ethanolic extract of *Moringa oleifera* leaf. *Int. J. Pharm. Bio Sci.* **2014**, *5*, 263–275.
47. Faizi, S.; Siddiqui, B.S.; Saleem, R.; Siddiqui, S.; Aftab, K. Isolation and structure elucidation of new nitrile and mustard oilglycosides from *Moringa oleifera* and their effect on blood pressure. *J. Nat. Prod.* **1994**, *57*, 1256–1261. [CrossRef]
48. Olagbemide, P.T.; Alikwe, P.C. Proximate analysis and chemical composi-tion of raw and defatted *Moringa oleifera* kernel. *Adv. Life Sci. Technol.* **2014**, *24*, 92–99.
49. Anwar, F.; Latif, S.; Ashraf, M.; Gilani, A.H. *Moringa oleifera*: A food plant with multiple medicinal uses. *Phyther. Res.* **2007**, *21*, 17–25. [CrossRef]

50. Abdulkarim, S.M.; Long, K.; Lai, O.M., Muhammad, S K.S.; Ghazali, H.M. Some physico-chemical properties of *Moringa oleifera* seed oil extracted using solvent and aqueous enzymatic methods. *Food Chem.* **2005**, *93*, 253–263. [CrossRef]
51. Moyo, B.; Masika, P.J.; Hugo, A.; Muchenje, V. Nutritional characterization of *Moringa* (*Moringa oleifera* Lam.) leaves. *Afr. J. Biotechnol.* **2011**, *10*, 12925–12933.
52. Alam, P.; Elkholy, S.F.; Mahfouz, S.A.; Alam, P.; Sharaf-Eldin, M.A. HPLC based estimation and extraction of rutin, quercetin and gallic acid in *Moringa oleifera* plants grown in Saudi Arabia. *J. Chem. Pharm.* **2016**, *8*, 1243–1246.
53. Mbikay, M. Therapeutic potential of *Moringa oleifera* leaves in chronic hyperglycemia and dyslipidemia: A review. *Front. Pharmacol.* **2012**, *3*, 24. [CrossRef]
54. Brilhante, R.S.N.; Sales, J.A.; Pereira, V.S.; Castelo, D.D.S.C.M.; de Aguiar Cordeiro, R.; de Souza Sampaio, C.M.; Paiva, M.D.A.N.; Dos Santos, J.B.F.; Sidrim, J.J.C.; Rocha, M.F.G. Research advances on the multiple uses of *Moringa oleifera*: A sustainable alternative for socially neglected population. *Asian Pac. J. Trop. Med.* **2017**, *10*, 621–630. [CrossRef] [PubMed]
55. Vongsak, B.; Sithisarn, P.; Mangmool, S.; Thongpraditchote, S.; Wongkrajang, Y.; Gritsanapan, W. Maximizing total phenolics, total flavonoids contents and antioxidant activity of *Moringa oleifera* leaf extract by the appropriate extraction method. *Ind. Crops Prod.* **2013**, *44*, 566–571. [CrossRef]
56. Balogun, T.A.; Buliamimu, K.D.; Chukwudozie, O.S.; Tiamiyu, Z.A.; Idowu, T.J. Anticancer Potential of *Moringa oleifera* on BRCA-1 Gene: Systems Biology. *Bioinform. Biol. Insights* **2021**, *15*, 11779322211010703. [CrossRef]
57. Ndong, M.; Uehara, M.; Katsumata, S.; Suzuki, K. Effects of oral administration of *Moringa oleifera* Lam on glucose tol-erance in Goto-KakizakiandWistar rats. *J. Clin. Biochem. Nutr.* **2007**, *40*, 229–233. [CrossRef]
58. Singh, B.N.; Singh, B.R.; Singh, R.L. Oxidative DNA damage protective activity, antioxidant and anti-quorum sensing potentials of *Moringa oleifera*. *Food Chem. Toxicol.* **2009**, *47*, 1109–1116. [CrossRef]
59. Riaz, A.; Rasul, A.; Hussain, G.; Zahoor, M.K.; Jabeen, F.; Subhani, Z.; Younis, T.; Ali, M.; Sarfraz, I.; Selamoglu, Z. Astragalin: A Bioactive Phytochemical with Potential Therapeutic Activities. *Adv. Pharmacol. Sci.* **2018**, *2018*, 9794625. [CrossRef]
60. Leone, A.; Spada, A.; Battezzati, A.; Schiraldi, A.; Aristil, J.; Bertoli, S. Cultivation, genetic, ethnopharmacology, phytochemistry and pharmacology of *Moringa oleifera* leaves: An overview. *Int. J. Mol. Sci.* **2015**, *16*, 12791–12835. [CrossRef]
61. Kaur, G.; Invally, M.; Sanzagiri, R.; Buttar, H.S. Evaluation of the antidepressant activity of *Moringa oleifera* alone and in combination with fluoxetine. *J. Ayurveda Integr. Med.* **2015**, *6*, 273–279. [CrossRef] [PubMed]
62. Korbecki, J.; Bajdak-Rusinek, K. The effect of palmitic acid on inflammatory response in macrophages: An overview of molecular mechanisms. *Inflamm. Res.* **2019**, *68*, 915–932. [CrossRef]
63. Rue, E.A.; Rush, M.D.; Van Breemen, R.B. Procyanidins: A comprehensive review encompassing structure elucidation via mass spectrometry. *Phytochem. Rev.* **2018**, *17*, 1–16. [CrossRef] [PubMed]
64. El Shehawi, A.M.; Alkafafy, M.; El Shazly, S.; Sayed, S.; Farouk, S.; Alotaibi, S.; Madkour, D.A.; Khalifa, H.K.; Ahmed, M.M. *Moringa oleifera* leaves ethanolic extract ameliorates high-fat diet-induced obesity in rats. *J. King Saud. Univ. Sci.* **2021**, *33*, 101552. [CrossRef]
65. Snehal, M.; Parag, G.; Jyotsna, W.; Satyanarayan, N.N. Intensified synthesis of structured lipids from oleic acid rich *Moringa* oil in the presence of supercritical CO_2. *Food Bioprod. Process.* **2020**, *112*, 86–95.
66. Chigurupati, S.; Almurikhy, A.; Almahmoud, S.A.; Almoshari, Y.; Ahmed, A.S.; Vijayabalan, S.; Felemban, S.G.; Palanimuthu, V.R. Molecular docking of phenolic compounds and screening of antioxidant and antidiabetic potential of *Moringa oleifera* ethanolic leaves extract from Qassim region, Saudi Arabia. *Saudi J. Biol. Sci.* **2022**, *29*, 854–859. [CrossRef]
67. Ercan, K.; Gecesefa, O.F.; Taysi, M.E.; Ali Ali, O.A.; Taysi, S. *Moringa Oleifera*: A review of its occurrence, pharmacological importance and oxidative stress. *Mini Rev. Med. Chem.* **2021**, *21*, 380–396. [CrossRef]
68. Caceres, A.; Saravia, A.; Rizzo, S.; Zabala, L.; De Leon, E.; Nave, F. Pharmacologic properties of *Moringa oleifera*. 2: Screening for antispasmodic, anti-inflammatory and diuretic activity. *J. Ethnopharmacol.* **1992**, *36*, 233–237. [CrossRef] [PubMed]
69. Mahajan, S.G.; Banerjee, A.; Chauhan, B.F.; Padh, H.; Nivsarkar, M.; Mehta, A.A. Inhibitory effect of n-butanol fraction of *Moringa oleifera* Lam. seeds on ovalbumin-induced airway inflammation in a Guinea pig model of asthma. *Int. J. Toxicol.* **2009**, *28*, 519–527. [CrossRef]
70. Das, N.; Sikder, K.; Ghosh, S.; Fromenty, B.; Dey, S. *Moringa oleifera* Lam. leaf extract prevents early liver injury and restores antioxidant status in mice fed with high-fat diet. *Indian J. Exp. Biol.* **2012**, *50*, 404–412.
71. Gupta, A.; Gautam, M.K.; Singh, R.K.; Kumar, M.V.; Rao, C.V.; Goel, R.K.; Anupurba, S. Immunomodulatory effect of *Moringa oleifera* Lam. extract on cyclophosphamide induced toxicity in mice. *Indian J. Exp. Biol.* **2010**, *48*, 1157–1160. [PubMed]
72. Upadhyay, P.; Yadav, M.K.; Mishra, S.; Sharma, P.; Purohit, S. *Moringa oleifera*: A review of the medical evidence for its nutritional and pharmacological properties. *Int. J. Res. Pharm. Sci.* **2015**, *5*, 12–16.
73. Padla, E.P.; Solis, L.T.; Levida, R.M.; Shen, C.C.; Ragasa, C.Y. Antimicrobial isothiocyanates from the seeds of *Moringa oleifera* Lam. *Z. Für Nat. C* **2012**, *67*, 557–564. [CrossRef] [PubMed]
74. Ahmadua, T.; Ahmad, K.; Ismail, S.I.; Rashed, O.; Asib, N.; Omar, D. Antifungal efficacy of *Moringa* oliefera leaves and seed extract against Botrytis cinerea causing graymold disease of tomato. *Braz. J. Biol.* **2020**, *81*, 1007–1022. [CrossRef] [PubMed]
75. Moodley, J.S.; Krishna, S.B.N.; Pillay, K. Green synthesis of silver nanoparticles from *Moringa oleifera* leaf extracts and itsantimicro-bial potential. *Adv. Nat. Sci. Nanosci. Nanotechnol.* **2018**, *9*, 015011. [CrossRef]

76. Mohd Fisall, U.F.; Ismail, N.Z.; Adebayo, I.A.; Arsad, H. Dichloromethane fraction of *Moringa oleifera* leaf methanolic extract selectively inhibits breast cancer cells (MCF7) by induction of apoptosis via upregulation of Bax, p53 and caspase 8 expressions. *Mol. Biol. Rep.* **2021**, *48*, 4465–4475. [CrossRef]
77. Singh, U.; Dwivedi, C.; Kulsum, U.; Verma, N.; Saraf, S.; Pradhan, D.K. Phytochemistry and medicinal uses of *Moringa oleifera*: An overview. *J. Drug Deliv. Ther.* **2017**, *7*, 104–116. [CrossRef]
78. Sutalangka, C.; Wattanathorn, J.; Muchimapura, S.; Thukhammee, W. *Moringa oleifera* mitigates memory impairment and neurodegeneration in animal model of age-related dementia. *Oxid. Med. Cell. Longev.* **2013**, *2013*, 695936. [CrossRef]
79. Kirisattayakul, W.; Wattanathorn, J.; Tong-Un, T.; Muchimapura, S.; Wannanon, P.; Jittiwat, J. Cerebroprotective effect of *Moringa oleifera* against focal ischemic stroke induced by middle cerebral artery occlusion. *Oxid. Med. Cell. Longev.* **2013**, *2013*, 951415. [CrossRef]
80. Hannan, M.A.; Kang, J.Y.; Mohibbullah, M.D.; Hong, Y.K.; Lee, H.; Choi, J.S.; Choi, I.S.; Moon, I.S. *Moringa oleifera* with promising neuronal survival and neurite outgrowth promoting potentials. *J. Ethnopharmacol.* **2014**, *152*, 142–150. [CrossRef]
81. Toppo, R.; Roy, B.K.; Gora, R.H.; Baxla, S.L.; Kumar, P. Hepatoprotective activity of *Moringa oleifera* against cadmium toxicity in rats. *Vet. World* **2015**, *8*, 537–540. [CrossRef]
82. Sharifudin, S.A.; Fakurazi, S.; Hidayat, M.T.; Hairuszah, I.; Aris Mohd Moklas, M.; Arulselvan, P. Therapeutic potential of *Moringa oleifera* extracts against acetaminophen-induced hepatotoxicity in rats. *Pharm. Biol.* **2013**, *51*, 279–288. [CrossRef]
83. Mishra, G.; Singh, P.; Verma, R.; Kumar, S.; Srivastav, S.; Jha, K.K.; Khosa, R.L. Traditional uses, phytochemistry and pharmacological properties of *Moringa oleifera* plant: An overview. *Der Pharm. Lett.* **2011**, *3*, 141–164.
84. Dinesha, B.L.; Nidoni, U.; Ramachandra, C.T.; Naik, N.; Sankalpa, K.B. Effect of extraction methods on physicochemical, nutritional, antinutritional, antioxidant and antimicrobial activity of *Moringa* (*Moringa oleifera* Lam.) seed kernel oil. *J. Appl. Nat. Sci.* **2018**, *10*, 287–295. [CrossRef]
85. Nandave, M.; Ojha, S.K.; Joshi, S.; Kumari, S.; Arya, D.S. *Moringa oleifera* leaf extract prevents isoproterenol-induced myocardial damage in rats: Evidence for an antioxidant, antiperoxidative, and cardioprotective intervention. *J. Med. Food.* **2009**, *12*, 47–55. [CrossRef]
86. Panda, S.; Kar, A.; Sharma, P.; Sharma, A. Cardioprotective potential of N,alpha-L-rhamnopyranosyl vincosamide, an indole alkaloid, isolated from the leaves of *Moringa oleifera* in isoproterenol induced cardiotoxic rats: In vivo and in vitro studies. *Bioorg. Med. Chem. Lett.* **2012**, *23*, 959–962. [CrossRef]
87. Khan, H.; Jaiswal, V.; Kulshreshtha, S.; Khan, A. Potential Angiotensin Converting Enzyme Inhibitors from *Moringa oleifera*. *Recent. Pat. Biotechnol.* **2019**, *13*, 239–248. [CrossRef]
88. Khan, H.; Hussain, T.; Kataria, M.; Seth, A.; Malik, M.; Dash, A.; Chand, S.; Khan, M. Role of selective Bioactive Compounds as an Angiotensin Converting Enzyme Inhibitor. *Res. Sq.* **2020**, *7*, 1–25.
89. Yadav, S.; Mathur, J. An updated review on Phytochemical constituent and pharmacological properties of *Moringa oleifera* Lam. *J. Phytopharm.* **2013**, *4*, 26–29. [CrossRef]
90. Akinyeye, A.J.; Solanke, E.O.; Adebiyi, I.O. Phytochemical and antimicrobial Evaluation of Leaf and Seed of *Moringa oleifera* Extracts. *IJRSMHS* **2014**, *4*, 1–10.
91. Adedapo, A.A.; Mogbojuri, O.M.; Emikpe, B.O. Safety evaluations of the aqueous extract of the leaves of *Moringa oleifera* in rats. *J. Med. Plant Res.* **2009**, *3*, 586–591.
92. Ajibade, T.O.; Arowolo, R.; Olayemi, F.O. Phytochemical screening and toxicity studies on the methanol extract of the seeds of *Moringa oleifera*. *J. Complement. Integr. Med.* **2013**, *10*, 11–16. [CrossRef]
93. Reddy, Y.R.R.; Lokanatha, O.; Ratnam, K.S.V.P.; Reddy, C.S.; Raju, I.S.; Reddy, C.D. Acute and Sub Acute Toxicity of *Moringa oleifera* Stem Bark Extract in Swiss Albino Mice. *IJLBPR* **2013**, *2*, 73–82.
94. Pareek, A.; Pant, M.; Gupta, M.M.; Kashania, P.; Ratan, Y.; Jain, V.; Pareek, A.; Chuturgoon, A.A. *Moringa oleifera*: An Updated Comprehensive Review of Its Pharmacological Activities, Ethnomedicinal, Phytopharmaceutical Formulation, Clinical, Phytochemical, and Toxicological Aspects. *Int. J. Mol. Sci.* **2023**, *24*, 2098. [CrossRef]

nutrients

MDPI

Review

Antitumor Effects of Resveratrol Opposing Mechanisms of *Helicobacter pylori* in Gastric Cancer

Daniela Trautmann [1,†], Francesca Suazo [1,†], Keila Torres [1,2,*] and Layla Simón [1,*]

[1] Nutrition and Dietetic School, Universidad Finis Terrae, Santiago 7501015, Chile; dtrautmannq@uft.edu (D.T.); fsuazom@uft.edu (F.S.)
[2] Department of Hematology and Oncology, School of Medicine, Pontificia Universidad Católica de Chile, Santiago 8331150, Chile
* Correspondence: keilatorresizarra@gmail.com (K.T.); lsimon@uft.cl (L.S.); Tel.: +56-22420-7340 (L.S.)
† These authors contributed equally to this work.

Abstract: Gastric cancer is an aggressive and multifactorial disease. *Helicobacter pylori* (*H. pylori*) is identified as a significant etiological factor in gastric cancer. Although only a fraction of patients infected with *H. pylori* progresses to gastric cancer, bacterial infection is critical in the pathology and development of this malignancy. The pathogenic mechanisms of this bacterium involve the disruption of the gastric epithelial barrier and the induction of chronic inflammation, oxidative stress, angiogenesis and metastasis. Adherence molecules, virulence (CagA and VacA) and colonization (urease) factors are important in its pathogenicity. On the other hand, resveratrol is a natural polyphenol with anti-inflammatory and antioxidant properties. Resveratrol also inhibits cancer cell proliferation and angiogenesis, suggesting a role as a potential therapeutic agent against cancer. This review explores resveratrol as an alternative cancer treatment, particularly against *H. pylori*-induced gastric cancer, due to its ability to mitigate the pathogenic effects induced by bacterial infection. Resveratrol has shown efficacy in reducing the proliferation of gastric cancer cells in vitro and in vivo. Moreover, the synergistic effects of resveratrol with chemotherapy and radiotherapy underline its therapeutic potential. However, further research is needed to fully describe its efficacy and safety in treating gastric cancer.

Keywords: polyphenol; natural product; antioxidant; anti-inflammatory; antitumor; gastric carcinoma

1. Introduction

Gastric cancer is a prevalent malignancy and constitutes the fourth cause of cancer-related mortality globally, exhibiting a median survival period of only 12 months in its advanced stages [1]. The progression of gastric cancer occurs over an extended period, sometimes developing after 20–30 years of exposure to carcinogenic agents, and evolving through different stages [1,2]. Initially, non-cancerous cells undergo abnormal growth leading to dysplasia. Subsequently, normal cells are transformed into cancer cells, developing carcinoma in situ, in which cancer is confined to the superficial mucosal layer of the stomach. Finally, cancer cells spread through the different layers of the stomach and affect other nearby organs, resulting in invasive carcinoma [2].

Gastric cancer is an aggressive and multifactorial disease that includes environmental and genetic risk factors. Environmental factors, more than genetic alterations, increase the possibility of developing gastric cancer. For instance, dietary habits with a high intake of fruit and vegetables are protective, whereas processed meals, smoked meat and salt-preserved food are risk factors. In addition, smoking and alcohol intake are associated with a high risk of gastric cancer. For that reason, early diagnosis, proper treatment and prevention with diets are alternative therapeutic efforts to reduce patient suffering [1].

Infection with *Helicobacter pylori* (*H. pylori*) is a major environmental risk factor for gastric cancer and is linked to the development of gastric ulcers. This association is largely attributed to the inflammatory response induced by the infection with this bacterium [3]. Conventional therapy involves proton pump inhibitors and antibiotics. However, the indiscriminate use of antibiotics has led to microbial resistance. As a result, new studies on alternative therapies for eradicating the bacterium have been proposed. These novel therapies consider sterols and polyphenols as potential inhibitors of the activity of *H. pylori* [3].

Resveratrol is a natural polyphenol present in nuts, apples, red fruits, black olives, grapes and red wines. This natural product has antioxidant, anti-inflammatory and antimicrobial properties due to its ability to interact with reactive oxygen species (ROS) and cytoplasmic and nuclear proteins within cells. For that reason, resveratrol has been used as an alternative and complementary therapy for metabolic and cardiovascular diseases [4] and has also been effectively used in treating gastric cancer [5]. This review aims to provide a comprehensive summary of resveratrol as a potential therapeutic alternative in the prevention and treatment of gastric cancer induced by *H. pylori*.

2. *Helicobacter pylori*

H. pylori is a Gram-negative bacterium that colonizes the human stomach and is associated with various gastrointestinal diseases such as peptic ulcer disease and gastric cancer. *H. pylori* infection is one of the most common bacterial diseases worldwide, with an estimated 4.4 billion individuals infected. Almost 50% of the population over the age of 50 are infected with the bacterium, though prevalence varies across different geographical regions and ethnic groups [6–9].

The transmission of this infection occurs via oral–oral or fecal–oral routes. The pathogen exhibits a repertoire of mechanisms that enable it to colonize the stomach. Among these mechanisms are its motility, its adherence to gastric epithelial cells, and the modulation of the gastric environment [3]. Moreover, *H. pylori* promotes inflammation and oxidative stress, facilitating infection and carcinogenesis.

2.1. *Mechanisms of Tumorigenesis Induced by H. pylori*

Although only some individuals infected with *H. pylori* will develop gastric cancer, the presence of the bacterium significantly increases the risk [10]. The mechanisms through which *H. pylori* can trigger the development of gastric cancer are associated with infection (adhesion and colonization), the disruption of the gastric epithelium, DNA damage, the alteration of repair mechanisms, the activation of the inflammatory cascade, oxidative stress, angiogenesis and metastasis [11]. Figure 1 summarizes these mechanisms and factors induced by *H. pylori* during colonization, infection and tumorigenesis within the gastric mucosa. For instance, virulence factors, adherence molecules and cytokines promote inflammation and angiogenesis (Figure 1, red box) which are related to the promotion of gastric cancer (Figure 1, light pink box) and mucosa infection (Figure 1, blue box). Moreover, γ-glutamyl transferase (GGT) and urease are colonization factors that induce oxidative stress and angiogenesis (Figure 1, yellow box), thereby also promoting gastric cancer (Figure 1, light pink box) and infection (Figure 1, blue box).

The presence of the bacterium activates the release of proinflammatory cytokines, such as tumor necrosis factor-alpha (TNF-α), transforming growth factor-beta (TGF-β) and interleukins (ILs), leading to the infiltration of inflammatory cells into the gastric tissue. In this sense, *H. pylori* induces a chronic inflammation that perpetuates the damage to the gastric mucosa and promotes abnormal cell proliferation by triggering the proliferation of inactive endothelium to synthesize new blood vessels, thereby promoting angiogenesis (Figure 1, red box) [12].

Adhesion molecules and virulence factors of *H. pylori* play a crucial role in its ability to colonize and produce damage in the stomach. Proteins such as the blood group antigen binding adhesin (BabA), sialic acid-binding adhesin (SabA), the adherence associated lipoprotein A (AlpA) and outer membrane porin HopQ and HopZ and facilitate *H. pylori* adherence to the gastric epithelium. Factors like the outer inflammatory protein (OipA), cytotoxin-associated gene A (CagA) and vacuolating cytotoxin A (VacA) induce cellular damage, promoting chronic inflammation and the development of gastric cancer (Figure 1, red and light pink boxes). Additionally, the activity of GGT contributes to oxidative stress, induces the release of pro-inflammatory proteins, and favors *H. pylori* pathogenicity and persistence in the acidic gastric environment (Figure 1, yellow box) [3,13–15].

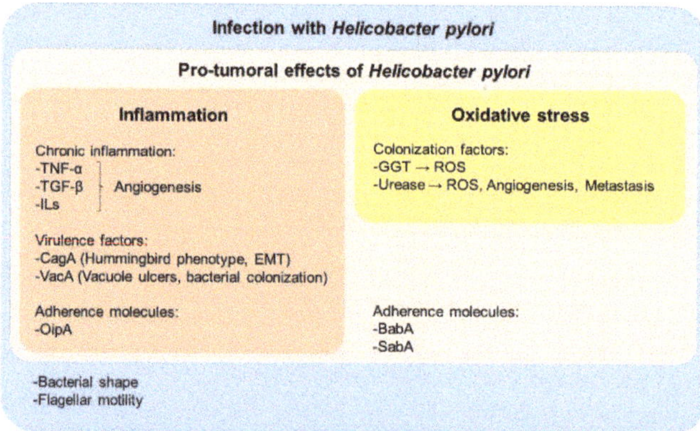

Figure 1. Mechanisms associated with *H. pylori* gastric infection (all, blue box) and the development of gastric cancer (light pink box). *H. pylori* presents adherence molecules and virulence factors such as CagA and VacA that alter the gastric epithelium. CagA reduces cell adhesion and promotes epithelial–mesenchymal transition (EMT). VacA induces bacterial incorporation into the host cell membrane and enhances bacterial colonization into the stomach. Additionally, gastric carcinogenesis is associated with inflammation, which induces angiogenesis (red box). Colonization factors such as GGT and urease promote the generation of reactive oxygen species (ROS), angiogenesis, and metastasis (yellow box).

In addition, the helix shape and flagellar motility of the bacterium are essential for the survival and colonization of the stomach (Figure 1, blue box). Moreover, the enzyme urease facilitates the conversion of urea into ammonia and carbon dioxide, establishing a nearly neutral microenvironment that safeguards the bacterium against gastric acidity. Meanwhile, carbon dioxide acts as a protective barrier against bactericidal agents. These mechanisms underline the complex relationship between *H. pylori* and the stomach environment, highlighting the diverse strategies the bacterium employs to ensure its survival and involvement in pathological processes for the host, including gastric cancer and duodenal ulcer (Figure 1, yellow box) [16–19].

2.2. *H. pylori-Induced Gastric Cancer*

Gastric cancer is a malignant disease that affects the stomach and is characterized by its ability to invade and destroy surrounding tissues [2]. In 2020, the global incidence of gastric cancer was documented at approximately 1.09 million new cases, with a total of 769,000 fatalities reported. In this sense, gastric cancer was one of the top five cancer types in terms of mortality [20].

Genetic and external factors can influence the alterations in tumor cells in gastric cancer. Among the latter are obesity, exposure to carcinogens, the consumption of alcohol and tobacco, radiation exposure, and dietary habits, such as a high intake of salt, smoked, and processed meals, coupled with a low intake of fruits and vegetables. Infections with viruses or bacteria, such as the Epstein–Barr virus or *H. pylori*, alterations in the gastrointestinal microbiota, gastroesophageal reflux disease, gastric ulcers, or previous gastric surgery, also play a role in gastric cancer development [2,21].

Infection with *H. pylori* in the gastric mucosa initiates a chronic inflammatory response, leading to gastritis, which can progress through a multi-step gastric tumorigenesis cascade, known as the Correa cascade [2,22]. The first step of this progression is atrophic gastritis, characterized by sustained inflammation that causes the loss of normal gastric glands. Furthermore, atrophic gastritis can lead to intestinal metaplasia, a process in which gastric epithelial cells lining the stomach transform into cells resembling those of the intestine, an adaptive response to chronic inflammation regarded as a precancerous stage. Intestinal metaplasia can progress to dysplasia, where metaplastic cells begin to exhibit dysplastic changes, i.e., precancerous alterations in their shape and organization. Classified as low- or high-grade, high-grade dysplasia is a direct step toward cancer. Adenocarcinoma represents the final and malignant form of gastric cancer, where cells have undergone oxidative stress, mutations, and transformations allowing for the uncontrolled growth and eventual invasion of neighboring tissues, leading to metastasis [10,23].

3. Treatments for Gastric Cancer

In the early stages of gastric cancer, endoscopic resection is the recommended technique for managing lesions with a low risk of lymph node metastasis. Minimally invasive surgical techniques are viable alternatives for early lesions unsuitable for endoscopic intervention [24]. In contrast, advanced stages of gastric cancer require more aggressive treatments such as surgery, chemotherapy and radiotherapy. These therapeutic modalities aim to control the spread of cancer and enhance the quality of life for patients [25].

3.1. Conventional Treatments for Gastric Cancer

Surgery is commonly employed for the removal of gastric tumors. While it can be curative in some cases of gastric cancer, it presents challenges in other cases, where achieving complete tumor resection is difficult. Moreover, it carries inherent risks and potential complications, such as infections, bleeding and impaired gastric function (Table 1) [26,27].

Table 1. Conventional Treatments for Gastric Cancer.

Treatment	Advantages	Disadvantages	References
Surgery	Curative in early stages of GC.	Complications: infections, bleeding, thrombus, impaired gastric function.	[26,27]
Chemotherapy: Fluorouracil, Leucovorin, Oxaliplatin and Docetaxel	Reduces tumor size before surgery. Eliminate remaining cells after surgery.	Side effects: nausea, vomiting, fatigue, hair loss, and suppression of the immune system. Drug resistance.	[27,28]
Molecular therapeutic agent: Apatinib, PD-1 inhibitors	Useful in refractory cases and metastatic gastric cancer.	Side effects: proteinuria and hypertension.	[27,29,30]
Radiotherapy	Metastatic GC. Useful as a palliative effect and for control of the bleeding from the primary tumor.	Side effects: nausea, diarrhea, loss of appetite, and fatigue. Resistance.	[31]

GC: Gastric cancer.

Chemotherapy is applied both before surgery (neoadjuvant) and after surgery (adjuvant) to reduce the tumor size or eliminate remaining cancer cells, respectively. The combination of Fluorouracil, Leucovorin (calcium folinic acid), Oxaliplatin and Docetaxel is successful in some patients with gastric cancer [27]. Although it can be effective in destroying cancer cells, it can also induce significant side effects, including nausea, vomiting, fatigue, hair loss and the suppression of the immune system. Furthermore, drug resistance may limit its long-term efficacy [28]. In this sense, molecular therapeutic targets such as anti-angiogenic factors are used in gastric cancer refractory cases. For instance, Apatinib is a tyrosine kinase inhibitor that targets vascular endothelial growth factor receptor 2 and prolongs the survival rates of patients with advanced gastric cancer for whom conventional chemotherapy fails [27,29]. Moreover, PD-1 inhibitors and chemo-anti-angiogenic agent combination therapy improve the effects of immunotherapy in metastatic gastric cancer [30].

Radiotherapy employs high-energy radiation to destroy cancer cells and reduce tumor size. Radiotherapy can be useful for controlling tumor growth, treating the bleeding from the primary tumor, and alleviating symptoms in patients with metastatic gastric cancer. However, radiotherapy can also harm healthy tissues near the treated area, leading to side effects such as nausea, diarrhea, loss of appetite and fatigue. Additionally, some gastric tumors may exhibit intrinsic resistance to radiotherapy [31].

3.2. *Polyphenols as a Potential Treatment for Gastric Cancer*

As shown in Table 1, conventional treatments for gastric cancer have some disadvantages such as complications, side effects and resistance. For that reason, looking for alternative therapies for the prevention and treatment of gastric cancer is mandatory. In this scenario, natural products, specifically, polyphenols, which can control inflammation and oxidative stress, emerge as candidates.

Bioinformatic analysis has described genes that contribute to inflammation and oxidative stress in gastric cancer (e.g., IL-2, IL-6, IL-8, IFN-γ and LOX). Moreover, treatment with a polyphenolic cocktail and maggot larvae reduces the expression of these markers in a mouse model of gastric cancer [32]. In addition, a phenolic-rich extract of the Cactaceae *Nopalea cochenillifera* attenuates gastric lesions by inhibiting inflammation and oxidative stress. Specifically, this extract, enriched in the bioactive compound isorhamnetin, reduces gastric lesions, inflammation (TNF-α and IL-1β levels), and oxidative stress (COX-2 and MDA levels) in rats when administered at 100 mg/kg [33]. Furthermore, 10 mg/kg of carvacrol, a dietary polyphenol from Lamiaceae plants, reduces inflammation (IL-1β, IL-6, TNF-α and TGF-β) and oxidative stress (oxidative stress index (OSI) = total oxidant status (TOS)/total antioxidant status (TAS)) in a rat model of gastric cancer [34].

Polyphenols are also efficient in the prevention and treatment of *H. pylori*-induced gastric cancer. For instance, ellagitannins (castalagin and vescalagin) from *Castanea sativa* impair the *H. pylori*-induced inflammation (IL-8 release and NF-κB signaling) in human gastric cells [35]. Furthermore, the extracts obtained from *Cistus* × *incanus* L. and *Castanea sativa* are rich in polyphenols such as tannins, procyanidins and flavonoids, which can reduce IL-8 and NF-κB induced by *H. pylori* [36]. Moreover, the pretreatment of cells and mice with silibinin mitigates the *H. pylori*-induced dysplasia, hyperplasia, inflammation (NF-κB and STAT3 activation) and oxidative stress (COX-2 and iNOS expression) [37]. Similarly, walnut polyphenol extracts suppress the activation of STAT3 induced by *H. pylori* infection in RGM-1 gastric mucosal cells, thereby inhibiting the inflammatory and mutagenic action of the bacterium [38].

4. Resveratrol

Resveratrol is a polyphenol found in the berry family, including mulberries (5 mg of resveratrol per 100 g), blueberries (0.38 mg per 100 g), and cranberries (1.92 mg of resveratrol per 100 g), as well as in grapes (0.24 to 1.25 mg per 160 g) and nuts, such as peanuts (1.12 mg of resveratrol per 100 g) and pistachios (0.11 mg of resveratrol per 100 g) (Figure 2). It is renowned for its anti-inflammatory and antioxidant properties and has also been reported to possess antimicrobial properties by inhibiting the growth of *Staphylococcus aureus*, *Escherichia coli*, *Candida albicans* and *H. pylori* strains [6,39–41].

The appropriate dosage of resveratrol varies depending on the use and specific medical condition. Typical doses range from 100 to 500 mg of resveratrol daily, though some studies have used higher doses [42]. Resveratrol can be administered in numerous supplements and fortified foods [43,44]. However, the oral bioavailability of resveratrol is low due to its rapid metabolism and elimination. Only 12% of digested resveratrol reaches the bloodstream and body tissues [39]. For instance, when comparing dietary-achievable (5 mg) or pharmacological (1 g) doses of resveratrol, the concentrations required in blood and tissues to prevent cell growth are difficult to achieve in humans (Figure 2) [43]. For this reason, pharmaceutical formulations have been developed to improve the bioavailability of resveratrol. Techniques such as encapsulation in controlled-release systems and combination with other ingredients are employed to enhance both its absorption and bioavailability [43,45].

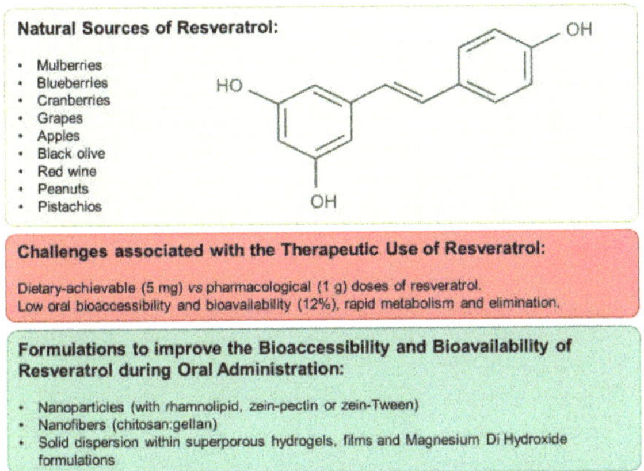

Figure 2. Resveratrol: natural sources, challenges associated with its therapeutic use, and formulations to improve its bioaccessibility and bioavailability during oral administration.

The co-encapsulation of resveratrol and Coenzyme Q10 into nanoparticles with rhamnolipid improves the chemical stability and release of resveratrol after in vitro gastrointestinal digestion [46]. Moreover, the encapsulation in nanoparticles with zein and pectin increases the solubility and the bioaccessibility of resveratrol in gastric and intestinal phases in vitro [47]. Nanoparticles with zein and Tween increase resveratrol bioaccessibility to 84% after the intestinal phase of in vitro digestion, compared with the low bioaccessibility of free resveratrol (13%) [48]. In addition, resveratrol loaded in chitosan–gellan nanofibers can deliver an equivalent to 840 μM of resveratrol with increased antioxidant capacity (Figure 2) [49].

The solid dispersion of resveratrol within superporous hydrogels based on blends of chitosan and polyvinyl alcohol sustains the drug release over 12 h in simulated gastric fluid [50]. Furthermore, the solid dispersion of resveratrol within films prepared of starch and chitosan has an efficient delivery of resveratrol (80% over 12 h), cytotoxic activity against human gastric cells, and anti-inflammatory effects against macrophage-like cells [51]. A solid dispersion of resveratrol supported by Magnesium di hydroxide has better solubility in gastric simulation fluid compared to pure resveratrol. In a clinical trial, human subjects consuming 180 mg of pure resveratrol, or the formulation supported by Magnesium di hydroxide, had a maximum plasma concentration of resveratrol of 2.2 and 6.3 μM, respectively, demonstrating a better bioavailability with the formulation (Figure 2) [45].

4.1. Properties of Resveratrol

Some properties of resveratrol are attributed to regulating various molecular mechanisms which are currently subjects of ongoing research regarding its therapeutic effects. Resveratrol has been suggested to modulate the activity of several enzymes and transcription factors, such as sirtuins, NF-κB and insulin-like growth factor 1 (IGF-1). These mechanisms involved oxidative stress, inflammation and tumor progression (Figure 3, all the mechanisms, light pink box) [52,53]. For instance, resveratrol has anti-inflammatory properties by reducing NF-κB, COX-2 and cytokines, in an *H. pylori*-opposite way (compare Figures 1 and 3, red boxes). In addition, resveratrol can scavenge free radicals and reduce oxidative stress, while *H. pylori* has the opposite effect (compare Figures 1 and 3, yellow boxes). In this sense, resveratrol inhibits *H. pylori* infection by reducing inflammation and oxidative stress (Figure 3, blue box). Moreover, resveratrol inhibits signaling pathways associated with cancer, such as mitogen-activated protein kinase (MAPK), AMP-activated protein kinase (AMPK) and protein kinase C (PKC). Also, resveratrol induces apoptosis and cell cycle arrest, but prevents angiogenesis, thereby exerting an antitumor effect (Figure 3, light pink box).

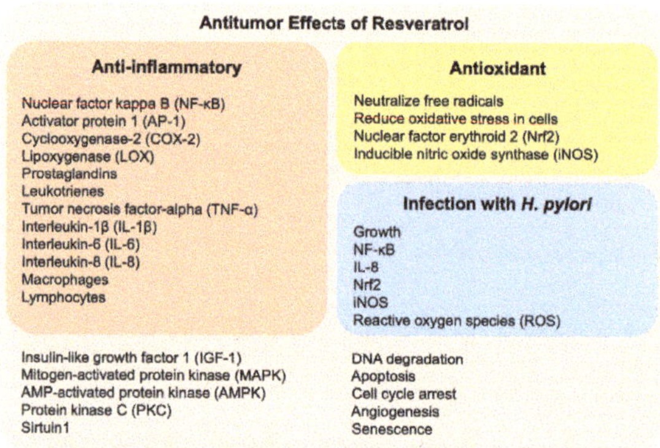

Figure 3. Mechanisms of resveratrol in preventing inflammation (red box), oxidative stress (yellow box), *H. pylori* infection (light blue box) and, thereby, cancer (all, light pink box).

Resveratrol plays an anti-inflammatory role in inhibiting the activation of pro-inflammatory transcription factors such as NF-κB and activator protein 1 (AP-1) (Figure 3, red box). Moreover, resveratrol blocks the production of inflammatory mediators, such as prostaglandins and leukotrienes, by inhibiting the activity of key enzymes involved in their synthesis, including cyclooxygenase-2 (COX-2) and lipoxygenase (LOX). Resveratrol decreases the production of pro-inflammatory cytokines, such as TNF-α, interleukin-1β (IL-1β) and interleukin-6 (IL-6), while increasing the production of anti-inflammatory cytokines, such as interleukin-10 (IL-10). Furthermore, resveratrol modulates the function of immune system cells, such as macrophages and lymphocytes. For instance, resveratrol inhibits macrophage activation and reduces the production of ROS and pro-inflammatory cytokines by these cells. By reducing oxidative stress, resveratrol also attenuates the inflammatory response associated with oxidative damage [39].

Resveratrol acts as a potent antioxidant (Figure 3, yellow box), neutralizing free radicals and reducing oxidative stress in cells. Moreover, resveratrol has been shown to protect against oxidative damage and cellular aging, which may have implications in preventing diseases associated with oxidative stress, such as cardiovascular, neurodegenerative diseases and cancer [52]. Resveratrol modulates several cellular signaling pathways involved in oxidative stress, such as the nuclear factor erythroid 2- related factor 2 (Nrf2). This pathway promotes the expression of antioxidant enzymes, thereby protecting cells against oxidative damage [54,55].

In this context, resveratrol protects against *H. pylori*-induced gastritis by suppressing inflammation and oxidative stress, inhibiting markers like IL-8, iNOS, NF-κB and Nrf2 (Figure 3, light blue box) [56]. Additionally, the treatment with 100 μM of resveratrol for 2 h reduces the levels of ROS and IL-8 in MKN-45 gastric cells infected with a CagA-positive *H. pylori* strain [57]. Resveratrol derivatives have antibacterial effects against *H. pylori* viability, biofilm formation and infection in an in vivo model using *Galleria mellonella* [58]. Chitosan nanoparticles containing resveratrol have bactericidal effects against *H. pylori*, also preventing biofilm and in vitro (AGS and MKN-74 cell lines) and in vivo infection (*Galleria mellonella* model) [59].

4.2. Properties of Resveratrol in Gastric Cancer

Resveratrol has a tumor-suppressing effect on several cancers, including gastric cancer [5]. Likewise, this molecule can trigger apoptosis in tumor cells (Figure 3, light pink box). This involves the activation of intracellular signaling cascades that lead to DNA degradation and the destruction of cancerous cells. Also, resveratrol reduces the proliferation of tumor cells by blocking cell cycle progression. Resveratrol interferes with the activity of certain key proteins that regulate the cell cycle (i.e., cyclin D1 and CDK4), resulting in a halt in cell growth [6,60,61] and showing efficacy in inhibiting cancer metastasis [62].

Additionally, resveratrol inhibits the formation of new blood vessels in the process of angiogenesis, which is essential for the supply of nutrients and oxygen to tumors. By blocking angiogenesis, resveratrol deprives tumors of the necessary resources for their growth and spread [63,64]. This polyphenol interferes with several cellular signaling pathways involved in the proliferation and survival of tumor cells. Resveratrol modulates the activity of proteins such as NF-κB, MAPK and AMPK, which are involved in cellular survival and growth (Figure 3, light pink box) [39].

Specifically, resveratrol has shown effects on gastric cancer [65] independent of *H. pylori* infection. In KATO-III and SNU-1 cells, resveratrol inhibits the activity of PKC, thereby reducing the growth of gastric adenocarcinoma cells via tumor suppression, cell cycle arrest, reduced proliferation and increased apoptosis (Figure 3, light pink box) [66,67]. In this sense, the exposure of SNU-1 cells to 100 μM resveratrol for 24 h induces cell death and cell cycle arrest [68]. Furthermore, 25 and 50 μM resveratrol inhibit the viability of gastric cancer cells, AGS, BGC-823 and SGC-7901, in a sirtuin1-dependent manner through the induction of senescence and cell cycle arrest [60]. Similarly, resveratrol has shown effects in an animal model of gastric cancer. Indeed, 40 mg/kg/day of resveratrol reduces gastric cancer development by decreasing the fractions of Ki67-positive proliferative cells in the tumor specimens of nude mice [6,60].

The treatment of human gastric adenocarcinoma SGC-7901 cells with 50–200 μM resveratrol for 48 h induces apoptosis and DNA damage attributed to an increased generation of ROS and cytotoxicity [69]. Wu et al. (2018) demonstrated that treating SGC-7901 cells with 200 μM resveratrol reduces viability, induces S phase arrest, and increases the Bax/Bcl-2 ratio. This suggests that resveratrol inhibits the proliferation of gastric cancer cells, induces apoptosis, and suppresses NF-κB pathway [70].

Moreover, the treatment of other gastric cancer cell lines, AGS and MKN45, with resveratrol results in reduced heparanase activity alongside increased superoxide dismutase activity, an antioxidant enzyme. The reduction in heparanase activity correlates with decreased NF-kB transcriptional activity and attenuates the invasion potential in gastric cancer cells [71]. Gao et al. (2015) reported that resveratrol effectively inhibits the invasion and metastatic potential of gastric cancer cells in vitro by targeting the hedgehog signaling pathway and suppressing epithelial-to-mesenchymal transition (EMT). These results suggest the potential of resveratrol as a promising therapeutic agent in the treatment of gastric cancer [72].

Likewise, pre-treatment with resveratrol effectively attenuates the enhanced motility of gastric cancer cells and reverses the EMT induced by gastric cancer-derived mesenchymal stem cells (GC-MSCs) within the tumor microenvironment. This effect is mediated through the inhibition of the Wnt/β-catenin signaling pathway and results in the downregulation of the expression and secretion of several pro-inflammatory cytokines and angiogenic factors, including IL-6, IL-8, MCP-1 and VEGF, at both the RNA and protein levels [73]. Resveratrol decreases HIF-1α protein levels induced by hypoxia in SGC-7901 cells, thereby mitigating the stimulation of cell proliferation, migrative and invasive capabilities, as well as the induction of EMT changes through Hedgehog pathway activation [74].

Su et al. (2022) reported that resveratrol inhibited miR-155-5p expression, a microRNA whose upregulation promotes the initiation and progression of the cell cycle. This inhibition subsequently modulated the expression levels of claudin 1, cyclin D1, c-Myc, Bcl-2 and caspase-3, thereby arresting cell cycle progression in gastric cancer cell lines [75]. Yang et al. (2022) demonstrated that resveratrol downregulated the expression of *MALAT1*, impacting proliferation, migration and invasion. Additionally, the regulation of the MALAT1/miR-383-5p/DDIT4 signaling pathway by resveratrol induces apoptosis in cell line SGC7901 [76].

Similarly, resveratrol inhibits proliferation, migration and invasion, while inducing apoptosis by inhibiting β-catenin and Bcl-2 but increasing Bax expression in MKN7 cells [77]. Also, resveratrol prevents IL-6-induced invasion of SCG-7901 and HSC-39 cells by reducing the Raf-MAPK signaling pathway and the metalloproteinases (MMPs) MMP2 and MMP9 expressions. In addition, resveratrol treatment (20 μM resveratrol intratumorally injected every four days for 3 weeks) inhibits metastasis in an in vivo model of HSC-39 cells injected into the tail vein of nude mice [78].

After therapy with 25 mg/kg/2d resveratrol for 20 days, the tumors, formed by SGC-7901 cells injected into BALB/c nude mice, reduced their volume and weight. These effects were attributed to the induction of apoptosis, a reduction in EMT, migration and invasion through the inhibition of Akt/mTOR, MAPK/ERK and Wnt/β-catenin pathways, and the modulation of lncRNA H19 [79]. Moreover, resveratrol prevents gastric intestinal metaplasia through the inhibition of the Akt pathway, and the activation of p-FoxO4 signaling. In this sense, the expression of p-FoxO4 is reduced in intestinal metaplasia compared with normal tissues [80] and suggests that resveratrol may prevent metaplasia in humans.

Resveratrol loaded in Mesoporous Silica Nanoparticles (Res-loaded MSN) exhibits superior suppressive efficacy on HGC-27 and AGS cells, as well as enhanced anticancer effects on gastric cancer in vivo, compared to treatment with resveratrol alone. These results suggest that mesoporous silica nanoparticles might be a promising drug delivery system for gastric cancer therapy [81].

Altogether, these findings suggest that resveratrol can control *H. pylori*-induced effects by suppressing infection, inflammation and oxidative stress. Additionally, resveratrol reduces the growth of cancer cells through several mechanisms, notably its role in signaling pathways, cell cycle, apoptosis and senescence. Given this, resveratrol represents a significant barrier against the initiation, development and progression of *H. pylori*-induced gastric cancer.

4.3. *Combination Therapy Strategies with Resveratrol*

Resveratrol has demonstrated synergy with various chemotherapeutic agents, such as 5-fluorouracil (5-FU) and doxorubicin, thereby enhancing their antitumor effects across several types of cancers [63,82]. Hu et al. (2019) reported the promising therapeutic potential of resveratrol, particularly when combined with ginkgetin, a biflavone, and 5-FU, resulting in the suppressed expressions of COX-2 and inflammatory cytokines and relieving the 5-fluorouracil-induced inflammatory response (Table 2). Likewise, ginkgetin and resveratrol inhibit VEGF-induced endothelial cell proliferation, migration, invasion and angiogenesis [63].

Resveratrol combined with doxorubicin regulates the SIRT1/β-catenin signaling pathway to reverse EMT, consequently inhibiting cell migration and promoting cell apoptosis, thereby enhancing their antitumor effects [82,83]. In an in vivo study involving nude mice with xenografts of doxorubicin-resistant subclones from a gastric cancer cell line (SGC7901), treatment with 3 mg/kg of doxorubicin and 50 mg/kg of resveratrol achieved a tumor volume reduction of 86.97%. Immunohistochemistry confirmed that the combination treatment significantly enhanced PTEN and caspase-3 expression while inhibiting vimentin and Ki67 expression, compared to individual treatments. Resveratrol can delay tumor growth by inhibiting EMT and promoting apoptosis, thereby reversing doxorubicin resistance in gastric cancer [84].

Resveratrol enhances the cytotoxic profile of Herceptin (trastuzumab) and exhibits synergistic interactions with it, resulting in a marked decrease in the gene expression of Bcl-xL, and thereby, the induction of apoptosis [85]. Kong et al. (2017) reported that the combination of resveratrol (5 μg/mL or 10 μg/mL) and paclitaxel (5 μg/mL) demonstrated synergistic growth inhibitory effects and increased apoptosis compared to separate treatments. This combinatory treatment significantly downregulates the mRNA and protein expressions of various key molecules involved in cancer progression, including COX-2, VEGF, MMP1, MMP2, MMP9, NF-κB, anti-apoptotic proteins (Bcl-2, Bcl-xL), procollagen I, collagen I, collagen III and CTGF, as well as pro-inflammatory cytokines (TNF-α, IL-1β) and iNOS, while upregulating the expression of anti-cancer genes (TIMPs—TIMP-1, TIMP-2, TIMP-3, IκB-α, p53, p21, caspases—caspase-3, caspase-8, caspase-9, Bax). These findings suggest that the combined treatment could serve as an effective enhancer of the anticancer properties of paclitaxel [86].

Türkmen et al. (2023) demonstrated that resveratrol effectively reduces both the expression of caspase-3 protein and the histopathological changes resulting from treatment with pembrolizumab (PEMB), a monoclonal antibody targeting the PD-1 surface protein and used as an anticancer agent. Moreover, resveratrol administration effectively mitigates the biochemical, immunological and histological alterations induced by PEMB [87]. A clinical trial revealed that the combination of resveratrol and copper reduces the toxicity of docetaxel chemotherapy in advanced gastric cancer. Specifically, resveratrol reduces the incidence of non-hematological toxicities such as hand–foot syndrome, diarrhea, and vomiting (13%) [88].

The cisplatin–resveratrol combination exhibits significant efficacy in suppressing metastasis. This treatment hinders proliferation and decreases cell invasion and telomerase activity while inducing ß-galactosidase activity. Additionally, the combination treatment leads to cell cycle arrest at the G0/G1 stage and promotes apoptosis and cell senescence by targeting the P38/P53 and P16/P21 pathways [89]. Additionally, resveratrol and cisplatin synergistically inhibit the proliferation of AGS gastric cancer cells by inducing endoplasmic reticulum stress-mediated apoptosis and G2/M phase cell cycle arrest [90].

Resveratrol safeguards against radiation-induced intestinal damage caused by radiotherapy by reducing oxidative stress and apoptosis through the SIRT1/FOXO3a and PI3K/Akt pathways in normal cells [91]. Moreover, resveratrol enhances the efficacy of radiotherapy by increasing the sensitivity of tumor cells to radiation and promoting apoptosis [64]. The radio-sensitizing effect of resveratrol is achieved by impairing DNA repair capacity in the early stages, inhibiting proliferation, inducing autophagy, and promoting apoptosis both in vitro and in vivo [92].

Table 2. Synergistic effects of resveratrol with chemotherapeutic agents and radiotherapy.

Therapy Agent	Effects of Combination with Resveratrol	References
5-Fluorouracil (5-FU)	Mitigating the inflammatory response induced by 5-FU	[63]
Doxorubicin	Inhibiting cell migration and EMT, promoting cell apoptosis	[82,83]
Trastuzumab (Herceptin)	Induction of apoptosis	[85]
Paclitaxel	Growth inhibitory effects and increased apoptosis	[86]
Pembrolizumab (PEMB)	Mitigating the biochemical, immunological, and histological alterations induced by PEMB	[87]
Docetaxel	A combination of resveratrol and copper reduces the toxicity of docetaxel chemotherapy	[88]
Cisplatin	Suppressing metastasis, promoting apoptosis and cell senescence, inhibiting proliferation, and causing cell cycle arrest	[89]
Radiotherapy	Safeguarding against radiation-induced intestinal damage, reducing oxidative stress and apoptosis in normal cells, increasing the sensitivity of tumor cells to radiation, promoting apoptosis, and inducing autophagy	[91]

On the other hand, resistance mechanisms to resveratrol treatment involve several factors, including the activation of alternative signaling pathways or survival mechanisms by cancer cells, which can counteract the effects of resveratrol [93]. Additionally, the efficacy of resveratrol is influenced by the metabolism of the compound; variations in the expression of drug-metabolizing enzymes may significantly affect therapeutic outcomes [94]. Furthermore, the modulation of transport proteins within cell membranes plays a crucial role in regulating the absorption and excretion of resveratrol [95,96].

5. Conclusions

Researching resveratrol as a promising therapeutic option for *Helicobacter pylori*-induced gastric cancer provides new insights and avenues for treatment. With its antioxidant, anti-inflammatory and antitumor properties, resveratrol could offer therapeutic benefits without the side effects and toxicity associated with conventional therapies. However, further research and clinical studies are essential to thoroughly evaluate its efficacy and safety in the context of gastric cancer and to determine the optimal dosages, formulations, administration routes and drug interactions to fully harness the therapeutic potential of resveratrol in gastric cancer. Finally, future perspectives for resveratrol as a treatment for gastric cancer include the development of more comprehensive clinical studies to validate its therapeutic potential. With further evidence, resveratrol could become a more widely accepted component in clinical practice due to its antitumor properties.

Author Contributions: Conceptualization, K.T. and L.S.; investigation, D.T., F.S., K.T. and L.S.; resources, L.S.; writing—original draft preparation, D.T., F.S., K.T. and L.S.; writing—review and editing, K.T. and L.S.; visualization, K.T. and L.S.; supervision, L.S.; project administration, L.S.; funding acquisition, L.S. All authors have read and agreed to the published version of the manuscript.

Funding: This research was funded by ANID-FONDECYT-Iniciación [11230112] (LS), Concurso de Investigación con Colaboración Internacional de la Universidad Finis Terrae (LS), ANID-FONDECYT-Postdoctorado [3201028] (KT).

Conflicts of Interest: The authors declare no conflicts of interest.

References

1. Machlowska, J.; Baj, J.; Sitarz, M.; Maciejewski, R.; Sitarz, R. Gastric Cancer: Epidemiology, Risk Factors, Classification, Genomic Characteristics and Treatment Strategies. *Int. J. Mol. Sci.* **2020**, *21*, 4012. [CrossRef]
2. Gullo, I.; Grillo, F.; Mastracci, L.; Vanoli, A.; Carneiro, F.; Saragoni, L.; Limarzi, F.; Ferro, J.; Parente, P.; Fassan, M. Precancerous Lesions of the Stomach, Gastric Cancer and Hereditary Gastric Cancer Syndromes. *Pathologica* **2020**, *112*, 166–185. [CrossRef] [PubMed]
3. De Brito, B.B.; da Silva, F.A.F.; Soares, A.S.; Pereira, V.A.; Santos, M.L.C.; Sampaio, M.M.; Neves, P.H.M.; Melo, F.F. de Pathogenesis and Clinical Management of *Helicobacter Pylori* Gastric Infection. *World J. Gastroenterol.* **2019**, *25*, 5578–5589. [CrossRef] [PubMed]
4. Berretta, M.; Bignucolo, A.; Di Francia, R.; Comello, F.; Facchini, G.; Ceccarelli, M.; Iaffaioli, R.V.; Quagliariello, V.; Maurea, N. Resveratrol in Cancer Patients: From Bench to Bedside. *Int. J. Mol. Sci.* **2020**, *21*, 2945. [CrossRef] [PubMed]
5. Rauf, A.; Imran, M.; Butt, M.S.; Nadeem, M.; Peters, D.G.; Mubarak, M.S. Resveratrol as an Anti-Cancer Agent: A Review. *Crit. Rev. Food Sci. Nutr.* **2018**, *58*, 1428–1447. [CrossRef] [PubMed]
6. Zulueta, A. Resveratrol: A Potential Challenger against Gastric Cancer. *World J. Gastroenterol.* **2015**, *21*, 10636. [CrossRef] [PubMed]
7. Ferreira, R.M.; Machado, J.C.; Figueiredo, C. Clinical Relevance of Helicobacter Pylori VacA and CagA Genotypes in Gastric Carcinoma. *Best. Pract. Res. Clin. Gastroenterol.* **2014**, *28*, 1003–1015. [CrossRef] [PubMed]
8. Hooi, J.K.Y.; Lai, W.Y.; Ng, W.K.; Suen, M.M.Y.; Underwood, F.E.; Tanyingoh, D.; Malfertheiner, P.; Graham, D.Y.; Wong, V.W.S.; Wu, J.C.Y.; et al. Global Prevalence of Helicobacter Pylori Infection: Systematic Review and Meta-Analysis. *Gastroenterology* **2017**, *153*, 420–429. [CrossRef] [PubMed]
9. Chen, Y.-C.; Malfertheiner, P.; Yu, H.-T.; Kuo, C.-L.; Chang, Y.-Y.; Meng, F.-T.; Wu, Y.-X.; Hsiao, J.-L.; Chen, M.-J.; Lin, K.-P.; et al. Global Prevalence of Helicobacter Pylori Infection and Incidence of Gastric Cancer Between 1980 and 2022. *Gastroenterology* **2024**, *166*, 605–619. [CrossRef]
10. Piscione, M.; Mazzone, M.; Di Marcantonio, M.C.; Muraro, R.; Mincione, G. Eradication of Helicobacter Pylori and Gastric Cancer: A Controversial Relationship. *Front. Microbiol.* **2021**, *12*, 630852. [CrossRef]
11. Salvatori, S.; Marafini, I.; Laudisi, F.; Monteleone, G.; Stolfi, C. Helicobacter Pylori and Gastric Cancer: Pathogenetic Mechanisms. *Int. J. Mol. Sci.* **2023**, *24*, 2895. [CrossRef] [PubMed]

12. Malespín-Bendaña, W.; Alpízar-Alpízar, W.; Figueroa-Protti, L.; Reyes, L.; Molina-Castro, S.; Une, C.; Ramírez-Mayorga, V. Helicobacter Pylori Infection Induces Gastric Precancerous Lesions and Persistent Expression of Angpt2, Vegf-A and Tnf-A in a Mouse Model. *Front. Oncol.* **2023**, *13*, 1072802. [CrossRef] [PubMed]
13. Sharndama, H.C.; Mba, I.E. Helicobacter Pylori: An up-to-Date Overview on the Virulence and Pathogenesis Mechanisms. *Braz. J. Microbiol.* **2022**, *53*, 33–50. [CrossRef] [PubMed]
14. Ansari, S.; Yamaoka, Y. Helicobacter Pylori Virulence Factors Exploiting Gastric Colonization and Its Pathogenicity. *Toxins* **2019**, *11*, 677. [CrossRef] [PubMed]
15. Wüstner, S.; Anderl, F.; Wanisch, A.; Sachs, C.; Steiger, K.; Nerlich, A.; Vieth, M.; Mejías-Luque, R.; Gerhard, M. Helicobacter Pylori γ-Glutamyl Transferase Contributes to Colonization and Differential Recruitment of T Cells during Persistence. *Sci. Rep.* **2017**, *7*, 13636. [CrossRef] [PubMed]
16. Talebi Bezmin Abadi, A. Strategies Used by *Helicobacter Pylori* to Establish Persistent Infection. *World J. Gastroenterol.* **2017**, *23*, 2870. [CrossRef] [PubMed]
17. Marcus, E.A.; Sachs, G.; Scott, D.R. Acid-regulated Gene Expression of *Helicobacter Pylori*: Insight into Acid Protection and Gastric Colonization. *Helicobacter* **2018**, *23*, e12490. [CrossRef] [PubMed]
18. Takeshita, H.; Watanabe, E.; Norose, Y.; Ito, Y.; Takahashi, H. Neutralizing Antibodies for *Helicobacter pylori* Urease Inhibit Bacterial Colonization in the Murine Stomach In Vivo. *Biomed. Res.* **2019**, *40*, 87–95. [CrossRef] [PubMed]
19. Baj, J.; Forma, A.; Sitarz, M.; Portincasa, P.; Garruti, G.; Krasowska, D.; Maciejewski, R. Helicobacter Pylori Virulence Factors—Mechanisms of Bacterial Pathogenicity in the Gastric Microenvironment. *Cells* **2020**, *10*, 27. [CrossRef]
20. Ferlay, J.; Colombet, M.; Soerjomataram, I.; Parkin, D.M.; Piñeros, M.; Znaor, A.; Bray, F. Cancer Statistics for the Year 2020: An Overview. *Int. J. Cancer* **2021**, *149*, 778–789. [CrossRef]
21. Yang, W.-J.; Zhao, H.-P.; Yu, Y.; Wang, J.-H.; Guo, L.; Liu, J.-Y.; Pu, J.; Lv, J. Updates on Global Epidemiology, Risk and Prognostic Factors of Gastric Cancer. *World J. Gastroenterol.* **2023**, *29*, 2452–2468. [CrossRef] [PubMed]
22. Correa, P. Human Gastric Carcinogenesis: A Multistep and Multifactorial Process--First American Cancer Society Award Lecture on Cancer Epidemiology and Prevention. *Cancer Res.* **1992**, *52*, 6735–6740. [PubMed]
23. Rawla, P.; Barsouk, A. Epidemiology of Gastric Cancer: Global Trends, Risk Factors and Prevention. *Gastroenterol. Rev.* **2019**, *14*, 26–38. [CrossRef] [PubMed]
24. Conti, C.B.; Agnesi, S.; Scaravaglio, M.; Masseria, P.; Dinelli, M.E.; Oldani, M.; Uggeri, F. Early Gastric Cancer: Update on Prevention, Diagnosis and Treatment. *Int. J. Environ. Res. Public Health* **2023**, *20*, 2149. [CrossRef] [PubMed]
25. Ye, S.; Wang, L.; Zuo, Z.; Bei, Y.; Liu, K. The Role of Surgery and Radiation in Advanced Gastric Cancer: A Population-Based Study of Surveillance, Epidemiology, and End Results Database. *PLoS ONE* **2019**, *14*, e0213596. [CrossRef] [PubMed]
26. Cunningham, D.; Allum, W.H.; Stenning, S.P.; Thompson, J.N.; Van de Velde, C.J.H.; Nicolson, M.; Scarffe, J.H.; Lofts, F.J.; Falk, S.J.; Iveson, T.J.; et al. Perioperative Chemotherapy versus Surgery Alone for Resectable Gastroesophageal Cancer. *N. Engl. J. Med.* **2006**, *355*, 11–20. [CrossRef] [PubMed]
27. Wang, Y.; Zhang, L.; Yang, Y.; Lu, S.; Chen, H. Progress of Gastric Cancer Surgery in the Era of Precision Medicine. *Int. J. Biol. Sci.* **2021**, *17*, 1041–1049. [CrossRef] [PubMed]
28. Wagner, A.D.; Syn, N.L.; Moehler, M.; Grothe, W.; Yong, W.P.; Tai, B.-C.; Ho, J.; Unverzagt, S. Chemotherapy for Advanced Gastric Cancer. *Cochrane Database Syst. Rev.* **2017**, *2017*, CD004064. [CrossRef]
29. Li, J.; Qin, S.; Xu, J.; Xiong, J.; Wu, C.; Bai, Y.; Liu, W.; Tong, J.; Liu, Y.; Xu, R.; et al. Randomized, Double-Blind, Placebo-Controlled Phase III Trial of Apatinib in Patients With Chemotherapy-Refractory Advanced or Metastatic Adenocarcinoma of the Stomach or Gastroesophageal Junction. *J. Clin. Oncol.* **2016**, *34*, 1448–1454. [CrossRef] [PubMed]
30. Gou, M.; Zhang, Y.; Wang, Z.; Dai, G. PD-1 Inhibitors-Based Second-Line Therapy for Metastatic Gastric Cancer. *Front. Immunol.* **2023**, *14*, 1136437. [CrossRef]
31. Chong, I.Y.; Chau, I. Is There Still a Place for Radiotherapy in Gastric Cancer? *Curr. Opin. Pharmacol.* **2023**, *68*, 102325. [CrossRef] [PubMed]
32. Kaviani, E.; Hajibabaie, F.; Abedpoor, N.; Safavi, K.; Ahmadi, Z.; Karimy, A. System Biology Analysis to Develop Diagnostic Biomarkers, Monitoring Pathological Indexes, and Novel Therapeutic Approaches for Immune Targeting Based on Maggot Bioactive Compounds and Polyphenolic Cocktails in Mice with Gastric Cancer. *Environ. Res.* **2023**, *238*, 117168. [CrossRef] [PubMed]
33. da Silva, E.C.S.; Bernardo Guerra, G.C.; de Araújo, E.R.D.; Schlamb, J.; da Silva, V.C.; de Aragão Tavares, E.; Dantas-Medeiros, R.; Abreu, L.S.; Fechine Tavares, J.; de Araújo Júnior, R.F.; et al. Phenolic-Rich Extract of *Nopalea Cochenillifera* Attenuates Gastric Lesions Induced in Experimental Models through Inhibiting Oxidative Stress, Modulating Inflammatory Markers and a Cytoprotective Effect. *Food Funct.* **2023**, *14*, 3242–3258. [CrossRef] [PubMed]
34. Gunes-Bayir, A.; Guler, E.M.; Bilgin, M.G.; Ergun, I.S.; Kocyigit, A.; Dadak, A. Anti-Inflammatory and Antioxidant Effects of Carvacrol on N-Methyl-N′-Nitro-N-Nitrosoguanidine (MNNG) Induced Gastric Carcinogenesis in Wistar Rats. *Nutrients* **2022**, *14*, 2848. [CrossRef]
35. Piazza, S.; Martinelli, G.; Fumagalli, M.; Pozzoli, C.; Maranta, N.; Giavarini, F.; Colombo, L.; Nicotra, G.; Vicentini, S.F.; Genova, F.; et al. Ellagitannins from Castanea Sativa Mill. Leaf Extracts Impair H. Pylori Viability and Infection-Induced Inflammation in Human Gastric Epithelial Cells. *Nutrients* **2023**, *15*, 1504. [CrossRef]

36. Martinelli, G.; Fumagalli, M.; Pozzoli, C.; Nicotra, G.; Vicentini, S.F.; Maranta, N.; Sangiovanni, E.; Dell'Agli, M.; Piazza, S. Exploring In Vitro the Combination of Cistus × Incanus L. and Castanea Sativa Mill. Extracts as Food Supplement Ingredients against H. Pylori Infection. *Foods* **2023**, *13*, 40. [CrossRef] [PubMed]
37. Cho, K.; Lee, H.G.; Piao, J.-Y.; Kim, S.-J.; Na, H.-K.; Surh, Y.-J. Protective Effects of Silibinin on *Helicobacter Pylori* -Induced Gastritis: NF-KB and STAT3 as Potential Targets. *J. Cancer Prev.* **2021**, *26*, 118–127. [CrossRef] [PubMed]
38. Park, J.M.; An, J.M.; Han, Y.M.; Surh, Y.J.; Hwang, S.J.; Kim, S.J.; Hahm, K.B. Walnut Polyphenol Extracts Inhibit Helicobacter Pylori-Induced STAT3;Tyr705 Phosphorylation through Activation of PPAR-γ and SOCS1 Induction. *J. Clin. Biochem. Nutr.* **2020**, *67*, 248–256. [CrossRef] [PubMed]
39. Meng, T.; Xiao, D.; Muhammed, A.; Deng, J.; Chen, L.; He, J. Anti-Inflammatory Action and Mechanisms of Resveratrol. *Molecules* **2021**, *26*, 229. [CrossRef]
40. Ren, B.; Kwah, M.X.-Y.; Liu, C.; Ma, Z.; Shanmugam, M.K.; Ding, L.; Xiang, X.; Ho, P.C.-L.; Wang, L.; Ong, P.S.; et al. Resveratrol for Cancer Therapy: Challenges and Future Perspectives. *Cancer Lett.* **2021**, *515*, 63–72. [CrossRef]
41. Almeida, T.C.; Seibert, J.B.; de Almeida, S.H.S.; Amparo, T.R.; de Teixeira, L.F.M.; Barichello, J.M.; Postacchini, B.B.; dos Santos, O.D.H.; da Silva, G.N. Polymeric Micelles Containing Resveratrol: Development, Characterization, Cytotoxicity on Tumor Cells and Antimicrobial Activity. *Braz. J. Pharm. Sci.* **2020**, *56*, e18411. [CrossRef]
42. Ahmadi, R.; Ebrahimzadeh, M.A. Resveratrol—A Comprehensive Review of Recent Advances in Anticancer Drug Design and Development. *Eur. J. Med. Chem.* **2020**, *200*, 112356. [CrossRef]
43. Cai, H.; Scott, E.N.; Britton, R.G.; Parrott, E.; Ognibene, T.J.; Malfatti, M.; Khan, M.; Steward, W.P.; Brown, K. Distribution and Metabolism of [14C]-Resveratrol in Human Prostate Tissue after Oral Administration of a "Dietary-Achievable" or "Pharmacological" Dose: What Are the Implications for Anticancer Activity? *Am. J. Clin. Nutr.* **2021**, *113*, 1115–1125. [CrossRef] [PubMed]
44. Ishida, T.; Takeda, T.; Koga, T.; Yahata, M.; Ike, A.; Kuramoto, C.; Taketoh, J.; Hashiguchi, I.; Akamine, A.; Ishii, Y.; et al. Attenuation of 2,3,7,8-Tetrachlorodibenzo-p-Dioxin Toxicity by Resveratrol: A Comparative Study with Different Routes of Administration. *Biol. Pharm. Bull.* **2009**, *32*, 876–881. [CrossRef] [PubMed]
45. Iannitti, R.G.; Floridi, A.; Lazzarini, A.; Tantucci, A.; Russo, R.; Ragonese, F.; Monarca, L.; Caglioti, C.; Spogli, R.; Leonardi, L.; et al. Resveratrol Supported on Magnesium DiHydroxide (Resv@MDH) Represents an Oral Formulation of Resveratrol With Better Gastric Absorption and Bioavailability Respect to Pure Resveratrol. *Front. Nutr.* **2020**, *7*, 570047. [CrossRef] [PubMed]
46. Wei, Y.; Yang, S.; Zhang, L.; Dai, L.; Tai, K.; Liu, J.; Mao, L.; Yuan, F.; Gao, Y.; Mackie, A. Fabrication, Characterization and in Vitro Digestion of Food Grade Complex Nanoparticles for Co-Delivery of Resveratrol and Coenzyme Q10. *Food Hydrocoll.* **2020**, *105*, 105791. [CrossRef]
47. Huang, X.; Liu, Y.; Zou, Y.; Liang, X.; Peng, Y.; McClements, D.J.; Hu, K. Encapsulation of Resveratrol in Zein/Pectin Core-Shell Nanoparticles: Stability, Bioaccessibility, and Antioxidant Capacity after Simulated Gastrointestinal Digestion. *Food Hydrocoll.* **2019**, *93*, 261–269. [CrossRef]
48. Zhang, J.; Zhang, X.; Wang, Q.; Wu, C. Changes of Physicochemical Properties and Bioactivities of Resveratrol-Loaded Core-Shell Biopolymer Nanoparticles during in Vitro Gastrointestinal Digestion. *Food Chem.* **2023**, *424*, 136444. [CrossRef]
49. Rostami, M.; Ghorbani, M.; Aman Mohammadi, M.; Delavar, M.; Tabibiazar, M.; Ramezani, S. Development of Resveratrol Loaded Chitosan-Gellan Nanofiber as a Novel Gastrointestinal Delivery System. *Int. J. Biol. Macromol.* **2019**, *135*, 698–705. [CrossRef]
50. Issarachot, O.; Bunlung, S.; Kaewkroek, K.; Wiwattanapatapee, R. Superporous Hydrogels Based on Blends of Chitosan and Polyvinyl Alcohol as a Carrier for Enhanced Gastric Delivery of Resveratrol. *Saudi Pharm. J.* **2023**, *31*, 335–347. [CrossRef]
51. Boontawee, R.; Issarachot, O.; Kaewkroek, K.; Wiwattanapatapee, R. Foldable/Expandable Gastro-Retentive Films Based on Starch and Chitosan as a Carrier For Prolonged Release of Resveratrol. *Curr. Pharm. Biotechnol.* **2022**, *23*, 1009–1018. [CrossRef]
52. Aggarwal, B.B.; Bhardwaj, A.; Aggarwal, R.S.; Seeram, N.P.; Shishodia, S.; Takada, Y. Role of Resveratrol in Prevention and Therapy of Cancer: Preclinical and Clinical Studies. *Anticancer. Res.* **2004**, *24*, 2783. [PubMed]
53. Ko, J.-H.; Sethi, G.; Um, J.-Y.; Shanmugam, M.K.; Arfuso, F.; Kumar, A.P.; Bishayee, A.; Ahn, K.S. The Role of Resveratrol in Cancer Therapy. *Int. J. Mol. Sci.* **2017**, *18*, 2589. [CrossRef] [PubMed]
54. Leonard, S.S.; Xia, C.; Jiang, B.-H.; Stinefelt, B.; Klandorf, H.; Harris, G.K.; Shi, X. Resveratrol Scavenges Reactive Oxygen Species and Effects Radical-Induced Cellular Responses. *Biochem. Biophys. Res. Commun.* **2003**, *309*, 1017–1026. [CrossRef] [PubMed]
55. Li, C.; Xu, X.; Tao, Z.; Wang, X.J.; Pan, Y. Resveratrol Dimers, Nutritional Components in Grape Wine, Are Selective ROS Scavengers and Weak Nrf2 Activators. *Food Chem.* **2015**, *173*, 218–223. [CrossRef] [PubMed]
56. Zhang, X.; Jiang, A.; Qi, B.; Ma, Z.; Xiong, Y.; Dou, J.; Wang, J. Resveratrol Protects against Helicobacter Pylori-Associated Gastritis by Combating Oxidative Stress. *Int. J. Mol. Sci.* **2015**, *16*, 27757–27769. [CrossRef] [PubMed]
57. Zaidi, S.F.H.; Ahmed, K.; Yamamoto, T.; Kondo, T.; Usmanghani, K.; Kadowaki, M.; Sugiyama, T. Effect of Resveratrol on Helicobacter Pylori-Induced Interleukin-8 Secretion, Reactive Oxygen Species Generation and Morphological Changes in Human Gastric Epithelial Cells. *Biol. Pharm. Bull.* **2009**, *32*, 1931–1935. [CrossRef] [PubMed]
58. Di Fermo, P.; Di Lodovico, S.; Amoroso, R.; De Filippis, B.; D'Ercole, S.; Di Campli, E.; Cellini, L.; Di Giulio, M. Searching for New Tools to Counteract the Helicobacter Pylori Resistance: The Positive Action of Resveratrol Derivatives. *Antibiotics* **2020**, *9*, 891. [CrossRef] [PubMed]

59. Spósito, L.; Fonseca, D.; Gonçalves Carvalho, S.; Sábio, R.M.; Marena, G.D.; Bauab, T.M.; Bagliotti Meneguin, A.; Parreira, P.L.; Martins, M.C.; Chorilli, M. Engineering Resveratrol-Loaded Chitosan Nanoparticles for Potential Use against Helicobacter Pylori Infection. *Eur. J. Pharm. Biopharm.* **2024**, *199*, 114280. [CrossRef]
60. Yang, Q.; Wang, B.; Zang, W.; Wang, X.; Liu, Z.; Li, W.; Jia, J. Resveratrol Inhibits the Growth of Gastric Cancer by Inducing G1 Phase Arrest and Senescence in a Sirt1-Dependent Manner. *PLoS ONE* **2013**, *8*, e70627. [CrossRef]
61. Yang, Z.; Xie, Q.; Chen, Z.; Ni, H.; Xia, L.; Zhao, Q.; Chen, Z.; Chen, P. Resveratrol Suppresses the Invasion and Migration of Human Gastric Cancer Cells via Inhibition of MALAT1-mediated Epithelial-to-mesenchymal Transition. *Exp. Ther. Med.* **2018**, *17*, 1569–1578. [CrossRef] [PubMed]
62. Song, B.; Wang, W.; Tang, X.; Goh, R.M.W.-J.; Thuya, W.L.; Ho, P.C.L.; Chen, L.; Wang, L. Inhibitory Potential of Resveratrol in Cancer Metastasis: From Biology to Therapy. *Cancers* **2023**, *15*, 2758. [CrossRef] [PubMed]
63. Hu, W.-H.; Chan, G.K.-L.; Duan, R.; Wang, H.-Y.; Kong, X.-P.; Dong, T.T.-X.; Tsim, K.W.-K. Synergy of Ginkgetin and Resveratrol in Suppressing VEGF-Induced Angiogenesis: A Therapy in Treating Colorectal Cancer. *Cancers* **2019**, *11*, 1828. [CrossRef] [PubMed]
64. Wang, Z.; Dabrosin, C.; Yin, X.; Fuster, M.M.; Arreola, A.; Rathmell, W.K.; Generali, D.; Nagaraju, G.P.; El-Rayes, B.; Ribatti, D.; et al. Broad Targeting of Angiogenesis for Cancer Prevention and Therapy. *Semin. Cancer Biol.* **2015**, *35*, S224–S243. [CrossRef]
65. Ashrafizadeh, M.; Rafiei, H.; Mohammadinejad, R.; Farkhondeh, T.; Samarghandian, S. Anti-Tumor Activity of Resveratrol against Gastric Cancer: A Review of Recent Advances with an Emphasis on Molecular Pathways. *Cancer Cell Int.* **2021**, *21*, 66. [CrossRef] [PubMed]
66. Atten, M.J.; Attar, B.M.; Milson, T.; Holian, O. Resveratrol-Induced Inactivation of Human Gastric Adenocarcinoma Cells through a Protein Kinase C-Mediated Mechanism. *Biochem. Pharmacol.* **2001**, *62*, 1423–1432. [CrossRef]
67. Atten, M.J.; Godoy-Romero, E.; Attar, B.M.; Milson, T.; Zopel, M.; Holian, O. Resveratrol Regulates Cellular PKC α and δ to Inhibit Growth and Induce Apoptosis in Gastric Cancer Cells. *Invest. New Drugs* **2005**, *23*, 111–119. [CrossRef] [PubMed]
68. Shin, K.-O.; Park, N.-Y.; Seo, C.-H.; Hong, S.-P.; Oh, K.-W.; Hong, J.-T.; Han, S.-K.; Lee, Y.-M. Inhibition of Sphingolipid Metabolism Enhances Resveratrol Chemotherapy in Human Gastric Cancer Cells. *Biomol. Ther.* **2012**, *20*, 470–476. [CrossRef]
69. Wang, Z.; Li, W.; Meng, X.; Jia, B. Resveratrol Induces Gastric Cancer Cell Apoptosis via Reactive Oxygen Species, but Independent of Sirtuin1. *Clin. Exp. Pharmacol. Physiol.* **2012**, *39*, 227–232. [CrossRef]
70. Wu, X.; Xu, Y.; Zhu, B.; Liu, Q.; Yao, Q.; Zhao, G. Resveratrol Induces Apoptosis in SGC-7901 Gastric Cancer Cells. *Oncol. Lett.* **2018**, *16*, 2949–2956. [CrossRef]
71. Rojo, D.; Madrid, A.; Martín, S.S.; Párraga, M.; Silva Pinhal, M.A.; Villena, J.; Valenzuela-Valderrama, M. Resveratrol Decreases the Invasion Potential of Gastric Cancer Cells. *Molecules* **2022**, *27*, 3047. [CrossRef] [PubMed]
72. Gao, Q.; Yuan, Y.; Gan, H.-Z.; Peng, Q. Resveratrol Inhibits the Hedgehog Signaling Pathway and Epithelial-Mesenchymal Transition and Suppresses Gastric Cancer Invasion and Metastasis. *Oncol. Lett.* **2015**, *9*, 2381–2387. [CrossRef] [PubMed]
73. Yin, L.; Zhang, R.; Hu, Y.; Li, W.; Wang, M.; Liang, Z.; Sun, Z.; Ji, R.; Xu, W.; Qian, H. Gastric-Cancer-Derived Mesenchymal Stem Cells: A Promising Target for Resveratrol in the Suppression of Gastric Cancer Metastasis. *Hum. Cell* **2020**, *33*, 652–662. [CrossRef] [PubMed]
74. Xu, Q.-H.; Xiao, Y.; Li, X.-Q.; Fan, L.; Zhou, C.-C.; Cheng, L.; Jiang, Z.-D.; Wang, G.-H. Resveratrol Counteracts Hypoxia-Induced Gastric Cancer Invasion and EMT through Hedgehog Pathway Suppression. *Anticancer Agents Med. Chem.* **2020**, *20*, 1105–1114. [CrossRef] [PubMed]
75. Su, N.; Li, L.; Zhou, E.; Li, H.; Wu, S.; Cao, Z. Resveratrol Downregulates MiR-155-5p to Block the Malignant Behavior of Gastric Cancer Cells. *Biomed. Res. Int.* **2022**, *2022*, 1–10. [CrossRef] [PubMed]
76. Yang, Z.; Xia, L. Resveratrol Inhibits the Proliferation, Invasion, and Migration, and Induces the Apoptosis of Human Gastric Cancer Cells through the MALAT1/MiR-383-5p/DDIT4 Signaling Pathway. *J. Gastrointest. Oncol.* **2022**, *13*, 985–996. [CrossRef] [PubMed]
77. Liu, H.; Zhang, X.; Fang, C.; Li, S. Resveratrol Induces the Growth Inhibition of CDX-Deficient Gastric Cancer Cells Using CDX2 and RUNX3 via the β-Catenin/TCF4 Signaling Pathway. *Transl. Oncol.* **2023**, *35*, 101727. [CrossRef] [PubMed]
78. Yang, T.; Zhang, J.; Zhou, J.; Zhu, M.; Wang, L.; Yan, L. Resveratrol Inhibits Interleukin-6 Induced Invasion of Human Gastric Cancer Cells. *Biomed. Pharmacother.* **2018**, *99*, 766–773. [CrossRef]
79. Li, T.; Zhang, X.; Cheng, L.; Li, C.; Wu, Z.; Luo, Y.; Zhou, K.; Li, Y.; Zhao, Q.; Huang, Y. Modulation of LncRNA H19 Enhances Resveratrol-inhibited Cancer Cell Proliferation and Migration by Regulating Endoplasmic Reticulum Stress. *J. Cell Mol. Med.* **2022**, *26*, 2205–2217. [CrossRef]
80. Lu, W.; Ni, Z.; Jiang, S.; Tong, M.; Zhang, J.; Zhao, J.; Feng, C.; Jia, Q.; Wang, J.; Yao, T.; et al. Resveratrol Inhibits Bile Acid-induced Gastric Intestinal Metaplasia via the PI3K/AKT/p-FoxO4 Signalling Pathway. *Phytother. Res.* **2021**, *35*, 1495–1507. [CrossRef]
81. Lin, M.; Yao, W.; Xiao, Y.; Dong, Z.; Huang, W.; Zhang, F.; Zhou, X.; Liang, M. Resveratrol-Modified Mesoporous Silica Nanoparticle for Tumor-Targeted Therapy of Gastric Cancer. *Bioengineered* **2021**, *12*, 6343–6353. [CrossRef]
82. Tomikoshi, Y.; Nomura, M.; Okudaira, N.; Sakagami, H.; Wakabayashi, H. Enhancement of Cytotoxicity of Three Apoptosis-Inducing Agents Against Human Oral Squamous Cell Carcinoma Cell Line by Benzoxazinotropone. *In Vivo* **2016**, *30*, 645–650.
83. Jin, X.; Wei, Y.; Liu, Y.; Lu, X.; Ding, F.; Wang, J.; Yang, S. Resveratrol Promotes Sensitization to Doxorubicin by Inhibiting Epithelial-mesenchymal Transition and Modulating SIRT1/B-catenin Signaling Pathway in Breast Cancer. *Cancer Med.* **2019**, *8*, 1246–1257. [CrossRef] [PubMed]

84. Xu, J.; Liu, D.; Niu, H.; Zhu, G.; Xu, Y.; Ye, D.; Li, J.; Zhang, Q. Resveratrol Reverses Doxorubicin Resistance by Inhibiting Epithelial-Mesenchymal Transition (EMT) through Modulating PTEN/Akt Signaling Pathway in Gastric Cancer. *J. Exp. Clin. Cancer Res.* **2017**, *36*, 19. [CrossRef] [PubMed]
85. Abdel-Latif, G.A.; Al-Abd, A.M.; Tadros, M.G.; Al-Abbasi, F.A.; Khalifa, A.E.; Abdel-Naim, A.B. The Chemomodulatory Effects of Resveratrol and Didox on Herceptin Cytotoxicity in Breast Cancer Cell Lines. *Sci. Rep.* **2015**, *5*, 12054. [CrossRef] [PubMed]
86. Kong, F.; Zhang, R.; Zhao, X.; Zheng, G.; Wang, Z.; Wang, P. Resveratrol Raises in Vitro Anticancer Effects of Paclitaxel in NSCLC Cell Line A549 through COX-2 Expression. *Korean J. Physiol. Pharmacol.* **2017**, *21*, 465. [CrossRef] [PubMed]
87. Türkmen, N.B.; Yüce, H.; Şahin, Y.; Taşlıdere, A.Ç.; Özek, D.A.; Ünüvar, S.; Çiftçi, O. Protective Effect of Resveratrol against Pembrolizumab-induced Hepatotoxicity and Neurotoxicity in Male Rats. *J. Biochem. Mol. Toxicol.* **2023**, *37*, e23263. [CrossRef] [PubMed]
88. Ostwal, V.; Ramaswamy, A.; Bhargava, P.; Srinivas, S.; Mandavkar, S.; Chaugule, D.; Peelay, Z.; Baheti, A.; Tandel, H.; Jadhav, V.K.; et al. A Pro-Oxidant Combination of Resveratrol and Copper Reduces Chemotherapy-Related Non-Haematological Toxicities in Advanced Gastric Cancer: Results of a Prospective Open Label Phase II Single-Arm Study (RESCU III Study). *Med. Oncol.* **2022**, *40*, 17. [CrossRef] [PubMed]
89. Rahimifard, M.; Baeeri, M.; Mousavi, T.; Azarnezhad, A.; Haghi-Aminjan, H.; Abdollahi, M. Combination Therapy of Cisplatin and Resveratrol to Induce Cellular Aging in Gastric Cancer Cells: Focusing on Oxidative Stress, and Cell Cycle Arrest. *Front. Pharmacol.* **2023**, *13*, 1068863. [CrossRef]
90. Ren, M.; Zhou, X.; Gu, M.; Jiao, W.; Yu, M.; Wang, Y.; Liu, S.; Yang, J.; Ji, F. Resveratrol Synergizes with Cisplatin in Antineoplastic Effects against AGS Gastric Cancer Cells by Inducing Endoplasmic Reticulum Stress-mediated Apoptosis and G2/M Phase Arrest. *Oncol. Rep.* **2020**, *44*, 1605–1615. [CrossRef]
91. Qin, H.; Zhang, H.; Zhang, X.; Zhang, S.; Zhu, S.; Wang, H. Resveratrol Attenuates Radiation Enteritis through the SIRT1/FOXO3a and PI3K/AKT Signaling Pathways. *Biochem. Biophys. Res. Commun.* **2021**, *554*, 199–205. [CrossRef]
92. Wang, L.; Long, L.; Wang, W.; Liang, Z. Resveratrol, a Potential Radiation Sensitizer for Glioma Stem Cells Both in Vitro and in Vivo. *J. Pharmacol. Sci.* **2015**, *129*, 216–225. [CrossRef] [PubMed]
93. Wang, Z.; Zhang, L.; Ni, Z.; Sun, J.; Gao, H.; Cheng, Z.; Xu, J.; Yin, P. Resveratrol Induces AMPK-Dependent MDR1 Inhibition in Colorectal Cancer HCT116/L-OHP Cells by Preventing Activation of NF-KB Signaling and Suppressing CAMP-Responsive Element Transcriptional Activity. *Tumor Biol.* **2015**, *36*, 9499–9510. [CrossRef] [PubMed]
94. Juan, M.E.; Alfaras, I.; Planas, J.M. Colorectal Cancer Chemoprevention by Trans-Resveratrol. *Pharmacol. Res.* **2012**, *65*, 584–591. [CrossRef] [PubMed]
95. Song, L.; Liu, H.; Ma, L.; Zhang, X.; Jiang, Z.; Jiang, C. Inhibition of Autophagy by 3-MA Enhances Endoplasmic Reticulum Stress-Induced Apoptosis in Human Nasopharyngeal Carcinoma Cells. *Oncol. Lett.* **2013**, *6*, 1031–1038. [CrossRef]
96. Pan, J.; Shen, J.; Si, W.; Du, C.; Chen, D.; Xu, L.; Yao, M.; Fu, P.; Fan, W. Resveratrol Promotes MICA/B Expression and Natural Killer Cell Lysis of Breast Cancer Cells by Suppressing c-Myc/MiR-17 Pathway. *Oncotarget* **2017**, *8*, 65743–65758. [CrossRef]

nutrients

MDPI

Systematic Review

Carotenoids Intake and Cardiovascular Prevention: A Systematic Review

Sandra Sumalla-Cano [1,2,3,*], Imanol Eguren-García [1], Álvaro Lasarte-García [1], Thomas A. Prola [4], Raquel Martínez-Díaz [1,2,3] and Iñaki Elío [1,5,6,*]

1 Research Group on Foods, Nutritional Biochemistry and Health, Universidad Europea del Atlántico, 39011 Santander, Spain; imanol.eguren@uneatlantico.es (I.E.-G.); alvaro.lasarte@alumnos.uneatlantico.es (Á.L.-G.); raquel.martinez@uneatlantico.es (R.M.-D.)
2 Faculty of Health Sciences, Universidade do Cuanza, Cuito EN250, Bié, Angola
3 Faculty of Health Sciences, Universidad de La Romana, La Romana 22000, Dominican Republic
4 Faculty of Social Sciences and Humanities, European University of the Atlantic, 39011 Santander, Spain; thomas.prola@uneatlantico.es
5 Faculty of Health Sciences, Universidad Internacional Iberoamericana, Arecibo, PR 00613, USA
6 Department of Health, Nutrition and Sport, Universidad Internacional Iberoamericana, Campeche 24560, Mexico
* Correspondence: sandra.sumalla@uneatlantico.es (S.S.-C.); inaki.elio@uneatlantico.es (I.E.)

Abstract: Background: Cardiovascular diseases (CVDs) encompass a variety of conditions that affect the heart and blood vessels. Carotenoids, a group of fat-soluble organic pigments synthesized by plants, fungi, algae, and some bacteria, may have a beneficial effect in reducing cardiovascular disease (CVD) risk. This study aims to examine and synthesize current research on the relationship between carotenoids and CVDs. **Methods:** A systematic review was conducted using MEDLINE and the Cochrane Library to identify relevant studies on the efficacy of carotenoid supplementation for CVD prevention. Interventional analytical studies (randomized and non-randomized clinical trials) published in English from January 2011 to February 2024 were included. **Results:** A total of 38 studies were included in the qualitative analysis. Of these, 17 epidemiological studies assessed the relationship between carotenoids and CVDs, 9 examined the effect of carotenoid supplementation, and 12 evaluated dietary interventions. **Conclusions:** Elevated serum carotenoid levels are associated with reduced CVD risk factors and inflammatory markers. Increasing the consumption of carotenoid-rich foods appears to be more effective than supplementation, though the specific effects of individual carotenoids on CVD risk remain uncertain.

Keywords: cardiovascular diseases (CVDs); carotenoids; systematic review; supplementation; inflammation; prevention

1. Introduction

Coronary artery disease (CAD), which includes angina, myocardial infarction, and heart failure; cerebrovascular disease, which includes stroke and transient ischemic attacks; peripheral arterial disease; and aortic atherosclerosis are the four primary categories of cardiovascular diseases (CVDs). These diseases encompass a range of conditions affecting the heart or blood vessels [1]. Despite advances in prevention and treatment, CVDs remain one of the leading causes of early mortality worldwide, with a 21.1% increase in prevalence observed between 2007 and 2017 [2].

Risk factors for CVDs are divided into non-modifiable and modifiable categories. Non-modifiable risk factors include age (over 55 years), male sex, ethnic origin, family history, and genetic markers [3]. Modifiable risk factors can be further classified as lifestyle factors and metabolic risk factors. Lifestyle factors include inadequate diet, smoking, sedentary behavior, alcohol intake, poor mental health, psychosocial stress, low socioeconomic status, and exposure to environmental toxins. Metabolic risk factors include abnormal blood lipid levels (total cholesterol, triglycerides, high-density lipoprotein, low-density lipoprotein), homocysteine, troponin T, inflammatory markers (C-reactive protein, IL-1, IL-6, IL-18, TNF-α, vascular and cellular adhesion molecules), and high blood pressure (BP), among others, as well as the presence of other conditions such as being overweight, obesity, diabetes, and hypertension [4]. Approximately 50% of CVDs are attributable to modifiable risk factors [5].

The complex relationship between diet and cardiovascular health has become a central focus in preventive medicine. Higher consumption of fruits and vegetables may reduce the risk of CVDs, lower BP, decrease pro-inflammatory markers, and improve insulin resistance, according to epidemiological studies [6]. The World Cancer Research Fund recommends consuming at least 400 g/day of a variety of non-starchy vegetables and fruits to prevent non-communicable chronic diseases, including CVDs [7]. Phytochemicals, bioactive compounds in addition to traditional macronutrients, appear to play a role in the cardiovascular protective effects of fruits and vegetables [8]. Among these phytochemicals, carotenoids have attracted significant interest for their potential in reducing cardiovascular disease (CVD) risk [9,10] (Figure 1).

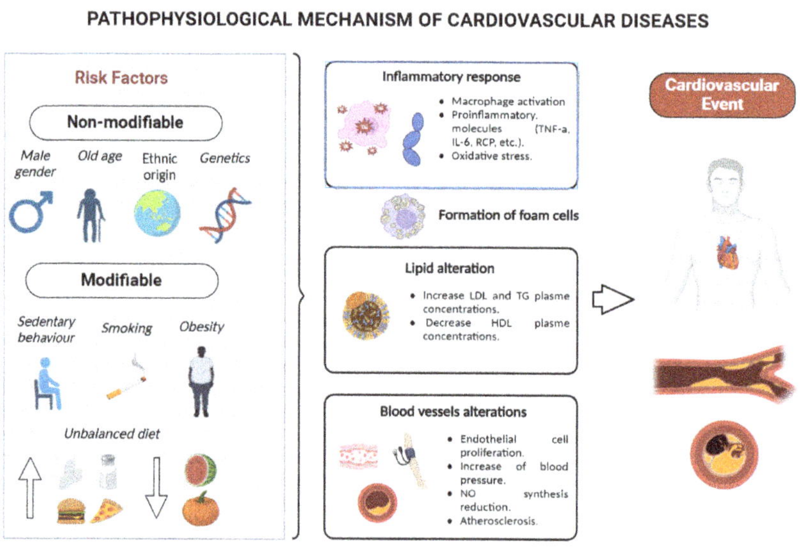

Figure 1. Pathophysiological mechanism of CVDs.

Carotenoids are a group of fat-soluble organic pigments synthesized in the chloroplasts of plants, fungi, algae, and some bacteria from an isopentenyl pyrophosphate molecule. As carotenoids consist of eight repeated isoprene units, they are categorized as isoprenoids [11,12].

Based on molecular composition, carotenoids are classified as either carotenes or xanthophylls. Carotenes are hydrocarbon molecules containing only hydrogen and carbon atoms without functional groups. This group includes lycopene, α-carotene, and β-carotene. In contrast, xanthophylls are hydrocarbons that also contain oxygen, including compounds such as β-cryptoxanthin, lutein, zeaxanthin, violaxanthin, neoxanthin, fucoxanthin, astaxanthin, capsanthin, bixin, and crocin [13].

Some carotenoids, including β-carotene, α-carotene, γ-carotene, and β-cryptoxanthin, serve as vitamin A precursors [11]. Vitamin A and its precursors are involved in vision, development, immunity, and the regulation of glucose and fat metabolism [14].

Humans cannot synthesize carotenoids, so they must be obtained through diet or supplements [15]. In Western diets, the most commonly consumed carotenoids are α-carotene and β-carotene, found in foods such as carrots, pumpkins, and spinach, and lycopene, present in tomatoes and watermelon. Certain animal foods, such as salmon and crustaceans, can also accumulate carotenoids [16] (Figure 2). The number of carotenoids ingested and their presence in blood plasma are established markers of fruit and vegetable intake [17,18].

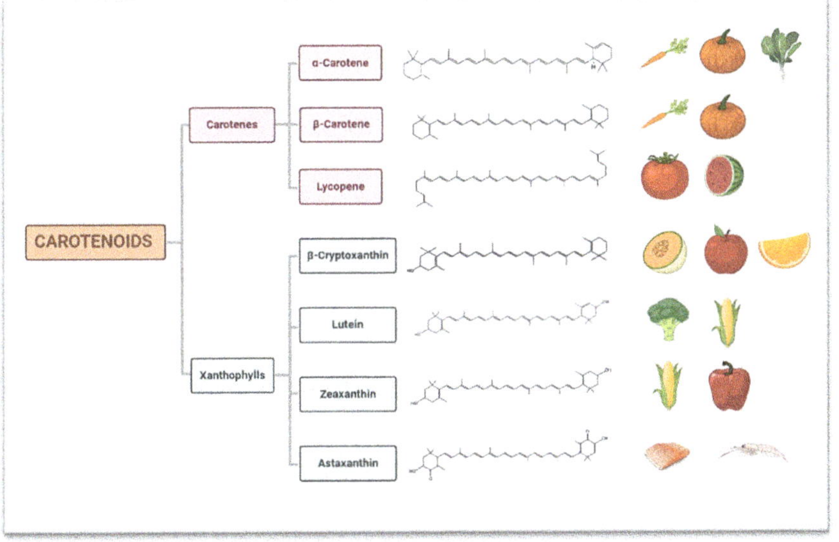

Figure 2. Classification of carotenoids and main sources in Western diet.

It is well known that all carotenoids have strong antioxidant properties that neutralize intracellular reactive oxygen species [19]. By reducing LDL oxidation in cardiovascular tissues, antioxidants contribute to slowing the atherogenesis process. While many carotenoids possess antioxidant qualities, they also improve endothelial function, reduce inflammatory markers, and enhance the lipid profile by mitigating several CVD risk factors through various molecular mechanisms [20].

Lycopene demonstrates anti-inflammatory properties by inhibiting the synthesis of IL-1, IL-6, and TNF-α. It also improves the lipid profile by reducing HDL and triglycerides (TG), inhibits LDL oxidation, and enhances endothelial function while maintaining nitric oxide (NO) levels [21]. Lutein inhibits the transcription of NF-kB and reduces molecules associated with inflammation, such as tumor necrosis factor-alpha (TNF-α), interleukin-6 (IL-6), prostaglandin E2 (PGE-2), monocyte chemoattractant protein-1 (MCP-1), and macrophage inflammatory protein-2 (MIP-2) [22]. It also aids in controlling systolic BP [23].

Recent studies have shown that lutein supplementation lowers some lipid markers, including low-density lipoprotein (LDL), and reduces inflammatory physiological responses. Zeaxanthin regulates the oxidative stress response by lowering oxidized glutathione and increasing intracellular reduced glutathione levels [24]. Higher zeaxanthin levels are also associated with reduced carotid intima-media stiffness (CIMT) [25]. β-carotene decreases LDL oxidation, regulates vascular nitric oxide (NO) bioavailability, lowers nuclear factor kappa-light-chain-enhancer of activated B cells (NF-kB) activation, and reduces the production of pro-inflammatory cytokines, vascular cell adhesion molecule-1 (VCAM-1), intercellular adhesion molecule-1 (ICAM-1), and e-selectin [6].

The objective of this study is to review and synthesize existing literature on the relationship between carotenoids and CVDs. Carotenoids are recognized for their biological activity and antioxidant properties, and they are associated with several physiological processes that influence cardiovascular health. Due to their anti-inflammatory properties and their ability to impact lipid metabolism and endothelial function, carotenoids may offer new avenues for preventing and treating CVDs [26].

This review aims to provide a comprehensive understanding of how carotenoid levels may influence cardiovascular risk factors and promote cardiovascular health by integrating data from epidemiological studies, clinical trials, and mechanistic investigations. By examining the complex relationships between carotenoids and cardiovascular health, this review seeks to provide insights that may inform clinical practice and public health initiatives, paving the way for a more refined approach to managing and preventing cardiovascular disease.

2. Materials and Methods

2.1. Study Design

This article is a systematic review conducted in accordance with the guidelines outlined in the PRISMA statements [27]. The review aims to answer the following research question: Is there evidence that carotenoid intake can prevent CVDs?

2.2. Search Strategy

To identify relevant scientific publications published in English between January 2011 and February 2024, we conducted a comprehensive literature search. A systematic review was performed to gather studies evaluating the effectiveness of carotenoid intake in the prevention of CVDs. The primary databases used in this study were the Cochrane Library and MEDLINE (PubMed).

The search strategy for the MEDLINE database included the following formula: ("carotenoids" OR "carotenoid") AND ("cardiovascular diseases") AND ("human" OR "person") AND ("intervention" OR "study" OR "trial").

In the Cochrane Library, papers in English were searched using the formula: ("carotenoids" OR "carotenoid") AND ("cardiovascular diseases") AND ("human" OR "person") AND ("intervention" OR "study" OR "trial").

2.3. Selection Criteria

Studies involving subjects aged 18 years or older were selected. Epidemiological observational studies, clinical trials, and randomized controlled trials (RCTs) were included in the analysis.

A detailed list of eligibility criteria, developed using the PICOS (Population, Intervention, Comparison, Outcome, Study Design) format, is presented in Table 1.

Table 1. PICOS table for inclusion of studies.

Parameters	Inclusion Criteria
Population	Age 18 years or older
Intervention	Carotenoid intake as CVD prevention
Comparison	Low carotenoids intake
Outcomes	Health and disease markers
Study design	Epidemiological observational studies, clinical trials, and RCTs

2.4. Exclusion Criteria

Clinical recommendations, reviews, protocols, preliminary research, and preclinical investigations were not included. Additionally, gray literature was excluded.

2.5. Classification of Selected Studies

There are several approaches to studying the effect of carotenoids on cardiovascular health. For this review, studies have been grouped into three main categories: (1) studies that examine the relationship between plasma levels of carotenoids and CVD risk;

(2) studies that investigate the effects of oral carotenoid supplementation; and (3) studies that analyze the intake of carotenoids through food or food concentrates. In each case, we assessed the effect of plasma carotenoid levels or carotenoid intake, which are closely related, on CVD markers such as total cholesterol (TC), High-Density Lipoprotein (HDL), LDL, and CIMT values.

3. Results

Study Selection

As shown in the PRISMA diagram (Figure 3), a total of 170 records were identified from the database searches (PubMed and Cochrane Library). After removing 32 duplicate articles, 138 studies were screened, with 81 excluded based on their titles and abstracts. A total of 57 eligible records underwent full-text screening, and 18 studies were excluded for not meeting the inclusion criteria. At the end of the selection process, 38 papers were included in the qualitative analysis. Seventeen epidemiological observational studies evaluated the relationship between carotenoids and CVDs [25,27–42], 9 studies examined the effect of carotenoid supplementation on CVDs [43–51], and 12 studies evaluated dietary interventions [52–63]. Of these, 7 studies provided fruit and vegetable juices [52,56,58–60,62,63], and 5 focused on increasing fruit and vegetable consumption [53–55,57,61].

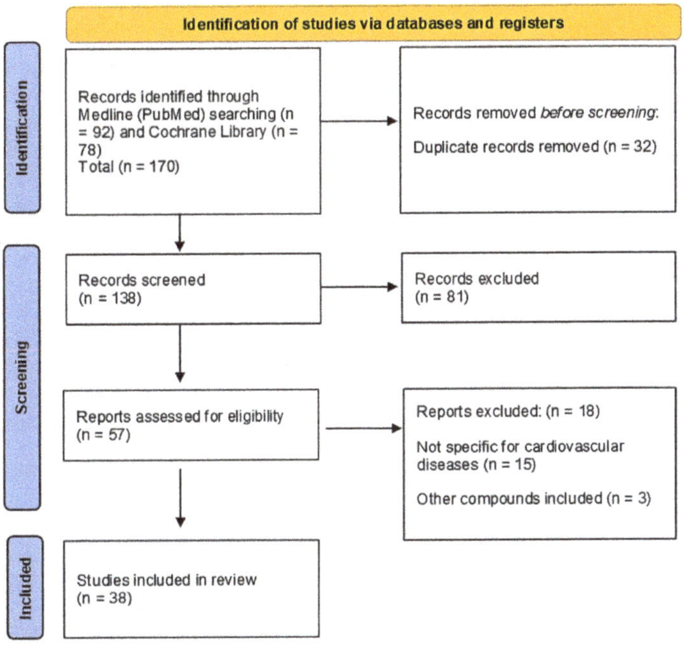

Figure 3. PRISMA flow chart of the systematic review literature search.

The studies included in this review were conducted across various countries, with the highest number performed in the United States (n = 9), followed by the UK (n = 6), China (n = 6), and Spain (n = 3). Two studies were conducted in Finland (n = 2), Israel (n = 2), and Japan (n = 2). Australia (n = 1), Brazil (n = 1), Germany (n = 1), the Netherlands (n = 1), Norway (n = 1), Singapore (n = 1), South Korea (n = 1), and Sweden (n = 1) each contributed one study.

4. Discussion

As previously noted, various fruits and vegetables contain carotenoids, which are among the compounds believed to contribute to the health benefits associated with fruit and vegetable consumption. Carotenoids have potential value in new approaches to preventing and treating CVDs due to their anti-inflammatory properties and their ability to influence lipid metabolism and endothelial function [26]. They are particularly promising as a preventive strategy for CVDs, given their widespread presence in the plant kingdom, offering similar health benefits to those of a plant-based or Mediterranean diet [6]. An increase in plasma carotenoid levels is strongly correlated with carotenoid intake, whether through supplementation or consumption of fruits and vegetables [64], making carotenoid consumption a recognized biomarker of fruit and vegetable intake [17].

4.1. Observational Epidemiological Studies

The 17 observational studies, summarized in Table 2, examine the relationship between serum carotenoid levels and CVD risk. Some studies indicate that high plasma carotenoid levels are associated with a reduction in CVD risk factors [27,29,30,38,39] and improvements in vascular function [25,27,33]. Furthermore, most of the observational studies reviewed [25,27,28,30–41] show that higher plasma carotenoid concentrations, or at least one carotenoid, are linked to a lower risk of developing CVDs, whereas lower carotenoid concentrations are associated with an increased risk [34,35]. Specifically, Prentice RL et al. [31] found that higher levels of α-carotene and β-carotene are associated with lower CVD risk, while lutein and zeaxanthin levels do not appear to affect CVD risk. Huang J, et al. [37] observed a reduced risk of developing CVDs with elevated β-carotene levels. In contrast, Shardell MD, et al. [35] found no association between β-carotene levels and a decreased occurrence of all-cause disease; only higher lycopene levels were related to a lower risk of developing CVDs and all-cause mortality. Matsumoto M. et al. [39] showed that maintaining high blood concentrations of total carotenoids is inversely associated with seven CVD risk biomarkers in men (brachial-ankle pulse wave velocity, systolic BP, diastolic BP, insulin resistance index (HOMA-IR), insulin, and HDL). Zhu X. et al. [40] examined the correlation between serum carotenoids and cardiovascular and all-cause mortality risk and found that lower levels of α-carotene, β-cryptoxanthin, and lycopene were linked to lower cardiovascular mortality, although β-carotene and lutein/zeaxanthin were not. Wang M. et al. [49] reported that the prevalence of CVDs, particularly heart attack and stroke, was inversely correlated with blood levels of lutein/zeaxanthin, α-carotene, lycopene, and β-cryptoxanthin. Lastly, Wang Y. et al. [34] identified a strong negative correlation between homocysteine levels and dietary intake of β-carotene, lycopene, and total carotenoids, as well as an inverse association between LDL serum levels and dietary intake of β-carotene and lutein/zeaxanthin. Additionally, they observed a positive correlation between HDL concentrations and dietary lutein/zeaxanthin intake.

Regarding cardiovascular function, Zou Z. et al. [25] found that lower serum lutein levels were associated with a higher CIMT, while lower levels of zeaxanthin and β-carotene were linked to increased stiffness in the right common carotid artery. Wang C. et al. [33] observed an inverse, dose-dependent association between serum carotenoid concentrations and mean CIMT. Among the carotenoids studied, β-carotene showed the strongest association, followed by total carotenoids, lutein/zeaxanthin, α-carotene, and β-cryptoxanthin, with lycopene exhibiting the weakest association. Huang Y. et al. [27] found that serum levels of α-carotene, all-trans-β-carotene, and lycopene were independently associated with higher heart rate variability (HRV).

One study [36] that examined the relationship between blood carotenoids and IL-6 levels, an inflammatory marker in patients with CAD, found that only lutein/zeaxanthin showed an inverse correlation with IL-6 in individuals with stable angina. The other carotenoids included in the study showed no correlation with lutein/zeaxanthin.

Table 2. Observational studies about carotenoids and CVDs.

Author, Publication Year	Country/Region	Type of Study/ Study Name	Follow-Up Period	Study Size	Carotenoids Evaluated	Findings
Wang, L. et al., 2008 [29]	USA	Case-control studies/Women's Health Study	1 year and 6 months	39,876	α-carotene, β-carotene, β-cryptoxanthin, lycopene, and lutein/zeaxanthin	Association of ↑ α-carotene, β-carotene, and lycopene with ↑ LDL. ↓ lycopene with ↑ of HDL and ↑ of HbA1c. ↓ β-carotene with ↑ of CRP.
Hozawa, A. et al., 2009 [30]	USA	Prospective, multicentre epidemiologic study/ Coronary Artery Risk Development in Young Adults Study	20 years	4412	α-carotene, β-carotene, lutein/zeaxanthin, cryptoxanthin, lycopene	Sum of 4 carotenoids was significantly inversely associated with HT. Lycopene was unrelated to HT in any model.
Prentice, RL. et al., 2019 [31]	USA	Randomized controlled Clinical Trial/Nutrition and Physical Activity Assessment Study	5 years	5488	α- and β-carotene, lutein + zeaxanthin (L+Z), and α-tocopherol	↑ levels of α-carotene, β-carotene with ↓ risk of CVDs. ↑ levels of L+Z shown not to affect CVDs.
Matos, A. et al., 2018 [32]	Brazil	Cross-sectional observational study	1 year	90	β-carotene	β-carotene diminished as the extent score rose of CAD, although this was not statistically significant.
Zou, Z. et al., 2011 [25]	China	Case-control study	Baseline	125	Lutein, zeaxanthin, β-carotene and lycopene	↓ levels serum lutein with ↑ CIMT. ↓ levels serum Zeaxanthina and β-carotene with ↑ carotid artery stiffness.
Wang, C. et al., 2018 [33]	China	Cross-sectional study/ Guangzhou Nutrition and Health Study	Baseline	2947	α-carotene, β-carotene, lutein + zeaxanthin, β-cryptoxanthin and lycopene	↑ carotenoid levels in diet and serum are associated with lower carotid CIMT values
Huang, Y. et al., 2021 [27]	USA	Cross-sectional analysis/Midlife in the United States	Baseline	1074	Lutein, zeaxanthin, β-cryptoxanthin, 13-cis-β-carotene, α-carotene, all-trans-β-carotene and lycopene	Blood α-carotene, all-trans-β-carotene and lycopene levels were independently associated with higher HRV, reducing the risk of CVDs.
Karppi, J. et al., 2012 [34]	Finland	Prospective cohort study/Kuopio Ischaemic Heart Disease Risk Factor	15.9-year follow-up	1031	Lycopene, α-carotene, β-carotene	Low serum concentrations of β-carotene were strongly related to an increased CVDs mortality risk after adjustment for confounders.
Shardell, D. et al., 2011 [35]	USA	Observational study, NHANES III	14.3 years	13,293	α-carotene, β-carotene, β-cryptoxanthin, lycopene, and lutein + zeaxanthin	Low α-carotene was associated with ↑ CVDs mortality. Very low serum of total carotenoid, α-carotene, and lycopene concentrations may be risk factors for mortality.
Chung, RWS. et al., 2017 [36]	Sweden	Cross-sectional and longitudinal study	3 months	193	Lutein + zeaxanthin, β-cryptoxanthin, lycopene, α- and β-carotene and IL-6	Inverse association between lutein and IL-6 in CAD patients.
Huang, J. et al., 2018 [37]	Finland	Prospective Cohort Study	5–8 years between 1985 and 1988	29,133	β-carotene	Higher β-carotene biochemical status is associated with lower overall CVDs, heart disease, stroke, and other causes of mortality.
Toh, DWK. et al., 2021 [38]	Singapore	Cross-sectional study	13 months	108	β-carotene, α-carotene, lycopene, lutein, zeaxanthin and β-cryptoxanthin	Skin carotenoids and plasma carotenoids were inversely associated with systolic BP and diastolic BP.
Matsumoto, M. et al., 2020 [39]	Japan	Resident-based cross-sectional study	Baseline	1350	Lutein, zeaxanthin, β-cryptoxanthin, α-carotene, β-carotene, and lycopene	Higher concentration of serum carotenoids in relatively healthy individuals was associated with better CVD markers.

Table 2. *Cont.*

Author, Publication Year	Country/Region	Type of Study/ Study Name	Follow-Up Period	Study Size	Carotenoids Evaluated	Findings
Zhu, X et al., 2023 [40]	China	Prospective study NHANES III	6 years	13,688	Lutein/zeaxantine, α-carotene, β-carotene, β-cryptoxanthin, lycopene	Higher concentrations of major serum carotenoids were associated with decreased risk of cardiovascular mortality.
Wang, M et al., 2023 [41]	China	Cross-sectional study	5 years	12,424	Lutein/zeaxantine, α-carotene, β-carotene, β-cryptoxanthin, lycopene	Serum carotenoids were negatively associated with the prevalence of CVDs.
Wang, Y. et al., 2014 [28]	USA	Cross-sectional study	3 years	2856	Individual dietary carotenoid intake	Significant inverse associations with LDL cholesterol were observed for dietary β-carotene and lutein + zeaxanthin, and with homocysteine for dietary β-carotene, lycopene and total carotenoids. Dietary lutein + zeaxanthin intake was also positively associated with HDL concentrations.
Qiu, Z. et al., 2022 [42]	USA	Prospective study	5 years (2001–2006)	3107	α-carotene, β-carotene, β-cryptoxanthin, lutein/zeaxanthin, and lycopene	The action of β-carotene on people with type 2 diabetes is unclear.

Some studies examined the relationship between plasma carotenoid levels and hypertension as an indicator of CVDs. Hozawa A. et al. [30] found that lycopene was not correlated with hypertension in any model, but four carotenoids—lutein/zeaxanthin, β-carotene, β-cryptoxanthin, and α-carotene—were significantly inversely correlated with hypertension. Toh DWK et al. [38] showed that plasma carotenoid levels were inversely associated with systolic and diastolic BP. Matsumoto M. et al. [39] reported similar results.

However, some authors have not found a relationship between carotenoid levels and a reduction in CVD risk and, in some cases, have observed an increase in certain markers. For example, Wang L. et al. [29] found that in middle-aged and older women, an increase in LDL was associated with higher plasma levels of α-carotene, β-carotene, and lycopene; an increase in HDL was associated with lower plasma lycopene levels; and an increase in CRP was associated with lower plasma β-carotene concentrations. Matos A. et al. [32] did not observe any significant correlation between β-carotene levels and CVDs. Additionally, Qiu Z. et al. [42] reported that, while other individual carotenoids (α-carotene, β-cryptoxanthin, lycopene, and lutein/zeaxanthin) were not significantly associated with cardiovascular mortality, higher serum β-carotene concentrations were significantly associated with an increased risk of cardiovascular mortality. It should be noted, however, that this study was conducted in individuals with type 2 diabetes.

Except for three studies [29,32,42], most of the recent observational studies generally indicate a correlation between blood carotenoid concentrations and a protective effect against CVDs. The most consistent correlations are observed with total carotenoid levels [30,33,35,38–41], though findings for specific carotenoids are more variable [25,27,29–32,34,35,37].

Most of these observational studies do not clarify whether the reduction in mortality is directly due to carotenoid effects, whether other dietary components in fruits and vegetables play a role in CVD development, or whether carotenoid intake is from supplements or carotenoid-rich foods.

Given that high fruit and vegetable intake is widely associated with elevated serum carotenoid levels, it remains uncertain whether carotenoids alone prevent CVDs or if they interact with other components of fruits and vegetables to produce these effects. Consequently, it would be valuable to examine findings from studies that provide carotenoid supplements to assess their effectiveness in CVD prevention.

4.2. Intervention Studies with Carotenoid Supplements

There are nine studies that examine the effect of carotenoid supplements on CVDs (Table 3). Gajendragadkar P. et al. [43] investigated the effects of two months of lycopene supplementation in patients with CVDs and in healthy volunteers. They found that lycopene improved endothelial function in patients with CVDs but had no effect on age-matched healthy volunteers. Wolak T. et al. [45] evaluated the effect of capsules containing a tomato nutrient complex with 15 mg and 30 mg of lycopene, comparing it to capsules with 15 mg of synthetic lycopene and a placebo. The study found that the tomato nutrient complex, containing both 15 mg and 30 mg of lycopene, effectively lowered systolic BP in healthy volunteers, whereas lower doses of pure lycopene did not produce comparable benefits. No statistically significant effect was observed on diastolic BP. Zou Z. et al. [47] assessed the effects of supplementing individuals with subclinical atherosclerosis with lutein (20 mg) alone and in combination with lycopene (20 + 20 mg). The combined lutein and lycopene treatment was more effective in preventing CIMT progression, while both treatments reduced CIMT. Xu XR et al. [44] examined the effects of three months of lutein supplementation (20 mg) on early atherosclerosis, focusing on inflammation biomarkers associated with CVDs (IL-6, MCP-1) and lipid profile (LDL, TG). They observed significant reductions in serum TG, LDL levels, and inflammatory cytokines. Stonehouse W. et al. [48] investigated the effects of an eight-week carotene supplementation (21 mg daily) on vascular function and CVD risk factors in adults at high risk of poor vascular function. No significant effects were found on vascular function, as measured by brachial artery flow-mediated dilatation, pulse wave velocity, atherogenic index, or circulating markers of vascular function. Additionally, no notable impact was observed on other CVD risk factors, including inflammatory markers, lipid profiles, BP, or glucose metabolism.

Kawashima A. et al. [49] examined the effects of four weeks of supplementation with a capsule containing dehydrated concentrates from various fruit and vegetable juices on DNA damage, oxidative stress indicators, and plasma homocysteine levels. While serum lipid peroxide levels decreased following the intervention, these results did not differ significantly from those of a placebo. Engelhard Y. et al. [50] administered one capsule daily of encapsulated tomato extract to subjects with grade 1 hypertension over eight weeks and found a significant reduction in both systolic and diastolic BP, as well as a decrease in lipid peroxidation products. However, the supplement did not affect blood lipids, lipoproteins, or homocysteine levels. Graydon R. et al. [56] conducted an eight-week intervention with middle-aged, healthy subjects who received either a mixed lutein and zeaxanthin supplement (containing 5 mg zeaxanthin and 10 mg lutein), a 15 mg β-carotene supplement, or a placebo. No changes were observed in macular pigment level (MPL) or in markers of endothelial activation, inflammation, or oxidation following supplementation with either spinach powder or carrot juice. However, an improvement in MPL was noted in the highest serum responders and in those with initially low MPL. Ryu N. et al. [51] evaluated the effects of 5 g per day of Chlorella powder tablets versus lactose powder tablets over four weeks in subjects with mild hypercholesterolemia. The Chlorella group showed significant reductions in total cholesterol and triglycerides. Improvement in serum lipids was supported by notable decreases in very low-density lipoproteins (VLDL), apolipoprotein, non-HDL, and the HDL/TG ratio, suggesting an inhibitory effect of Chlorella on the intestinal absorption of dietary and endogenous lipids. The authors propose that these changes in serum lipids were related to changes in serum carotenoid levels.

Lastly, Schwab S. et al. [46] investigated the association between carotenoid supplement use and changes in HbA1c levels, a biomarker of CVDs, over ten years in non-diabetic individuals. They found that carotenoid intake above 6.8 mg/day was associated with a smaller increase in HbA1c levels compared to no carotenoid intake, but this effect was observed only in non-smokers.

Table 3. Intervention studies with carotenoid supplementation.

Author, Publication Year	Country/ Region	Type of Study/Study Name	Follow-Up Period	Study Size	Carotenoids Supplemented	Findings
Gajendragadkar, Pr. et al., 2014 [43]	UK	Randomized, double-blind trial	2 months	72	Lycopene	Lycopene supplementation improves endothelial function in CVDs but not in healthy volunteers.
Xu, XR et al., 2013 [44]	China	Randomized, double-blind, placebo-controlled intervention trial	3 months	65	Lutein	After 3 months of supplementation with lutein ↓ IL-6, MCP-1, LDL, and TG levels.
Wolak, T. et al., 2019 [45]	Israel	Double-blind, randomized, placebo-controlled study	2 months	61	Tomato nutrient complex (5, 15 and 30 mg lycopene) vs. 15 mg of synthetic lycopene	Carotenoid levels achieved by the tomato nutrient complex (TNC) dose of 15 mg lycopene or higher correlate to a beneficial effect on systolic BP in hypertensive subjects, while lower doses and lycopene alone do not.
Schwab, S. et al., 2015 [46]	Germany	Two population-based cohorts/Monitoring of Trends and Determinants in Cardiovascular Diseases and Cooperative Health Research in the Region of Augsburg	10 years	2774	Carotenes	High carotenoid intake could be one strategy for the prevention of cardiovascular complications in non-diabetic people. ↓ HbA1c levels.
Zou, Z. et al., 2014 [47]	China	Randomized, double-blind, placebo-controlled trial.	12 months	144	Lutein and lycopene	The mean values of CAIMT decreased significantly in the lutein and combination groups at month 12. The change in CIMT was inversely associated with the increase in serum lutein concentrations in both the active treatment groups and with that in serum lycopene concentrations in the combination group.
Stonehouse, W. et al., 2016 [48]	Australia	A randomized, placebo-controlled, double-blind study	2 months	90	Carotenes	Carotenes had no effects on vascular function or CVD risk factors.
Kawashima, A. et al., 2007 [49]	USA	Double-blinded placebo controlled randomized study	1 month	60	Juice	Serum lipid peroxides and urine concentrations of 8-OHdG decreased significantly but were not significantly different than a placebo.
Engelhard YN. et al., 2006 [50]	Israel	Double-blinded, placebo-controlled pilot study	8 weeks	31	Tomato extract	Reduced systolic and diastolic BP in patients with grade 1 hypertension. No significant changes were found in lipid parameters.
Ryu, NH. et al., 2014 [51]	South Korea	Double-blinded, randomized, placebo-controlled study	4 weeks	63	5 g Chlorella powder a day	Chlorella group exhibited remarkable changes in TC, TG, lutein/zeaxanthin, and α-carotene.

Overall, it appears that combinations of carotenoids [45–47,50,51] are more effective than supplementing a single carotenoid [43,44], although the results are generally more modest than those observed in epidemiological studies, as the same carotenoids are not always supplemented and do not consistently produce the expected effect. However, at comparable dosages to those used in other studies, two studies [48,49] reported no effect of carotenoid supplementation.

4.3. Dietary Intervention Studies

Finally, 12 studies that utilized dietary interventions to increase carotenoid consumption were analyzed: seven studies provided vegetable and fruit juices (Table 4), and five studies focused on increasing fruit and vegetable intake (Table 5).

Table 4. Intervention studies with dietetic carotenoids providing vegetable and fruit juices.

Author, Publication Year	Country/Region	Type of Study/ Study Name	Follow-Up Period	Study Size	Dietary Intervention	Findings
Takagi, T. et al., 2020 [52]	Japan	Randomized, double-blinded, controlled clinical trial	8-weeks	28	High lycopene + high lutein, high lycopene + low lutein, low lycopene + high lutein, and low lycopene + low lutein by vegetable beverages	Daily beverage-intake significantly decreased the visceral fat level, and CoQ10 oxidation rate was decreased in all the groups.
Graydon, R. et al., 2012 [56]	UK	Randomized placebo-controlled trial	8-week	52	Dried spinach powder (lutein and zeaxanthin-rich food) or carrot juice (α and β-carotene rich food)	Lutein and zeaxanthin had no significant effect on MPL or serological markers of endothelial activation, inflammation and oxidation in healthy volunteers.
Colmán-Martínez, M. et al., 2017 [58]	Spain	Retrospective, randomized, cross-over, and controlled clinical trial	4 weeks	28	200 mL (LD) or 400 mL (HD) of tomato juice	Trans-lycopene reduced the concentration of important adhesion molecules ICAM-1, and VCAM-1, related to atherosclerosis.
Paterson, E. et al., 2006 [59]	UK	Single blind, randomized, controlled, crossover dietary intervention study.	4 weeks	36	During the test intervention period, the subjects were asked to consume 1 soup (500 mL) plus 1 juice (300 mL) or shot (fruit and vegetable preparation made from concentrated juices and purees) (100 mL) per day	Consumption of the carotenoid-rich soups and beverages only decreased the plasma homocysteine concentration by 8.8%.
Bub, A. et al., 2000 [60]	The Netherlands	Clinical trial	8 weeks	23	330 mL/d of a tomato juice (40 mg lycopene) in addition to their meals or 330 mL carrot juice (15.7 mg a-carotene and 22.3 mg b-carotene) daily	Tomato juice consumption reduced plasma thiobarbituric acid reactive substances (TBARS) and lipoprotein oxidizability in terms of an increased lag time. Carrot juice and spinach powder had no effect on lipid peroxidation.
Tomás, A. et al., 2021 [62]	Spain	Clinical trial	4 weeks	12	Orange-carrot juice, tomato juice, and boiled spinach, providing 415 mg of total carotenoids/week (carotenes, cryptoxanthin, lycopene, and lutein + zeaxanthin)	Significant decrease in LDL and atherogenic index, and an increase in HDL were observed.
Biddle, MJ. et al., 2015 [63]	USA	Two-group, randomized controlled intervention pilot study	30 days	40	11.5 ounces of a juice of vegetables (29.4 mg of lycopene; 70 calories; 140 mg of sodium; vitamins A and C; 820 mg of potassium; 2% of the recommended daily allowance for iron and magnesium; and 3 g of fiber	No differences on CRP levels.

Table 5. Intervention studies with dietetic carotenoids by increasing fruit and vegetable intake.

Author, Publication Year	Country/Region	Type of Study/ Study Name	Follow-Up Period	Study Size	Dietary Intervention	Findings
Daniels, JA. et al., 2014 [53]	UK	Randomized, double-blinded, controlled clinical trial	8-weeks	80	Randomized to a 1- or ≥6-portion/day fruit and vegetables diet	≥6- vs. 1-portion post-intervention comparisons, carotenoids increased in serum, HDL2 and particularly HDL3, as did the activities of PON-1 and LCAT in HDL3.
Wallace, I. et al., 2013 [54]	UK	Randomized controlled trial	12-week	89	One to two, four, or seven portions of FandVs	No significant difference was found in measures of whole-body, peripheral, or hepatic IR or adiponectin multimers.

Table 5. *Cont.*

Author, Publication Year	Country/Region	Type of Study/ Study Name	Follow-Up Period	Study Size	Dietary Intervention	Findings
Hurtado-Barroso, S. et al., 2019 [55]	Spain	Clinical trial	1 day	22	Single portion of sofrito (240 g/70 kg bodyweight) in a state of fasting	Significant decrease in CRP and TNF-α was observed, but only TNF-α was inversely correlated with an increase in TPE (total polyphenol excretion) and plasma β-carotene.
Thies, F. et al., 2012 [57]	UK	Single-blind, randomized controlled trial	12 weeks	225	Diet low in tomato-based foods, a high-tomato-based diet, or a control diet supplemented with lycopene capsules (10 mg/d)	High daily consumption of tomato-based products or lycopene supplements is ineffective at reducing conventional CVD risk markers.
Svendsen M. et al., 2007 [61]	Norway	Randomized, controlled trial	3 months	138	Consumption of vegetables to at least 400 g/day, and fruit to at least 300 g/day	Weight reduction and reduced systolic and diastolic BP. No effect on antioxidant defence measured with FRAP.

4.3.1. Vegetable and Fruits Juices

Takagi T. et al. [52] analyzed the effects of an eight-week intake of a vegetable drink rich in carotenoids, specifically lycopene or lutein, in men with a body mass index (BMI) over 25 kg/m^2. They observed a reduction in visceral adiposity and oxidative stress, specifically in the CoQ10 oxidation rate. Colmán-Martínez M. et al. [58] investigated the effects of providing subjects at high risk for CVDs with either 200 mL or 400 mL of tomato juice or a placebo for four weeks. They found that trans-lycopene from tomato juice may reduce CVD risk by lowering the concentration of inflammatory molecules associated with atherosclerosis, such as adhesion molecules ICAM-1, VCAM-1, and IL-8. These markers were not significantly reduced by other carotenoids. Paterson E. et al. [59] studied the effect of consuming one soup (500 mL) plus one juice (300 mL) or one shot (100 mL of a concentrated fruit and vegetable preparation) daily for one month in healthy subjects. They observed a significant reduction in plasma homocysteine concentrations following the dietary intervention, although other risk markers remained unaffected. Bub A. et al. [60] examined the effects of daily consumption of 330 mL of tomato juice, followed by 330 mL of carrot juice and 10 g of spinach powder, each consumed for two weeks in healthy men. The results showed that tomato juice reduced plasma thiobarbituric acid reactive substances and lipoprotein oxidisability by increasing lag time, whereas carrot juice and spinach powder had no effect on lipid peroxidation. Additionally, water-soluble antioxidants, ferric-reducing antioxidant power (FRAP), and activities of glutathione peroxidase and reductase remained unchanged throughout the study periods. Biddle M. et al. [63] supplemented 11.5 ounces of low-sodium vegetable juice daily for one month in patients with heart failure and found no difference in CRP levels between the control and intervention groups. Tomás A. et al. [62] observed statistically significant changes in serum levels of LDL, VLDL, HDL, triglycerides, and atherogenic index after administering orange–carrot juice, tomato juice, and boiled spinach for four weeks to perimenopausal and postmenopausal women with cardiometabolic risk factors but no prior CVDs symptoms. Lastly, Graydon R. et al. [56] conducted an eight-week intervention with middle-aged, healthy subjects who consumed either 131 mL of carrot juice or 10.4 g of dried spinach powder daily. No changes were observed in macular pigment levels (MPL) or in markers of endothelial activation, inflammation, or oxidation following supplementation with spinach powder or carrot juice. However, MPL improvements were noted in the highest serum responders and those with initially low MPL.

Contradictory findings are apparent regarding the impact of carotenoid consumption through fruit and vegetable juices. Effects tend to be more noticeable in individuals with existing cardiovascular symptoms or risk factors [52,58,62]. Although some studies found no impact [63], certain studies have shown minor benefits on inflammatory markers in healthy individuals [59,60]; however, Graydon R. et al. [56] identified improvements only in those with low baseline carotenoid levels (Table 4).

4.3.2. Increased Consumption of Fruit and Vegetable

In this section, we review studies that have directly increased fruit and vegetable consumption as an intervention. Daniels J. et al. [53] randomly assigned obese subjects with type 2 diabetes to a diet of either one or six or more portions of fruits and vegetables daily for eight weeks. They found that the carotenoid content in HDL2 and HDL3 increased, especially for α-carotene, β-cryptoxanthin, lutein, and lycopene in HDL3, indicating an enhancement in HDL's antioxidant properties. Wallace I. et al. [54] studied the effects of consuming one, two, four, or seven portions of fruits and vegetables per day over 12 weeks in subjects with a CVD risk of 20% or higher and a mean age of 56 years but found no significant changes in whole-body, peripheral, or hepatic insulin resistance (IR) or adiponectin multimers. Svendsen M. et al. [61] examined the effects of consuming 400 g/day of vegetables and 300 g/day of fruit over three months in obese subjects with sleep-related breathing disorders. The intervention group showed reductions in weight and BP but no changes in antioxidant defences, as measured by FRAP. In contrast, Hurtado-Barroso S. et al. [55] investigated the acute effects of a single dose of sofrito sauce (240 g/70 kg body weight) in fasting healthy volunteers. They observed improvements in inflammatory biomarkers, specifically CRP and TNF-α, although IL-6 was unaffected. An inverse relationship was found between β-carotene levels and the reduction in TNF-α. Lastly, Thies F. et al. [57] analyzed the effects of a low tomato-based foods diet, a high tomato-based diet, or a control diet supplemented with lycopene capsules (10 mg/day) for 12 weeks in healthy, middle-aged subjects. They found no changes in systemic markers (CRP, IL-6, ICAM-1, oxidized LDL, HOMA-IR) or in the quantitative insulin-sensitivity check index after the dietary intervention. Additionally, lipid concentrations and arterial stiffness were unaffected by the interventions.

There is ongoing debate over the impact of increasing the consumption of carotenoid-rich fruits and vegetables, as some research has yielded inconclusive results [54,57]. While some studies have reported reductions in weight and BP in obese individuals [61], most research has examined improvements in antioxidant capacity, showing that higher carotenoid intake leads to significant improvements [53,55] (Table 5).

4.4. Final Analysis

In summary, epidemiological research has shown more promising results than intervention studies. Key findings regarding the impact of carotenoid intake on CVDs are compiled in Figure 4. Unlike intervention studies, which typically involve short-term interventions lasting one to three months, epidemiological studies span from one to twenty years and consider long-term dietary patterns, so some observed outcomes may be time-dependent [25,27,29–35,37–42]. An exception to this trend is the study by Schwab S. et al. [46], which examined the effects of carotenoid supplementation over a ten-year period and found a cardioprotective effect, and the study by Zou Z. et al. [47], which demonstrated that lutein or lutein/lycopene supplementation can effectively prevent CIMT progression. This suggests that the timing of carotenoid intake assessment may be critical in evaluating its impact on CVD risk indicators and actual risk reduction. Several studies examining short-term antioxidant capacity [44,53,55,59,60] have yielded encouraging results, suggesting that sustained intake over time could translate into physiological benefits. However, short-term effects appear more pronounced in individuals with existing CVDs than in healthy individuals [43–45,50–52]. Based on the reviewed data, the combined effect of all carotenoids appears to offer greater cardiovascular benefits than any single carotenoid. In fact, studies supplementing with a single carotenoid [43,45,47] tend to show less favourable outcomes than those using multiple carotenoids or a single plant extract [45,46,50,51]. Most clinical trials included in this review are short in duration, and although improvements in controlling CVD risk factors or inflammation markers are observed, the extent to which these improvements reduce the risk of developing CVDs remains unclear, as none of the clinical trials have directly assessed this relationship. It is also important to note that each study evaluates different carotenoids or combinations of carotenoids, and supplement dosages vary, making it challenging to compare findings across studies.

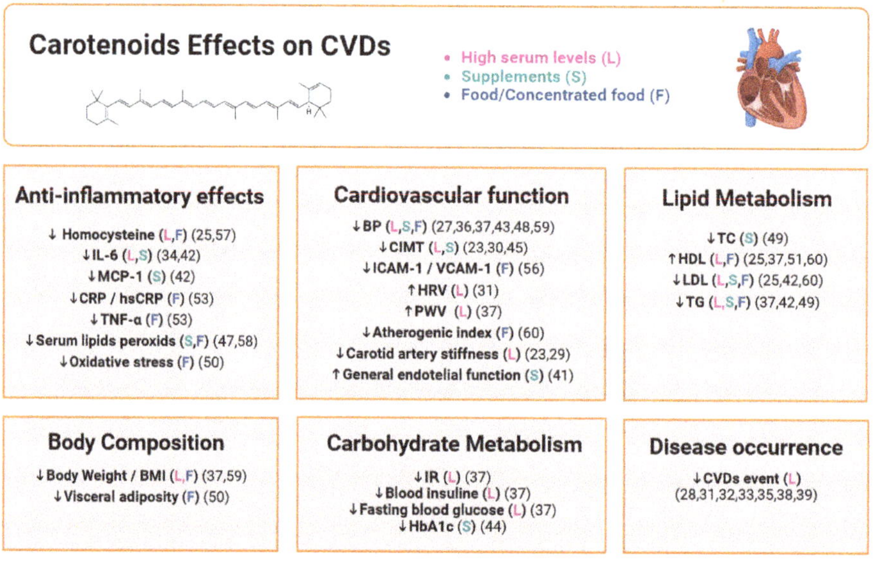

Figure 4. Summary of the effects of the carotenoids on CVDs.

4.5. Limitations of the Study

This review is limited by the well-known variability in clinical trials, which affects both the carotenoids examined and the CVD risk factors assessed. The comparison of the effects on CVD risk reduction between dietary supplements, carotenoid-rich foods, and concentrated carotenoid sources is particularly challenging due to the different carotenoid's combinations, and the significant differences in de dosages of carotenoids used in these interventions. Moreover, many of the included studies do not account for baseline consumption of fruits and vegetables, both before and during the intervention period, nor do they assess the overall diet quality of participants. These dietary factors may contain additional bioactive compounds that interact with carotenoids and, therefore, could collectively influence the reduction of CVD risk factors.

Another limitation is the lack of clarity regarding the molecular mechanisms through which carotenoids contribute to the reduction of various CVD risk factors. This gap complicates the ability to establish definitive conclusions about the biological pathways involved.

Moreover, although some studies have found reductions in the risk factors for CVDs, it is challenging to ascertain if these modifications result in long-term decreases in the incidence of CVDs due to the brief duration of interventions.

Future studies should address the gaps by standardizing carotenoids combinations and dosages and sources to allow for more accurate comparisons of their effects on CVD risk factors. Longer intervention periods are necessary to assess the long-term impact of carotenoids on actual CVD incidence. Additionally, comprehensive dietary assessments, including baseline fruit and vegetable intake and overall diet quality, should be incorporated to better isolate the effects of carotenoids. Research should also explore the molecular mechanisms through which carotenoids influence CVD risk and include diverse populations to determine their efficacy across different demographic groups. Finally, RCTs with larger sample sizes and the investigation of synergistic effects with other nutrients are needed to strengthen the evidence and provide more definitive conclusions.

5. Conclusions

This review provides an overview how carotenoids intake from diet and supplements affects the development and course of CVDs. Elevated blood carotenoid levels are associated with reduced CVD risk factors and inflammatory markers, potentially lowering the likelihood of cardiovascular events. Increasing the consumption of carotenoids rich foods seems more effective than supplementation in reducing inflammatory markers and CVD risk indicators. Natural sources of carotenoids, which contain a combination of carotenoids and other phytocompounds, may enhance or modify the effects of carotenoids on CVD risk. Consequently, the effect of individual carotenoids on CVD risk remains unclear. Additionally, the short duration of most clinical trials limits the ability to assess the long-term impact of carotenoids intake on CVD risk reduction. Despite these limitations, it is evident that consuming a diverse range of carotenoids, mostly through food, may delay the onset and progression of CVDs.

As already mentioned in the limitations of the study, future research should focus on longer-term clinical trials to explore the direct relationship between carotenoid intake and the actual occurrence of CVDs, going beyond the mere assessment of risk factors or markers.

Author Contributions: Conceptualization, S.S.-C. and I.E.; methodology, S.S.-C., I.E., I.E.-G., Á.L.-G. and R.M.-D.; validation, S.S.-C., I.E. and T.A.P.; investigation S.S.-C., I.E., I.E.-G., Á.L.-G. and R.M.-D.; writing—original draft preparation, S.S.-C., I.E., I.E.-G. and Á.L.-G.; writing—review and editing, S.S.-C., I.E., I.E.-G., Á.L.-G. and T.A.P.; supervision, S.S.-C., R.M.-D., T.A.P. and I.E. All authors have read and agreed to the published version of the manuscript.

Funding: This research received no external funding.

Informed Consent Statement: Not applicable.

Data Availability Statement: Not applicable.

Acknowledgments: Sandra Conde-González for her support during the review process and Jorge Daniel Ayala Cruz for his thorough revision of the English language.

Conflicts of Interest: The authors declare no conflicts of interest.

References

1. Olvera Lopez, E.; Ballard, B.D.; Jan, A. Cardiovascular Disease. In *StatPearls*; StatPearls Publishing: Treasure Island, FL, USA, 2024.
2. GBD 2017 Causes of Death Collaborators Global, Regional, and National Age-Sex-Specific Mortality for 282 Causes of Death in 195 Countries and Territories, 1980–2017: A Systematic Analysis for the Global Burden of Disease Study 2017. *Lancet* **2018**, *392*, 1736–1788. [CrossRef] [PubMed]
3. 2021 ESC Guidelines on Cardiovascular Disease Prevention in Clinical Practice | European Heart Journal | Oxford Academic. Available online: https://academic.oup.com/eurheartj/article/42/34/3227/6358713?login=false (accessed on 22 July 2024).
4. Lacey, B.; Herrington, W.G.; Preiss, D.; Lewington, S.; Armitage, J. The Role of Emerging Risk Factors in Cardiovascular Outcomes. *Curr. Atheroscler. Rep.* **2017**, *19*, 28. [CrossRef]
5. Magnussen, C.; Ojeda, F.M.; Leong, D.P.; Alegre-Diaz, J.; Amouyel, P.; Aviles-Santa, L.; De Bacquer, D.; Ballantyne, C.M.; Bernabe-Ortiz, A.; Bobak, M.; et al. Global Impact of Modifiable Risk Factors on Cardiovascular Disease and Mortality. *N. Engl. J. Med.* **2023**, *389*, 1273–1285. [CrossRef] [PubMed]
6. Gammone, M.A.; Riccioni, G.; D'Orazio, N. Carotenoids: Potential Allies of Cardiovascular Health? *Food Nutr. Res.* **2015**, *59*, 26762. [CrossRef] [PubMed]
7. Diet, Nutrition and the Prevention of Chronic Diseases: Report of a Joint WHO/FAO Expert Consultation, Geneva, 28 January–1 February 2002. Available online: https://www.who.int/publications-detail-redirect/924120916X (accessed on 20 December 2023).
8. Pagliaro, B.; Santolamazza, C.; Simonelli, F.; Rubattu, S. Phytochemical Compounds and Protection from Cardiovascular Diseases: A State of the Art. *BioMed Res. Int.* **2015**, *2015*, 918069. [CrossRef]
9. Mozos, I.; Stoian, D.; Caraba, A.; Malainer, C.; Horbańczuk, J.O.; Atanasov, A.G. Lycopene and Vascular Health. *Front. Pharmacol.* **2018**, *9*, 521. [CrossRef]

10. Protective Effect of Lycopene on Serum Cholesterol and Blood Pressure: Meta-Analyses of Intervention Trials. In *Database of Abstracts of Reviews of Effects (DARE): Quality-Assessed Reviews [Internet]*; Centre for Reviews and Dissemination: York, UK, 2011.
11. González-Peña, M.A.; Ortega-Regules, A.E.; Anaya de Parrodi, C.; Lozada-Ramírez, J.D. Chemistry, Occurrence, Properties, Applications, and Encapsulation of Carotenoids—A Review. *Plants* **2023**, *12*, 313. [CrossRef]
12. Sandmann, G. Carotenoids and Their Biosynthesis in Fungi. *Molecules* **2022**, *27*, 1431. [CrossRef]
13. Milani, A.; Basirnejad, M.; Shahbazi, S.; Bolhassani, A. Carotenoids: Biochemistry, Pharmacology and Treatment. *Br. J. Pharmacol.* **2017**, *174*, 1290–1324. [CrossRef]
14. Chen, G. The Interactions of Insulin and Vitamin A Signaling Systems for the Regulation of Hepatic Glucose and Lipid Metabolism. *Cells* **2021**, *10*, 2160. [CrossRef]
15. Eggersdorfer, M.; Wyss, A. Carotenoids in Human Nutrition and Health. *Arch. Biochem. Biophys.* **2018**, *652*, 18–26. [CrossRef] [PubMed]
16. Saini, R.K.; Prasad, P.; Lokesh, V.; Shang, X.; Shin, J.; Keum, Y.-S.; Lee, J.-H. Carotenoids: Dietary Sources, Extraction, Encapsulation, Bioavailability, and Health Benefits—A Review of Recent Advancements. *Antioxidants* **2022**, *11*, 795. [CrossRef]
17. Burrows, T.L.; Williams, R.; Rollo, M.; Wood, L.; Garg, M.L.; Jensen, M.; Collins, C.E. Plasma Carotenoid Levels as Biomarkers of Dietary Carotenoid Consumption: A Systematic Review of the Validation Studies. *J. Nutr. Intermed. Metab.* **2015**, *2*, 15–64. [CrossRef]
18. Henning, T.; Wagner, P.; Gedat, E.; Kochlik, B.; Kusch, P.; Sowoidnich, K.; Vastag, M.; Gleim, J.; Braune, M.; Maiwald, M.; et al. Evaluation of Modern Approaches for the Assessment of Dietary Carotenoids as Markers for Fruit and Vegetable Consumption. *Nutrients* **2023**, *15*, 1665. [CrossRef]
19. Fiedor, J.; Burda, K. Potential Role of Carotenoids as Antioxidants in Human Health and Disease. *Nutrients* **2014**, *6*, 466–488. [CrossRef] [PubMed]
20. Stringham, N.T.; Green, M.; Roche, W.; Prado-Cabrero, A.; Mulcahy, R.; Nolan, J. Lutein, Zeaxanthin, and Meso-Zeaxanthin Supplementation Attenuates Inflammatory Cytokines and Markers of Oxidative Cardiovascular Processes in Humans. *Nutr. Metab. Cardiovasc. Dis.* **2024**, *34*, 1976–1983. [CrossRef]
21. Przybylska, S.; Tokarczyk, G. Lycopene in the Prevention of Cardiovascular Diseases. *Int. J. Mol. Sci.* **2022**, *23*, 1957. [CrossRef]
22. Ahn, Y.J.; Kim, H. Lutein as a Modulator of Oxidative Stress-Mediated Inflammatory Diseases. *Antioxidants* **2021**, *10*, 1448. [CrossRef]
23. Hajizadeh-Sharafabad, F.; Ghoreishi, Z.; Maleki, V.; Tarighat-Esfanjani, A. Mechanistic Insights into the Effect of Lutein on Atherosclerosis, Vascular Dysfunction, and Related Risk Factors: A Systematic Review of in Vivo, Ex Vivo and in Vitro Studies. *Pharmacol. Res.* **2019**, *149*, 104477. [CrossRef]
24. Murillo, A.G.; Hu, S.; Fernandez, M.L. Zeaxanthin: Metabolism, Properties, and Antioxidant Protection of Eyes, Heart, Liver, and Skin. *Antioxidants* **2019**, *8*, 390. [CrossRef]
25. Zou, Z.; Xu, X.; Huang, Y.; Xiao, X.; Ma, L.; Sun, T.; Dong, P.; Wang, X.; Lin, X. High Serum Level of Lutein May Be Protective against Early Atherosclerosis: The Beijing Atherosclerosis Study. *Atherosclerosis* **2011**, *219*, 789–793. [CrossRef] [PubMed]
26. Crupi, P.; Faienza, M.F.; Naeem, M.Y.; Corbo, F.; Clodoveo, M.L.; Muraglia, M. Overview of the Potential Beneficial Effects of Carotenoids on Consumer Health and Well-Being. *Antioxidants* **2023**, *12*, 1069. [CrossRef] [PubMed]
27. Huang, Y.; Chen, H.; Su, Y.; Liu, H.; Hu, J.; Hong, K. Increased Blood Alpha-Carotene, All-Trans-Beta-Carotene and Lycopene Levels Are Associated with Beneficial Changes in Heart Rate Variability: A CVD-Stratified Analysis in an Adult Population-Based Study. *Nutr. J.* **2021**, *20*, 43. [CrossRef]
28. Wang, Y.; Chung, S.-J.; McCullough, M.L.; Song, W.O.; Fernandez, M.L.; Koo, S.I.; Chun, O.K. Dietary Carotenoids Are Associated with Cardiovascular Disease Risk Biomarkers Mediated by Serum Carotenoid Concentrations. *J. Nutr.* **2014**, *144*, 1067–1074. [CrossRef]
29. Wang, L.; Gaziano, J.M.; Norkus, E.P.; Buring, J.E.; Sesso, H.D. Associations of Plasma Carotenoids with Risk Factors and Biomarkers Related to Cardiovascular Disease in Middle-Aged and Older Women. *Am. J. Clin. Nutr.* **2008**, *88*, 747–754. [CrossRef] [PubMed]
30. Hozawa, A.; Jacobs, D.R.; Steffes, M.W.; Gross, M.D.; Steffen, L.M.; Lee, D.-H. Circulating Carotenoid Concentrations and Incident Hypertension: The Coronary Artery Risk Development in Young Adults (CARDIA) Study. *J. Hypertens.* **2009**, *27*, 237–242. [CrossRef]
31. Prentice, R.L.; Pettinger, M.; Neuhouser, M.L.; Tinker, L.F.; Huang, Y.; Zheng, C.; Manson, J.E.; Mossavar-Rahmani, Y.; Anderson, G.L.; Lampe, J.W. Application of Blood Concentration Biomarkers in Nutritional Epidemiology: Example of Carotenoid and Tocopherol Intake in Relation to Chronic Disease Risk. *Am. J. Clin. Nutr.* **2019**, *109*, 1189–1196. [CrossRef]
32. Matos, A.; Gonçalves, V.M.d.S.; Souza, G.; Cruz, S.P.d.; Cruz, S.; Ramalho, A. Vitamin A Nutritional Status in Patients with Coronary Artery Disease and Its Correlation with the Severity of the Disease. *Nutr. Hosp.* **2018**, *35*, 1215–1220. [CrossRef]
33. Wang, C.; Qiu, R.; Cao, Y.; Ouyang, W.-F.; Li, H.-B.; Ling, W.-H.; Chen, Y.-M. Higher Dietary and Serum Carotenoid Levels Are Associated with Lower Carotid Intima-Media Thickness in Middle-Aged and Elderly People. *Br. J. Nutr.* **2018**, *119*, 590–598. [CrossRef]
34. Karppi, J.; Laukkanen, J.A.; Mäkikallio, T.H.; Ronkainen, K.; Kurl, S. Low β-Carotene Concentrations Increase the Risk of Cardiovascular Disease Mortality among Finnish Men with Risk Factors. *Nutr. Metab. Cardiovasc. Dis.* **2012**, *22*, 921–928. [CrossRef]

35. Shardell, M.D.; Alley, D.E.; Hicks, G.E.; El-Kamary, S.S.; Miller, R.R.; Semba, R.D.; Ferrucci, L. Low Serum Carotenoid Concentrations and Carotenoid Interactions Predict Mortality in US Adults: The Third National Health and Nutrition Examination Survey (NHANES III). *Nutr. Res.* **2011**, *31*, 178–189. [CrossRef] [PubMed]
36. Chung, R.W.S.; Leanderson, P.; Lundberg, A.K.; Jonasson, L. Lutein Exerts Anti-Inflammatory Effects in Patients with Coronary Artery Disease. *Atherosclerosis* **2017**, *262*, 87–93. [CrossRef] [PubMed]
37. Huang, J.; Weinstein, S.J.; Yu, K.; Männistö, S.; Albanes, D. Serum Beta Carotene and Overall and Cause-Specific Mortality. *Circ. Res.* **2018**, *123*, 1339–1349. [CrossRef]
38. Toh, D.W.K.; Sutanto, C.N.; Loh, W.W.; Lee, W.Y.; Yao, Y.; Ong, C.N.; Kim, J.E. Skin Carotenoids Status as a Potential Surrogate Marker for Cardiovascular Disease Risk Determination in Middle-Aged and Older Adults. *Nutr. Metab. Cardiovasc. Dis.* **2021**, *31*, 592–601. [CrossRef]
39. Matsumoto, M.; Waki, N.; Suganuma, H.; Takahashi, I.; Kurauchi, S.; Sawada, K.; Tokuda, I.; Misawa, M.; Ando, M.; Itoh, K.; et al. Association between Biomarkers of Cardiovascular Diseases and the Blood Concentration of Carotenoids among the General Population without Apparent Illness. *Nutrients* **2020**, *12*, E2310. [CrossRef]
40. Zhu, X.; Cheang, I.; Tang, Y.; Shi, M.; Zhu, Q.; Gao, R.; Liao, S.; Yao, W.; Zhou, Y.; Zhang, H.; et al. Associations of Serum Carotenoids with Risk of All-Cause and Cardiovascular Mortality in Hypertensive Adults. *J. Am. Heart Assoc.* **2023**, *12*, e027568. [CrossRef] [PubMed]
41. Wang, M.; Tang, R.; Zhou, R.; Qian, Y.; Di, D. The Protective Effect of Serum Carotenoids on Cardiovascular Disease: A Cross-Sectional Study from the General US Adult Population. *Front. Nutr.* **2023**, *10*, 1154239. [CrossRef]
42. Qiu, Z.; Chen, X.; Geng, T.; Wan, Z.; Lu, Q.; Li, L.; Zhu, K.; Zhang, X.; Liu, Y.; Lin, X.; et al. Associations of Serum Carotenoids with Risk of Cardiovascular Mortality Among Individuals with Type 2 Diabetes: Results From NHANES. *Diabetes Care* **2022**, *45*, 1453–1461. [CrossRef]
43. Gajendragadkar, P.R.; Hubsch, A.; Mäki-Petäjä, K.M.; Serg, M.; Wilkinson, I.B.; Cheriyan, J. Effects of Oral Lycopene Supplementation on Vascular Function in Patients with Cardiovascular Disease and Healthy Volunteers: A Randomised Controlled Trial. *PLoS ONE* **2014**, *9*, e99070. [CrossRef]
44. Xu, X.-R.; Zou, Z.-Y.; Xiao, X.; Huang, Y.-M.; Wang, X.; Lin, X.-M. Effects of Lutein Supplement on Serum Inflammatory Cytokines, ApoE and Lipid Profiles in Early Atherosclerosis Population. *J. Atheroscler. Thromb.* **2013**, *20*, 170–177. [CrossRef]
45. Wolak, T.; Sharoni, Y.; Levy, J.; Linnewiel-Hermoni, K.; Stepensky, D.; Paran, E. Effect of Tomato Nutrient Complex on Blood Pressure: A Double Blind, Randomized Dose-Response Study. *Nutrients* **2019**, *11*, E950. [CrossRef] [PubMed]
46. Schwab, S.; Zierer, A.; Heier, M.; Fischer, B.; Huth, C.; Baumert, J.; Meisinger, C.; Peters, A.; Thorand, B. Intake of Vitamin and Mineral Supplements and Longitudinal Association with HbA1c Levels in the General Non-Diabetic Population—Results from the MONICA/KORA S3/F3 Study. *PLoS ONE* **2015**, *10*, e0139244. [CrossRef] [PubMed]
47. Zou, Z.-Y.; Xu, X.-R.; Lin, X.-M.; Zhang, H.-B.; Xiao, X.; Ouyang, L.; Huang, Y.-M.; Wang, X.; Liu, Y.-Q. Effects of Lutein and Lycopene on Carotid Intima–Media Thickness in Chinese Subjects with Subclinical Atherosclerosis: A Randomised, Double-Blind, Placebo-Controlled Trial. *Br. J. Nutr.* **2014**, *111*, 474–480. [CrossRef] [PubMed]
48. Stonehouse, W.; Brinkworth, G.D.; Thompson, C.H.; Abeywardena, M.Y. Short Term Effects of Palm-Tocotrienol and Palm-Carotenes on Vascular Function and Cardiovascular Disease Risk: A Randomised Controlled Trial. *Atherosclerosis* **2016**, *254*, 205–214. [CrossRef] [PubMed]
49. Kawashima, A.; Madarame, T.; Koike, H.; Komatsu, Y.; Wise, J.A. Four Week Supplementation with Mixed Fruit and Vegetable Juice Concentrates Increased Protective Serum Antioxidants and Folate and Decreased Plasma Homocysteine in Japanese Subjects. *Asia Pac. J. Clin. Nutr.* **2007**, *16*, 411–421.
50. Engelhard, Y.N.; Gazer, B.; Paran, E. Natural Antioxidants from Tomato Extract Reduce Blood Pressure in Patients with Grade-1 Hypertension: A Double-Blind, Placebo-Controlled Pilot Study. *Am. Heart J.* **2006**, *151*, 100. [CrossRef]
51. Ryu, N.H.; Lim, Y.; Park, J.E.; Kim, J.; Kim, J.Y.; Kwon, S.W.; Kwon, O. Impact of Daily Chlorella Consumption on Serum Lipid and Carotenoid Profiles in Mildly Hypercholesterolemic Adults: A Double-Blinded, Randomized, Placebo-Controlled Study. *Nutr. J.* **2014**, *13*, 57. [CrossRef]
52. Takagi, T.; Hayashi, R.; Nakai, Y.; Okada, S.; Miyashita, R.; Yamada, M.; Mihara, Y.; Mizushima, K.; Morita, M.; Uchiyama, K.; et al. Dietary Intake of Carotenoid-Rich Vegetables Reduces Visceral Adiposity in Obese Japanese Men—A Randomized, Double-Blind Trial. *Nutrients* **2020**, *12*, E2342. [CrossRef]
53. Daniels, J.-A.; Mulligan, C.; McCance, D.; Woodside, J.V.; Patterson, C.; Young, I.S.; McEneny, J. A Randomised Controlled Trial of Increasing Fruit and Vegetable Intake and How This Influences the Carotenoid Concentration and Activities of PON-1 and LCAT in HDL from Subjects with Type 2 Diabetes. *Cardiovasc. Diabetol.* **2014**, *13*, 16. [CrossRef]
54. Wallace, I.R.; McEvoy, C.T.; Hunter, S.J.; Hamill, L.L.; Ennis, C.N.; Bell, P.M.; Patterson, C.C.; Woodside, J.V.; Young, I.S.; McKinley, M.C. Dose-Response Effect of Fruit and Vegetables on Insulin Resistance in People at High Risk of Cardiovascular Disease: A Randomized Controlled Trial. *Diabetes Care* **2013**, *36*, 3888–3896. [CrossRef]
55. Hurtado-Barroso, S.; Martínez-Huélamo, M.; Rinaldi de Alvarenga, J.F.; Quifer-Rada, P.; Vallverdú-Queralt, A.; Pérez-Fernández, S.; Lamuela-Raventós, R.M. Acute Effect of a Single Dose of Tomato Sofrito on Plasmatic Inflammatory Biomarkers in Healthy Men. *Nutrients* **2019**, *11*, E851. [CrossRef] [PubMed]

56. Graydon, R.; Hogg, R.E.; Chakravarthy, U.; Young, I.S.; Woodside, J.V. The Effect of Lutein- and Zeaxanthin-Rich Foods v. Supplements on Macular Pigment Level and Serological Markers of Endothelial Activation, Inflammation and Oxidation: Pilot Studies in Healthy Volunteers. *Br. J. Nutr.* **2012**, *108*, 334–342. [CrossRef] [PubMed]
57. Thies, F.; Masson, L.F.; Rudd, A.; Vaughan, N.; Tsang, C.; Brittenden, J.; Simpson, W.G.; Duthie, S.; Horgan, G.W.; Duthie, G. Effect of a Tomato-Rich Diet on Markers of Cardiovascular Disease Risk in Moderately Overweight, Disease-Free, Middle-Aged Adults: A Randomized Controlled Trial. *Am. J. Clin. Nutr.* **2012**, *95*, 1013–1022. [CrossRef] [PubMed]
58. Colmán-Martínez, M.; Martínez-Huélamo, M.; Valderas-Martínez, P.; Arranz-Martínez, S.; Almanza-Aguilera, E.; Corella, D.; Estruch, R.; Lamuela-Raventós, R.M. Trans-Lycopene from Tomato Juice Attenuates Inflammatory Biomarkers in Human Plasma Samples: An Intervention Trial. *Mol. Nutr. Food Res.* **2017**, *61*, 1600993. [CrossRef]
59. Paterson, E.; Gordon, M.H.; Niwat, C.; George, T.W.; Parr, L.; Waroonphan, S.; Lovegrove, J.A. Supplementation with Fruit and Vegetable Soups and Beverages Increases Plasma Carotenoid Concentrations but Does Not Alter Markers of Oxidative Stress or Cardiovascular Risk Factors. *J. Nutr.* **2006**, *136*, 2849–2855. [CrossRef]
60. Bub, A.; Watzl, B.; Abrahamse, L.; Delincée, H.; Adam, S.; Wever, J.; Müller, H.; Rechkemmer, G. Moderate Intervention with Carotenoid-Rich Vegetable Products Reduces Lipid Peroxidation in Men. *J. Nutr.* **2000**, *130*, 2200–2206. [CrossRef]
61. Svendsen, M.; Blomhoff, R.; Holme, I.; Tonstad, S. The Effect of an Increased Intake of Vegetables and Fruit on Weight Loss, Blood Pressure and Antioxidant Defense in Subjects with Sleep Related Breathing Disorders. *Eur. J. Clin. Nutr.* **2007**, *61*, 1301–1311. [CrossRef]
62. Tomás Luiz, A.; Martín Pozuelo, G.; González Navarro, I.; Elvira Torales, L.; Ponce, H.; González Barrio, R.; García Alonso, J.; Periago, M.J. Influence of dietary carotenoids on biomarkers of cardiometabolic risk in peri- and post-menopausal women. *Nutr. Hosp.* **2021**, *38*, 993–1001. [CrossRef]
63. Biddle, M.J.; Lennie, T.A.; Bricker, G.V.; Kopec, R.E.; Schwartz, S.J.; Moser, D.K. Lycopene Dietary Intervention: A Pilot Study in Patients with Heart Failure. *J. Cardiovasc. Nurs.* **2015**, *30*, 205–212. [CrossRef]
64. Böhm, V.; Lietz, G.; Olmedilla-Alonso, B.; Phelan, D.; Reboul, E.; Bánati, D.; Borel, P.; Corte-Real, J.; de Lera, A.R.; Desmarchelier, C.; et al. From Carotenoid Intake to Carotenoid Blood and Tissue Concentrations—Implications for Dietary Intake Recommendations. *Nutr. Rev.* **2020**, *79*, 544–573. [CrossRef]

MDPI AG
Grosspeteranlage 5
4052 Basel
Switzerland
Tel.: +41 61 683 77 34

Nutrients Editorial Office
E-mail: nutrients@mdpi.com
www.mdpi.com/journal/nutrients

www.ingramcontent.com/pod-product-compliance
Lightning Source LLC
Chambersburg PA
CBHW041945260926
51850CB00018B/821

9783725864065